Handbook
Cardiovasc
Emergenci

CW00344645

Handbook of Cardiovascular Emergencies

Edited by

James W. Hoekstra, M.D.

Associate Professor of Emergency Medicine, Ohio State
University College of Medicine; Attending Physician,
Department of Emergency Medicine, The University
Hospitals, Columbus, Ohio

Little, Brown and Company
Boston   New York   Toronto   London

Library of Congress Cataloging-in-Publication Data

Handbook of cardiovascular emergencies / edited by James W. Hoekstra.
   p. cm.
  Includes bibliographical references and index.
  ISBN 0-316-36760-5
  1. Cardiovascular emergencies—Handbooks, manuals, etc.
 I. Hoekstra, James W.
  [DNLM: 1. Cardiovascular Diseases—therapy—handbooks.
 2. Emergencies—handbooks. WG 39 H23575 1996]
 RC675.H36   1996
 616.1025—dc20
 DNLM/DLC
 for Library of Congress   96-28913
                                              CIP

Printed in the United States of America

COM

Editorial: Tammerly J. Booth, Deeth K. Ellis
Production Services: Textbook Writers Associates, Inc.
Copyeditors: Joyce Churchill, Seth Maislin, Susan Zorn
Indexer: Michael Loo
Cover Designer: Mike Burggren

Contents

VII. Hemodynamic Alterations

Preface

Emergency medicine and critical care are fields that often require rapid diagnosis and intervention for specific emergent conditions. These critical interventions can be lifesaving or severely debilitating depending on their appropriateness and timeliness. It's no wonder that medical students, interns, and non–emergency medicine residents often find the emergency department and intensive care unit to be very intimidating places. Critically ill patients can cause significant anxiety for these individuals, especially when rapid intervention is needed. The limited time allowed in these situations to access reference material makes the *Handbook of Cardiovascular Emergencies* crucial.

Of the patients who commonly present to emergency departments and intensive care units, those with cardiovascular emergencies are often the most challenging. Patients with cardiac arrest, shock, myocardial infarction, or pulmonary embolus require rapid and efficient diagnosis and critical interventions to avoid complications of their disease processes. Emergency physicians and intensivists must be able to quickly recognize patients with these conditions, stabilize them with rapid and appropriate therapy, and triage them to appropriate care settings. Failure to do so can often lead to devastating results.

This handbook is designed to address these difficulties. It is meant to be an easily accessible, readable, organized pocket reference guide to assist medical students, interns, and residents with the care of patients with cardiovascular emergencies. It is written from an emergency medicine point of view, stressing the initial diagnosis, stabilization, management, and disposition of patients as if they are presenting acutely "off the street." It also includes some prehospital emergency medical service considerations that are more germane to emergency medicine than to any other medical specialty. This handbook has usefulness beyond the scope of emergency medicine, however. It may be helpful as a quick reference to medical students, residents, intensivists, and non–emergency medicine practitioners, who may, during the course of their practice, come into contact with patients with acute cardiovascular emergencies. This handbook is not meant to be comprehensive, especially with regard to epidemiology and pathophysiology. It is meant to be a clinically oriented quick reference to disease processes, diagnostic considerations, and appropriate pharmacologic therapy in the emergent setting.

The first part of the handbook (Chaps. 1–8) deals with the topics of cardiac resuscitation, prehospital care, airway management, vascular access, and hemodynamic monitoring. These chapters are meant to be reference material not only for cardiac arrest management but also for many procedures and resuscitation techniques that are crucial to the management of all cardiovascular emergencies. Many subsequent chapters refer to these introductory chapters for certain procedures and techniques.

The second part of the handbook (Chaps. 9–13) is devoted to the diagnosis and care of the patient with acute myocardial infarction. This relatively common cardiovascular emergency is emphasized because appropriate therapy is crucial to provide an adequate outcome and avoid the cardiovascular complications delineated in the third part of the handbook (Chaps. 14–19). It is only fair that a significant portion of the book is devoted to the diagnosis and treatment of myocardial infarction and its complications.

The remainder of the handbook is devoted to a number of non-myocardial infarction cardiovascular emergencies: Cardiac emergencies, toxicologic emergencies, disorders of the vascular system, and disorders of hemodynamics are discussed in separate sections.

J. W. H.

Contributing Authors

Eric Anderson, M.D.
Quality Review Officer, Department of Emergency Medicine, Cleveland Clinic Foundation, Cleveland

Misty E. Arnold, M.D.
Resident, Department of Emergency Medicine, The University Hospitals, Ohio State University College of Medicine, Columbus, Ohio

Ralph Battels, M.D.
Resident, Department of Emergency Medicine, The University Hospitals, Ohio State University College of Medicine, Columbus, Ohio

Aaron L. Bender, M.D.
Resident, Department of Emergency Medicine, The University Hospitals, Ohio State University College of Medicine, Columbus, Ohio

Philliph I. Bialecki, M.D.
Chief Resident, Department of Emergency Medicine, The University Hospitals, Ohio State University College of Medicine, Columbus, Ohio

William J. Brady Jr., M.D.
Assistant Professor of Emergency Medicine, University of Virginia School of Medicine; Clinical Director, Department of Emergency Medicine, University of Virginia Hospital, Charlottesville, Virginia

Gerard X. Brogan Jr., M.D.
Assistant Professor of Clinical Emergency Medicine, State University of New York at Stony Brook Health Sciences Center School of Medicine; Associate Director of Clinical Faculty, Department of Emergency Medicine, University Hospital, Stony Brook, New York

Jonathan Brooks, M.D.
Assistant Professor of Clinical Emergency Medicine, Ohio State University College of Medicine, Columbus, Ohio

Steven C. Carleton, M.D., Ph.D.
Assistant Professor of Emergency Medicine, University of Cincinnati College of Medicine; Staff Physician, Center for Emergency Care, University Hospital, Cincinnati

Marcel J. Casavant, M.D.
Assistant Professor of Emergency Medicine, Ohio State University College of Medicine; Attending Physician, Department of Emergency Medicine, Division of Clinical Pharmacology/Toxicology, Children's Hospital, Columbus, Ohio

David P. Chan, M.D.
Assistant Professor of Pediatrics, Ohio State University College of Medicine; Pediatric Cardiologist, Division of Cardiology, Children's Hospital, Columbus, Ohio

Daniel M. Cohen, M.D.
Associate Professor of Pediatrics, Ohio State University
College of Medicine; Attending Physician, Department of
Emergency Medicine, Children's Hospital, Columbus, Ohio

Stephanie H. Conwell, M.D.
Attending Emergency Physician, Department of Emergency
Medicine, Fairview General Hospital, Cleveland

Ellen C. Corey, M.D.
EMS Medical Director, Department of Emergency Medicine,
Fairview Health Systems, Cleveland

Daniel J. DeBehnke, M.D.
Associate Professor and Director of Research, Department of
Emergency Medicine, Medical College of Wisconsin; Senior
Attending Staff, Department of Emergency Medicine and
Trauma Center, Froedtert Memorial Lutheran Hospital,
Milwaukee

Michael Dick, M.D.
Assistant Professor of Emergency Medicine, Ohio State
University College of Medicine, Columbus; Director,
Department of Emergency Medicine, Lima Memorial
Hospital, Lima, Ohio

Eric Drobny, M.D.
Resident, Department of Emergency Medicine, The
University Hospitals, Ohio State University College of
Medicine, Columbus, Ohio

Michelle A. Flemmings, M.D.
Resident, Department of Emergency Medicine, The
University Hospitals, Ohio State University College of
Medicine, Columbus, Ohio

W. Brian Gibler, M.D.
Richard C. Levy Professor and Chairman, Department of
Emergency Medicine, University of Cincinnati College of
Medicine; Director, Center for Emergency Care, University
Hospital, Cincinnati

Fred Ginsburg, M.D.
Resident, Department of Emergency Medicine, St. Vincent
Hospital and Medical Center, Toledo, Ohio

Alan G. Gora, M.D.
Clinical Instructor in Emergency Medicine, Ohio State
University College of Medicine; Attending Physician,
Department of Emergency Medicine, Mount Carmel Medical
Center, Columbus, Ohio

Diane L. Gorgas, M.D.
Assistant Professor of Emergency Medicine, Ohio State
University College of Medicine, Columbus, Ohio

Andrew T. Guertler, M.D.
Assistant Professor of Emergency Medicine, University of
Virginia School of Medicine, Charlottesville, Virginia

Christina E. Hantsch, M.D.
Chief Resident, Department of Emergency Medicine,
Medical College of Wisconsin; Chief Resident, Department of

Emergency Medicine, Froedtert Memorial Lutheran
Hospital, Milwaukee

Karla R. Haversperger, M.D.
Fellow, Department of Emergency Medicine, Children's
Hospital, Columbus, Ohio

Judd E. Hollander, M.D.
Assistant Professor of Clinical Emergency Medicine and
Internal Medicine, State University of New York at Stony
Brook Health Sciences Center School of Medicine; Attending
Physician, Department of Emergency Medicine, University
Hospital, Stony Brook, New York

Colin G. Kaide, M.D.
Clinical Instructor, Department of Emergency Medicine,
Ohio State University College of Medicine; House Staff, The
University Hospitals, Columbus, Ohio

Michael T. Kelley, M.D.
Associate Professor of Emergency Medicine, Ohio State
University College of Medicine; Director, Central Ohio
Poison Center, Children's Hospital, Columbus, Ohio

Robert L. Levine, M.D.
Associate Professor of Emergency Medicine, Ohio State
University College of Medicine, Columbus, Ohio; Director of
Education, Department of Emergency Medicine, Cleveland
Clinic Foundation, Cleveland

Charles Little, D.O.
Assistant Professor of Emergency Medicine, Ohio State
University College of Medicine, Columbus, Ohio

Charles J. Love, M.D.
Assistant Professor of Clinical Medicine, Ohio State
University College of Medicine, Columbus, Ohio

Robert F. McCurdy, M.D.
Resident, Department of Surgery, Section of Emergency
Medicine, University Hospital, University of Michigan
Medical School, Ann Arbor, Michigan

Steve Marso, M.D.
Senior Resident, Department of Internal Medicine,
University of Virginia Hospital, University of Virginia School
of Medicine, Charlottesville, Virginia

Daniel R. Martin, M.D.
Associate Professor of Emergency Medicine, Ohio State
University College of Medicine; Director, Emergency
Medicine Residency Program, The University Hospitals,
Columbus, Ohio

Vicki Mazzorana, M.D.
Resident, Department of Emergency Medicine, Froedtert
Memorial Lutheran Hospital, Milwaukee

Joseph J. Moellman, M.D.
Chief Resident, Department of Emergency Medicine,
University Hospital, University of Cincinnati College of
Medicine, Cincinnati

Bruce K. Neely, M.D.
Clinical Instructor in Emergency Medicine, Ohio State
University College of Medicine, Columbus, Ohio; Attending
Physician, Department of Emergency Medicine, Providence
Medical Center, Seattle

Richard N. Nelson, M.D.
Associate Professor of Emergency Medicine, Ohio State
University College of Medicine; Medical Director,
Department of Emergency Medicine, The University
Hospitals, Columbus, Ohio

W. Frank Peacock IV, M.D.
Director of Clinical Operations, Department of Emergency
Medicine, Cleveland Clinic Foundation, Cleveland

Erica E. Remer, M.D.
Assistant Staff, Department of Emergency Medicine,
Cleveland Clinic Foundation, Cleveland

David Reyes, M.D.
Attending Physician, Department of Emergency Medicine,
Hazel Hawkins Memorial Hospital, Hollister, California

Daniel G. Rowland, M.D.
Assistant Professor of Pediatrics, Ohio State University
College of Medicine; Pediatric Cardiologist, Division of
Cardiology, Children's Hospital, Columbus, Ohio

Daniel J. Scherzer, M.D.
Associate Professor of Pediatrics, Ohio State University
College of Medicine; Attending Physician, Department of
Emergency Medicine, Children's Hospital, Columbus, Ohio

Michael P. Sotak, M.D.
Attending Physician, Department of Emergency Medicine,
University of California, Davis, Medical Center; Attending
Physician, Department of Emergency Medicine, Woodland
Memorial Hospital, Woodland, California

John M. Strayer, M.D.
Clinical Instructor in Emergency Medicine, Ohio State
University College of Medicine; House Staff, Department of
Emergency Medicine, The University Hospitals, Columbus,
Ohio

Gary L. Swart, M.D.
Assistant Professor of Emergency Medicine, Medical College
of Wisconsin; Senior Attending Staff Physician, Department
of Emergency Medicine, Froedtert Memorial Lutheran
Hospital, Milwaukee

J. Chadwick Tober, M.D.
Assistant Professor of Vascular Surgery, Ohio State
University College of Medicine; Attending Physician,
Department of Surgery (Vascular), The University Hospitals,
Columbus, Ohio

Carlos A. A. Torres, M.D.
Fellow, Department of Emergency Medicine, Ohio State
University College of Medicine; Fellow, Department of
Emergency Medicine, The University Hospitals, Columbus,
Ohio

Michael D. Waite, M.D.
Chief Resident, Department of Emergency Medicine, The University Hospitals, Ohio State University College of Medicine, Columbus, Ohio

Howard A. Werman, M.D.
Associate Professor of Emergency Medicine, Ohio State University College of Medicine; Attending Physician, Department of Emergency Medicine, The University Hospitals, Columbus, Ohio

Brian J. Zink, M.D.
Assistant Professor of Surgery and Emergency Medicine, University of Michigan Medical School; Attending Physician, Department of Surgery, Section of Emergency Medicine, University Hospital, Ann Arbor, Michigan

Introduction: Approach to the Patient with a Cardiovascular Emergency

Patients who present with cardiovascular emergencies do not fit into any one typical case scenario or clinical pattern. They can present with anything from cardiac arrest with unconsciousness and cardiac standstill to an asymptomatic state. The diagnosis of cardiovascular emergencies, therefore, often boils down to pattern recognition. Certain constellations of symptoms, physical signs, and laboratory and diagnostic test results should indicate specific cardiovascular emergencies to the astute physician. As a result, this handbook is written from the standpoint of **patient presentation** (historical and physical findings) and **patient assessment** (pertinent laboratory and diagnostic test results). If a given diagnosis is suspected because of a certain pattern of historical, physical, and laboratory findings, it can be referenced in this handbook. The physical and historical findings can be verified, and the appropriate **patient management** and **patient disposition** can be followed as outlined.

Aside from the patient with cardiac arrest (where the cardiovascular emergency is obvious), certain symptoms can alert the physician to the diagnosis of an occult cardiovascular emergency. These symptoms include chest pain, shock, syncope, shortness of breath, and palpitations. Whereas this list is not comprehensive, the majority of patients with cardiovascular emergencies will exhibit one of these symptoms. The differential diagnosis and brief initial workup of each of these is discussed below.

Chest Pain

Chest pain can be the presenting symptom for a wide range of diseases with either benign or catastrophic prognoses. Failure to recognize certain cardiovascular emergencies in patients with chest pain can lead to significant morbidity and mortality for the patient as well as to medicolegal ramifications for the physician. Missed myocardial infarctions, for instance, are responsible for 20% of the malpractice awards against emergency physicians.

Physical findings in patients with chest pain are often absent, subtle, or nonspecific. The physician must therefore elicit a thorough history to differentiate the benign causes of chest pain from the catastrophic. The character, location, radiation, chronology, associated symptoms, aggravating factors, and alleviating factors should be thoroughly explored. Risk factors for certain cardiovascular diseases should also be documented. Once these historical factors are sorted through, specific patterns can be recognized. Chest pain can often be categorized anatomically, given the history and physical findings, as outlined in Table I-1. The principal organs in the chest that cause pain include the heart, great vessels, the esophagus, the lungs and bronchi, and the chest wall. The pleura, pericardium, and mediastinum are often included in this list, but irritation of these structures is often due to pathology in the adjacent organs, not the serosal surfaces themselves.

Once the history is obtained and the physical examination

Table I-1. Chest pain: Historical description based on anatomic location

Organ system	Pain character	Location	Radiation	Associated symptoms	Aggravating/ alleviating factors
Heart	Dull, tightness, squeezing	Substernal, left chest	Left shoulder, left arm, neck, jaw	Shortness of breath, diaphoresis, nausea, vomiting, anxiety	Worse with exercise if angina
Great vessels	Tearing, sharp, severe, acute onset	Substernal, migratory	Back	Diaphoresis, syncope, shortness of breath, stroke symptoms, extremity ischemia	None
Esophagus	Burning, aching	Substernal	Neck, epigastric region	Nausea, belching, occasional vomiting	Worse with eating, drinking, belching, lying down; better with antacids
Lungs	Sharp, acute onset	Localized to area of pathology	Posterior shoulder if diaphragm is involved, abdomen if lower lung fields	Shortness of breath, fever, cough, sputum production if pneumonia	Worse with inspiration, cough; leg swelling with deep vein thrombosis or pulmonary embolus
Bronchi	Dull, burning	Substernal	Throat or neck	Cough, fever, sputum production, shortness of breath	Worse with inspiration, cough
Chest wall	Sharp	Localized to area of pathology	None	None	Worse with movement, cough, deep breath; reproduced with palpation

completed, certain ECG, laboratory, and x-ray studies can be used to confirm the diagnosis. When these tests are used, it is important to use them to rule out the cardiovascular emergencies first. Benign causes of chest pain should be diagnoses of exclusion, once the catastrophic causes of chest pain have been ruled out. The cardiovascular emergencies that cause chest pain can often be recognized by their patterns of historical, physical, and laboratory findings as shown in Table I-2. These represent the classic presentations for these cardiovascular emergencies. Each of these emergencies is discussed in detail in specific chapters in this handbook.

Shock

Shock has a number of etiologies, but the common result of shock is tissue hypoperfusion and ischemia secondary to circulatory failure. The etiologies of shock include hypovolemia, pump failure, loss of vascular tone, and mechanical causes that inhibit cardiac filling. The differential diagnosis of shock is listed in Table I-3. The specific causes of shock listed in Table I-3 are covered in detail in specific chapters in this handbook.

Patients in shock present with a wide range of symptoms including syncope, shortness of breath, lethargy, weakness, nausea, anxiety, abdominal pain, and chest pain. The vital signs are often abnormal, with low blood pressure as a late but universal finding irrespective of the etiology of shock. In hemorrhagic shock, however, up to 25% of the blood volume may be lost before the blood pressure is affected. Cardiovascular drug effects and extremes of age may mask the vital sign changes typically seen with shock of certain etiologies. Beta-blocker therapy, for instance, will often blunt the tachycardia that is expected with hypovolemic or septic shock. Despite these qualifications, the etiologies of shock noted in Table I-3 tend to produce certain clinical patterns that can often be recognized by the clinician and used to classify the cause of shock. These classic patterns of physical findings are illustrated in Table I-4 and described in detail in specific chapters in this handbook. Central venous pressure, pulmonary venous pressure, cardiac output, and systemic vascular resistance, which can be determined by invasive monitoring techniques, can be used to further clarify the etiology of shock. These patterns are discussed in the chapter on hemodynamic monitoring as well as in the chapters on specific causes of shock.

Syncope

Syncope, the episodic loss of consciousness followed by awakening, can be the presenting complaint in many cardiovascular emergencies. The common causes of syncope are listed in Table I-5. Of these, cardiovascular disorders that can cause syncope include cardiac syncope due to pump failure or arrhythmias, peripheral vascular syncope due to vasodilatation or vascular obstruction, and hypovolemic syncope due to hemorrhage or dehydration. Pulmonary embolus is included in the latter category because it causes relative hypovolemia due to limitation of left heart filling pressure. These etiologies are discussed in detail in specific chapters in the handbook. There is significant overlap of these etiologies with the causes of shock listed in Table I-3, since temporary shock or positional shock can cause hypoperfusion of the central nervous system, which in turn precipitates unconsciousness. Syncope is especially

Table I-2. Cardiovascular emergencies presenting with chest pain

Diagnosis	Classic history	Laboratory findings	ECG findings	Chest x-ray	Definitive testing
Myocardial infarction	Substernal chest pain, tightness, squeezing Lasting >1 hr Cardiac risk factors	Myoglobin elevates 3–6 hr CK-MB, troponin elevate 6–12 hr Lactic dehydrogenase elevates 24+ hr	Transmural: ST elevation 2 contiguous leads, bundle-branch block Subendocardial: ST depression, T-wave inversion	Nonspecific, but congestive heart failure may be present	Coronary angiography consistent with arterial occlusion
Unstable angina	Like myocardial infarction pain but lasts <1 hr Occurring at rest or with less than usual exertion Cardiac risk factors	Nonspecific Troponin elevated in minority of patients	May be normal if no pain ST depression, T-wave inversion, strain patterns	Nonspecific	Coronary angiography shows arterial narrowing Positive stress testing when appropriate

Pulmonary embolus	Sudden onset of sharp pleuritic pain Shortness of breath Risk factors for pulmonary embolus	Elevated arterial-alveolar oxygen gradient	Nonspecific, often tachycardia $S_1Q_3T_3$ pattern Right heart strain	Nonspecific Atelectasis, elevated diaphragm, or localized infiltrate	V/Q scan positive Pulmonary angiogram specific
Aortic dissection	Sharp severe chest pain, radiates to back History of hypertension Stroke or ischemia symptoms	Nonspecific	Nonspecific May show transmural myocardial infarction if coronary artery involved	Widening of mediastinum	Chest CT for screening Transesophageal echocardiography Angiogram definitive
Pericarditis	Sharp pleuritic chest pain Shock if tamponade present	Nonspecific	Diffuse ST elevation, PR depression	Nonspecific Enlarged heart shadow with effusions	Echocardiography to rule out effusion, tamponade

Table I-3. Etiologies of shock

General classification		Specific etiologies
Hypovolemia	Hemorrhagic shock	Gastrointestinal bleeding Ruptured ectopic pregnancy Traumatic hemorrhage
	Dehydration	Vomiting, diarrhea Insensible losses Diuretic use
	Extravascular pooling	Pancreatitis Cirrhosis Multiorgan system failure
Loss of vascular tone	Septic shock	Urinary tract infections Intraabdominal infections Pneumonia
	Anaphylactic shock	Bee stings Allergic reactions
	Spinal shock	Spinal cord injury
	Drug toxicity	Vasodilators Calcium channel blockers
Pump failure	Cardiogenic shock	Myocardial infarction Cardiac arrhythmias Cardiomyopathies Valvular disease Myocarditis
	Drug toxicity	Tricyclic antidepressants Beta blockers Digitalis
Mechanical causes	Decreased cardiac filling	Cardiac tamponade Tension pneumothorax Pulmonary embolus Constrictive pericarditis

prevalent with orthostatic changes in blood pressure due to dehydration, hemorrhage, or drug effects.

When evaluating a patient with syncope, it is important to rule out the cardiovascular emergencies as the cause of the syncope. Assuming that a patient has vasovagal or factitious syncope, discharging him to home can cause significant mortality or morbidity in a patient with a true cardiovascular emergency. The former diagnoses should be diagnoses of exclusion after cardiovascular causes have been ruled out. Certain clinical patterns of historical and physical findings can guide decisions regarding the etiology of syncope. Table I-6 describes the classic clinical patterns of syncope due to the more common cardiovascular and neurologic disorders. Cardiovascular diagnoses discussed in this handbook that can cause syncope include myocardial ischemia, atrial and ventricular arrhythmias, the various shock states, and pacemaker failure. Syncope due to vasodilating and cardiotoxic drugs is covered in specific chapters on beta blockers and calcium channel blockers, digitalis, cocaine, tricyclic antidepressants, and miscellaneous drugs and toxins.

Table I-4. Clinical patterns of shock

Etiology	Blood pressure	Heart rate	Skin	Lungs	Neck veins	Miscellaneous
Hemorrhagic shock	Decreased	Increased	Pale, cool, clammy	Clear	Flat	Bleeding source
Septic shock	Decreased	Increased early, variable late	Warm, pink	Clear	Flat	Fever Source of infection
Cardiogenic shock	Decreased	Variable	Pale, cool, clammy	Rales	Variable	Chest pain Cardiac arrhythmias
Anaphylactic shock	Decreased	Increased	Warm, pink	Clear	Flat	Urticarial rash Wheezing Laryngeal stridor
Spinal shock	Decreased	Unchanged	Warm, pink	Clear	Flat	Paralysis
Mechanical causes	Decreased	Increased	Pale, cool, clammy	Clear	Distended	Decreased heart sounds with tamponade Unilateral decreased breath sounds with tension pneumothorax

Table I-5.   Causes of syncope

Cardiovascular	
Cardiac	Arrhythmias
	Bradycardia
	Myocardial ischemia
	Pacemaker failure
Alterations of vascular tone	Vasovagal syncope
	Carotid sinus hypersensitivity
	Vasodilating drugs
Hypovolemia	Orthostatic syncope
	Ruptured abdominal aortic aneurysm
	Ruptured ectopic pregnancy
	Gastrointestinal hemorrhage
	Pulmonary embolus
Neurologic	
Central nervous system	Seizures
	Transient ischemic attacks
	Subarachnoid hemorrhage
	Occult head trauma
Peripheral nervous system	Autonomic neuropathy with orthostatic hypotension
Metabolic	Hypoglycemia
	Drug and alcohol intoxication
Psychiatric	Hyperventilation
	Factitious fainting
Miscellaneous	Micturition syncope
	Cough syncope
	Pregnancy
	Valsalva, defecation

Shortness of Breath

Shortness of breath, or dyspnea, is defined as an elevation of the respiratory rate. The causes of shortness of breath are many, involving not only the pulmonary and cardiovascular systems but also the central nervous system, the neuroendocrine axis, and the musculoskeletal system. As a result, the differential diagnosis of the patient who presents with acute shortness of breath can be exhausting. Common causes of acute shortness of breath, including common cardiovascular causes, are listed in Table I-7. A number of the common cardiovascular causes of shortness of breath are discussed in this handbook, including myocardial ischemia, congestive heart failure, and the various shock states. Pulmonary, chest wall, metabolic, and toxic causes are not considered cardiovascular emergencies and are therefore not included in this text.

Palpitations

Palpitations can be defined as the perception of an abnormal beating of the heart. Patients often describe their hearts as jumping, skipping, fluttering, racing, or pounding. Palpitations are a relatively common complaint, and up to 90% of patients with palpitations will have a cardiac dysrhythmia as the cause of their

Table I-6. Clinical patterns of common causes of syncope

Etiology	Historical findings	Physical findings	ECG findings	Laboratory findings
Cardiac arrhythmia	Associated chest pain Palpitations Sudden onset Cardiac risk factors Pacemaker	Irregular pulse or tachycardia May be normal	May be normal or ischemic Arrhythmias or warning arrhythmias Pacemaker failure	Nonspecific
Hypovolemia	History of volume loss, nausea, vomiting, or diuretic use Orthostatic symptoms	Signs of dehydration Orthostatic hypotension Hypotension, tachycardia if severe	Nonspecific or tachycardia	Nonspecific Uremia if severe Hypokalemic alkalosis if vomiting or diuretic use
Acute hemorrhage	Blood loss externally Hematemesis, hematochezia Acute abdominal pain or back pain	Orthostatic hypotension Pallor Tachycardia, hypotension	Normal or tachycardia	Anemia if subacute or chronic blood loss Lactic acidosis if shock
Vasovagal syncope	Preceding weakness, pallor, diaphoresis, and nausea Stressor Past fainting history	Normal or bradycardia	Normal	Normal
Seizure	Sudden onset Toxic-clonic activity Urination, tongue biting Postictal state History of seizures	Postictal state	Normal	Lactic acidosis if early postictal EEG positive at times

Table I-7. Common causes of acute shortness of breath

Cardiac	Myocardial infarction
	Myocardial ischemia
	Congestive heart failure
	Cardiac tamponade
	Cardiogenic shock
Pulmonary	Pneumonia
	Asthma
	Chronic obstructive pulmonary disease
	Pulmonary embolus
	Pneumothorax
	Noncardiac pulmonary edema
	(adult respiratory distress syndrome)
	Pulmonary contusion
	Pleurisy
	Toxic inhalations
Cardiovascular	Septic shock
	Neurogenic shock
Musculoskeletal	Chest wall injuries
	Costochondritis
Upper airway	Croup
	Epiglottitis
	Angioedema
	Foreign body
	Tracheal/laryngeal trauma
Metabolic/toxic	Acidosis
	Salicylates
	Thyrotoxicosis
	Cyanide
	Carbon monoxide
Neurologic	Psychogenic hyperventilation
	Uncal herniation
	Cheyne-Stokes respiration
Allergic	Anaphylaxis

symptoms. The key for the clinician is determining whether the dysrhythmias are benign or life threatening. Often this determination must be made without witnessing the dysrhythmias on a cardiac monitor. The clinician must base decisions on the potential causes of the dysrhythmias, and whether or not these causes are life threatening. The common causes of dysrhythmias and palpitations are listed in Table I-8. Many of the cardiac and toxic causes of palpitations are discussed in this handbook.

Of the causes listed, myocardial ischemia and myocardial infarction have perhaps the most potential for morbidity and mortality. Therefore the evaluation of the patient with palpitations often centers around eliminating myocardial ischemia as the cause of the symptoms. And patients with chest pain or risk factors for coronary disease must be evaluated seriously if they present with palpitations. In addition, patients with associated syncope, chest pain,

Table I-8. Common causes of dysrhythmias and palpitations

Cardiac	
Atrial dysrhythmias	Preexcitation syndromes
	Sick sinus syndrome
	Mitral valve prolapse
	Mitral stenosis/insufficiency
	Atrial ischemia
Ventricular dysrhythmias	Myocardial ischemia
	Myocardial infarction
	Cardiomyopathies
	Myocarditis
	Valvular disease
Metabolic	Thyrotoxicosis
	Hypokalemia
	Hypoxia
	Pheochromocytoma
Toxic	Stimulants
	Cocaine
	Digitalis
Infectious	Sepsis
Psychogenic	Anxiety

shortness of breath, or shock must be evaluated to rule out serious cardiovascular disease as outlined earlier.

J. W. H.

Cardiac Resuscitation

Basic Life Support and CPR

Fred Ginsburg

Basic life support (BLS) incorporates (1) prevention of respiratory or circulatory arrest via prompt recognition and intervention and (2) ventilatory and circulatory support for the victim of cardiorespiratory arrest. Cardiopulmonary resuscitation (CPR) provides ventilatory support via forced ventilations and circulatory support via chest compressions. In BLS an infant is less than 1 year old, a child is from 1 to 8 years old, and anyone over 9 is considered an adult.

I. **General emergency procedures.** The medical professional may be called upon to render care outside the standard work area. In this situation the rescuer should consider the following basic emergency concepts.
   A. **Rescuer personal safety.** The rescuer's safety is critical because if the rescuer becomes incapacitated, he or she will not only fail in assisting the victim but will also split the resources of the response team by becoming an additional victim.
   B. **Scene assessment.** Upon arriving on the scene, the rescuer should, without spending excess time, survey the scene for threats to self and to the victim. Environmental threats such as power lines, fires, carbon monoxide, and traffic should be considered. Bystanders should be evaluated for threats, especially if the injury involves weapons.
   C. **Activating the emergency medical system (EMS).** A nonresponsive adult victim can be assumed to be having a lethal cardiac arrhythmia. **Defibrillation is the most critical action** in these patients. If only one rescuer is present, upon discovering a nonresponsive adult it is imperative to activate EMS before proceeding with any other intervention. The 911 number should be used, if available, or the local EMS number or in-house "code" number can be used when applicable. The following information should be offered: (1) location with cross streets and landmarks; (2) call-back phone number; (3) nature of the event, for example, medical emergency or trauma; (4) number of victims; (5) conditions of victims; and (6) resources already on the scene. The need for defibrillation should be emphasized to ensure that the appropriate resources are dispatched. Exceptions to the call-first rule include the following: (1) the victim is a child (respiratory etiology most common); (2) available EMS activation (i.e., telephone) is over 10 minutes away; and (3) the victim has an exsanguinating hemorrhage that should receive immediate treatment first.
   D. **Patient positioning.** When CPR is performed, the victim must be supine on a firm surface. A trauma victim normally should not be moved except for safety reasons, unless spontaneous respirations cannot be detected. When a rescuer evaluates a scene, he or she should quickly consider the physical constraints of performing

advanced cardiac life support (ACLS) including CPR, intubation, IV access, and cardiac monitoring and if possible position the patient to make best use of available space before the victim becomes "fixed" at a location.

E. Legal considerations. Good Samaritan laws are intended to protect those engaged in emergency care outside a medical facility from civil liability. Although these laws vary among jurisdictions, they generally cover those who have no duty to respond, who perform in good faith, and who are not grossly negligent in their response.

F. Patient disposition. BLS continues until one of the following conditions occurs: (1) the patient regains a spontaneous pulse and respirations; (2) ACLS is initiated; (3) the rescuer is too exhausted to continue; or (4) the patient is declared dead by appropriate personnel. The emotional needs of the victim's family, especially with a pediatric victim, need to be taken into consideration before the resuscitation effort is terminated.

II. Adult cardiac arrest. One million deaths per year can be attributed to cardiovascular disease, with approximately half of those due to coronary artery disease, most of whom present with sudden death. Two-thirds of the sudden death victims suffer arrest outside the home within 2 hours after the onset of symptoms. Drowning, electrocution, drug intoxication, and trauma are other etiologies of sudden death. The time from onset of cardiorespiratory arrest to the initiation of CPR and subsequent administration of ACLS is critical to patient outcome. Since the earliest possible time to start CPR is in the field by layperson bystanders, BLS training should be available to as many persons within a community as possible in addition to those most likely to encounter a cardiac emergency.

A. The ABCs of adult CPR. In each step of the BLS process, the rescuer must perform an adequate assessment before proceeding to the next, more invasive, step. **In the initial assessment,** the victim is assessed for unresponsiveness. Tapping or gently shaking the victim while asking, "Are you OK?" is appropriate. If the victim gives no response, EMS should be activated. The patient should then be positioned supine on a firm surface so that the rescuer can proceed with the following ABCs of CPR.

1. **Airway.** The victim's tongue and epiglottis are elevated from the posterior pharynx by the head tilt–chin lift maneuver. One hand is used to lift the chin upward while the other hand is used to tilt the head backward by placing pressure on the forehead (Fig. 1-1).

2. **Breathing.** After kneeling next to the victim, the rescuer places his or her ear next to the victim's mouth and looks toward the victim's chest. Respirations are detected by hearing air exchange, feeling airflow on the ear, or seeing the chest rise and fall. This evaluation should last 3 to 5 seconds. If the victim is breathing, he or she should be placed on the side in the "recovery" position (Fig. 1-2). If no spontaneous respirations are detected, forced ventilations must be supplied via rescue breathing as follows.

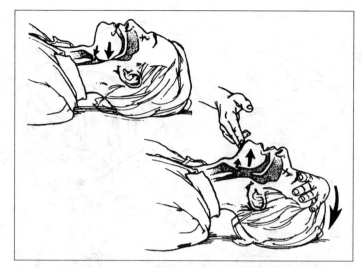

Fig. 1-1.   The "head tilt–chin lift" method of opening the airway. (From Emergency Cardiac Care Committee and Subcommittees, AHA. Guidelines for CPR and ECC. *JAMA* 268:2186, 1992. Copyright 1992, American Medical Association.)

   a. Mouth-to-mouth ventilation. While maintaining the head tilt–chin lift, the rescuer pinches the victim's nose while placing his or her mouth over the victim's mouth and giving two slow rescue breaths, verifying that the chest rises and falls with each respiration. If ventilation is not possible, the victim's head should be repositioned and ventilation reattempted. If ventilation is still not possible, then the victim is considered to have a foreign body airway obstruction (FBAO) (see sec. **V.**). The patient should be ventilated 10 to 12 times a minute. Each breath should last for 1½ to 2 seconds (Fig. 1-3).
   b. Mouth-to-mask ventilation. The use of a mask provides a sanitary seal to the rescuer while allow-

Fig. 1-2.   The "recovery position." (From Emergency Cardiac Care Committee and Subcommittees, AHA. Guidelines for CPR and ECC. *JAMA* 268:2187, 1992. Copyright 1992, American Medical Association.)

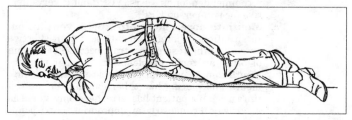

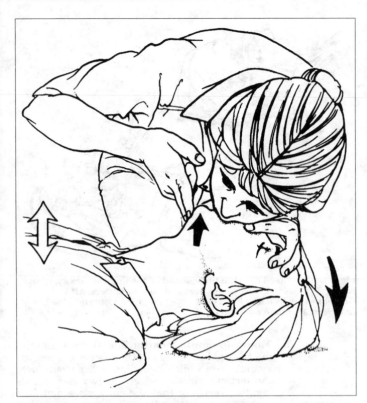

Fig. 1-3.   Rescue breathing. (From Emergency Cardiac Care Committee and Subcommittees, AHA. Guidelines for CPR and ECC. *JAMA* 268:2188, 1992. Copyright 1992, American Medical Association.)

ing for adjunctive oxygen application and enhanced C-spine control. The key to mask use is to **make a complete seal on the victim's face**. The mask is placed with the point of the tear over the victim's nose. A thumb is placed over each side of the mask as the rescuer lifts up on the jaw with his or her fingers at the angle of the mandible. C-spine control can be maintained by placing the palms on each side of the victim's head. Mouth to mask is not recommended for one-person CPR but is very effective for two-person CPR.

c. **Mouth-to-nose, mouth-to-stoma ventilation.** In situations where the mouth is not an effective entry into the respiratory tract because of trauma or other anatomic problems, the rescuer may try mouth-to-nose ventilation by closing the victim's mouth and placing his or her mouth over the victim's nose. If a patient has a tracheostomy stoma as an airway, it can also be an appropriate entry point.

  d. Modified jaw thrust. In the case of suspected trauma, the rescuer should establish the airway and C-spine control by placing a hand on each side of the victim's head. Each hand is then used to lift up on the angle of the mandible to open the victim's mouth and establish an airway. The victim's nose or mouth can then be occluded with the rescuer's mouth for ventilations.

3. **Circulation.** After two adequate ventilations are completed, the patient is assessed for a palpable carotid pulse. Two fingers are placed over the larynx and slid toward the rescuer into the groove between the trachea and the sternocleidomastoid (SCM) muscle to attempt to palpate the carotid pulse (Fig. 1-4). This effort should be limited to 5 to 10 seconds. If a pulse is palpated, then rescue breathing is continued until spontaneous breathing begins. The pulse should be reassessed every few minutes. If no pulse is palpated, circulation must be established by using external chest compressions as follows.

  a. The rescuer kneels with his or her knees next to the chest of the victim.

  b. The chest of the victim should be exposed as much as possible to assist with the location of landmarks and to reduce restriction of movement. Minimal time should be lost in this effort.

  c. Two fingers are run up the lower sternal border to the substernal notch. Using this point as a guide, the rescuer moves up the sternum two finger widths. The heel of the rescuer's other hand is placed against the finger guide along the sternum (Fig. 1-5).

  d. The rescuer's other hand is placed on top of the first and the fingers are interlocked. Fingers should be kept off the ribs to reduce breakage.

  e. The rescuer should align his or her shoulder, the heels of his or her hands, and the victim's sternum and spinal cord in a single line. Bending at the hips and keeping the elbows locked, the rescuer can then compress the sternum 1½ to 2 inches deep at a rate of 80 to 100 compressions a minute for 15 compressions (see Fig. 1-5).

  f. After 15 compressions, the rescuer can move to the victim's head to deliver two rescue breaths of 1½ to 2 seconds each. This is followed by another 15 chest compressions.

  g. After four cycles of two rescue breaths and 15 chest compressions, the victim is reevaluated for pulse or spontaneous respirations. If the pulse has returned, the rescuer need only perform rescue breaths, checking for a pulse every few minutes. If the victim is breathing spontaneously, he or she should be put in the recovery position (see Fig. 1-2). If the victim still has no pulse, CPR should be continued, with the pulse rechecked every few minutes.

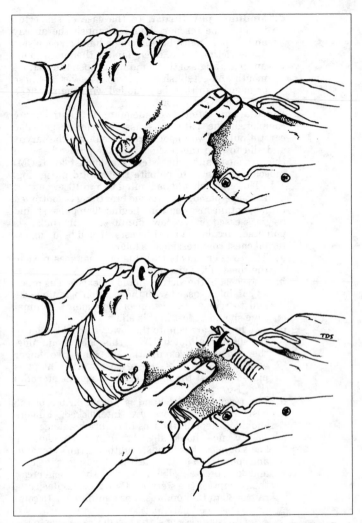

Fig. 1-4.   Palpation of the carotid pulse. (From Emergency Cardiac Care Committee and Subcommittees, AHA. Guidelines for CPR and ECC. *JAMA* 268:2189, 1992. Copyright 1992, American Medical Association.)

   B. Two-rescuer CPR. When two rescuers are available, one
       manages the head and airway while performing ventila-
       tions. The second rescuer performs chest compressions,
       pausing now and then to allow for ventilations. In two-
       rescuer CPR, a 5:1 ratio of compressions to ventilations is
       used. When the person doing chest compressions tires, he
       or she may call for a switch of positions. At this time the
       patient should be reevaluated for pulse and spontaneous
       respirations.

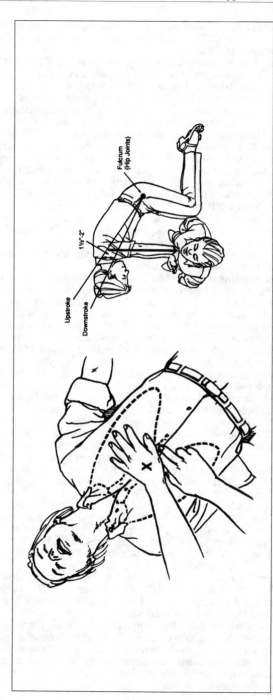

Fig. 1-5. Proper hand positioning for chest compressions. (From Emergency Cardiac Care Committee and Subcommittees, AHA. Guidelines for CPR and ECC. *JAMA* 268:2190, 1992. Copyright 1992, American Medical Association.)

C. **Alternative methods of CPR.** Multiple adjunctive methods of CPR are being evaluated to increase the effectiveness of CPR.
1. **Active compression-decompression CPR** (ACD-CPR) involves the use of a hand-held suction cup device (resembling a plumber's helper) to actively expand the chest by pulling up during the relaxation phase of chest compressions. Initial research has been promising, and the technology is inexpensive.
2. **Interposed abdominal compression CPR** (IAC-CPR) requires three rescuers. One rescuer performs ventilations, the second performs chest compressions, and the third presses on the abdomen during the relaxation phase of chest compressions. Animal studies have documented improved blood flow using IAC-CPR.
3. **Vest CPR** uses the thoracic pump theory to increase intrathoracic pressure in an attempt to increase blood flow during the compression phase. This method requires a large, somewhat cumbersome, inflatable vest that inflates around the patient during each compression phase to assist CPR.

III. **Child cardiac arrest.** The most likely etiology of a child's cardiac arrest is respiratory arrest caused by a preventable accident. Primary cardiac arrests in children are rare. As such, the first priority in child CPR should be to establish an airway and assist ventilation. Activation of EMS to initiate ACLS care is secondary. After unconsciousness is established, the ABCs of CPR are initiated. Only after 1 minute of CPR is EMS activated.
A. **Airway.** Elevation of the tongue and epiglottis from the posterior pharynx is accomplished by the head tilt–chin lift maneuver. Unlike with the adult, the child's head is tilted into a neutral to slightly extended position.
B. **Breathing.** The rescuer kneels next to the victim, placing his or her ear next to the victim's mouth while looking toward the victim's chest. Respirations are detected by hearing air exchange, feeling air flow on the ear, or seeing the chest rise and fall. The evaluation should last 3 to 5 seconds. If no spontaneous respirations are detected, the rescuer must supply forced ventilations via rescue breathing. Maintaining the head tilt–chin lift, the rescuer pinches the victim's nose while placing his or her mouth over the victim's mouth and giving two slow rescue breaths, verifying that the chest rises and falls with each respiration. If ventilation is not successful, the victim's head is repositioned and ventilation is reattempted. If ventilation is still not possible, the rescuer must assume that the child has an FBAO (see sec. **V.**). The patient should be ventilated 20 times a minute. Each breath should last for 1 to 1½ seconds.
C. **Circulation.** After the completion of two adequate ventilations, the victim is assessed for a palpable carotid pulse. If a pulse is palpated, then rescue breathing is continued. The pulse should be reassessed every few minutes. If no pulse is palpated, then circulation must be established using external chest compressions as follows.

1. The rescuer kneels next to the child's chest.
2. The child's chest is exposed to assist in finding landmarks.
3. The substernal notch is visualized or located by the rescuer running his or her finger up the bottom of the rib cage. The rescuer's hand is placed for compressions two finger widths up from the substernal notch. The other hand remains at the child's head to maintain head positioning (Fig. 1-6).
4. Compressions are made to a depth of 1 to 1½ inches at a rate of 100 compressions a minute.
5. The ratio of compressions to ventilations is 5:1.
6. After 20 cycles of 5:1 compressions to ventilations, the victim is reevaluated for pulse or spontaneous respirations. If the pulse has returned, the rescuer need only perform rescue breaths, rechecking for pulse every few minutes. EMS should be activated at this time. If there is no pulse, then CPR is continued while rechecking for a pulse every few minutes.

IV. Infant cardiac arrest. As with child cardiac arrest, infant cardiac arrest is usually of respiratory etiology. As such, once unconsciousness is established, early attempts should

Fig. 1-6. Proper hand positioning for CPR in a child. (From Emergency Cardiac Care Committee and Subcommittees, AHA. Guidelines for CPR and ECC. *JAMA* 268:2193, 1992. Copyright 1992, American Medical Association.)

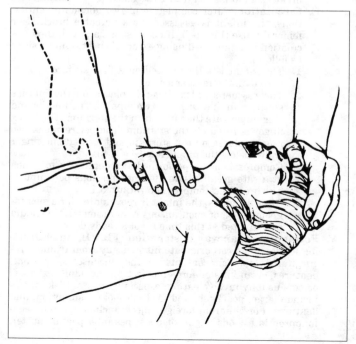

center on the establishment of airway and ventilation. EMS should be activated after 1 minute of CPR. Infants can be placed on a table or the floor, or they can be carried on the rescuer's forearm. The rescuer may be able to carry the baby while performing CPR so that EMS can be activated without losing any resuscitation time. Consideration of the parents must be included in the decision to start or stop CPR on an infant. It may be best to start CPR even though a significant time has elapsed since the onset of arrest.

A. **Airway.** Unlike the adult's, the infant's head is placed in the **neutral position**.

B. **Breathing.** The rescuer places his or her ear next to the baby's mouth and looks toward the chest. Respirations are detected by hearing air exchange, feeling air flow on the ear, or watching the chest rise and fall. This evaluation should last 3 to 5 seconds. If the baby is breathing, then further investigation is required to discover the reason for the reduced level of consciousness. If no spontaneous respirations are detected, then the rescuer must supply positive pressure ventilations via rescue breathing. The rescuer places his or her mouth over the baby's mouth and nose and delivers "puffs" of air. If ventilation is not successful, the infant is repositioned and ventilation is reattempted. If ventilation is still not possible, then the infant is considered to have an airway obstruction (see sec. **V.**). The baby should be ventilated 20 times a minute. Each breath should last for 1 to 1½ seconds.

C. **Circulation.** After completion of two adequate ventilations, the infant is assessed for a palpable brachial or femoral pulse (Fig. 1-7). If no pulse is palpated, then circulation is established using external chest compressions as follows.

1. The infant is either placed on a firm surface or supported on the rescuer's arm.

2. The rescuer's index finger is placed on the infant's sternum in line with the two nipples. The middle and ring fingers are then placed on the sternum. The index finger is lifted off the sternum. The net result is two fingers placed on the sternum and located one finger width below the nipple line (Fig. 1-8).

3. Compressions are performed at a depth of ½ to 1 inch at a rate greater than 100 compressions per minute.

4. The breath-to-compression ratio is 5:1.

5. After 20 cycles, the infant is reevaluated for a spontaneous pulse or spontaneous respirations. EMS should be activated at this time if not already done.

V. **Foreign body airway obstruction (FBAO).** An obstructing foreign body can originate intrinsically from trauma, regurgitated stomach contents in the unconscious patient, dentures, or an inhaled foreign object. In the adult, extrinsic objects usually involve eating, especially meats. Risk factors include large, poorly chewed food, alcohol consumption, and dentures. For children, foreign objects include not only age-inappropriate foods (e.g., hot dogs, peanuts, peanut butter,

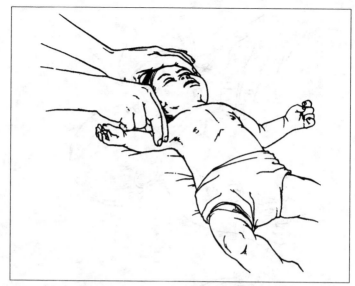

Fig. 1-7. Palpation of a brachial pulse in an infant. (From Emergency Cardiac Care Committee and Subcommittees, AHA. Guidelines for CPR and ECC. *JAMA* 268:2193, 1992. Copyright 1992, American Medical Association.)

grapes, and popcorn) but also small objects, including coins, beads, thumbtacks, and marbles. Nearly 4000 persons a year die from foreign body obstructions.

A. **Presentation. A choking infant** may have severe respiratory distress, be cyanotic, and be desperately using accessory muscles to breathe. If there is still air exchange, the infant may cough or wheeze. With complete blockage the baby will stop breathing and lose consciousness. A **child or adult** victim may be coughing forcefully enough to dislodge the object and still maintain good air exchange. With more complete obstruction the victim may start wheezing or crowing while developing cyanosis. The victim may bring his or her hands up to the neck to indicate the universal choking sign. Ultimately, the victim will stop breathing and become unconscious. In all ages, the initial presentation of foreign body obstruction may be unconsciousness. Infectious etiology of the obstruction should be considered if evidenced by history, fever, and clinical presentation.

B. **Management of an FBAO in a conscious child or adult.** While the victim maintains adequate air exchange and is actively trying to expel the object, the rescuer should not interfere by trying to reach for the object or slapping the victim on the back. Activation of 911 may be considered at this time. When the victim fails to maintain adequate air exchange and so is unable to continue attempts at expelling the object, then the rescuer must in-

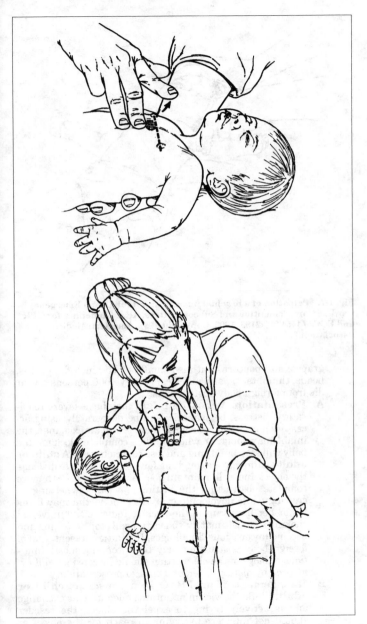

Fig. 1-8.   Proper hand positioning for CPR in an infant. (From Emergency Cardiac Care Committee and Subcommittees, AHA. Guidelines for CPR and ECC. *JAMA* 268:2255, 1992. Copyright 1992, American Medical Association.)

tervene. Subdiaphragmatic abdominal thrusts are used to compress the air in the lungs, thereby ejecting the object (the "Heimlich maneuver").

1. The rescuer should introduce himself or herself to the victim for reassurance. This step is especially important with larger victims.
2. The rescuer should position himself or herself behind the victim, make a fist, and then place the side of the thumb into a spot above the victim's umbilicus but below the xyphoid process. A larger victim may be seated for better control. A smaller victim or a child can lie over the rescuer's fist to take better advantage of gravity.
3. Diaphragmatic thrusts are quickly produced inward and upward into the victim's abdomen (Fig. 1-9).
4. This action is continued until the victim either ejects the object or becomes unconscious.
5. The rescuer must be prepared to support the victim's transition to unconsciousness. Since the rescuer's

Fig. 1-9. Abdominal thrusts to dislodge a foreign body airway obstruction in a conscious victim (Heimlich maneuver). (From Emergency Cardiac Care Committee and Subcommittees, AHA. Guidelines for CPR and ECC. *JAMA* 268:2256, 1992. Copyright 1992, American Medical Association.)

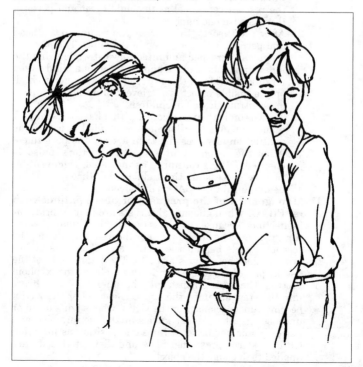

arms are already under the victim, this is best accomplished by supporting the victim while walking backward to ease the transition. Care must be exercised to ensure that the victim's head does not make a hard impact with the floor.

6. Once the patient is on the floor, a finger sweep is attempted on the adult patient by lifting up on the tongue and mandible while sweeping to the back of the pharynx. On a child, this maneuver should not be attempted unless the object is visible. Continue the process described for the unconscious victim.

C. **Management of an FBAO in an unconscious child or adult.** The typical scenario for unconscious FBAO unfolds when the rescuer finds an unconscious victim in whom ventilation is not possible despite repositioning. There may or may not be a history of choking. Since the victim is unconscious, the only way to know that a patent airway has been established is by a successful ventilation. Removal of the suspected FBAO is attempted as follows.

1. The hips of the adult victim are straddled and the heel of one of the rescuer's hands is placed on the victim's abdomen midway between the xyphoid process and the umbilicus. The other hand is placed on top of the first, and up to five abdominal thrusts are directed upward toward the diaphragm (Fig. 1-10). For the child, the rescuer can kneel at the child's feet and perform thrusts with one hand.

2. After the thrusts, the rescuer can return to the head and perform a finger sweep in the adult. The jaw and tongue are grasped and lifted upward while using the index finger of the other hand to attempt a blind sweep for any object from the posterior pharynx. For a child, only a visible object is retrieved; blind finger sweeps are contraindicated in children.

3. The victim is then positioned with a head tilt–chin lift maneuver and ventilation is attempted twice. If one ventilation is successful, then a second is performed. After the second ventilation, the victim's pulse is checked. CPR is continued as indicated. If no ventilation is successful, then abdominal thrusts are repeated until the FBAO is dislodged.

D. **Management of the pregnant or obese patient with an FBAO.** When abdominal thrusts are inappropriate or ineffectual because of excess abdominal mass, chest thrusts should be attempted. For the standing victim, the rescuer stands behind the victim and places his or her arms under the victim's armpits. The lateral side of the fist is placed on the sternum well above the xyphoid process. The fist is grasped with the other hand and thrust into the sternum until the object is ejected or the victim becomes unconscious. For the victim who is lying down or unconscious, the rescuer kneels at the victim's side and places his or her hand in the same position as for doing CPR chest compressions. Slow and distinct thrusts are applied to dislodge the object.

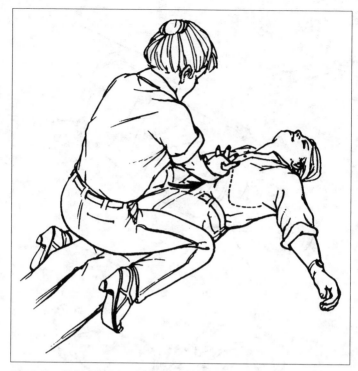

Fig. 1-10. Abdominal thrusts in an unconscious victim. (From Emergency Cardiac Care Committee and Subcommittees, AHA. Guidelines for CPR and ECC. *JAMA* 268:2257, 1992. Copyright 1992, American Medical Association.)

E. **Management of the infant with an FBAO.** The infant presenting with sudden stridor, wheezing, gagging, or cyanosis with no cry may be suffering from an FBAO. An unconscious infant's blocked airway may be discovered upon attempts to ventilate. The management of an infant differs from that of the adult and child because of the differences in relative anatomy and the ability of the rescuer to manipulate the entire infant.

1. The infant is rested prone on the rescuer's forearm with the head lower than the body. The infant's head is supported by maintaining a firm grip on the jaw with the supporting hand. Up to five back blows are then delivered firmly between the infant's shoulder blades.

2. By sandwiching the infant between the rescuer's two arms, with one hand supporting the jaw and the other supporting the back of the head, the rescuer can quickly turn over the infant so that he or she is resting supine on the rescuer's other forearm, with the head supported by the rescuer's hand.

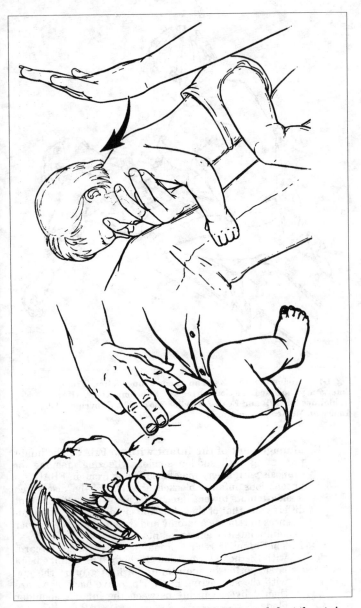

Fig. 1-11.   Proper hand positioning for back blows and chest thrusts in an infant. (From Emergency Cardiac Care Committee and Subcommittees, AHA. Guidelines for CPR and ECC. *JAMA* 268:2258, 1992. Copyright 1992, American Medical Association.)

3. Up to five quick chest thrusts are then delivered. Two fingers are placed in line with the sternum one finger width below the intramammary line for chest compressions. This is the same location as for chest compressions during infant CPR (Fig. 1-11).
4. If the infant is conscious, back blows and chest thrusts are continued until the object dislodges, as recognized by the infant crying or making other noises indicating a cleared airway. If the child is unconscious, ventilations are attempted between chest and abdominal thrust sequences to check for a patent airway. While cradling the infant on his or her forearm, the rescuer inspects the infant's mouth for foreign bodies and attempts to retrieve the objects if possible. Ventilation is again attempted. If that fails, the rescuer returns to doing back blows and chest thrusts, checking for the foreign object, and attempting to ventilate.

Bibliography

Chandra NC, Hazinski MF (eds.). *Textbook of Basic Life Support for Healthcare Providers.* Dallas: American Heart Association, 1994.

Cummins RO (ed.). *Textbook of Advanced Cardiac Life Support.* Dallas: American Heart Association, 1994.

Emergency Cardiac Care Committee and Subcommittees. American Heart Association guidelines for cardiopulmonary resuscitation and emergency cardiac care. *JAMA* 268:2172–2298, 1992.

Airway Management

Jonathan Brooks

Ensuring adequate ventilation and oxygenation should be the first priority of physicians when faced with a cardiovascular emergency. Airway management is a vital skill in caring for critically ill patients. Expertise in the oral, nasal, and surgical approaches of securing an airway can only be obtained through proper training and practice. The ability to recognize which approach is optimal for a given clinical situation requires sound clinical judgment.

Cardiovascular emergencies are among the most common causes of airway compromise (Table 2-1). Many cardiovascular emergencies present with airway compromise, whereas others are the result of it, with poor oxygenation or ventilation causing acidosis, tissue hypoxia, and subsequent cardiovascular collapse.

I. **Assessment of the airway.** The evaluation of a patient with respiratory distress should begin with a brief history (when obtainable), general inspection, rapid examination of the chest, assessment of cardiovascular function, the level of consciousness, and vital signs (Table 2-2). If the patient is in such distress that he or she is unable to speak (especially if symptoms have developed over a short period of time), then airway management should proceed with haste. Use of pulse oximetry, arterial blood gas analysis, and a chest x-ray will guide therapy for patients who are in less distress.

   A. **History.** The history should include a brief questioning period regarding recent illness and preceding symptoms, medications, last oral intake, allergies, and previous need for intubation. If the history is unobtainable, physical assessment and airway management should proceed rapidly.

   B. **General inspection.** A general inspection should be performed with attention to patient size and anatomic abnormalities, the presence of head or facial trauma, neck masses, or tracheostomy scars. Respiratory effort and change in skin color such as paleness, mottling, or cyanosis should also be assessed.

   C. **Physical exam.** The physical exam of the lungs should include "looking" for symmetric chest excursion, "listening" for air exchange, rales, wheezes or rhonchi, and "feeling" for air escape through the nose or mouth.

   D. **Cardiovascular assessment.** Assessment of cardiovascular function should include auscultation of the heart tones and abnormal sounds such as murmurs, rubs, and gallops. The quality and nature of pulses and capillary refill should also be assessed.

   E. **Level of consciousness.** Alterations in the level of consciousness manifested by restlessness, agitation, drowsiness, disorientation or coma often are the result of hypoxia or hypercarbia. Conversely, alteration of consciousness due to CNS dysfunction or trauma can also result in the loss of

Table 2-1.   Causes of respiratory failure

Cardiovascular
Myocardial infarction
Dysrhythmias
Congestive heart failure
Thoracic and abdominal aneurysms
Cardiogenic shock
Pulmonary edema

Trauma
Head Injury
Maxillofacial and mandible injury
Neck injury (blunt or penetrating)
  Cervical spine injury
  Laryngotracheal injury
Chest trauma (blunt or penetrating)
Hypovolemic shock
Inhalation injury

Upper airway obstruction
Foreign body
Infections (e.g., epiglottitis, abscess)
Tumors
Angioneurotic edema
Laryngospasm
Anaphylaxis
Sleep apnea

Pulmonary
Pneumonia
Embolus
Asthma
Chronic obstructive pulmonary
  disease
Pulmonary edema

Toxicologic
Drugs (e.g., tricyclic antidepressants, narcotics)
Organophosphates
Carbon monoxide
Toxins (e.g., botulism)

Neurologic
Cerebrovascular accidents
Meningitis and encephalitis
Status epilepticus
Myasthenia gravis
Guillain-Barré syndrome
Cerebral edema
Tumors

Metabolic (e.g., uremia and diabetic ketoacidosis)

Endocrine (e.g., Addison's disease and hypothyroidism)

Table 2-2.   Initial airway assessment

History
General inspection
Physical exam of lungs
Cardiovascular exam
Level of consciousness
Respiratory rate and pattern
Pulse oximetry
Arterial blood gas
Chest x-ray

airway control, necessitating airway management. Assessment of the gag reflex has always been advocated as a method of assessing airway control in the unconscious patient. Unfortunately, stimulating the back of the pharynx to elicit a gag reflex can also induce vomiting with subsequent aspiration. As a result, this maneuver is no longer recommended.

F. Respiratory rate. The respiratory rate is the vital sign that is least accurately assessed, although it most often provides clues to systemic diseases. Tachypnea is common with many disease states whereas bradypnea occurs with much less frequency. (Tables 2-3 and 2-4) Patients with rapid shallow breathing and little air exchange will often require emergent airway intervention.

G. Pulse oximetry. Pulse oximetry is useful as a guide to the oxygenation of arterial blood. It measures the saturation of hemoglobin by oxygen in the peripheral circulation. Because hyperventilation can elevate the PO_2, patients with an elevated alveolar to arterial oxygen gradient can have normal oxygen saturation, giving the evaluating physician a false sense of security. Pulse oximetry does not reflect the adequacy of ventilation or the PCO_2 tension. When a patient is severely hypoxemic (saturation below 90%) or hypoventilation is suspected, arterial blood gas measurement is indicated. In addition, patients in shock or with low flow states often have poor peripheral perfusion, resulting in low tissue hemoglobin saturation and falsely depressed pulse oximetry readings. In general, pulse oximetry is only useful in normotensive subjects.

H. Arterial blood gas. Arterial blood gas analysis is the best objective test to document respiratory failure. An arterial PO_2 less than 60 mm Hg (on 100% O_2) or a PCO_2 greater than 50 mm Hg are diagnostic for respiratory

Table 2-3. Causes of tachypnea

Acute respiratory failure	Metabolic acidosis
Increased metabolic rate	Diabetic ketoacidosis
Fever	Uremia
Infection	Lactic acidosis
Hyperthyroidism	Poisonings
Exertion	Methanol
Stress	Ethylene glycol
Pain	Salicylates
Cardiac dysfunction	Amphetamines
Abdominal distention	Psychogenic
Ascites	Anemia
Bowel obstruction	Shock
Pregnancy	
Central nervous system dysfunction	

Table 2-4. Causes of bradypnea

Chronic obstructive pulmonary disease with CO_2 retention
Central nervous system dysfunction
Poisonings
   Sedative-hypnotics
   Barbiturates
   Narcotics
   Alcohol intoxication
Endocrine
   Cushing's syndrome
   Adrenal dysfunction
   Myxedema (hypothyroidism)
Hypothermia
Metabolic alkalosis

failure. If the arterial blood pH is less than 7.3, with an elevated PCO_2, then acute respiratory failure is present and emergent airway management is indicated unless aggressive therapy can reverse the acidosis. The combination of arterial blood gas analysis and pulse oximetry can help direct supplemental oxygen therapy and decisions regarding intubation.

I. **Chest x-ray.** If time permits, the chest x-ray can provide valuable diagnostic information that might influence the immediate management of the airway. Aggressive therapy for reversible causes of airway compromise such as pneumothorax, congestive heart failure, or asthma can alleviate the need for invasive airway management.

II. **Management of the compromised airway.** There are five general indications for securing an airway by endotracheal intubation. These include **respiratory insufficiency, airway obstruction, inability to protect the airway,** a **need for hyperventilation,** and **anticipated or impending airway compromise** (Table 2-5).

A. **Initial airway management**

1. Management of the unconscious, apneic patient begins with opening the airway. An **oropharyngeal exam** will reveal any foreign bodies that should be manually removed with the assistance of a rigid-tipped suction or Magill forceps under direct vision.

2. The **head tilt** with the **chin lift** or **jaw thrust** maneuver prevents obstruction of the airway by the tongue, which can occlude the airway at the level of the pharynx. The head tilt [contraindicated with suspected cervical spine (C-spine) fracture] places the patient in the "sniffing" position with the neck flexed in relation to the thorax and the head extended in relation to the neck (Fig. 2-1). The chin lift is performed by placing fingers under the symphysis of the mandible and lifting forward. The jaw thrust is the method of

Table 2-5. Indications for intubation

Respiratory failure
Apnea
Hypoxemia
Hypercapnea

Airway obstruction
Foreign body
Trauma
Blood, secretions, emesis
Tumor
Edema
Abscess

Airway protection
Altered mental status
Loss of airway reflexes

Need for hyperventilation
Head trauma
Metabolic acidosis in critical illness

Impending airway compromise
Shock
Multiple trauma

Fig. 2-1. Opening the airway. Top: Airway obstruction produced by tongue and epiglottis. Bottom: Relief by head tilt–chin lift. (Reproduced with permission. *Textbook of Advanced Cardiac Life Support*, 1994. Copyright American Heart Association.)

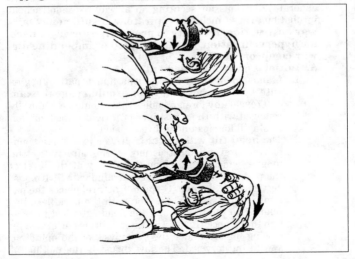

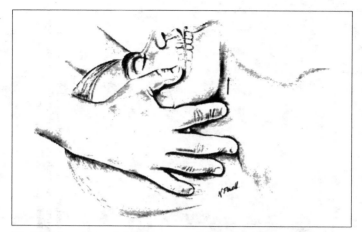

Fig. 2-2. **In an obtunded or comatose patient, the soft tissues of the oropharynx become relaxed and may obstruct the upper airway. Obstruction can be alleviated by placing the thumbs on the maxilla with the index fingers under the ramus of the mandible and rotating the mandible forward with pressure from the index fingers (*arrow*). This maneuver will bring the soft tissues forward and therefore frequently reduce the airway obstruction. (From Kaur S, Heard SO. Airway management and endotracheal intubation. In Rippe JM, Irwin RS, Fink MP, Cerra FB (eds.), *Intensive Care Medicine* (3rd ed.). Boston: Little, Brown, 1996.)**

choice when a C-spine fracture is suspected and involves grasping the angles of the mandible and lifting forward without tilting the head (Fig. 2-2).

3. If the patient remains apneic, ventilation should be initiated with a **bag-valve-mask device** and **supplemental high flow oxygen** while preparation for endotracheal intubation is initiated. The bag-valve-mask device includes a self-inflating bag with oxygen reservoir and a nonrebreathing valve. It is attached to a clear face mask with a pliable border to enhance the seal. To deliver 100% oxygen, the reservoir must be at least as large as the bag. Ventilation is performed utilizing the chin lift or jaw thrust technique and is more easily performed by two persons. This technique is best used in conjunction with an oral airway (see below). The positive pressure generated by bag-valve-mask ventilation will lead to gastric distention and increase the risk of aspiration. Cricoid pressure (the **Sellick maneuver**), which compresses the esophagus posteriorly, should be performed to reduce this risk.

4. An **oropharyngeal airway** is a semicircular device that lifts the base of the tongue off the hypopharynx (Fig. 2-3A). In addition to facilitating ventilation with the bag-valve-mask device, it can be used as a bite block to prevent occlusion of the endotracheal tube in the orally intubated patient. Insertion is performed

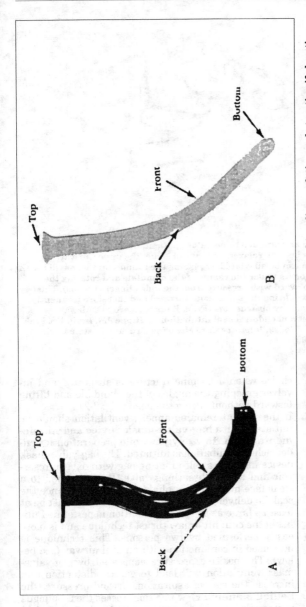

Fig. 2-3. Oropharyngeal (A) or nasopharyngeal (B) airways can be used to relieve soft tissue obstruction if elevating the mandible proves ineffective. (From Kaur S, Heard SO. Airway management and endotracheal intubation. In Rippe JM, Irwin RS, Fink MP, Cerra FB (eds.), *Intensive Care Medicine* (3rd ed.). Boston: Little, Brown, 1996.)

with a tongue blade to move the tongue out of the way or by placing the oropharyngeal airway backwards as it enters the mouth and rotating it when it approaches the posterior pharynx. If the oropharyngeal airway is inserted incorrectly, the tongue may be pushed backwards, worsening the obstruction. Since the oropharyngeal airway can stimulate the gag reflex, precipitating vomiting and aspiration, it should only be used in the unconscious patient without protective airway reflexes.

5. In the semiconscious patient who will not tolerate the oropharyngeal airway, the **nasopharyngeal airway** is a better choice. It is a soft-rubber uncuffed tube with internal diameter of 6–9 mm (Fig. 2-3B). After lubrication with anesthetic jelly, it should be inserted through the least obstructed nostril, close to the midline, along the floor of the nasal passage until it bypasses the tongue into the posterior pharynx. Complications include injury to the nasal mucosa with bleeding or inadvertent insertion into the esophagus causing gastric distention (often seen if too long a tube is used).

6. In the patient with adequate respiratory effort, the application of **high-flow oxygen** should coincide with initial airway clearing techniques. A **nasal cannula** with flow rates up to 6 liter/min can provide a patient with up to 40% inspired oxygen concentration. Patients in severe respiratory distress usually require higher concentrations of oxygen. A **face mask** equipped with a **reservoir** and a **nonrebreathing valve** with flow rates of 10 liter/min can deliver oxygen concentrations close to 100% if a tight seal is maintained.

B. **Esophageal obturator and related devices**
1. The **esophageal obturator airway** (EOA) and similar devices are used in the prehospital setting as temporary alternatives to endotracheal intubation, to protect the airway and to provide ventilation. The blind insertion technique for an EOA does not require manipulation of the cervical spine (Fig. 2-4). Because of a high rate of complications, its use is somewhat controversial. There is probably no role for the use of these devices in the emergency department or hospital setting.

The EOA is a 34 cm semirigid tube with a rounded occluded distal lumen with an inflatable cuff. At the proximal end of the tube is a face mask to provide occlusion at the face. The proximal hollow portion of the EOA has multiple side openings at the level of the hypopharynx to provide ventilation. The EOA is inserted blindly into the esophagus and the distal cuff is inflated to occlude the esophagus, which prevents regurgitation. Ventilation through the mask then provides oxygen to the region of the trachea (Fig. 2-5).

2. The **esophageal gastric tube airway (EGTA)** is an EOA with an added hollow esophageal tube that allows passage of a nasogastric tube and decompression

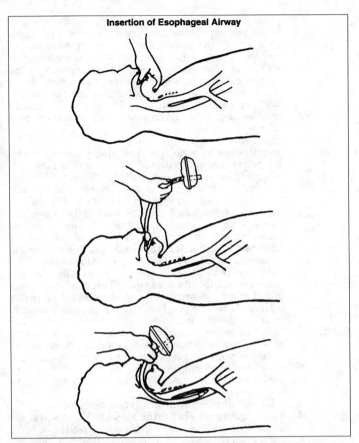

Insertion of Esophageal Airway

Fig. 2-4.   An obturator is introduced into the esophagus by elevating the tongue and jaw from the corner of the mouth with one hand, with head and neck flexed forward. (Reproduced with permission. *Textbook of Advanced Cardiac Life Support,* 1994. Copyright American Heart Association.)

of the stomach. Otherwise it is identical to the standard EOA (Fig. 2-6).

3. The **esophageal trachael combitube (ETC)** (Fig. 2-7) and the **pharyngeal tracheal lumen airway (PTLA)** allow ventilation in a similar fashion to the EOA. They are different in that neither has a face mask as the proximal occluding device. They have balloons that occlude the airway above and below the trachea. Ventilation is provided through perforations in the tube between the two balloons. Tube location and confirmation of placement is often difficult in the field setting.

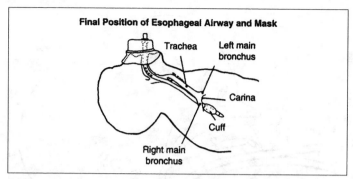

Fig. 2-5. Properly positioned obturator airway. The rim of the face mask must be sealed tightly against the face to effect an airtight seal. (Reproduced with permission. *Textbook of Advanced Cardiac Life Support*, 1994. Copyright American Heart Association.)

4. **Complications** of the EOA and related devices include esophageal injury or perforation, aspiration, inadequate seal of the face mask, and pharyngeal or tracheal trauma (Table 2-6). **Contraindications** to the use of these devices include awake or semiconscious individuals, infants, children or individuals shorter than 120 cm, and suspected esophageal injury or caustic ingestion.

5. A patient presenting to the emergency department with the EOA or related device in place should have it

Fig. 2-6. Esophageal gastric tube airway (EGTA). The gastric tube can be passed through the lumen of the airway. Ventilation is carried out by standard mask technique, with the mask held securely against the face. (Reproduced with permission. *Textbook of Advanced Cardiac Life Support*, 1994. Copyright American Heart Association.)

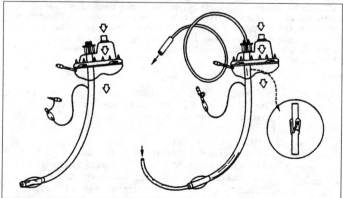

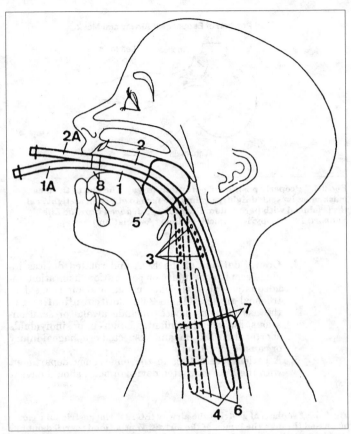

Fig. 2-7.   Cross section of the esophageal tracheal Combitude (ETC) in esophageal (*continuous lines*) and tracheal (*dotted lines*) position. 1: 'Esophageal' lumen. 1A: Longer, blue connector leading to lumen 1. 2: 'Tracheal' lumen. 2A: Shorter, clear connector leading to lumen 2. 3: Perforations of lumen 1. 4: Distal blocked end of lumen 1. 5: Pharyngeal balloon. 6: Distal open end of lumen 2. 7: Distal cuff (for sealing of either the esophagus or the trachea). 8: Printed rings indicating depth of insertion. (From Comparison of ventilatory pressure curves. *J Trauma* 29:1477, 1989.)

replaced by an endotracheal tube as soon as possible. The tube should be **removed under direct laryngoscopic visualization** after intubation of the trachea.

C. **Principles of intubation**

1. **Endotracheal intubation** is the definitive form of airway management. The advantages to endotracheal intubation include isolating the airway and maintaining patency, reducing the risk of aspiration, allowing suctioning of the trachea, ensuring the delivery of high

Table 2-6. Complications of esophageal airways

Tracheal intubation
Tracheal injury or perforation
Esophageal perforation
Aspiration
Respiratory acidosis
Pneumothorax
Pneumomediastinum
Mediastinitis
Inadequate mask to face seal
Emesis on removal

concentrations of oxygen and adequate ventilation, and providing a route for administration of drugs. The process of endotracheal intubation should be carried out under controlled conditions as much as possible, with appropriate equipment available. Universal precautions including gown, gloves, mask, and face shield should be used as often as possible.

2. A **preintubation evaluation** should be performed in even the most emergent situations for the purpose of rapidly assessing the airway anatomy and choosing the appropriate route of intubation. **Cervical spine mobility** (in the absence of trauma) can be assessed by flexion and extension of the neck. Conditions affecting mobility include degenerative arthritis, previous trauma, and age over 70 years. **Temporomandibular joint function** should be tested. It can be limited by any form of arthritis and conditions that cause a receding mandible. Normal adults can open their mouths 50–60 mm (this corresponds to 3 finger widths held vertically in the midline). If the opening is less than 40 mm, a difficult intubation should be expected. **Examination of the oral cavity** is mandatory. Dentures and removable bridgework should be taken out and any loose, missing, or chipped teeth noted. Examination of the soft palate, uvula, and facial pillars with the mouth open and tongue protruded provides a useful clinical test to evaluate the airway. The fewer the visible structures the more likely a difficult intubation will occur (Fig. 2-8).

3. **Orotracheal intubation,** which permits direct visualization of the glottis, is the preferred method of intubation for most patients. It provides the best assurance of correct tube placement because the tube is seen passing between the vocal cords into the trachea. If there is a contraindication to orotracheal intubation or attempts are unsuccessful, then alternative methods including **blind techniques** and **surgical techniques** can be used (Table 2-7). These techniques will

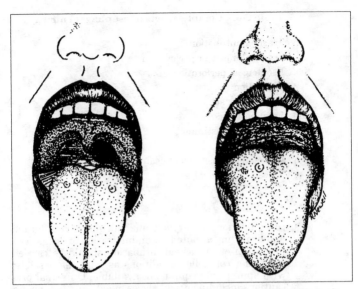

Fig. 2-8.   The facial pillars, soft palate, and uvula are not visible in the patient on the right. One should expect difficulty in orotracheal intubation. (From Kaur S, Heard SO. Airway management and endotracheal intubation. In Rippe JM, Irwin RS, Fink MP, Cerra FB (eds.), *Intensive Care Medicine* (3rd ed.). Boston: Little, Brown, 1996.)

be discussed below, with the relative indications and complications of each individual procedure.

4. Once intubation has been performed, assessment of tube position and **confirmation of placement** is imperative (Table 2-8). Tube position can be verified by auscultation of the lungs, inspection of the chest rising with inspiration, and visualization of vapor in the tube with each exhalation. The reliability of **end tidal CO_2 detectors** for confirmation of tube placement in patients not in cardiac arrest have become the standard of care. The endotracheal tube should be secured by taping about the head and neck. Patients should be restrained to prevent accidental extubation. The chest x-ray is used to confirm position above the carina.

5. Most patients will require frequent suctioning with

Table 2-7.   Alternative methods of intubation

Blind techniques	Surgical techniques
Nasotracheal	Retrograde translaryngeal
Light wand guided	Cricothyroidotomy
Fiberoptic bronchoscope	Percutaneous transtracheal ventilation
Tactile oral	Tracheostomy

Table 2-8. Confirmation of endotracheal tube placement

Direct visualization during placement
Chest x-ray
Auscultation of lung fields
Auscultation of epigastrium (absent breath sounds)
Observation of chest rise
Observation of the escape of air or moisture (clouding of tube)
Palpation of cuff insufflation at second tracheal ring
Pulse oximetry
End tidal CO_2 detector

flexible suction catheters designed for endotracheal tubes. Close observation for complications of intubation and positive pressure ventilation that might occur in the immediate postintubation period is important (see Chap. 5).

III. **Intubation techniques**
   A. **Oral endotracheal intubation**
      1. **Indications.** The indications for endotracheal intubation have been discussed previously (see Table 2-5).
      2. **Contraindications.** There are a few relative contraindications to orotracheal intubation including severe maxillofacial trauma, continuous bleeding or excessive secretions in the hypopharynx, mechanical obstruction, unusual anatomic features, or wiring of the jaw as in patients with jaw fractures. Most experts do not consider the need for cervical spine immobilization a contraindication as long as in-line head stabilization is maintained during the procedure.
      3. **Equipment.** All equipment should be ready prior to attempting intubation (Table 2-9). The tip of the endotracheal tube should be lubricated with lidocaine jelly, and a stylet should be inserted. The endotracheal balloon should be tested to assure patency. The functioning suction catheter, bag-valve-mask device, laryngoscope, and endotracheal tube with balloon-inflating-syringe should be at hand prior to intubation attempts. Universal precautions should be followed. There are two types of **laryngoscope blades,** the straight (Miller) and curved (Macintosh) blades (Fig. 2-9). Individual preference usually guides blade choice.
      4. **Patient preparation.** One of the most important aspects of the technique is proper patient positioning. Alignment of the oral, pharyngeal, and laryngeal axes is accomplished by placing the patient in the sniffing position. (Fig. 2-10). Preoxygenation can be attained with a bag-valve-mask device or a 100% oxygen mask in the breathing patient.
      5. **Intubation technique.** After patient positioning is attained, endotracheal intubation is attempted. The laryngoscope is held in the left hand and inserted into

Table 2-9.   Equipment for intubation

Oxygen supply
Face mask (100% nonrebreather)
Bag-valve-mask device
Suction equipment
   Rigid "tonsil" tip
   Flexible suction catheters
Oral and nasal airways
Tongue depressors
Magill forceps
Vasoconstrictors and local anesthetics
Endotracheal tubes (various sizes)
Stylets
Laryngoscope handle and blades
   Curved and straight (various sizes)
Syringe for cuff inflation
Tape and tincture of benzoin

the right side of the patient's mouth, displacing the tongue to the left. The straight blade is inserted over the epiglottis whereas the curved blade is inserted in the vallecula. With the blade in place, force is directed upward and away from the body (in the direction of the handle) in a plane 45 degrees from horizontal to expose the vocal cords. The handle should not be used with a prying motion nor the upper teeth used as a fulcrum. The endotracheal tube is inserted in the right corner of the mouth and advanced under direct vision through the vocal cords until the proximal end of the cuff is below the cords. In the average-size adult, tube position at the level of the incisors should be the 23-cm mark for men or the 21-cm mark for women. The cuff is then inflated and the position of the tube is confirmed. Attempts at intubation should last **no more than 30 seconds.** Bag-valve-mask ventilation and reoxygenation for 2 to 3 minutes should occur between attempts.

    6. Complications. Complications of oral intubation include trauma to the mouth (teeth, lips, tongue, pharynx) resulting in bleeding or hematoma, esophageal intubation, esophageal perforation, vomiting and aspiration of gastric contents, arytenoid or vocal cord injury, right mainstem bronchus intubation, hypertension, tachycardia or cardiac arrhythmia (Table 2-10).

B. Nasotracheal intubation

    1. Indications. Indications for nasotracheal intubation are similar to those for orotracheal intubation with a few exceptions. The prime candidate for nasotracheal intubation is the awake, spontaneously breathing patient who requires airway control and might otherwise require sedation and muscle paralysis to facilitate

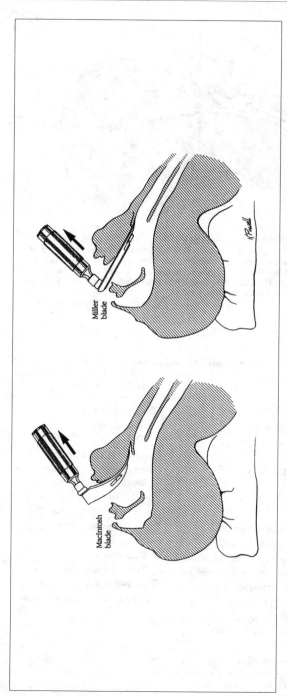

Fig. 2-9. The two basic types of laryngoscope blades, Macintosh (*left*) and Miller (*right*). The Macintosh blade is curved. The blade tip is placed in the vallecula and the handle of the laryngoscope pulled forward at a 45-degree angle. The Miller blade is straight. The tip is placed posterior to the epiglottis, pinning the epiglottis between the base of the tongue and the straight laryngoscope blade. The motion on the laryngoscope handle is the same as that used with the Macintosh blade. (From Kaur S, Heard SO. Airway management and endotracheal intubation. In Rippe JM, Irwin RS, Fink MP, Cerra FB (eds.), *Intensive Care Medicine* (3rd ed.). Boston: Little, Brown, 1996.)

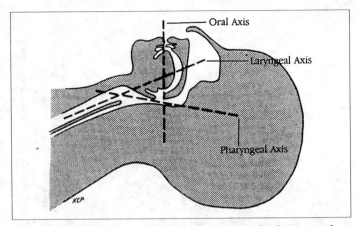

Fig. 2-10.   In the supine patient, the axes of the mouth, pharynx, and larynx lie in divergent directions. To facilitate intubation, the axes of these three regions must be brought into close approximation. (From Kaur S, Heard SO. Airway management and endotracheal intubation. In Rippe JM, Irwin RS, Fink MP, Cerra FB (eds.), *Intensive Care Medicine* (3rd ed.). Boston: Little, Brown, 1996.)

Table 2-10.   Complications of intubation

Early (during procedure)	Late (tube in place)
Spinal cord injury	Tube obstruction
Mandible dislocation	Secretions
Mouth soft-tissue injury	Kinking
Dental fractures	Accidental extubation
Perforation or laceration of:	Ulceration of lips, pharynx, or
pharynx	vocal cord
larynx	Vocal cord paralysis
trachea	Pneumothorax
Arytenoid dislocation or avulsion	Pneumomediastinum
Vocal cord spasm or injury	Infections
Right mainstem bronchus intubation	Pneumonia
Esophageal intubation or perforation	Tracheobronchitis
Vomiting and aspiration	Tracheoesophageal fistula
Cardiovascular problems	Tracheal ulceration or stenosis
Hypertension or hypotension	
Bradycardia or tachycardia	
Dysrhythmia	
Excessive delay of CPR	

orotracheal intubation. Other indications include non-apneic patients who have trismus or an inability to open their mouths because of facial fractures, temporomandibular joint disease, oropharyngeal infections, or congenital malformations. Patients with limited motion of the neck as a result of degenerative joint disease are also included. Some experts prefer the nasotracheal route in the patient with suspected or unstable cervical spine injuries. Recent cadaver studies, however, demonstrate spinal cord movement even with careful nasotracheal attempts. The selection of nasotracheal intubation over orotracheal intubation is often dependent on the experience and preference of the physician. Available clinical data do not clearly establish one procedure as superior to the other.

2. **Contraindications.** Nasotracheal intubation does have several definite contraindications. Patients with a coagulopathy or anticoagulant therapy are at risk for massive bleeding from the nose with nasotracheal intubation. Midface fractures and basilar skull fractures create the risk of penetration of the cribriform plate into the brain substance with attempts at the nasal route. Patients with acute epiglottitis, upper airway foreign body, abscess or tumor should be intubated under direct vision or by a surgical route. Patients with very shallow breathing or apnea should be intubated by alternative measures.

3. **Intubation technique.** The technique of **blind nasotracheal intubation** begins by positioning the patient with the neck extended in the sniffing position, either sitting upright or supine. Both nostrils should be sprayed with a topical vasoconstrictor like phenylephrine 0.5–1.0% (neosynephrine). The nostril to be intubated can then be anesthetized by placement of a nasopharyngeal airway coated with lidocaine jelly. This also assures patency of the nasopharynx. Selection of an endotracheal tube 1 mm smaller than would be used for the oral route in recommended, however an 8 mm tube can be used for most adult males. The tube is initially advanced through the nasopharynx with the bevel of the tube facing the septum (to avoid trauma to Kiesselbach's plexus), perpendicular to the floor. Gentle pressure and slight rotation of the tube are required until a release is felt as the tube rounds the posterior pharyngeal wall. Once positioned in the oropharynx, the tube is easily advanced toward the glottis while the physician carefully listens for breath sounds. If breath sounds are lost at any point, the tube should be pulled back several centimeters until they are heard again. The tube can be rotated slightly prior to advancement. Maximal breath sounds occur when the tube is just proximal to the glottis. At this point the tube is swiftly advanced past the vocal cords during **inspiration.** Correct placement is often confirmed by coughing and the inability to speak. The

cuff is inflated and proper placement is confirmed as described above. Use of a trigger-type endotracheal tube (a wire connects the distal tip with a proximal loop to control tube flexion) is helpful in directing the endotracheal tube anteriorly facilitating tracheal placement.

   4. **Complications.** In addition to the complications described for oral endotracheal intubation, nasotracheal intubation carries the additional risk of epistaxis. Retropharyngeal perforation, nasal necrosis, and damage to the adenoid tissue can result from intubation trauma. Patients intubated longer than 5 days are at increased risk of developing paranasal sinusitis.

C. **Fiberoptic bronochoscope guided intubation**
   1. **Indications.** Patients who need intubation of the trachea with a flexible fiberoptic bronchoscope or laryngoscope are patients who have had known or suspected difficult intubations and who are awake and spontaneously breathing (Table 2-11).
   2. **Contraindications.** Contraindications include the uncooperative patient, profuse bleeding in the upper airway, or severe hypoventilation or hypoxia.
   3. **Intubation technique.** The technique involves initial preparation of the nasopharynx as described for a nasotracheal intubation with vasoconstrictors and anesthetics. A well-lubricated bronchoscope is inserted in an endotracheal tube and guided through the nasopharynx until the glottis is visualized. The endotracheal tube is then advanced partway into the nares to facilitate further advancement of the bronchoscope. Under direct vision the bronchoscope is passed through the vocal cords confirming placement by identifying tracheal rings. The endotracheal tube slides over the bronchoscope into the trachea.
   4. **Complications.** Complications of this procedure are similar to other techniques of endotracheal intubation, including nasal trauma and epistaxis.

Table 2-11.   Indications for fiberoptic bronchoscope guided intubation

Known or suspected difficult intubation
    Congenital craniofacial abnormalities
    Severe burns to face or upper airway
    Head and neck disease
    Trismus
    Maxillofacial trauma
Cervical spine injury
Morbid obesity
Risk of adverse reaction to neuromuscular blockers

D. Other techniques for intubation of the difficult airway

1. **Tactile oral intubation** is an alternative for the **apneic** patient when direct visualization of the glottis by laryngoscopy fails because of massive bleeding, vomitus, or excessive secretions in the airway. The endotracheal tube (with stylet in place) is grasped near the cuff with the index and middle fingers and inserted in the mouth with the palm facing the tongue. The fingers contact the posterior portion of the epiglottis, identifying the glottic structures, and guide the endotracheal tube through the vocal cords. Long fingers are required, and this technique works best in patients lacking teeth.

2. **Retrograde translaryngeal intubation** is an alternative when blind nasotracheal intubation is unsuccessful or is not possible in the **spontaneously breathing** patient. The cricothyroid membrane is punctured with a needle and a j-wire or catheter is inserted through the needle cephalad into the oropharynx. An endotracheal tube then is guided blindly over the wire into the larynx. A standard epidural catheter, which contains a wire within the catheter, can also be used. If there are excessive secretions or blood in the mouth, air can be injected through the catheter and the bubbles seen will identify its location in the oropharynx.

3. **Light-wand–guided intubation** via the oral or nasal route is another method used in the difficult airway as an alternative to blind nasotracheal intubation. An endotracheal tube is inserted over the light wand, which acts as a stylet. It is guided into the trachea by visualizing transillumination in the midline of the neck. Darkening the room and forward traction on the tongue can help facilitate this procedure.

IV. **Surgical airway alternatives**

A. **Cricothyroidotomy**

1. **Indications.** A surgical cricothyroidotomy is indicated for airway control when less invasive means are contraindicated or unsuccessful. Often it is required in patients with severe facial trauma, hemorrhage, or upper airway obstruction. A cricothyroidotomy is easier to perform and has less complications than a tracheostomy in an emergency situation and is the surgical airway of choice in adults.

2. **Contraindications.** The procedure is contraindicated in children less than 10 years of age and in patients with laryngeal trauma. Other situations where alternative means of airway management should be considered include trauma to the neck, thereby altering the anatomic landmarks and the presence of a coagulopathy.

3. **Intubation technique.** The technique begins with rapid **preparation** of the skin with antiseptic solution. The **anatomic landmarks** and location of the cricothyroid membrane (CTM) should be identified.

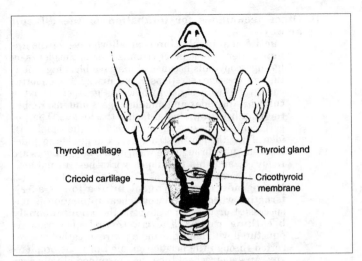

Fig. 2-11. Landmarks for locating the cricothyroid membrane. (Reproduced with permission. *Textbook of Advanced Cardiac Life Support,* **1994. Copyright American Heart Association.)**

The CTM is located between the thyroid cartilage superiorly and the cricoid cartilage inferiorly, approximately 1 cm below the vocal cords (Fig. 2-11). The usual size is 10 mm high by 22 mm wide. The location of the hyoid bone and the laryngeal prominence (Adam's apple) below it is identified first. The CTM is usually 1 to 1½ finger widths below the laryngeal prominence in the midline. The cricoid cartilage should be easily palpated below the CTM. Once the CTM is identified, the larynx should be immobilized with the left hand (for right-hand-dominant individuals) by grasping the thyroid cartilage with the thumb and long fingers and letting the index finger rest on the CTM. A **vertical incision** through the skin, subcutaneous tissue, and fascia is made in the midline measuring 2–3 cm using a No. 11 scalpel blade. **Reindentification** of the CTM by palpation with the left index finger confirms proper location. An **horizontal incision** then is made through the lower third of the CTM measuring 1.5 cm in length. The scalpel is removed and the left index finger inserted in the incision. A **tracheal hook** is inserted to assist in immobilizing the larynx and a **trousseau dilator** is inserted and opened in the vertical direction. If a dilator is not available, the scalpel handle can be used instead. A No. 6 cuffed endotracheal tube or tracheostomy tube is inserted through the incision, the tracheal hook is removed, and confirmation of placement is performed.

4. **Complications.** Acute complications from cricothyroidotomy include hemorrhage, false passage of the tube, and airway obstruction with blood or secretions. Subglottic stenosis has been reported as a long-term complication. If prolonged intubation is required, early conversion to a tracheostomy is recommended.

B. **Percutaneous transtracheal ventilation**

1. **Indications.** The indications for percutaneous transtracheal ventilation (PTV) via needle cricothyroidotomy are similar to those listed for surgical cricothyroidotomy. The technique may be considered when surgical cricothyroidotomy has failed or is contraindicated. PTV is a **temporary** means of establishing ventilation and should be used for only 30–45 minutes while a definitive airway is being secured. It may also be useful in selected pediatric patients, but because of the lack of research on the safety and efficacy in this population, it cannot be routinely recommended. In the very young child or infant, PTV may be harmful because of the difficulty in localizing the cricothyroid membrane and the lack of airway support.

2. **Contraindications.** PTV is contraindicated in patients with complete upper airway obstruction because of the risk of rapid increases in intrapulmonary pressures leading to barotrauma. In cases of partial airway obstruction, extreme caution should be exercised if PTV is attempted, utilizing a lower frequency of insufflation.

3. **Ventilation technique.** The technique involves the delivery of oxygen under high pressure into the airway via a plastic catheter placed through the CTM. After preparation of the skin, a 12- to 16-gauge angiocath is inserted in the midline through the lower half of the CTM angled caudally at 30 to 45 degrees (Fig. 2-12). An attached syringe is aspirated continuously until free flow of air confirms entrance into the trachea. The catheter is then advanced as the needle is withdrawn, and the catheter attached to a high-pressure oxygen source (50 psi) that is linked by an apparatus to control oxygen delivery. The apparatus should consist of **non-collapsible tubing** and a **valve** or **stopcock** to allow intermittent flow of oxygen (Fig. 2-13). Ventilation is accomplished with 1- to 2-second breaths and a 4- to 5-second exhalation time. Alternatively a Saunders-type jet ventilator may be used. The patient should be assessed for chest rise during oxygen insufflation. An ambu-bag and adapter attached to the catheter do not provide adequate ventilation and should not be used.

4. **Complications.** Most complications are secondary to barotrauma or chinking of the catheter. Pneumothorax and pneumomediastinum can occur rarely; patients with chronic lung disease or emphysema are more susceptible. Chinking of the catheters can be avoided if chink-resistant catheters are used. Aspira-

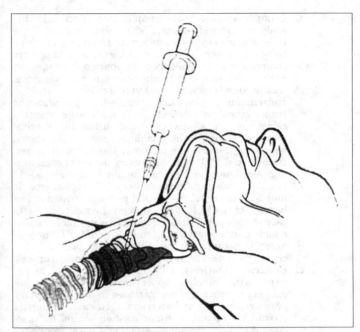

Fig. 2-12.   Insertion of a catheter with an attached syringe into the trachea across the cricothyroid membrane. (Reproduced with permission. *Textbook of Advanced Cardiac Life Support,* 1994. Copyright American Heart Association.)

Fig. 2-13.   Attachment of a transtracheal ventilation system to an intratracheal catheter. (Reproduced with permission. *Textbook of Advanced Cardiac Life Support,* 1994. Copyright American Heart Association.)

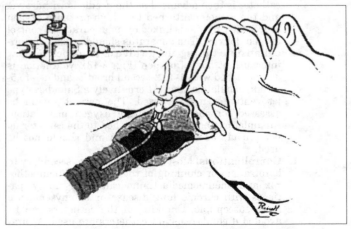

tion of secretions, blood or emesis is a potential complication because the airway is unprotected between insufflations.

V. **Pharmacological aids to intubation.** Some patients in the emergency setting require pharmacologic therapy to facilitate endotracheal intubation. Patients with seizures, agitation, combativeness, and inadequate muscle relaxation create difficulties in airway management. Prevention of the cardiovascular response to laryngoscopy and intubation is often desired. The use of pharmacologic adjuncts can, in select situations, reduce the difficulty of intubation and speed control of the airway. The ability to obtain a surgical airway if intubation attempts fail is a prerequisite to using drugs that produce apnea. Only clinicians with expertise and experience in airway management should use these agents.

A. **Rapid sequence induction**

1. **Rapid sequence induction (RSI)** is a specific method of inducing general anesthesia with the use of sedation and muscle relaxation to facilitate orotracheal intubation in the emergency setting. If properly performed it can reduce the risk of vomiting, prevent aspiration, and blunt both the cardiovascular response to intubation and elevations in intracranial pressure.

2. **Indications.** The indications for RSI include patients who are agitated or have altered mental status and require orotracheal intubation. The completely unresponsive, relaxed patient does not require RSI.

3. **Contraindications** include patients in whom orotracheal intubation is not likely to be successful or patients with contraindications to specific drugs used in RSI. Once a patient becomes paralyzed, the neurologic exam is obscured. Thus, for patients with status epilepticus, head trauma, or CVAs, there must be alternative plans to assess their neurologic condition.

4. **RSI technique.** The RSI technique is outlined in Table 2-12. Bag-valve-mask ventilation should only be used for patients with bradypnea or hypoventilation to avoid gastric distention. Premedication with atropine is beneficial in the pediatric patient to prevent bradycardia caused by vagal stimulation. A prefasciculating dose of muscle relaxants must be given 1–3 minutes prior to succinylcholine to be effective. Intravenous lidocaine is recommended especially for patients with cardiac arrhythmias or head injury and should be given at the same time as a prefasciculating dose of muscle relaxants. Administration of succinylcholine should follow immediately after injection of the induction agent. At this point cricoid pressure should be maintained until the completion of intubation.

B. **Neuromuscular blocking agents**

1. **Succinylcholine** is a depolarizing neuromuscular blocking agent that is the drug of choice for intubation in the emergency setting because of a rapid onset (30–60 seconds) and short duration of action (4–6 minutes). It is contraindicated in patients with penetrat-

Table 2-12   Rapid sequence intubation

Preoxygenate with 100% oxygen (use bag-valve-mask only if necessary)

Atropine (.02mg/kg, 1mg/kg maximum)

  For pediatric patients; optional for adults with bradycardia

Defasciculating dose (optional)

  Vecuronium 0.01mg/kg

Intravenous lidocaine 1.0–1.5mg/kg (optional)

Sedative/induction agent by rapid IV injection (problem specific)

  Etomidate 0.1–0.3mg/kg

  Thiopental 3–5mg/kg (0.5–1.0mg/kg if unstable)

  Ketamine 1–2 mg/kg

  Midazolam 0.1–0.3mg/kg

  Fentanyl 1–5μg/kg

Cricoid pressure initiated upon sedation

Succinylcholine 1.0–1.5 mg/kg by rapid IV injection

Intubate when full relaxation achieved

Confirm tube position

Inflate cuff and initiate ventilation

Relax cricoid pressure

---

     ing ocular trauma, patients at risk for hyperkalemia or malignant hyperthermia, and patients with a history of pseudocholinesterase deficiency.

2. **Vecuronium** is the nondepolarizing neuromuscular blocking agent that has minimal cardiovascular effects, a relatively short duration of action (20–40 minutes), and a rapid onset (within 2–3 minutes). Recently **mivacurium,** which has a similar profile to vecuronium but a duration of only 15–20 minutes, has become the nondepolarizing agent of choice when succinylcholine is contraindicated.

C. **Sedative/induction agents**

1. **Etomidate** is a nonbarbiturate, non-narcotic sedative hypnotic induction agent with no analgesic properties. Onset is less than 1 minute and the duration of action is 4–6 minutes. When given as a single injection, it has minimal cardiovascular effect and little respiratory depression. It may actually stimulate ventilation, which makes it an ideal choice for RSI. Like barbiturates, it causes a dose-dependent reduction in cerebral blood flow that can reduce intracranial pressure. Side effects reported in surgical cases include transient myoclonus and a transient suppression of endogenous cortisol production.

2. **Thiopental** is a short-acting barbiturate sedative with a rapid onset (10–20 seconds) and short duration (5–20 minutes). Beneficial effects include a reduction in intracranial pressure and a protective effect on the brain, making it useful in the head-injured patient. Because

thiopental can cause hypotension from vasodilatation and cardiac depression, it should be avoided in the patient with myocardial dysfunction, hypotension, or hypovolemia. Other problems with thiopental include poor analgesia and a dose-dependent respiratory depression.

3. **Ketamine** is a phenylcyclidine derivative producing a dissociative anesthetic state with rapid onset (1 minute) and short duration (5–15 minutes). It possesses sedative, hypnotic, analgesic, and amnestic properties. Ketamine increases systemic blood pressure through sympathomimetic stimulation, causes bronchodilation, and has minimal effects on airway reflexes. Disadvantages include elevation of intracranial and intraocular pressures, hallucinations, excessive secretions, and laryngospasm. Avoidance is recommended in patients with suspected coronary artery disease or irritability of the myocardium because of increased myocardial oxygen demands. Ketamine is a good agent for the patient with status asthmaticus or hypotension not related to coronary artery disease.

4. **Midazolam** is a potent benzodiazepine that provides anxiolysis, amnesia, and sedation. To be used as an induction agent, high doses are required (up to 0.3 mg/kg). Onset is within 1–2 minutes and duration of action is 30–60 minutes. At lower doses it has minimal cardiovascular effects, but at induction doses it can decrease cardiac contractility and reduce mean arterial pressure. In addition, it causes significant respiratory depression. The use of midazolam as the sole induction agent is not recommended, but at sedative doses it can serve as a useful adjunct to RSI and other airway procedures.

5. **Fentanyl** is a potent, narcotic analgesic with a short onset (1 minute) and short duration (30–60 minutes). The dose required to produce anesthesia varies from 2 to 20 µg/kg, which creates difficulties when used as an induction agent. It has minimal cardiovascular effects, but at higher doses may cause hypotension. It causes significant respiratory depression. Fentanyl blunts the intracranial pressure response to intubation and is most useful for sedation and analgesia after intubation.

VI. **Pediatric airway management.** Respiratory failure and respiratory arrest are the most common causes of cardiac arrest in children. A rapid evaluation of respiratory function with continuous monitoring of the pediatric patient for signs of deterioration is necessary to avoid adverse outcomes. The causes of respiratory failure include infections (e.g., croup, epiglottitis, pneumonia), asthma, head injury, toxic ingestions, and foreign body ingestion (Table 2-13). Management of the pediatric airway follows the same general principles as those for the adult airway. There are both anatomic and physiologic differences in the pediatric patient that alter the decision making and determine the procedure the physician uses in securing an airway.

Table 2-13. Causes of respiratory failure in pediatric patients

Epiglottitis
Croup
Foreign body
Trauma
Laryngospasm
Congenital abnormalities
Pneumonia
Asthma
Pneumothorax
Pulmonary edema
Head injury
Toxic ingestion
Sepsis

A. **Initial assessment of the pediatric airway.** Evaluation of the child begins with assessment of the respiratory rate, work of breathing, skin color, pulses and level of consciousness. A combination of clinical findings and arterial blood gas results are considered when making the diagnosis of respiratory failure (Table 2-14).

1. A slow **respiratory rate** can be indicative of impending respiratory failure. Tachypnea not only may represent respiratory distress but also can be secondary to

Table 2-14. Indicators of respiratory failure

Clinical finding	
General:	Limpness
	Loss of ability to cry
Pulmonary:	Decreased breath sounds with vigorous effort
	Weakening respiratory effort
	Chest retractions, grunting
Cardiovascular:	Severe bradycardia or tachycardia
	Peripheral collapse, cyanosis
Neurologic:	Agitation, severe restlessness
	Coma
Laboratory/Arterial blood gases	
PaO$_2$	<40–50 mm Hg (newborn)
	<50–60 mm Hg (older child)
PaCO$_2$	>60–65 mm Hg (newborn)
	>55–60 mm Hg (older child)

metabolic acidosis, shock, diabetic ketoacidosis, fever, or anxiety.

2. The **work of breathing** is a more sensitive indicator of respiratory distress. Nasal flaring, suprasternal, intercostal and subcostal retractions are indicative of hypoxia. The presence of inspiratory stridor denotes upper airway obstruction requiring immediate intervention. Auscultation of the lungs may reveal wheezes, rales, or decreased breath sounds that provide a clue to the diagnosis.

3. **Cyanosis,** which is best seen on mucous membranes of the mouth and nail beds when present, is indicative of severe distress.

4. **Cardiovascular dysfunction** manifest by dysrhythmias and hypotension is often a result of respiratory failure.

5. **Mental status changes:** Patients with hypoxia will often present with restlessness and agitation. Hypercapnia will manifest itself as drowsiness or unresponsiveness.

6. **Pulse oximetry** should be used on all seriously ill children to monitor oxygen saturation. However, pulse oximetry provides little information about ventilation, and patients in severe distress require arterial blood gas analysis.

B. **Management of the pediatric airway. Anatomic** and **physiologic** differences in the pediatric airway require equipment and technique modifications (Table 2-15).

1. **Equipment** for the pediatric airway differs from that for the adult. Different sizes of face masks, bag-valve-

Table 2-15. Anatomic and physiologic differences of the pediatric airway

The infant's head is relatively larger in proportion to the body.

The neck is naturally flexed and more supple from a greater proportion of cartilaginous support tissue.

The nares, oral cavity, and mandible are smaller, resulting in increased airway resistance and susceptibility to obstruction.

The tongue and lymphoid tissue (tonsils and adenoids) are relatively large.

The larynx is more anterior on direct laryngoscopy.

The epiglottis is larger and floppier.

The narrowest portion of the airway is the cricoid cartilage rather than the larynx as in the adult.

The muscosa is softer, looser, and more friable compared to the adult and is more prone to edema and disruption.

The chest wall is thinner, and both gastric and airway sounds radiate easily making auscultation less reliable.

Increased oxygen consumption (6–8 mL/kg/min instead of 3–4 mL/kg/min in the adult) makes infants susceptible to hypoxia.

mask units, oral and nasal airways, laryngoscope blades, and endotracheal tubes need to be readily available. Uncuffed endotracheal tubes should be used in children less than 8 years of age (the cricoid cartilaginous ring creates a physiologic seal). The size of the tube can be estimated by the formula: tube size in ml is equal to (16 + patient's age in years)/4. You also can choose the size of the endotracheal tube by comparing the child's little finger to the diameter of the tube. Table 2-16 lists a guide to intubation equipment. In children less than 4 years of age, use of a straight blade is recommended because of the large size of the epiglottis.

2. **Initial airway management** of the unconscious child is the same as for the adult. The alert child will choose the position of greatest airway patency, and if sitting upright the child should not be forced to lie down. Oral and nasal airways are less useful in children because they often stimulate emesis or laryngospasm if reflexes are intact. Placement can also traumatize the tonsillar and adenoidal mucosa, resulting in bleeding.

3. **Bag-valve-mask** ventilation is usually very effective in ventilating children. Do not rely on auscultation to assess adequacy of ventilation. Instead, chest wall movement should be observed. Failure of the ability to ventilate with a bag-valve-mask may indicate foreign body obstruction. In this situation, laryngoscopy to inspect the upper airway is required.

4. **Indications for endotracheal intubation** are the same in the pediatric patient as in the adult. **Orotracheal intubation** is the preferred route since blind nasotracheal intubation is technically more difficult in the child because of the anterior position of the larynx and the risk of trauma to lymphoid tissue. Because of severe bradycardia during intubation, all children

Table 2-16.   Pediatric intubation equipment

Age	Weight (kg)	Tube size (mm)	Suction catheter (F_r)
Premature	<2.5	2.5	6
Premature	2.5	2.5–3.5	6
Newborn	3.5	3.0–3.5	8
1 yr	10	4.0	8
2 yr	12	4.5	8
4 yr	16	5.0	10
6 yr	20	5.5	10
8 yr	25	6.0	10
10 yr	30	6.5	10
12 yr	40	6.5–7.0	10
14 yr	45	7.5	10

should be given atropine 0.01–0.02 mg/kg as premedication. Older infants may require sedation and muscle relaxation. The rapid sequence induction as described for adults should be followed. The technique itself is more difficult because of changes related to the anatomy described above, and assistance in stabilizing the head and neck is mandatory.

5. After intubation, **confirmation of proper tube placement** occurs along the same guidelines as in adults. Auscultation alone is unreliable in distinguishing esophageal and endotracheal intubation.

Bibliography

Benumoff JL. Management of the difficult adult airway. *Anesthesiology* 75:1087–1110, 1991.

Blackstock D. Respiratory failure. In Baldwin GA (ed.) *Handbook of Pediatric Emergencies.* Boston: Little, Brown, 1994.

Bogdonoff DL, Stone DJ. Emergency management of the airway outside the operating room. *Can J Anaesth* 39:1069–1089, 1992.

Einarsson D, Rochester CC, Rosenbaum S. Airway management in respiratory emergencies. *Clin Chest Med* 15:13–34, 1994.

Kauer S, Herd SO. Airway management and endotracheal intubation. In Ripp JM, Irwin RS, Fink MP, et al. (eds.). *Procedures and Techniques in Intensive Care Medicine.* Boston: Little, Brown, 1995.

Vascular Access

W. Frank Peacock IV

I. **Principles of vascular access.** Indications for vascular access are volume replacement and the delivery of medications directly into central circulation. Vascular access is needed before an emergency that requires circulatory access occurs. Vascular access is a prerequisite for many of the intensive care monitoring techniques and is a route for nutritional supplementation.

Fluid dynamics determine catheter selection. Flow via a catheter is directly related to the lumen diameter and inversely related to length. For maximal flow rates, catheters should be as short and fat as the vessel will allow. A number of catheter types are available. Physicians should be familiar with those types at their facility.

II. **Intravenous catheter types.** The simplest vascular access device, a **butterfly,** is a needle on a piece of clear plastic tubing. After insertion into the vein, a flashback of blood into the tubing indicates correct placement. The needle is then taped in place. Because movement can easily dislodge the needle, butterflies are difficult to maintain for long periods.

Over-the-needle catheters (Fig. 3-1) consist of a needle with an overlying plastic catheter. After the needle is introduced into the vessel, a flashback of blood is seen in the proximal chamber. The catheter is slipped over the needle into the lumen, and the needle is discarded. To prevent catheter embolus, the needle should not be reinserted once it has been removed. Lastly, the catheter is attached to the IV line. Because of their short length, these catheters are not suitable for central venous access lines.

Through-the-needle catheters (Fig. 3-2) consist of a large needle inserted into the vessel with a plastic catheter advanced through the needle. The catheter should *never* be withdrawn through the needle, lest catheter disruption and embolization occur. The needle is withdrawn partially, and a plastic guard is snapped over the needle.

The **Seldinger technique** (Fig. 3-3) requires a needle on a syringe that is inserted into the vessel. After blood flashback, the syringe is removed, and a J wire is advanced through the needle. The J wire should not be forced if it does not pass easily. A constant grip should be kept on the wire to prevent its embolization. The needle is removed, and the catheter is advanced over the wire. It is necessary sometimes to enlarge the puncture by placing a nick in the skin with a scalpel prior to advancing the catheter. Once the catheter is passed, the J wire can be removed and discarded. Blood samples are obtained, and the IV line position is checked. Some systems require an introducer-dilator, for rigidity, to be inserted over the wire before catheter placement. The introducer then is advanced over the wire, followed by catheter placement over the introducer.

All IV lines should be checked for correct placement prior to use. IV fluid should run freely, and no irritating solution

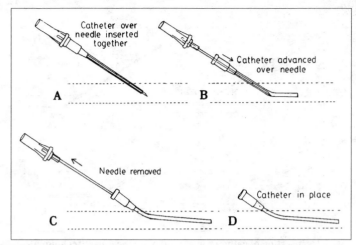

**Fig. 3-1. Insertion of catheter over needle. (Reproduced with
permission. *Textbook of Advanced Cardiac Life Support*, 1994. Copyright
American Heart Association.)**

should be used. Signs of extravasation should be watched for
and anticipated. When the IV line is properly placed, lowering
the IV bag below the patient should result in a flow of blood
"downhill." This is easily visualized in the IV tubing and confirms correct placement (assuming that no one-way valves are
present in the IV tubing).

Antibiotic ointment can be placed at the insertion site. The
catheter should be taped in place in such a manner that ex-

**Fig. 3-2. Insertion of catheter through needle. (Reproduced with
permission. *Textbook of Advanced Cardiac Life Support*, 1994. Copyright
American Heart Association.)**

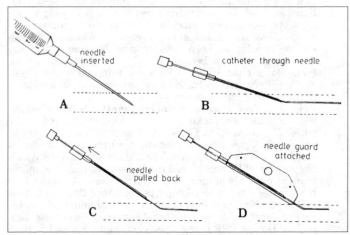

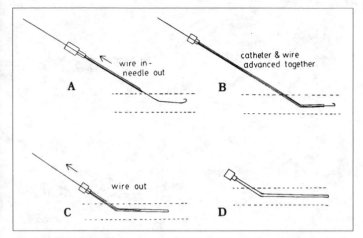

Fig. 3-3.   Insertion of catheter over guidewire (Seldinger technique). (Reproduced with permission. *Textbook of Advanced Cardiac Life Support,* **1994. Copyright American Heart Association.)**

travasation can be detected. Central venous catheters should be sutured in place. A gauze or film barrier dressing should be placed over the insertion site. Catheter sites should be checked daily and changed every 48 hours.

III. **Complications of vascular access.** The complications of vascular access are divided into those occurring immediately during the procedure and those that are delayed. Immediate complications include pain, bleeding, local infiltration of IV fluids, catheter part embolization, and air embolus. Delayed complications include infection (cellulitis and sepsis), phlebitis, and tissue damage from subcutaneous infiltration of sclerosing agents. Fluid overload can result as a complication of vascular access. Other problems are site dependent, based on those anatomic structures at risk. See Table 3-1 for a list of complications associated with central circulation vascular access. Air embolism is preventable. Whenever accessing the circulation, keep a finger over the open end of any catheter to avoid air being "sucked" into the venous circulation. Gloves should always be worn. Infection of the physician/ancillary staff by blood-borne pathogens is an avoidable complication of vascular access.

IV. **Prioritization of vascular access methods.** When selecting the route for vascular access, the decision is based on the patient's clinical state. Critically ill patients require immediate access. The time needed to perform a procedure is weighed against the relative risks and the success rate. A simple peripheral IV line, placed rapidly with minimal complications, is probably of more value than a venous cutdown that has greater risks and a longer performance time. Note that central circulation delivery times in hemodynamically stable patients are similar for peripheral versus central access techniques. During CPR using a peripheral line, a 20-ml flush (5

Table 3-1. Complications of subclavian venipuncture

Pulmonary
Pneumothorax
Hemothorax
Hydrothorax
Hemomediastinum
Hydromediastinum
Tracheal perforation
Endotracheal tube cuff puncture
Intrathoracic catheter fragmentation

Vascular
Air embolus
Subclavian artery puncture
Pericardial tamponade
Thrombophlebitis
Catheter embolus
Volume depletion
Arteriovenous fistula
Superior vena cava obstruction
Thoracic duct laceration
Local hematoma
Mural thrombus formation

Infectious
Generalized sepsis
Local cellulitis
Osteomyelitis
Septic arthritis

Neurologic
Phrenic nerve injury
Brachial plexus injury
Cerebral infarct

Miscellaneous
Dysrythmias
Ascites
Catheter knotting
Catheter malposition
Chest pain

Source: Reproduced with permission from Dronen SC, Central venous catheterization. In Roberts JR, Hedges JR (eds.), *Clinical Procedures in Emergency Medicine.* Philadelphia: Saunders, 1991.

ml in children) insures prompt delivery of medication to the central circulation.

Most patients requiring vascular access should have an initial attempt at a peripheral line. The progression for access procedures begins with the peripheral line and advances to increasingly more invasive and risky procedures. If a peripheral attempt fails, the external jugular vein should be evaluated for access. This is followed by the femoral vein, the neck and chest vessels (internal jugular or subclavian veins), and lastly a peripheral venous cutdown. In critical emergencies of the pediatric age group, an intraosseous line should be considered early in the algorithm. Multiple attempts may be performed simultaneously.

V. **Vascular access techniques**

A. **Peripheral venous cannulation and catheter (heparin) lock.** Peripheral venous cannulation is the simplest method of vascular access. It has the lowest complication risk of all the access procedures.

1. **Indications.** Peripheral venous access should be the first choice for most patients. Only the unusual patient, or a patient with permanently available vascular access, is not eligible for peripheral access as a first resort. Indications include volume replacement and drug access.

A **catheter lock** is used for patients not requiring IV fluids but in whom there is a potential need for vascular access. Examples include patients who require monitoring for cardiac arrhythmias, patients who may require IV medications, and patients in whom IV fluids are relatively contraindicated (renal failure, congestive heart failure). A catheter lock is a cost-effective technique and requires much less monitoring time.

2. **Contraindications.** Since peripheral access traverses the skin and utilizes the venous circulation, these two structures must be intact and not infected. Major extremity trauma, massive edema, overlying cellulitis, and thrombophlebitis are contraindications for use of the affected extremity. Line placement in the lower extremities of diabetics is a relative contraindication due to difficulties with healing and infection.

3. **Equipment needed.** Gloves, tourniquet, povidone-iodine or isoprophyl alcohol swabs for skin preparation, gauze sponges, antibiotic ointment, tape, and an intravenous catheter are needed to perform peripheral venous cannulation.

4. **Method of insertion.** Vein selection is the most important determinant of success (Figs. 3-4 and 3-5). A large straight vein, not on a joint surface, in the nondominant extremity, is ideal. Some practitioners prefer inserting the catheter into the fork of adjoining veins. Adjuncts for vein localization include venous tourniquet placement, muscular pumping of the extremity by the patient, tapping lightly over the vein, placing the extremity in a dependent position, or placing warm towels for a few minutes over the potential site. In the adult patient, $\frac{1}{4}$ in. of 2% nitroglycerin

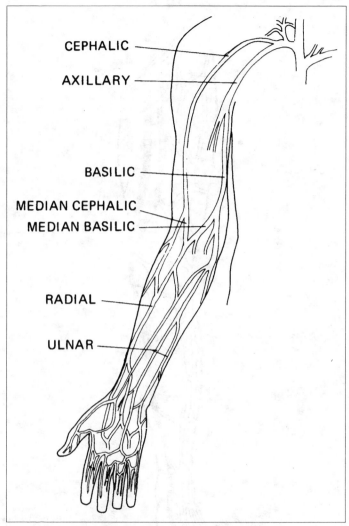

Fig. 3-4. Anatomy of veins of upper extremity. (Reproduced with permission. *Textbook of Advanced Cardiac Life Support,* 1994. Copyright American Heart Association.)

paste, spread over 1 in.^{2}, at the anticipated insertion site, may help cannulate small veins. Nitroglycerin paste should be removed after a few minutes, prior to catheter insertion.

A tourniquet (Penrose drain, sphygmomanometer cuff) is placed 5 cm proximal to the planned site of insertion. It should be of sufficient tightness to occlude

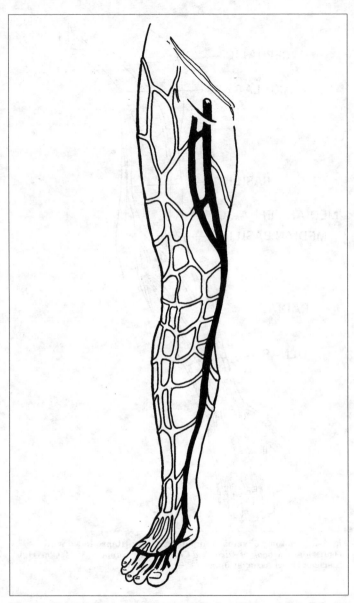

Fig. 3-5. Superficial venous anatomy of the leg. (Redrawn from Roberts JR, Hedges JR (eds.), *Clinical Procedures in Emergency Medicine.* Philadelphia: Saunders, 1991.)

the veins but not to exceed arterial pressure. Skin is prepared with either isopropyl alcohol or povidone-iodine. For most peripheral catheter insertions, anesthesia is not required.

Lidocaine (Xylocaine), 1%, is an effective anesthetic, but it should be used in volumes that do not distort the insertion site (0.1–0.2 cc).

To insert an over-the-needle catheter, the skin is pulled taut and the needle introduced at approximately 30 degrees (Fig. 3-6). Once through the skin, the needle is advanced parallel with the vein until a pop is felt, or until the catheter chamber fills with blood.

The catheter is advanced over the needle to the hub. If the catheter is felt to be in the lumen but fails to advance, the needle can be removed, an IV line attached, and IV fluid run in slowly while cautiously advancing the catheter. After the catheter is placed, it can be capped and flushed with saline to convert it to a catheter lock. A heparin flush does not improve the patency rate of a catheter lock.

5. **Complications.** Complications of peripheral line placement are rarely life threatening. They are predominately pain at the site of insertion, bleeding or hematoma formation, and local infiltration of IV fluid. Poor technique may lead to embolization of either air or catheter parts, and the lack of aseptic technique increases the risk of infection. Phlebitis may occur.

Fig. 3-6. Antecubital venipuncture. (Reproduced with permission. *Textbook of Advanced Cardiac Life Support,* **1994. Copyright American Heart Association.)**

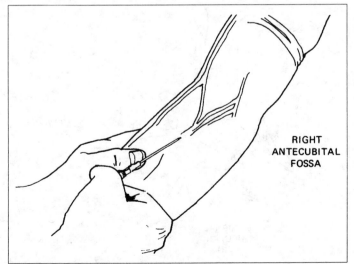

RIGHT
ANTECUBITAL
FOSSA

B. **External jugular (EJ) vascular access**
   1. **Indications.** The indication for EJ vein cannulation
      is the need for vascular access when peripheral access
      attempts have failed or are contraindicated. This tech-
      nique's advantages include a success rate exceeding
      75%, easily visualized landmarks (Fig. 3-7), and a site
      amenable to direct pressure should the attempt fail.
      Additionally, this procedure avoids the complications
      of other central venous access techniques that include
      pneumothorax or carotid artery puncture.
   2. **Contraindications.** Contraindications are similar to
      those for peripheral venous access since the EJ vein is
      essentially an anatomically constant peripheral vein.
      If the vessel is not visualized, another site of vascular
      access should be chosen. Because of the EJ vein's tor-
      tuosity and valves, direct access to the central circula-
      tion from the EJ vein is difficult without a guidewire.
      The anticipated need for central pressure monitoring
      mitigates an alternative procedure.
          Finally, this mode of vascular access can be difficult
      to keep in place. In agitated, violent, or uncooperative
      patients, another more secure method may be re-
      quired. Turning the patient's head often kinks the IV
      line, making this IV site very positional.
   3. **Equipment needed.** The same equipment is needed
      as that for peripheral venous access.

Fig. 3-7.   Anatomy of external jugular vein. (Reproduced with
permission. *Textbook of Advanced Cardiac Life Support*, 1994. Copyright
American Heart Association.)

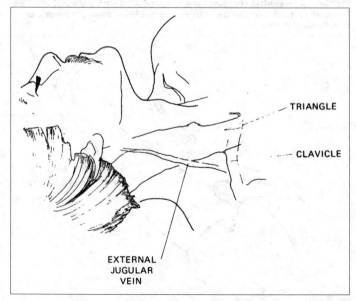

4. **Method of insertion.** The patient is placed in the Trendelenburg position to distend the EJ vein and decrease the risk of air embolus. The site is prepared as for a peripheral line. Distention of the vein is aided by applying pressure with a finger just above the clavicle. If the patient can cooperate, a Valsalva maneuver can cause vessel distention. The head is turned away from the insertion site (Fig. 3-8). The skin is pulled taut and the catheter is introduced until the pop of vessel entry is felt. A blood flashback may be noted in the catheter chamber, but it can be difficult to determine appropriate cannulation. Lowering the IV bag below the level of the patient will demonstrate immediate back blood flow if the catheter is in the lumen. The catheter should be taped in place and treated in the same fashion as a peripheral IV line. Looping the IV tubing over the ear before taping it down, will help to prevent dislodging the catheter.
5. **Complications.** The complications of EJ cannulation are similar to those of peripheral access.
C. **Infraclavicular and supraclavicular subclavian vein access**
1. **Indications.** The infraclavicular and supraclavicular routes are common approaches to the subclavian vein. Historically, the infraclavicular route is the more utilized, despite a slightly higher complication rate compared to the supraclavicular method. The indications for subclavian catheter placement include failed peripheral vascular IV line placement and a specific need for access to the central circulation. This procedure is one of several where fixed anatomic landmarks allow placement to be performed in a "blind" fashion. The choice of cannulation method should be strongly biased by the operator's experience. The supraclavicular approach is

Fig. 3-8.   External jugular venipuncture. (Reproduced with permission. *Textbook of Advanced Cardiac Life Support*, **1994. Copyright American Heart Association.)**

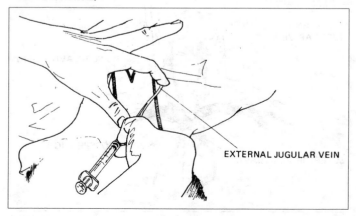

EXTERNAL JUGULAR VEIN

easier to perform during cardiopulmonary resuscitation, since it does not interfere with chest compression.

2. **Contraindications.** Contraindications to subclavian vein cannulation are anatomic deformity to the chest wall or clavicle, trauma to these structures, a history of radiation therapy to the region, a history of long-term subclavian catheterization, extremes of weight, and vasculitis. Because needle injury to the subclavian vessels cannot be directly compressed, this route should not be used in patients with suspected coagulopathies, on anticoagulants, or if thrombolytics are anticipated. Finally, this procedure is risky in agitated patients.

3. **Equipment needed.** The choice of catheter systems determines the supplies needed. Proprietary kits may contain all that is required to place a central line. This includes drapes, povidone-iodine, gauze sponges, 1% Lidocaine, 25-gauge needle, 10-ml locking syringe, catheter, 4-0 suture material, needle driver, suture scissors, antibiotic ointment, and tape. Various combinations of through-the-needle, over-the-needle, and Seldinger-technique catheter systems are available.

4. **Method of insertion.** A thorough knowledge of the significant anatomic landmarks is a prerequisite for any attempt at subclavian puncture (Fig. 3-9). The patient is placed in the supine Trendelenburg position to decrease the risk of air embolism. To decrease the possibility of injury to the left-side thoracic duct, the right subclavian vein is most frequently used. Since pneumothorax is a complication of this procedure, if the patient is known to have one, the catheter should be placed ipsilaterally. If the attempt follows a previous

Fig. 3-9.   Anatomy of the subclavian vein. (Reproduced with permission. *Textbook of Advanced Cardiac Life Support,* **1994. Copyright American Heart Association.)**

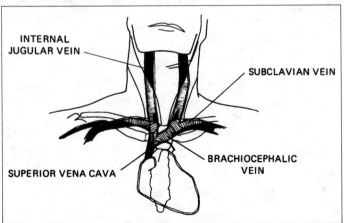

failed procedure for central venous access, the same side should be used, thereby preventing bilateral complications.

The site is prepared in sterile fashion, with povidone-iodine, and draped. Local anesthesia with 1% Xylocaine is placed in the skin and subcutaneous tissues of the conscious patient. With the infraclavicular approach, anesthesia is injected to the clavicular periosteum.

a. **Infraclavicular approach.** The thumb and forefinger are placed, as indicated (Fig. 3-10), to serve as a guide. A syringe makes needle control easier and provides the opportunity to obtain blood specimens. The needle-catheter system is introduced at the junction of the middle and proximal thirds of the clavicle. Care should be taken to maintain meticulous control of the needle tip. The needle is advanced, maintaining constant suction, aimed immediately above and posterior to the forefinger (Fig. 3-11). A blood flashback indicates vessel lumen penetration. Do not penetrate the posterior vessel wall. Arterial cannulation is indicated by bright red or pulsatile flow. When removing the syringe from the needle, a finger is kept over the hub to prevent an air embolism.

b. **Supraclavicular approach.** A 3-cm, 22-gauge needle may be used as a "locator" to assist in find-

Fig. 3-10. Hand placement during infraclavicular subclavian vein catheterization. (Redrawn from Roberts JR, Hedges JR (eds.), *Clinical Procedures in Emergency Medicine*. Philadelphia: Saunders, 1991.)

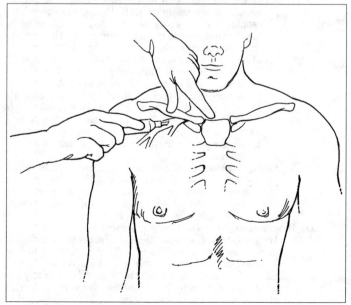

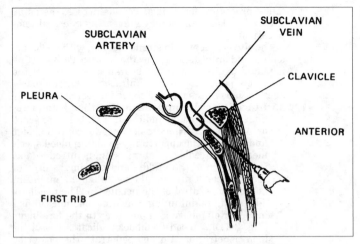

**Fig. 3-11.   Sagittal section through medial third of clavicle.
(Reproduced with permission. *Textbook of Advanced Cardiac Life
Support*, 1994. Copyright American Heart Association.)**

ing the vessel before the larger catheter-needle
system is introduced. The needle is placed at a
point 1 cm lateral to the clavicular head of the sternocleidomastoid, and 1 cm posterior to the clavicle,
in the supraclavicular fossa. It is aimed just caudal
to the contralateral nipple (the axis of the needle
should be approximately 10–15 degrees above horizontal). The needle is then advanced along a
course that bisects the angle formed by the clavicle
and the sternocleidomastoid (Fig. 3-12). Suction
should be maintained throughout the attempt. A
flashback of blood, indicating vessel lumen penetration, should be seen at a depth of 2–3 cm. Even
if unsuccessful, the chest should be auscultated after the procedure, and a stat chest radiograph
should be obtained to exclude pneumothorax and
assure correct line placement. To prevent arrhythmias, the catheter tip should not extend into the
right ventricle.

5. **Complications.** Complications from subclavian
placement are listed in Table 3.1. Pneumothorax is
most common acutely. If after several attempts the
vessel is not cannulated, consider a different route or
have a colleague attempt the procedure.

D. **Internal jugular vein vascular access**
1. **Indications.** The indications for internal jugular (IJ)
vein catheter placement are similar to those of the
subclavian vein. The IJ vein may be accessed during
CPR. The choice of technique should be strongly biased by the operator's experience. Since the vascular
structures of the neck are easily compressed, this

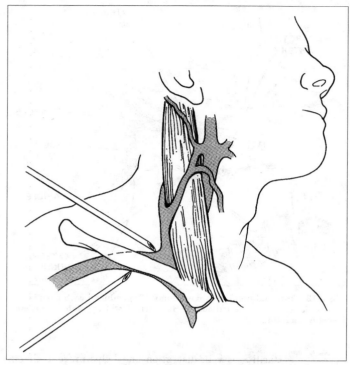

Fig. 3-12.   Supraclavicular and infraclavicular subclavian vein approaches. Note the needle bevel position, which may assist in correct catheter placement. (Redrawn from Roberts JR, Hedges JR (eds.), *Clinical Procedures in Emergency Medicine.* **Philadelphia: Saunders, 1991.)**

route should be considered over the subclavian in patients with coagulopathies.

2. **Contraindications.** Cervical trauma and anatomic distortions are contraindications to IJ cannulation. If carotid puncture occurs during an attempt at IJ placement, contralateral attempts should be avoided. This limits the possibility of bilateral neck hematomas and associated airway compromise. Finally, carotid arterial disease is a relative contraindication. If accidental carotid puncture occurs, it can lead to plaque emboli.

3. **Equipment needed.** The same equipment is needed as that for subclavian placement.

4. **Method of insertion.** The IJ vein is accessed by the anterior, central, or posterior approaches. A thorough anatomic knowledge should preface any attempts at line placement (Fig. 3-13). The IJ vein is located anterolaterally to the carotid, within the carotid sheath. In all approaches, the patient should be in the Trendelenburg position. If possible, a Valsalva maneuver

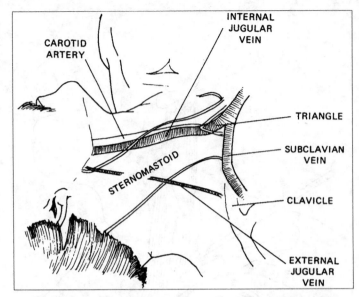

Fig. 3-13.   Internal jugular vein anatomy. (Reproduced with permission. Textbook of Advanced Cardiac Life Support, 1994. Copyright American Heart Association.)

facilitates vein distention and helps prevent air embolism. The head should be turned slightly away from the insertion site. The right IJ vein is preferred, since the course to the superior vena cava is straighter on this side, and trauma to the thoracic duct is not possible, as it is on the left.

The area is prepped with povidone-iodine, and in the conscious patient, local anesthesia may be obtained with 1% Lidocaine. If time permits, a 22-gauge "locator needle" is used to preface the attempt with the larger catheter needle. This aids in finding the vein while minimizing damage to deep neck structures. Once the jugular is located, the procedure is repeated with the catheter. Carotid puncture is indicated by bright red or pulsatile blood flow. If this occurs, the attempt is terminated, the needle withdrawn, and direct pressure applied.

a.   Anterior approach. After carotid identification, the needle enters the skin at the midpoint of the medial border of the sternocleidomastoid, angled at 30–45 degrees, and aimed at the ipsilateral nipple (Fig. 3-14). Cannulation, without carotid puncture, may be difficult.

b.   Central approach. Just lateral to the carotid, within a triangle formed by the heads of the sternocleidomastoid and clavicle, the needle is advanced caudally, at an angle of 30 degrees, parallel to the

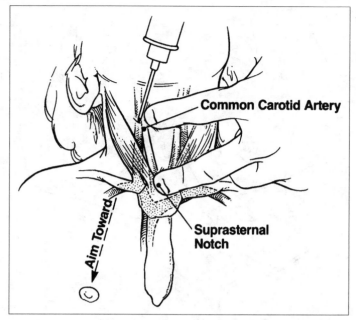

Common Carotid Artery

Suprasternal Notch

Aim Toward

Fig. 3-14. Anterior approach to the internal jugular vein. (Reproduced with permission. *Textbook of Pediatric Advanced Life Support*, 1994. Copyright American Heart Association.)

carotid (Fig. 3-15). Constant suction is maintained. Penetration should be limited to 5 cm. To prevent lacerating deep structures, if multiple attempts are required, withdraw the needle to the subcutaneous tissue before reinserting. Directing the needle toward the ipsilateral nipple may be used if the initial attempt fails.

c. **Posterior approach.** The needle should enter the skin one third of the way from the clavicle to the mastoid, just lateral to the posterior border of the sternocleidomastoid muscle. While maintaining suction, the needle is directed medially and caudally, just under the sternocleidomastoid, aiming for the sternal notch, until blood is aspirated (Fig. 3-16).

5. **Complications.** Complications of IJ catheterization are similar to those of the subclavian, with the addition of neck hematoma and carotid perforations. An isolated carotid puncture is treated by pressure and rarely results in dysfunction unless there is severe carotid atherosclerotic disease. As with any chest or neck catheterization, a chest x-ray is required to exclude pneumothorax and verify line placement. Lastly, arteriovenous fistula at the insertion site have been reported.

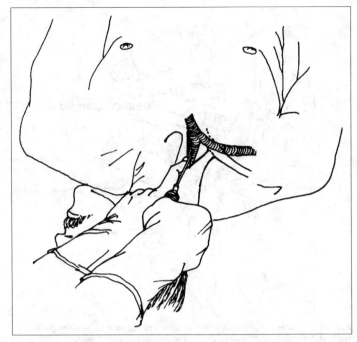

Fig. 3-15. Central approach to the internal jugular vein. (Reproduced with permission. *Textbook of Advanced Cardiac Life Support*, 1994. Copyright American Heart Association.)

E. **Femoral vein vascular access**
1. **Indications.** The indication for femoral line placement is failure to obtain peripheral line access.
2. **Contraindications.** Contraindications are similar to those of peripheral vascular access, with the addition of intra-abdominal trauma. A concurrent femoral hernia is a relative contraindication.
3. **Equipment needed.** The same equipment is needed as that required for subclavian vein catheterization.
4. **Method of insertion.** The site should be prepared with povidone-iodine, and 1% Lidocaine local anesthesia is used in the conscious patient. The needle is inserted 5–15 mm medial to the femoral pulse, while maintaining suction, until a blood flashback is seen (Fig. 3-17). Various catheter systems are available, with specific techniques described above. If central access is desired, the catheter may be presized by comparing it to the patient's body and estimating the distance from skin entrance to right atrium. If the catheter accesses the chest, a post-procedure x-ray should verify the position.

   If the femoral pulse is absent (e.g., during cardiac arrest), a blind attempt may be necessary. The femoral

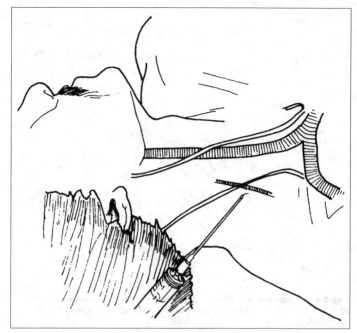

Fig. 3-16. Posterior approach to the internal jugular vein. (Reproduced with permission. *Textbook of Advanced Cardiac Life Support*, 1994. Copyright American Heart Association.)

artery crosses at the midpoint of a line connecting the public symphysis with the anterior superior iliac crest (Fig. 3-18). Punctures should be distal to this line so that, in the event of arterial laceration, direct pressure can be applied. During the chest compressions of CPR, the femoral vein may pulsate. If an initial attempt aiming medial to the pulse fails, aiming at the pulsations during CPR may result in successful cannulation.

5. **Complications.** Complications are similar to those for peripheral vascular access. In addition, femoral arterial puncture, arteriovenous fistula, femoral nerve injury, retroperitoneal hemorrhage, psoas abscess, and bowel or bladder puncture have been reported.

F. **Saphenous vein cutdown vascular access**
   1. **Indications.** There are no absolute indications for saphenous vein cutdown. Because it is a time-consuming procedure, a cutdown is considered only after other methods of vascular access have failed. It may be required in chronically ill patients, those with a history of multiple recent IV lines, the morbidly obese patient, and intravenous drug abusers.
   2. **Contraindications.** Contraindications to saphenous vein cutdown are similar to those of peripheral vascular access.

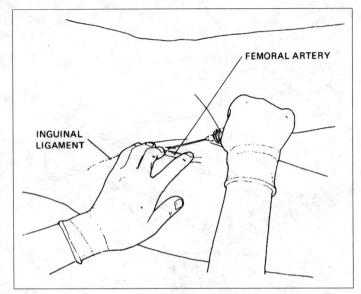

Fig. 3-17.   Femoral vein access. (Reproduced with permission. *Textbook of Advanced Cardiac Life Support,* **1994. Copyright American Heart Association.)**

3. **Equipment needed.** Instruments should be available on a sterile tray prior to the procedure. Povidone-iodine, 1% Lidocaine, Kelly hemostat, Mosquito hemostat, scalpel with blade, 4-0 silk suture ties, iris scissors, catheter, 4-0 nylon skin sutures, antibiotic ointment, gauze sponges, and tape are required.

4. **Method of insertion.** The site is prepped and draped with povidone-iodine. One percent local Lidocaine is needed in the conscious patient. If nonemergent, both exsanguination of the extremity, by raising it above the level of the heart for 5 minutes, and the placement of a tourniquet proximal to the cutdown site can limit bleeding.

   The greater saphenous vein runs subcutaneously anteromedially up the leg (see Fig. 3-5). The common site for cutdown is 1 cm anterior to the medial malleolus, where the vessel is adjacent to the tibial periosteum (Fig. 3-19). It is accompanied by the saphenous nerve supplying sensation to the medial foot.

   A transverse skin incision is made over the vessel. Using the curved hemostat, blunt dissection parallel to the course of the vessel will free it from local fat and connective tissue. Approximately 1–3 cm of vein is mobilized and isolated from the surrounding tissue. Proximal and distal silk ties are passed under the vein. The distal ligature may be tied.

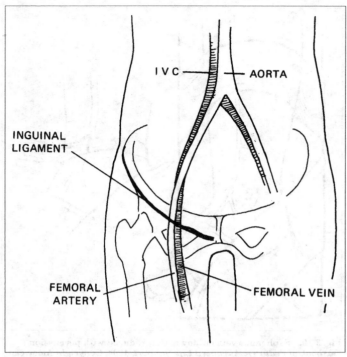

Fig. 3-18. Femoral vein anatomy. (Reproduced with permission.
Textbook of Advanced Cardiac Life Support, **1994. Copyright American Heart Association.)**

      If a through-the-needle catheter is to be used, it may be placed into the vein under direct visualization. When using a cannula, the vessel should be elevated and transversely incised 30%–50% of its diameter. The cannula is passed into the vein. Once the catheter/cannula is in place, the proximal ligature is tied tightly around the vessel wall and intraluminal device. The catheter is sutured in place, and the skin is closed. The extremity is immobilized to prevent accidentally dislodging the line.

    5. Complications. Bleeding, infection, sepsis, hematoma, phlebitis, embolization, and saphenous nerve injury are reported complications of saphenous vein cutdown.

VI. Pediatric vascular access techniques. Many of the IV access techniques in the pediatric patient are similar to those in the adult; however, correctly sized equipment is required. Generally, the largest catheter that can be inserted into the vessel is used (Table 3-2).

  A. Scalp vein vascular access

    1. Indications, contraindications, and complications. In the young pediatric age group, scalp veins are easily cannulated peripheral veins. Their use has

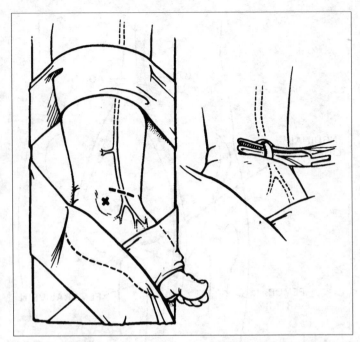

Fig. 3-19.   Saphenous vein cutdown. (Reproduced with permission. *Textbook of Pediatric Advanced Life Support,* **1994. Copyright American Heart Association.)**

the same indications, contraindications, and complications as any other peripheral IV access.

2. **Equipment needed.** The same equipment is needed as that required for peripheral IV access, as well as appropriately sized catheters, a razor to shave the site, and a rubber band to serve as a tourniquet.

3. **Method of insertion.** A rubber band is placed around the head as a tourniquet, and a vein is selected (Fig. 3-20). Veins are less tortuous than arteries, and their flow is toward the heart. Shave and prepare the site. Insert the catheter as described in peripheral venous access (see sec. **V.A.4.**), inserting the catheter in a direction toward the heart. The rubber band is carefully removed, and the catheter is secured. A cup may be taped over the catheter to prevent displacement (Fig. 3-21).

B. **Saphenous vein cutdown**
1. **Indications, contraindications, and equipment needed.** A cutdown has the same indications, contraindications, and equipment requirements as in the adult (see sec. **VI.A.2.**). Catheters should be appropriately sized.

2. **Method of insertion.** The saphenous vein may be used for cutdown anywhere along its course. The

Table 3-2. Appropriate sizes of pediatric vascular access equipment

Age (yr)	Weight (kg)	Butterfly needles (gauge)	Over-the-needle catheters (gauge)	Venous catheters				Catheter introducers			
				French size	Length (cm)	Wire diameter [mm (in.)]	Needle (gauge)	French size	Length (cm)	Wire diameter [mm (in.)]	Needle (gauge)
<1	<10	21, 23, 25	20, 22, 24	3.0	8	0.46 (.018)	21	4.0	6	0.53 (.021)	20
								4.5	6	0.53 (.021)	20
1–12	10–40	16, 18, 20	16, 18, 20	4.0	12	0.53 (.021)	20	5.0	13	0.64 (.025)	19
								5.5	13	0.64 (.025)	19
								6.5	13	0.64 (.025)	19
>12	>40	16, 18, 20	14, 16, 18	5.0	20	0.89 (.035)	18	7.0	13	0.89 (.035)	18
				6.3	20		18	8.0	13	0.89 (.035)	18

Source: Reproduced with permission. *Textbook of Pediatric Advanced Life Support*. 1994. Copyright American Heart Association.

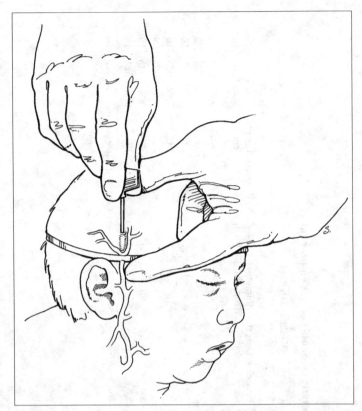

Fig. 3-20.   Procedure of scalp vein cannulation. (Redrawn from Roberts JR, Hedges JR (eds.), *Clinical Procedures in Emergency Medicine.* Philadelphia: Saunders, 1991.)

common location is at the ankle, although the knee and groin are also used.

The ankle is accessed 1–2 cm anterior and proximal to the medial malleolus (see Fig. 3-19). The groin site is just distal to a line joining the anterior superior iliac spine and the pubic tubercle, along the medial edge of the middle one-third of the thigh (Fig. 3-22). The knee site is 1–4 cm (5–10 cm in the adult) below the joint line, along the medial ridge of the tibia. The technique is the same as in the adult. The patient may require restraint. In conscious or uncooperative patients, the extremity should be immobilized prior to the cutdown attempt. Due to smaller vessel size, a vein introducer or an 18-gauge needle with the tip bent to 90 degrees, may aid in the passage of the catheter into the lumen.

3. **Complications.** Bleeding, infection, sepsis, hematoma,

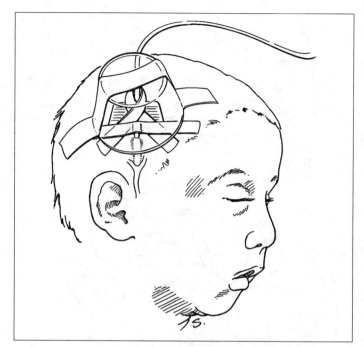

Fig. 3-21. Protecting the site with a plastic cup. (Redrawn from Engle WA, Rescorla FJ. Vascular access and blood sampling. In Roberts JR, Hedges JR (eds.), *Clinical Procedures in Emergency Medicine*. Philadelphia: Saunders, 1991.)

phlebitis, embolization, and saphenous nerve injury are complications of saphenous vein cutdown.

C. Intraosseous infusion

    1. Indications. Any drug or solution, administered intravenously, can be given intraosseously. The bone marrow is a noncollapsible vascular plexus with direct communication to the circulation. It is particularly useful in situatioins where vascular access is difficult (e.g., cardiac arrest, shock). In an emergency, only a few minutes should be given to attempt the placement of a peripheral IV line before moving to the intraosseous route. It is considered even earlier in cardiac arrest, particularly in children less than 6 years of age.

    2. Contraindications. There is no role for intraosseous access in the routine or elective placement of an IV line. Other contraindications include penetrating bony trauma (inclusive of multiple intraosseous attempts) or concurrent fracture of the extremity. Areas of overlying cellulitis or osteomyelitis at the desired site exclude attempts at intraosseous placement. Although

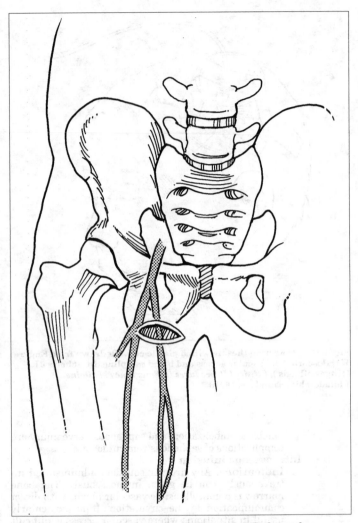

Fig. 3-22.   Proximal saphenous vein cutdown site. (Redrawn from Dronen SC, Yee AS, Tomlanovich MC. Proximal saphenous vein cutdown. *Ann Emerg Med* **10:328, 1981.)**

there is no well-defined cutoff, intraosseous placement becomes more difficult with increasing age.

3. **Equipment needed.** Povidone-iodine, gauze sponges, hemostat, tape, and a needle are required. Commercially available intraosseous needles are easiest to use; however, bone marrow biopsy and spinal needles are alternatives. In premature infants or neonates, a 19- or 21-gauge butterfly may suffice. However, without a stylet the lumen may plug with bone.

4. **Method of insertion.** The most common site for intraosseous infusion is the proximal tibia 1 cm below the tibial tuberosity, medially, on the tibial plateau (Fig. 3-23). The ankle malleoli, the midline distal femur 1 cm above the patella, and the iliac crests at the inferior aspect of the iliac spine are alternatives.

   The area is prepped with povidone-iodine. A reasonable amount of force is required to place the needle. (For the novice, practice with a chicken bone is an excellent simulation.) As the needle is advanced, a back-and-forth twisting motion eases insertion. The needle is angled away from the growth plate. A distinctive pop is felt when the marrow cavity is entered. Correctly placed, the needle should stand unsupported. To verify position, bone marrow can be aspirated and IO fluid should flow easily without extravasation.

   Flushing the needle may be needed if bone marrow results in obstruction. Intraosseous infusion fails for a number of reasons (Fig. 3-24). A hemostat, perpendicularly grasping the needle where it enters the skin, may be taped to the leg to help hold the needle in place. A paper cup, taped over the needle, may serve as a guard. A dressing should be placed and the extremity immobilized. Alternative vascular access should be obtained as soon as possible, since many of the complications can be avoided by the temporally short usage of this method.

5. **Complications.** Compartment syndrome, iatrogenic fracture, and osteomyelitis have been reported. Bone

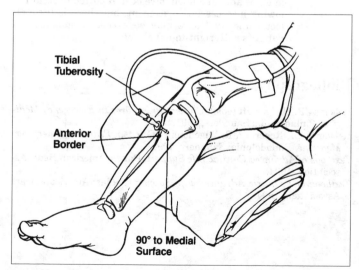

Tibial Tuberosity

Anterior Border

90° to Medial Surface

Fig. 3-23. Intraosseous cannulation. (Reproduced with permission. *Textbook of Pediatric Advanced Life Support*, 1994. Copyright American Heart Association.)

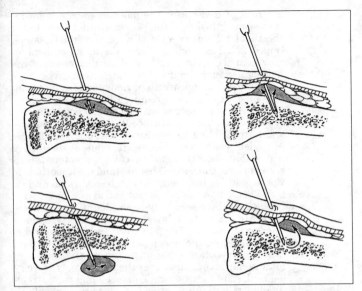

Fig. 3-24. Problems with intraosseous insertion: (top left) incomplete penetration, (top right) complete penetration of the bone (bottom left) extravasation, and (bottom right) leakage from previous puncture. (Redrawn from Spivey WH. Intraosseous infusion. In Roberts JR, Hedges JR (eds.), *Clinical Procedures in Emergency Medicine.* Philadelphia: Saunders, 1991.)

marrow and fat emboli have been reported to occur following intraosseous placement, but there is little effect clinically. There may be a risk of embolism in patients with right-to-left shunts.

Bibliography

Roberts JR, Hedges JR (eds.). *Clinical Procedures in Emergency Medicine.* Philadelphia: Saunders, 1991.

Reisdorff EJ, Roberts MR, Wigenstein JG (eds.). *Pediatric Emergency Medicine.* Philadelphia: Saunders, 1993.

Textbook of Advanced Cardiac Life Support. Dallas: American Heart Association, 1994.

Textbook of Pediatric Advanced Life Support. Dallas: American Heart Association, 1994.

Prehospital Cardiac Arrest Management

Bruce K. Neely

Sudden death due to coronary artery disease is the most prominent medical emergency in the United States. Nearly 1 million deaths each year are due to cardiovascular disease, and approximately 500,000 of those deaths are from sudden cardiac death. Collapse usually occurs outside the hospital, and death is frequent within 1 to 2 hours of the onset of symptoms, despite prehospital intervention. Over the past 30 years many advances have been made in the care of patients suffering cardiac arrest outside the hospital, and survival from prehospital cardiac arrest has risen from 5%–10% to nearly 30% in some locations. An understanding of prehospital care and treatment of cardiovascular emergencies is vital to the in-hospital care of these emergencies. No understanding of the prehospital environment is complete without an understanding of the systems and personnel involved.

HISTORIC PERSPECTIVE

Most of the advances in prehospital care of cardiac arrest have been made through the development of emergency medical services (EMS) systems. This development can be traced to the Napoleonic Wars, when Baron Dominique Jean Larrey introduced the concept of using light carriages to remove wounded soldiers from the battlefield. Further advances in prehospital care were made in each successive war up to Vietnam. The concept of using a mobile hospital on wheels to care for victims of cardiac disease can be traced to Pantridge in Belfast in 1967. At about the same time, Warren in Columbus, Ohio, and Cobb in Seattle, Washington, also developed mobile cardiac care centers, which were initially staffed with physicians. Since that time, the education and training of prehospital care providers, or emergency medical technicians (EMTs), have further extended the hospital into the community.

SINGLE- VERSUS TWO-TIERED SYSTEMS

EMS has evolved into a complex system integrating laypersons, EMTs, nurses, and physicians. Two major types of response systems are in widespread use today. One type is known as a single-tiered response. In these systems, whenever a call for help is received, a single type of vehicle is dispatched. This vehicle generally is equipped with advanced life support supplies and is staffed by two or more paramedics. This type of system has the advantage of providing the most highly trained prehospital personnel to each patient. A drawback of the single-tiered system is that these highly trained personnel may be committed to the care of non-life-threatening conditions and may be unavailable for other potentially life-threatening conditions.

In contrast, a two-tiered response system incorporates prehospital care providers with different levels of training into one system. In these systems, when a call for help is received, a first tier of personnel is dispatched. This first level of response is usually staffed by basic or advanced EMTs, police, or fire personnel. If the patient is found to have a potentially critical or life-threatening illness or injury, a second level of response is requested. This second level of response is generally made up of paramedics. The two-tiered system has the advantage of shortening initial response times and allowing paramedics to be reserved for only the more critically ill or injured. Thus, paramedics are available to a greater number of patients, even though there may be fewer of them than in a single-tiered system.

MEDICAL CONTROL

All EMS systems operate under the medical control of a physician. Two types of medical control systems are commonly used in the United States today. The first control system is termed on-line medical control. In an on-line control system, the prehospital providers give care mostly under preestablished protocols, but at a given point in the protocols, contact is made with the medical control physician via radio or telephone. The physician then gives further orders and instructions to the prehospital personnel for the ongoing care of the patient. These orders usually have to do with the administration of drugs, cardioversion, and transport and triage decisions, depending on the preestablished protocols. In an off-line medical control system, the EMS system is under the overall direction of a physician medical director. The medical director is responsible for developing system protocols and standing orders. These protocols and standing orders cover treatment, transport, triage, and administrative issues that may arise. The medical director is also responsible for system quality assurance. In an off-line control system the prehospital care providers do not need to contact a physician prior to treatment or transport of patients, but they do contact the receiving hospital to give a report of the patient and his or her condition.

   I. **Capabilities of EMTs and paramedics.** Before a discussion of prehospital cardiac arrest management begins, a definition of the training, capabilities, and equipment of the prehospital personnel is needed.

   Various levels of EMT training and education exist. The most basic level is EMT-Basic or EMT-Ambulance (EMT-A). These EMTs have completed a course of learning that includes didactic and clinical instruction. An EMT-A is trained in simple assessment of a patient and in skills that include immobilization, splinting, and basic life support. An EMT-A may choose to undergo additional training to perform more detailed patient assessment and other procedures. These persons are referred to as EMT-Intermediates (EMT-I). Additional training may include the use of a defibrillator, initiation of IV lines, and airway management. The EMT-I can be trained in one or more of the above areas. The highest level of EMT training is the EMT-Paramedic (EMT-P). An EMT-P (also commonly known as a paramedic or medic) is trained in recognition and treatment of cardiac dysrhythmias, initiation of IV lines, defibrillation, endotracheal intubation, basic trauma life support, complex patient assessment and management, and advanced cardiac life support.

   EMTs carry with them different equipment depending on

their level of training. Basic EMTs may only carry oxygen, basic wound care and immobilization devices, and simple airway adjuncts, whereas EMT-Is may carry with them, in addition to the supplies carried by EMT-As, IV supplies and defibrillators. EMT-Ps generally are well equipped with advanced airway capabilities, IV supplies, monitors and defibrillators, and cardiac resuscitation drugs (Tables 4-1 and 4-2).

II. **Management of prehospital cardiac arrest.** Management of prehospital cardiac arrest is a complex process involving the lay public, prehospital providers, and physicians. The "chain of survival" concept as described by the American

Table 4-1. Equipment commonly carried by paramedics

Airway management
  Oropharyngeal airway
  Nasopharyngeal airway
  Intubation supplies
    Endotracheal tubes (variety of sizes)
    Laryngoscope (variety of blade types and sizes)
Breathing management
  Oxygen delivery systems
    Nasal cannula
    Venturi masks
    Rebreathing masks
    Nonrebreathing masks
Circulation management
  IV catheters (variety of sizes)
  IV extension tubing (variety of sizes)
  Pressure infusion bags
  IV infusion pumps (optional)
Patient assessment tools
  Stethoscope
  Blood pressure cuff
  Penlight or flashlight
  Heavy scissors
Patient monitoring tools
  Monitor/defibrillator
  External pacer
  Noninvasive blood pressure monitoring
Other supplies
  Splinting supplies
  Traction splints
  Backboards
  Cervical collars
  MAST pants
  Assortment of bandages, tape, gauze

Table 4-2.   Medications commonly carried by paramedics

Resuscitation medications
  Oxygen
  Epinephrine (1:10,000 and 1:1000)
  Atropine
  Sodium bicarbonate
  Calcium chloride
  Lidocaine (2% and 20% solutions)
  Bretylium
  Procainamide
Cardiac medications
  Aspirin
  Nitroglycerin (tablets, paste, and IV infusion)
  Nifedipine
Other medications
  Glucose (both IV and oral)
  Insulin
  Albuterol for nebulization
  Paralytic agents (succinylcholine, vecuronium) (carried by
    some agencies)
  Diazepam
  Lorazepam
  Midazolam
  Morphine

Heart Association can be used as an outline of the management of prehospital cardiac arrest. The chain of survival incorporates four links to increase the rate of survival from cardiac arrest: (1) early access to EMS, (2) early CPR, (3) early defibrillation, and (4) early advanced care.

A. **Activation of EMS.** Activation of the EMS system in a timely manner is one simple way to help increase the chance of survival from sudden cardiac arrest. Since the greatest risk of death occurs in the first 2 hours after symptom onset, the public must be educated in recognizing the common signs and symptoms of a heart attack. In addition, the public must be educated in how to gain access to the local EMS system. Many communities in the United States now have the 911 emergency access number, and public awareness of this number is vital to ensuring that the EMS system is activated in a timely fashion. The person calling should be prepared to give a minimal amount of information, including (1) what prompted the call, (2) how many persons need help, (3) the location of the emergency, (4) what care has already been given or is currently ongoing, and (5) what is the condition (e.g., unconscious, not breathing, having severe chest pain) of the patient in need of help. The person calling for help should not hang up after giving the above information, but should remain on the line to answer any questions that the EMS dispatcher or provider may ask. In addition, if the victim is not responsive and the person calling does not know how to perform CPR, the EMS personnel may be able to give instruction over the phone until help arrives.

B. **First-responder/Bystander CPR.** The second link in the chain of survival is early CPR. If possible, this should be initiated immediately after collapse. In the ideal situation, it should be started in conjunction with activation of the EMS system. In adults, activating the EMS system takes precedence over initiating CPR, since cardiac dysrhythmias that only respond to paramedic-initiated defibrillation are often the causative event in the collapse. The best person to initiate CPR is the person witnessing the collapse or the first to discover the collapsed patient. Numerous studies have shown that survival rates are increased when bystander CPR was initiated before the arrival of any medical personnel. The number of persons trained in CPR will vary from location to location, and in cities where a greater number of citizens are trained in CPR, survival rates from cardiac arrest have been shown to be higher. In many cases, however, there is no bystander CPR, and EMS systems rely on first-responders to initiate CPR. First-responders are usually firefighters or police officers who are trained in basic life support, and who respond to 911 calls for suspected cardiac arrest. These persons are strategically placed within a community to allow for a very short response time to the patient, hopefully within 4 minutes. On arrival, they are responsible for initiating CPR and continuing it until more personnel with advanced training arrive. The goal of the first-responder is to provide adequate coronary and cerebral circulation so that attempts at early defibrillation have a greater chance at success.

C. **EMT/First-responder defibrillation.** The next link to increase the chance of survival from cardiac arrest is early defibrillation. Until the mid to late 1980s, only paramedics were trained and equipped to perform defibrillation. With the development of the automatic external defibrillator (AED), first-responders, basic EMTs, and laypersons can now safely perform defibrillation. Several studies have been performed to evaluate whether the use of an AED by first-responders increases the survival rate for out-of-hospital cardiac arrest. In one large study of 1287 patients, the survival rate was nearly doubled by first-responder AED use. Several other studies, however, have not shown the same increase in survival rates. Early CPR appears to be a necessary ingredient for first-responder or EMT defibrillation to be effective. Studies have shown that in communities where bystander CPR is common, successful early defibrillation is also common. Likewise, in communities where bystander CPR is uncommon, successful early defibrillation is less effective. Early CPR and first-responder defibrillation set the stage for the next step in prehospital care: the second-tier or paramedic response.

D. Second-tier or paramedic response. The second-tier or paramedic response allows for early administration of advanced cardiac life support prior to reaching the hospital. Potentially life-threatening postresuscitation dysrhythmias can be recognized and treated with the proper medications. In addition, paramedics can provide invasive airway management and other advanced treatments, including transcutaneous cardiac pacing, if needed. Paramedics are also trained to assess and treat other manifestations or cardiac disease, including ongoing chest pain, congestive heart failure, and cardiogenic shock. With their advanced training and capabilities, paramedics should be thought of, and respected as, invaluable members of the health care team.

E. EMS stabilization prior to transport. After the arrival of the second tier (paramedics), attempts are made to stabilize the patient as much as possible before transport. This entails a complete assessment and initiation of treatment. In most cases definitive airway management, initiation of an IV line, oxygenation, and administration of cardiac drugs take place prior to transport. When the time it would take to perform the above procedures is considerably greater than the time it would take to reach the nearest appropriate hospital, the patient may be transported without definitive attempts at stabilization.

III. Ethics of prehospital cardiac arrest management. The ethics of prehospital care are founded on two basic principles: (1) do no harm, and (2) treat others as you would have them treat you. These two concepts may seem simple, but they provide the ethical foundation of doing what is in the best interest of the patient. At times what is best for the patient may not be the most convenient or comfortable for the prehospital care provider, but ethically there is an obligation to do what is best for the patient. This may cause conflict with patients' families, especially when the patient is obviously dead and the family insists on resuscitative efforts, or when a resuscitation has been ongoing without success for an extended period of time. In these cases the prehospital personnel must do what they think is in the best interest of the patient, taking into account the ethical and legal obligations placed upon them.

In-field termination of resuscitative efforts. The question of when efforts to resuscitate a patient should cease is cause for great concern and debate within the EMS community. In many states EMTs are not allowed to stop resuscitation once it has been started. In general, EMT-As and EMT-Is are not allowed to pronounce death and must continue efforts at resuscitation until personnel with a higher level of training arrive. Paramedics are allowed to pronounce death in some states but only in the following circumstances: (1) evidence of obvious death (e.g., rigor mortis, dependent lividity), (2) decapitation, and (3) decomposition. The obvious question that arises is, "Are there circumstances where paramedics should be allowed to cease resuscitation?" In an effort to answer this question, several studies have been performed to evaluate outcomes and develop criteria for in-field termination. The consensus is that, except in cases of persistent ventricular fibrillation, patients who do not respond to prehospital advanced cardiac life support (ACLS) have an extremely low survival rate, and those who do survive have devastating neurologic outcomes. It has been proposed that if there is no return of spontaneous circulation after 25 minutes of ongoing ACLS, unless persistent ventricular fibrillation is present, efforts at resuscitation can be terminated. Until these criteria are verified in further trials and gain widespread acceptance, prehospital providers will be expected to continue resuscitation until they reach the hospital or unless directed to stop by an on-line medical control physician.

IV. **Medical-legal aspects of prehospital cardiac arrest management.** The laws concerning the practice of prehospital care vary from state to state. These laws address training, medical control, continuing education, and other issues. In addition, the laws regulate the scope of practice of prehospital providers. This defines the capabilities and limits to the practice of medicine by EMTs of all levels of training. In addition, many, if not all, states have developed "Good Samaritan laws" to protect people who come to the aid of others in a nonprofessional capacity and without the expectation of reimbursement. The goal of these laws is to encourage people to provide aid to others in need without the fear of legal action. In this fashion the government is helping to promote rapid access to CPR by sheltering those who come to the aid of others in good will.

V. **Outcome of prehospital cardiac arrest.** Despite advances in the prehospital management of cardiac arrest, mortality remains high. When CPR is begun by bystanders for witnessed cardiac arrests due to ventricular fibrillation, the rates for survival to hospital discharge range from 13% to 43%. Delaying the start of CPR greatly decreases the survival rate to hospital discharge. When CPR is begun late—more than 4 minutes after a witnessed arrest—the survival rate ranges from 2% to 21%. If spontaneous return of circulation has not been regained prior to arriving at the hospital, survival to hospital discharge rates are dismal, ranging from 0.0% to 0.6%. In view of these figures, attention must be focused on early recognition of warning signs and symptoms, early access to the EMS system, early CPR, and early advanced life support in order to achieve the highest possible survival rates.

Bibliography

American Heart Association, ACLS Subcommittee and ECC Committee. Improving survival from sudden cardiac arrest: the chain of survival concept. *Circulation* 83:1832–1847, 1991.

Bonnin MJ, Pepe PE, Kimball KT, et al. Distinct criteria for termination of resuscitation in the out-of-hospital setting. *JAMA* 270:1457–1462, 1993.

Emergency Cardiac Care Committees and Subcommittees. Guidelines for CPR and emergency cardiac care. *JAMA* 268:2117–2183, 1992.

Gray WA, Capone RJ, Most AS. Unsuccessful emergency medical resuscitation—are continued efforts in the emergency department justified? *N Engl J Med* 325:1393–1398, 1991.

Kellerman AL, Hackman BB, Somes G. Predicting the outcome of unsuccessful prehospital advanced cardiac life support. *JAMA* 270:1433–1436, 1993.

Kellerman AL, Hackman BB, Somes G, et al. Impact of first-responder defibrillation in an urban emergency medical services system. *JAMA* 270:1708–1713, 1993.

Vukov LF, White RD, Bachman JW, et al. New perspectives on EMT defibrillation. *Ann Emerg Med* 17:318–321, 1988.

Weaver WD, Hill D, Fahrenbruch CE, et al. Use of the automatic external defibrillator in the management of out-of-hospital cardiac arrest. *N Engl J Med* 319:661–666, 1988.

Advanced Cardiac Life Support

Gary L. Swart and Vicki Mazzorana

In the clinical setting, few situations provoke more anxiety than the management of a patient in cardiac arrest. In the physician's favor, the myriad of potential etiologies of cardiac arrest lead to a handful of final common pathways classified by cardiac rhythm. Advanced Cardiac Life Support (ACLS), both conceptually and as an educational curriculum developed by the American Heart Association (AHA), involves strategies or algorithms of care based on these final common pathways. Although the final common pathways remain the same, the world of resuscitation medicine continues to change, reflecting new understandings of pathophysiology and responses to pharmacologic and methodologic interventions. This chapter reflects the current standard of care as recommended in 1992 by the Emergency Cardiac Care Committee of the AHA.

I. **The etiology of cardiac arrest.** Cardiac arrest is the final common pathway to death in both cardiovascular disease (CVD) and non-cardiovascular-related illness and injury. Reported survival-to-hospital discharge rates have varied from 2% to 33% in both out-of-hospital nontraumatic cardiac arrest and in-hospital cardiac arrest.

   A. **Coronary heart disease.** CVD is responsible for approximately 1 million or nearly 50% of all deaths annually in the United States. Almost one half of these deaths can be attributed to coronary heart disease (CHD), one half of which occur as sudden cardiac deaths. The morbidity of CHD dropped 30% in the United States from 1979 to 1989, probably as a result of improved therapy and a healthier lifestyle. In 1989 more than 6 million people in the United States were estimated to have the suspected presence of CHD, with atherosclerotic coronary artery disease (CAD) being a subset of CHD.

   B. **Sudden cardiac death.** Although definitions vary, sudden cardiac death (SCD) is best defined as an unexpected collapse in a victim with or without known preexisting heart disease that occurrs within 1 hour of cardiac symptom onset. SCD is the presenting symptom in 20% of victims later found to have CHD. Approximately two thirds of SCDs occur outside the hospital. The relationship of atherosclerotic CAD to SCD is strong. Although present, the relationship of acute coronary thrombosis or spasm and resultant myocardial ischemia to SCD is less well defined.

   C. **Cardiac causes not related to CHD.** Table 5-1 shows categories of non-CHD cardiac causes of SCD.

   D. **Non-cardiac related causes.** Table 5-1 also shows categories of non-cardiac causes of SCD.

II. **Dysrhythmia recognition**

   A. **Identifying dysrhythmias.** Correct identification of cardiac rhythms is based on evaluation of the rhythm strip or 12-lead ECG as outlined below. All of the rhythm identifi-

Table 5-1.   Causes of sudden cardiac death (SCD)

 I. Coronary Heart Disease (CHD)—discussed in text
 II. Cardiac causes not related to CHD
   A. Structural abnormalities of the myocardium or valves
   B. Myocardial hypertrophy
   C. Congenital anomalies
   D. Acute and chronic heart failure
   E. Conduction system disease
   F. Infectious diseases of the myocardium or valves
   G. Infiltrative or inflammatory processes
 III. Noncardiac causes
   A. Dissection or rupture of the thoracic or abdominal aorta
   B. Pulmonary embolism
   C. Traumatic or atraumatic cardiac tamponade
   D. Blunt or penetrating chest/cardiac trauma
   E. Tension pneumothorax
   F. Metabolic/electrolyte derangement
   G. Hypoxia
   H. Electrical injury
   I. Drug or poison intoxication

cation critera do not apply to all of the dysrhythmias associated with cardiac arrest. Careful rhythm identification is important, however. If decisions are based solely on the monitor without evaluating a patient's airway, breathing, circulation, and level of consciousness, errors will be made.

1. **Rate determination** (Fig. 5-1). A quick method to determine rate is to find two consecutive R waves on the rhythm strip, the first of which peaks on a heavy vertical grid line. The position of the second QRS in relationship to the next heavy vertical grid line determines the rate, as shown in Fig. 5-1. For rates greater than 300 or less than 50, the rate can be determined by counting the number of complexes within a 6-second strip and multiplying by 10.

2. **Pattern regularity.** To determine regularity, note the distance between any two R waves in consecutive QRS complexes. If the R-R interval between any two complexes is constant, the rhythm is regular. Irregular rhythms suggest multiple foci of electrical activity. Disorganized electrical activity implies no coordinated depolarization of the ventricles.

3. **P-wave presence.** The presence of a P wave indicates electrical activity in the atria. The shape of the P wave may vary depending on the origin of the atrial depolarization. An upright P wave in lead II means that depolarization originated either in or near the sinoatrial node.

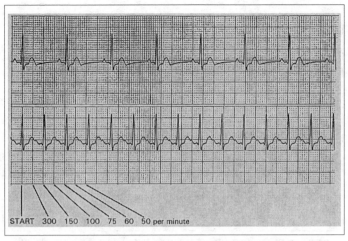

Fig. 5-1. Rate determination. In the top rhythm strip the rate is approximately 75/min; in the bottom rhythm strip the rate is approximately 150/min.

4. **Width of the ventricular complex.** The QRS complex is the electrical representation of ventricular depolarization and is normally less than 0.12 seconds wide. If a QRS complex is of normal width, its origin is supraventricular. If a QRS complex is wide, the depolarization may have originated in the ventricle or was conducted to the ventricle aberrantly. Aberrant conduction occurs if the electrical conduction system of the heart is affected by structural abnormality, ischemic damage, drug or toxin effects, or metabolic abnormalities.

5. **Relationship of P to QRS.** In the normal relationship the P wave occurs before the QRS with a PR interval of 0.12 to 0.2 seconds. A short PR interval, or P waves within or following the QRS complex, suggests that the origin of depolarization was below the atria and conducted to the atria in a retrograde fashion, whereas a long PR interval suggests partial atrioventricular block. No fixed relationship between P and QRS suggests complete atrioventricular block.

B. **Ventricular fibrillation (VF)** (Fig. 5-2)

1. **Electrical mechanism.** VF is the prototype of disorganized electrical activity with numerous foci within the ventricles in various states of depolarization and repolarization simultaneously. There is no cardiac output because the myocytes do not contract as a unit. VF is the most common dysrhythmia associated with cardiac arrest, and often results from myocardial ischemia or infarction.

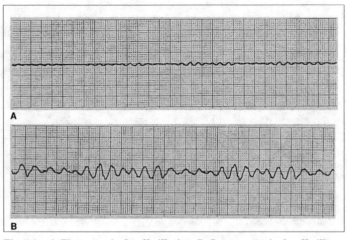

Fig. 5-2.   *A.* Fine ventricular fibrillation. *B.* Coarse ventricular fibrillation.

2. **Summary of identification criteria for VF**
   a. **Rate.** Rate is greater than 300/minute but is too disorganized to count.
   b. **Pattern.** There are higher amplitude and lower frequency waveforms in course VF and diminished amplitude and higher frequency waveforms in fine VF, with progression from course to fine over time.
   c. **Other.** Waveforms are of variable width and regularity with no identifiable P waves or QRS complexes.
3. **Confounding issues in correct identification.** Fine VF can be almost indistinguishable from asystole. Checking leads I, II, and III may help to distinguish fine VF from asystole. If in doubt, treat as ventricular fibrillation. Electrical interference on a normal rhythm strip can give the appearance of VF.
C. **Ventricular tachycardia (VT)** (Fig. 5-3)
   1. **Electrical mechanism.** VT consists of three or more organized ventricular depolarizations occurring at a

Fig. 5-3.   **Ventricular tachycardia.**

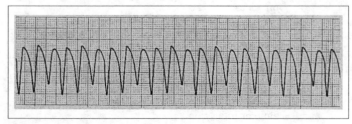

rate greater than 100/minute. The degree of hemodynamic compromise with VT is dependent on the degree of myocardial dysfunction and on the rate of VT. VT may occur in the setting of ischemic heart disease, angina, infarction, cardiomyopathy, prolonged QT syndrome, mitral valve prolapse, drug toxicity, and metabolic disorders.

2. **Summary of identification criteria for VT**

   a. **Rate.** Rate is greater than 100/minute but less than 200/minute.

   b. **Pattern.** Pattern is usually regular but may be irregular.

   c. **P waves.** P waves are often not recognizable except in slower VT.

   d. **Width of the ventricular complex.** The QRS complex is greater than 12 seconds and may be uniform (unifocal) or multiform (multifocal). The ST and T wave deflection is in the direction opposite to the major QRS deflection.

   e. **Relationship of P to QRS.** There is usually no fixed relation between the P wave and the QRS complex. In some instances, retrograde ventricular-atrial conduction may occur, resulting in a fixed QRS-P relationship.

   f. **Torsades de pointes.** Torsade de pointes is an unusal form of ventricular tachycardia in which the QRS complex amplitude fluctuates in a sinusoidal pattern. It is usually due to medication toxicity or an idiosyncratic reaction to Type 1A antiarrhythmic agents or other agents that prolong the QT interval to greater than 0.40 seconds.

3. **Confounding issues in correct identification.** If retrograde ventricular-atria conduction occurs, there will be a relationship between the QRS complex and the retrograde P wave. In this instance, differentiation from SVT with aberrant atrial-ventricular conduction can be difficult. If in doubt, treat as VT.

D. **Pulseless electrical activity (PEA)** (Fig. 5-4)

1. **Electrical mechanism.** The absence of a palpable pulse with the presence of any organized cardiac electric activity that is not VF or VT is PEA. PEA, therefore, has no defined rhythm, only a defined mechanism.

Fig. 5-4. Pulseless electrical activity.

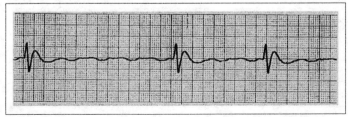

Electrical activity in PEA may be associated with no mechanical contraction [electromechanical dissociation (EMD)], or with mechanical contraction insufficient to produce a blood pressure obtainable by noninvasive means (pseudo-EMD). Other terms such as idioventricular rhythm and bradyasystole also fall under PEA. PEA may result from underlying etiologies such as hypovolemia, hypoxia, cardiac tamponade, tension pneumothorax, hypothermia, pulmonary embolism, drug overdose, metabolic derangements, and myocardial infarction. It is almost uniformly fatal unless the underlying etiology is identified and corrected.

2. **Summary of identification criteria for PEA**
    a. **Rate.** Rate is profoundly bradycardic to tachycardic.
    b. **Pattern.** Pattern is regular or irregular.
    c. **P waves.** P waves may or may not be present based on rhythm origin.
    d. **Width of the ventricular complex.** QRS complexes will be narrow to profoundly widened.
    e. **Relationship of P to QRS.** The relationship of P to QRS is variable depending on rhythm origin.
3. **Confounding issues in correct identification.** It is difficult to detect a palpable blood pressure using noninvasive methods in patients with a systolic blood pressure less than 60 mm Hg. Bloodflow may be detected by Doppler flow, echocardiography, or invasive arterial monitoring. If flow can be detected with the presenting rhythm, then the patient should be treated for severe hypotension with volume expansion or vasopressor agents.

E. **Ventricular asystole** (Fig. 5-5)
    1. **Electrical mechanism.** Asystole is defined as the lack of cardiac electrical activity. Asystole typically is seen in patients with underlying cardiac disease or metabolic abnormalities. It may occur as a primary event or it may follow VF or PEA. It is almost uniformly associated with a poor outcome.
    2. **Summary of identification criteria for asystole**
        a. **Rate.** There is no rate.
        b. **Pattern.** The pattern is a flat line.

Fig. 5-5.   Ventricular asystole.

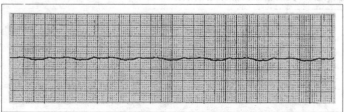

  c. **P waves.** P waves may occasionally occur spontaneously.

  d. **Width of the ventricular complex.** No QRS
   complexes are present.

  e. **Relationship of P to QRS.** There is no relationship of P to QRS.

 3. **Confounding issues in correct identification.**
  Asystole can be difficult to distinguish from fine VF.
  Therefore, the rhythm should be confirmed in ECG
  leads I, II, and III prior to therapeutic decision making. Also, electrical interference may make asystole
  look like VF. If there is any doubt about the rhythm, it
  should be treated as VF. A monitor with no input will
  display a flat line similar to asystole.

III. Electrical therapy of arrythmias

 A. Principles of electrical therapy. Cardioversion and defibrillation involve the therapeutic application of electrical current to simultaneously depolarize the entire heart.

 1. **Cardioversion.** Cardioversion is used to correct supraventricular rhythms as well as pulsatile VT. It is synchronized to the native cardiac rhythm and requires lower
  energy levels than defibrillation.

 2. **Defibrillation.** Defibrillation is used in situations of cardiac arrest with VF and pulseless VT. It is not synchronized to the underlying cardiac rhythm and requires
  higher energy levels than cardoversion. CPR may help to
  bridge the gap of time by providing a small degree of cardiac and cerebral blood flow until defibrillation is available. However, defibrillation remains the only effective
  therapy for VF and VT. Defibrillation is time dependent in
  its application because the probability of successful defibrillation after cardiac arrest diminishes rapidly over time.
  Prolonged ischemia results in an acidotic and energy-
  depleted heart, which may not respond to defibrillation or
  which may respond with post-defibrillation PEA or asystole. Without defibrillation, VT will decompensate spontaneously to VF, and VF to PEA or asystole.

 B. Dosing of electric therapy. The success of defibrillation
 depends on providing transmyocardial current flow that is
 sufficient to depolarize the entire myocardium and terminate the dysrhythmia but that is not high enough to cause
 myocardial damage.

 1. **Transthoracic resistance.** Transthoracic resistance
  to current flow decreases with repeated shocks, large
  surface contact area, appropriate paddle-chest contact
  pressure, the use of an electrically conductive paddle-
  chest interface, and full lung expiration. Therefore,
  higher current is generated with properly applied repeated shocks, even at the same energy level.

 2. **Defibrillation energy.** For defibrillation of VF or
  pulseless VT, the recommended energy level for the
  first shock is 200 joule, the second shock 200–300
  joule, and the third and subsequent shocks 360 joule.
  When a given energy level has successfully terminated
  a dysrhythmia, that energy level should be used if a

subsequent shock is required. Shock energies should
be increased when a shock fails to terminate VF/VT.
Once 360 joule of energy has been reached, subsequent
shocks can be stacked 360 joule × 3 to take advantage
of decreased transthoracic resistance with repeated
shocks.

C. Equipment. The equipment needed to perform defibrillation includes a monitor/defibrillator with associated leads
and paddles, and material to provide a paddle-to-chest
conductive interface. Most monitor/defibrillators can detect cardiac rhythm using the paddles as surrogate monitor leads. The monitor leads also can be placed on the
chest with self-adhesive patches to provide continuous
monitoring. The conducting material can be self-adhesive
electrode pads or gel.

D. Paddle placement (Fig. 5-6). One paddle, designated anterior or sternum, should be placed along the upper right
sternal border below the clavicle. The second paddle, designated apex, is placed lateral to the left nipple in the mid-
axillary line. This configuration maximizes current flow
through the myocardium. Approximately 25 pounds of
pressure should be used while the paddles are held to the
chest. The paddles must be well separated to avoid arcing
between paddles, and there must be no conducting material between the paddles.

Fig. 5-6.   Defibrillator paddle placement.

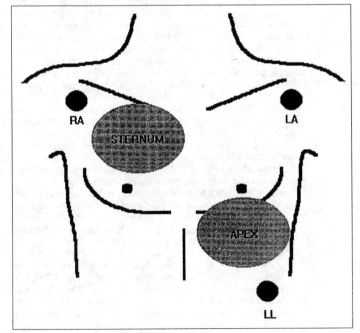

Table 5-2.   Defibrillation procedure

1 Place the patient in a safe environment away from water or metal surfaces.

2 Apply conductive material to the paddles or use conductive pads.

3 Turn on the monitor/defibrillator, and place the paddles in the anterior-apex location to use as monitor leads and confirm VF/VT.

4 Verify that the the unsynchronized mode is selected.

5 Select energy level; 200 joule is recommended as initial shock for VF or pulseless VT.

6 Press "Charge" to charge capacitor

7 Ensure paddle placement on the chest wall in the anterior-apex location as described in step 3.

8 Apply firm (25 lbs) pressure on paddles diminishing transthoracic resistance.

9 Make sure paddles are not too close to or in contact with extraneous conducting material.

10 Make sure no one is touching the patient. Call "All clear."

11 Deliver shock by pressing both paddle discharge buttons simultaneously.

12 Reassess rhythm; if unchanged, recharge defibrillator to 300 joule and deliver second shock.

13 Reassess rhythm; if unchanged, recharge defibrillator to 360 joule and deliver third shock.

14 Reassess rhythm; follow ACLS algorithms; repeat steps as needed for subsequent defibrillation attempts.

       E. Procedure (Table 5-2). Table 5-2 shows the basic steps used in the defibrillation of VF or pulseless VT.

IV. Management of cardiac arrest

    A. Patient presentation. The cardiac arrest victim will present as unresponsive, pulseless, and nonbreathing. Other presenting factors will be related to the events leading up to collapse and subsequent interventions. The five factors that affect survival in prehospital cardiac arrest victims are: (1) the etiology of arrest, (2) the presenting cardiac rhythm, (3) whether the arrest was witnessed, (4) the time to initiation of bystander CPR, and (5) the time to initiation of ACLS.

    B. Patient assessment. The tried-and-true method of patient assessment in any critical situation, including cardiac arrest, is to consider, in order: **responsiveness and the ABCs—A̲irway, B̲reathing, and C̲irculation** of basic life support.

        1. Responsiveness. Determine the level of responsiveness by stimulating the patient with both verbal and tactile stimuli. Responsiveness may be graded as AVPU—A̲lert, responsive to V̲erbal stimuli, responsive to P̲ainful stimuli, or U̲nresponsive.

        2. Airway. Secure an unobstructed passage through which the patient may breathe or be assisted in breathing. **Foreign body removal, the chin lift–jaw thrust maneuver, and the placement of a nasal or oral airway or endotracheal tube** are the skills required to successfully manage the airway. The potential for cervical spine injury must be considered and appropriate cautions taken in each case.

3. **Breathing.** Determine whether spontaneous breathing is occurring by looking, listening, and feeling. If there is no spontaneous breathing, the patient must be assisted. **Mouth-to-mouth, mouth-to-mask, bag-valve-mask, or bag-valve-endotracheal tube ventilation** are the skills required to provide breathing support.

4. **Circulation.** Pulses should be palpated at the carotid artery, since this is the location most likely to reveal a pulse pressure by noninvasive means. **CPR, intravenous cannulation, and a working knowledge of shock, fluid management, and use of pressor agents** are the skills required to manage abnormalities of circulation.

C. **Initiation of cardiopulmonary resuscitation**
   1. **Indications for the initiation of CPR** include unresponsiveness, the lack of spontaneous breathing, and the absence of a palpable pulse at the carotid artery.
   2. **Indication for the initiation of ACLS** is rhythm dependent as follows.

D. **ACLS treatment algorithms**
   1. **Classification of therapeutic interventions.** In each algorithm, therapeutic interventions are classified according to the strength of scientific evidence supporting their use. Notice that each algorithm is a process of assessment, intervention, reassessment, and further intervention.
      a. **Class I interventions** are usually indicated, always acceptable, and considered useful and efficacious.
      b. **Class IIa interventions** are acceptable but controversial; however, evidence is in favor of use.
      c. **Class IIb interventions** have less well-established evidence of efficacy but are not harmful.
      d. **Class III interventions** are inappropriate and may be harmful.
   2. **Universal algorithm for adults** (Fig. 5-7). The universal algorithm represents an approach to the patient. Responsiveness and the ABCs are considered, EMS is activated, and basic life support is initiated. The universal algorithm precedes other ACLS algorithms in most scenarios.
   3. **Ventricular fibrillation and pulseless ventricular tachycardia** (Fig. 5-8). Treatment begins in this algorithm with CPR until a monitor/defibrillator is available. Three stacked countershocks of 200 joule, 200–300 joule, and 360 joule are performed immediately after confirmation of VF/VT denoting that early defibrillation is the only reliable treatment for these rhythms. CPR is performed between defibrillation at-

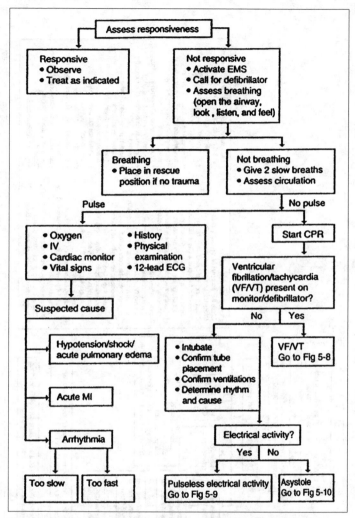

Fig. 5-7. ACLS universal algorithm for adult emergency cardiac care. (From American Heart Association Emergency Cardiac Care Committee. Guidelines for cardiopulmonary resuscitation and emergency cardiac care. *JAMA* 268:2216, 1992. Copyright 1992, American Medical Association. With permission.)

tempts, and endotracheal intubation and IV access are obtained if initial defibrillation fails. Epinephrine is given to improve myocardial blood flow during CPR, and defibrillation is attempted again. Lidocaine and/or bretylium are used for their antiarrhythmic properties with the expectation that they may help to maintain a spontaneous rhythm if defibrillation is successful.

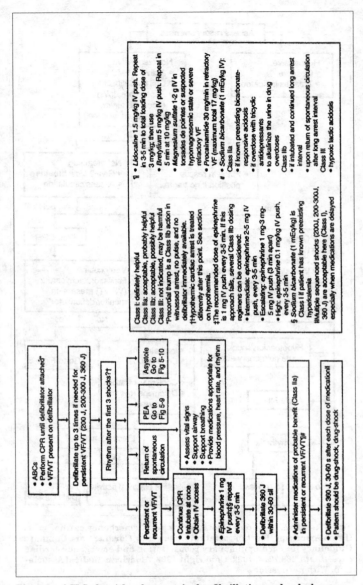

Fig. 5-8. ACLS algorithm for ventricular fibrillation and pulseless ventricular tachycardia. (From American Heart Association Emergency Cardiac Care Committee. Guidelines for cardiopulmonary resuscitation and emergency cardiac care. *JAMA* 268:2217, 1992. Copyright 1992, American Medical Association. With permission.)

These drugs do not defibrillate the heart spontaneously. There are three potential outcomes to a defibrillation attempt.

a. **Return of spontaneous circulation.** The resuscitator must consider what is required to maintain
the spontaneous rhythm. The underlying etiology
of VF/VT must be considered. Antiarrhythmics
must also be considered, particularly if they aided
in successful resuscitation.

b. **Recurrent VF/VT.** The resuscitator must consider what further therapy could potentially be
beneficial. A different antiarrhythmic may be considered, as may magnesium or bicarbonate based
on algorithm criterion. Appropriate airway management, oxygenation, and ventilation must be re-
confirmed. Brief unsustained rhythms that occur
in response to defibrillation may give clues to appropriate therapies. Tachycardias prior to refibril-
lation may benefit from beta-blocking drugs,
whereas bradycardias may benefit from atropine.
Suspected electrolyte abnormalities may also be
treated, such as hyperkalemia with calcium chloride (4 mg/kg) or hypokalemia with potassium and
magnesium.

c. **Asystole/PEA** as the result of defibrillation suggests a dismal outcome; however, their individual
algorithms should be followed if they occur.

4. **Pulseless electrical activity** (Fig. 5-9). Unlike the
VF/VT algorithm, the PEA algorithm begins with CPR
and immediate endotracheal intubation and IV access.
The myriad causes of PEA are then considered along
with therapeutic interventions. Hypovolemia is the
most common reversible cause of PEA, often related to
hemorrhage. Other reversible causes are shown in the
algorithm in Fig. 5-9. Epinephrine is given routinely
to patients experiencing PEA to improve myocardial
contractility. Atropine is used if the electrical activity
occurs at a rate of less than 60 complexes per minute.
Although the outcome from PEA is generally poor, a
reversible cause of this rhythm can be treated with
success and must not be missed. There are three potential outcomes in PEA.

a. **Treatment of a reversible cause with return
of spontaneous circulation** must be followed by
definitive care of the inciting cause of PEA.

b. **Change to another rhythm disturbance such
as asystole or VF** should be treated according to
the appropriate algorithm.

c. **Continued and unresolving PEA** following consideration and treatment for potentially reversible
causes and use of epinephrine or atropine portends
death.

5. **Asystole** (Fig. 5-10). The asystole algorithm begins
with CPR and immediate intubation and IV access.
Asystole must be confirmed in more than one ECG
lead to assure that it is not mistaken for fine VF.

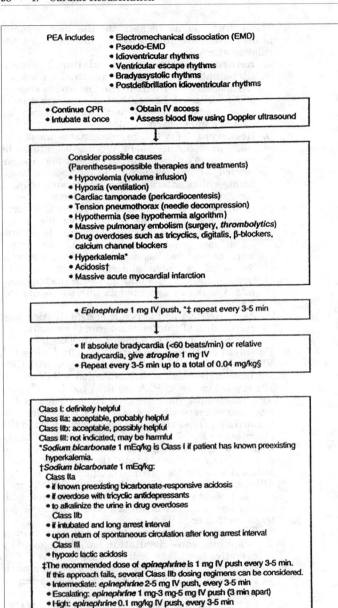

PEA includes
- Electromechanical dissociation (EMD)
- Pseudo-EMD
- Idioventricular rhythms
- Ventricular escape rhythms
- Bradyasystolic rhythms
- Postdefibrillation idioventricular rhythms

- Continue CPR
- Intubate at once
- Obtain IV access
- Assess blood flow using Doppler ultrasound

Consider possible causes
(Parentheses=possible therapies and treatments)
- Hypovolemia (volume infusion)
- Hypoxia (ventilation)
- Cardiac tamponade (pericardiocentesis)
- Tension pneumothorax (needle decompression)
- Hypothermia (see hypothermia algorithm)
- Massive pulmonary embolism (surgery, *thrombolytics*)
- Drug overdoses such as tricyclics, digitalis, β-blockers, calcium channel blockers
- Hyperkalemia*
- Acidosis†
- Massive acute myocardial infarction

- *Epinephrine* 1 mg IV push, *‡ repeat every 3-5 min

- If absolute bradycardia (<60 beats/min) or relative bradycardia, give *atropine* 1 mg IV
- Repeat every 3-5 min up to a total of 0.04 mg/kg§

Class I: definitely helpful
Class IIa: acceptable, probably helpful
Class IIb: acceptable, possibly helpful
Class III: not indicated, may be harmful
Sodium bicarbonate 1 mEq/kg is Class I if patient has known preexisting hyperkalemia.
†*Sodium bicarbonate* 1 mEq/kg:
  Class IIa
- if known preexisting bicarbonate-responsive acidosis
- if overdose with tricyclic antidepressants
- to alkalinize the urine in drug overdoses
  Class IIb
- if intubated and long arrest interval
- upon return of spontaneous circulation after long arrest interval
  Class III
- hypoxic lactic acidosis
‡The recommended dose of *epinephrine* is 1 mg IV push every 3-5 min. If this approach fails, several Class IIb dosing regimens can be considered.
- Intermediate: *epinephrine* 2-5 mg IV push, every 3-5 min
- Escalating: *epinephrine* 1 mg-3 mg-5 mg IV push (3 min apart)
- High: *epinephrine* 0.1 mg/kg IV push, every 3-5 min
§ Shorter *atropine* dosing intervals are possibly helpful in cardiac arrest (Class IIb).

Fig. 5-9. ACLS algorithm for pulseless electrical activity. (Adapted from American Heart Association Emergency Cardiac Care Committee. Guidelines for cardiopulmonary resuscitation and emergency cardiac care. *JAMA* 268:2219, 1992. Copyright 1992, American Medical Association. With permission.)

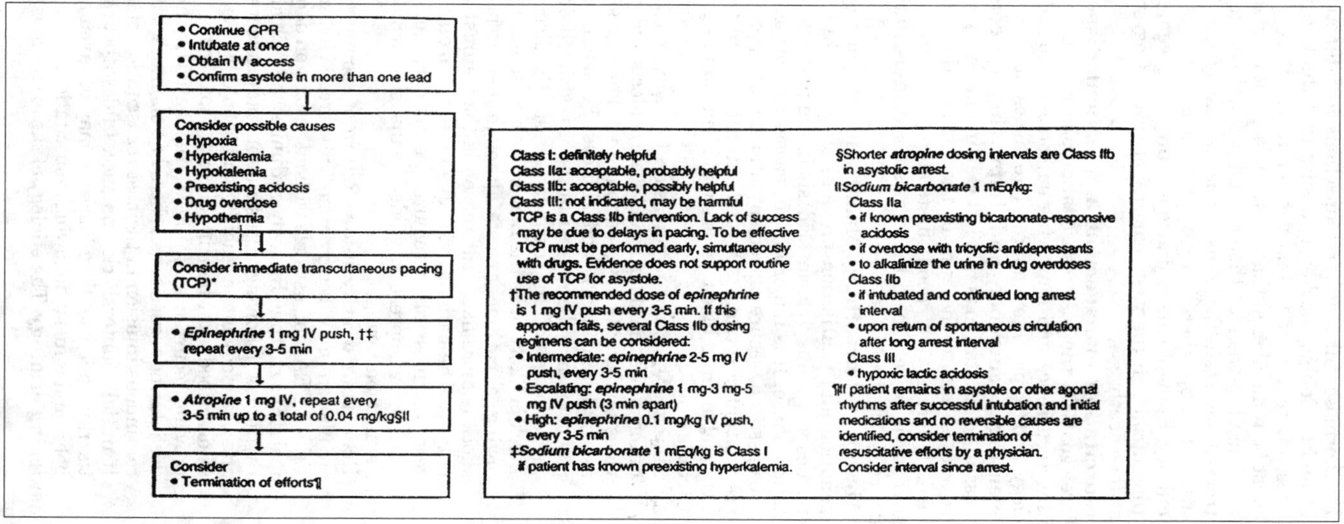
• Continue CPR
• Intubate at once
• Obtain IV access
• Confirm asystole in more than one lead
Consider possible causes
• Hypoxia
• Hyperkalemia
• Hypokalemia
• Preexisting acidosis
• Drug overdose
• Hypothermia
Consider immediate transcutaneous pacing (TCP)*
• *Epinephrine* 1 mg IV push, †‡ repeat every 3-5 min
• *Atropine* 1 mg IV, repeat every 3-5 min up to a total of 0.04 mg/kg§||
Consider
• Termination of efforts¶
Class I: definitely helpful
Class IIa: acceptable, probably helpful
Class IIb: acceptable, possibly helpful
Class III: not indicated, may be harmful
*TCP is a Class IIb intervention. Lack of success may be due to delays in pacing. To be effective TCP must be performed early, simultaneously with drugs. Evidence does not support routine use of TCP for asystole.
†The recommended dose of *epinephrine* is 1 mg IV push every 3-5 min. If this approach fails, several Class IIb dosing regimens can be considered:
• Intermediate: *epinephrine* 2-5 mg IV push, every 3-5 min
• Escalating: *epinephrine* 1 mg-3 mg-5 mg IV push (3 min apart)
• High: *epinephrine* 0.1 mg/kg IV push, every 3-5 min
‡*Sodium bicarbonate* 1 mEq/kg is Class I if patient has known preexisting hyperkalemia.
§Shorter *atropine* dosing intervals are Class IIb in asystolic arrest.
||*Sodium bicarbonate* 1 mEq/kg:
Class IIa
• if known preexisting bicarbonate-responsive acidosis
• if overdose with tricyclic antidepressants
• to alkalinize the urine in drug overdoses
Class IIb
• if intubated and continued long arrest interval
• upon return of spontaneous circulation after long arrest interval
Class III
• hypoxic lactic acidosis
¶If patient remains in asystole or other agonal rhythms after successful intubation and initial medications and no reversible causes are identified, consider termination of resuscitative efforts by a physician. Consider interval since arrest.

Fig. 5-10. ACLS asystole treatment algorithm. (From American Heart Association Emergency Cardiac Care Committee. Guidelines for cardiopulmonary resuscitation and emergency cardiac care. *JAMA* 268:2220, 1992. Copyright 1992, American Medical Association. With permission.

Furthermore, all monitor connections and functions should be double checked to assure that the flat line does not represent technical error in monitoring. It must be remembered that asystole does not represent a rhythm but the lack thereof, and it is unlikely to be treated successfully. Transcutaneous pacing may be attempted, but there is little scientific evidence of its efficacy. Epinephrine and atropine are also given, but the outcome in the vast majority of cases of asystole will be death.

V. **Post-resuscitation management and patient disposition.** Three goals for the post-resuscitation phase include: (1) preventing recurrence and improving outcome, (2) considering etiology, and (3) providing appropriate disposition.

A. **Preventing recurrence and improving outcome.** Successful resuscitation is the first step in improving outcome and is due to the sum of the interventions performed. Therefore, a good first step in preventing recurrence is to return to the first step of resuscitation and reconsider the ABCs.

   1. **Airway and breathing.** Maintaining adequate oxygenation and ventilation provides oxygen to hypoxic tissues and helps to clear acidosis in the post-resuscitation phase. It is important to reassess endotracheal tube position, secure placement, and choose appropriate ventilator settings. Oxygen saturation, end tidal CO_2, and arterial blood gases should be monitored.

   2. **Circulation**

      a. **Shock.** Persistent hypotension following resuscitation slows the clearing of tissue acidosis and provides inadequate oxygenation to vital organs such as the brain, heart, and kidneys. Persistent hypotension may be related to the arrest itself or to the etiology of the cardiac arrest. Cardiogenic shock is likely to be the reason for hypotension following a cardiac arrest, although hemorrhagic shock is more likely the reason in the traumatized patient. The patient in shock following cardiac arrest will most often require a careful balance of fluid and vasopressors guided by invasive hemodynamic monitoring.

      b. **Recurrent dysrhythmia.** Return of spontaneous circulation may occur from the arrest rhythms, VF/VT, PEA, and asystole without resolution of normal sinus rhythm. Bradydysrythmias and tachydysrhythmias following resuscitation may adversely affect hemodynamic stability and should be treated as described elsewhere in this text. Furthermore, to prevent recurrence of VF/VT, the antiarrhythmic used during resuscitation should be maintained as a continuous infusion in the post-resuscitation phase. If initial countershock was successful without antiarrhythmic use, then lidocaine may be given as a bolus and infusion following resuscitation.

B. **Considering etiology.** The etiology of the arrest must be considered and should guide further therapy in the post-resuscitation phase. Myocardial ischemia or infarction must be carefully considered. Every patient must be monitored following arrest with repeat ECGs and cardiac enzyme analysis. Patients with post-resuscitation ECGs that show evidence of myocardical infarction are still candidates for thrombolytic therapy, although this must be weighed against the available history to preclude contraindications and the duration and severity of the resuscitation attempt. Toxins, metabolic derangement, and injury also must be considered as potential etiologies and must be treated appropriately in the post-resuscitation phase.

C. **Providing appropriate disposition.** All patients resuscitated following a cardiac arrest must be transported to a hospital emergency department and admitted to an appropriately equipped intensive care unit. An institution receiving cardiac arrest and resuscitated patients from the prehospital setting must consider its ability to provide adequate or necessary care to the patient in the post-arrest phase. If this care cannot be provided, interhospital transport of the patient should meet the following criteria: (1) the transport should be made by a carrier able to provide advanced cardiac life support care, (2) arrangements for continued care should be made with an identified receiving physician who will accept responsibility for the patient, and (3) the patient or family should understand the need for and agree to the transfer.

D. **Considerations in the unsuccessful resuscitation**
   1. **Ceasing resuscitative efforts.** More resuscitation attempts in cardiac arrest will fail than be successful. Still, the decision to cease resuscitative efforts must be made on a case-by-case basis based on sound medical judgment and careful consideration of all potential etiologies of the arrest. If the proper considerations have been made, then a failed resuscitation should not be perceived as a failure on the part of the resuscitation team. A well-documented no code order available in hand at the time of resuscitation also may be used to justify cessation of resuscitative efforts, although regulations regarding this vary according to local and state statutes.
   2. **Informing the family.** Informing the family of a death may be difficult for the physician but sets the tone for the grief process and makes a lasting impression on the family. Several important considerations can aid in this process.
      a. **Know the victim's name** and the events leading to death. Also know the process that will follow death regarding removal of the body and signing of the death certificate.
      b. **Address the family** with a small group that includes a member of the resuscitation team and a social worker or member of the clergy who have

been made familiar with the case. Do not inform the family alone.

c. **Introduce yourself,** sit down, and address the closest relative to the deceased.

d. **Briefly describe** the events leading to death. Use the words death, dying, or dead rather than euphemistic phrases such as "passed away."

e. **Provide comfort** to the family with eye contact and touching, and allow enough time for all questions to be answered. Make yourself and your co-workers available to aid the family with further arrangements and to answer questions.

Bibliography

American Heart Association Emergency Cardiac Care Committee. Guidelines for cardiopulmonary resuscitation and emergency cardiac care. *JAMA* 268:2171–2302, 1992.

Hoekstra JW. Cardiac Resuscitation. In Gibler WB, Aufderheide TP (eds.), *Emergency Cardiac Care.* St. Louis: Mosby, 1994.

Myerburg RJ, Castellanos A. Cardiovascular Arrest and Sudden Cardiac Death. In Braunwald E (ed.), *Heart Disease: A Textbook of Cardiovascular Medicine* (3d ed.). Philadelphia: Saunders, 1988.

Roberts JR, Hedges JR (eds.), *Clinical Procedures in Emergency Medicine* (2d ed.). Philadelphia: Saunders, 1991.

Rosenthal R. Adult Cardiopulmonary Arrest. In Rosen P, Barkin RM (eds.), *Emergency Medicine: Concepts and Clinical Practice* (3d ed.). St. Louis: Mosby, 1992.

Neonatal Resuscitation

Daniel M. Cohen and Daniel J. Scherzer

Neonatal resuscitation mandates attention because of the vulnerable transition from fetus to neonate. "Neonates" typically refer to infants less than 4 weeks old; however, for resuscitation, newborn infants need specific focus. Between 6% to 10% of newborns require resuscitation. Even routine deliveries require a degree of resuscitation, such as drying and stimulation. Deliveries that are anticipated and attended by an obstetric and neonatal team in the delivery room are the safest scenarios; however, 1% of infants are not born in a hospital setting. Suboptimal settings are associated with factors contributing to morbidity and mortality, such as (1) poor prenatal care, (2) maternal illness, (3) premature delivery, (4) chorioamnionitis, (5) placental abruption or previa, and (6) trauma-induced delivery. Emergency physicians must be prepared for neonatal resuscitation. This includes recognizing and treating respiratory distress syndrome, sepsis, meconium aspiration, and hypovolemic shock of the newborn.

I. **Preparation for resuscitation.** Inadequately resuscitated neonates asphyxiate rapidly. Time spent organizing personnel and materials well in advance of a crisis is requisite. Trained staff and well-maintained, commercially available equipment can avert disaster. The staff must keep equipment organized, stocked, and easily accessible. Contacting the newborn nursery may help to obtain necessary staff or equipment. Check the equipment prior to the delivery.

   A. **Personnel.** Optimally, a newborn resuscitation team includes a team leader, a nurse, a respiratory therapist, and a pharmacist. The team leader must designate defined roles to each participant, prior to delivery. Certification in the Neonatal Resuscitation Program (American Heart Association/American Academy of Pediatrics) is highly recommended for physicians who attend deliveries.

   B. **Equipment.** Emergency departments must be stocked with medication and equipment in a range of sizes for neonatal resuscitation (Table 6-1).

   1. **Airway and breathing** support supplies must be readily accessible.

      a. **Suction catheters.** Catheters in sizes 8 and 10 should be on hand. Wall suction pressure must never exceed 100 mm Hg; duration should not exceed 10 seconds. To prevent disease transmission, do not suction by mouth (e.g., Delee suction).

      b. **Masks.** Face masks in sizes 0 and 1 will fit most newborns. Measure the mask on the neonate's face to assure a tight fit over the chin and nose (not over the eyes).

      c. **Bags.** For positive pressure ventilation, self-inflating bags (volume <500 ml) are recommended and safest for those unfamiliar with anesthesia bags. Pop-off valves reduce the risk of barotrauma.

Table 6-1. Neonatal resuscitation equipment and drugs

Equipment
Radiant warmer
Cardiorespiratory monitor
Pulse oximeter
Small electrocardiographic leads
Suction equipment
Suction catheters (5 to 10 Fr)
Oxygen with flow meter
De Lee suction apparatus
Self-inflating resuscitation bag (500 ml) with oxygen reservoir or anesthesia bag with manometer
Face masks (sizes 00, 0, 1, 2)
Oral airways (sizes 000, 00, 0)
Endotracheal tube (2.5, 3.0, 3.5, 4.0 mm) and small stylet
Laryngoscope and straight blades (No. 0, 1)
Umbilical catheters (3.5 and 5.0 Fr)
Three-way stopcocks
Nasogastric tube
Sterile umbilical catheter tray
Chest tubes (8 and 10 Fr)
Magill forceps (small)
Resuscitation chart

Drugs
Atropine 0.5 mg/ml
Sodium bicarbonate 0.5 mEq/ml
Calcium chloride 10%
Dextrose in water 10%, 25%
Epinephrine 1:10,000
Albumisol 5% solution or plasmanate
Naloxone 0.02 mg/ml

Source: From Fleisher GR, Ludwig S. *Textbook of Pediatric Emergency Medicine* (3rd ed.). Baltimore: Williams & Wilkins, 1993.

At times initial ventilatory pressures may require depression of the valve.

d. **Laryngoscopes.** Miller laryngoscope blades, size 0, are appropriate for most neonates; 1-Miller blades can be used for larger newborns.

e. **Endotracheal tubes (ETTs).** For estimating size, one rule of thumb is that small (1 kg), medium (2 kg), and large (3 kg) neonates require 2.5, 3.0, and 3.5 ETTs, respectively. For orotracheal intubation the depth of tube placement can be approximated with the "7-8-9" rule: At the lip the ETT is located at 7 cm for small (1 kg) neonates, at 8 cm for medium (2 kg) neonates, and at 9 cm for large (3 kg) neonates. These guidelines must be applied individually.

2. Three additional pieces of equipment should be highlighted: warmers, manometers, and umbilical lines.

   a. Maintaining a warm, dry environment for newborns is critical. Thermoneutrality decreases glucose consumption, acidosis, and hypoxia. Radiant **warmers** provide both warmth and access to the neonate. Heating lamps can be used as a temporizing measure but are suboptimal.

   b. **Manometers** are extremely useful in monitoring ventilation. Neonates may initially require high opening pressures; however, subsequent high ventilatory pressures may cause iatrogenic pneumothoraces. In-line airway pressure manometers help to assess pulmonary status and prevent problems.

   c. **Umbilical catheters** (3.5 and 5 French) should be stocked routinely. Umbilical venous cannulation, a 30-second procedure, is facile and lifesaving. Intraosseous cannulation is a feasible alternative if an umbilical vessel or peripheral vein cannot be cannulated (see Chap. 7, sec. **III.D.2.**).

II. Patient assessment

A. **Focused history.** A brief focused history should be obtained prior to delivery if time permits. Minimally, ask the following three questions:

1. Is the labor preterm? Estimate equipment sizes and potential for resuscitation.

2. Is this a multiple gestation pregnancy? Establish staffing and equipment requirements (e.g., twins require double the amount of supplies).

3. Is there meconium-stained fluid? Plan approach to airway management (see sec. **V.B.**).

B. **Additional history.** Maternal problems increase the risk of neonatal morbidity and mortality. These include diabetes, hypertension, toxemia, vaginal bleeding, infection, substance abuse, premature rupture of membranes, trauma, and previous difficult labor and delivery. Prematurity is abnormal; attempt to ascertain the etiology with a thorough maternal history.

C. **Physical assessment.** Perform the initial assessment and resuscitation simultaneously; reassess continuously (see sec. **III.** for details).

1. **Respiration.** Assess respiratory rate, chest rise, and air movement.

   a. Loud cry—no intervention.

   b. Slow, shallow breathing—stimulation and 100% oxygen.

   c. Gasping, apnea—positive pressure ventilation (PPV) with 100% oxygen.

2. **Heart rate.** Palpate umbilical, brachial, or femoral pulses, or auscultate apical heart.

   a. Rate greater than 100 bpm with spontaneous respirations—no intervention.

   b. Rate less than 100 bpm—PPV with 100% oxygen.

       c. Rate <80 bpm and falling despite PPV with 100% oxygen—chest compressions.

       d. Rate <60 bpm—PPV with 100% oxygen and chest compressions.

    3. Color. Differentiate peripheral versus central cyanosis.

       a. Peripheral (acrocyanosis) is normal in neonates.

       b. Central cyanosis (tongue/gums) is abnormal. Ensure that the oxygen supply, airway, ventilation, and heart rate are adequate. Provide 100% oxygen until the cause can be determined and addressed.

  D. Apgar scores

    1. Apgar scores are adjunctive, time-consuming, and **not** used for resuscitative decisions. They can be used for documentation of the newborn's progress.

    2. Apgar scores assess neonates at 1, 5, 10, or more minutes (Table 6-2).

III. Management. Neonatal resuscitation is different than either pediatric or adult resuscitation; the unique stepwise approach is illustrated in Figs. 6-1 and 6-2. The vast majority of neonates can be resuscitated with ventilatory support. The key to successful resuscitation is intervention with ongoing reassessment of respiration, heart rate, and color. One common exception to the inverted pyramid approach is in the event of thick meconium aspiration, which is discussed in sec. **V.B.**

  A. Dry, warm, position, suction, stimulate

    1. Wet infants rapidly develop hypothermia, which undermines resuscitative efforts. Gentle towel-drying and placement under a radiant warmer is sufficient stimulation.

    2. Position the baby on his or her back with the neck slightly extended. Do not hyperextend the infant's neck.

    3. Oral followed by nasal suctioning clears the airway. Suction the mouth before the nose. Nasal suctioning elicits grimacing, gasping, and crying. These behaviors precipitate aspiration of oral contents, contributing to transitional difficulties.

Table 6-2.   Apgar score

Sign	0	1	2
Heart rate per minute	Absent	Slow (less than 100)	Greater than 100
Respirations	Absent	Slow, irregular	Good, crying
Muscle tone	Limp	Some flexion	Active motion
Reflex irritability (catheter in nares)	No response	Grimace	Cough or sneeze
Color	Blue or pale	Pink body with blue extremities	Completely pink

Source: Reproduced with permission. From *Textbook of Pediatric Advanced Life Support*, 1994. Copyright American Heart Association.

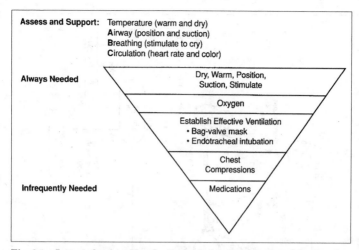

Assess and Support: Temperature (warm and dry)
Airway (position and suction)
Breathing (stimulate to cry)
Circulation (heart rate and color)

Always Needed

Dry, Warm, Position,
Suction, Stimulate

Oxygen

Establish Effective Ventilation
• Bag-valve mask
• Endotracheal intubation

Chest
Compressions

Infrequently Needed

Medications

Fig. 6-1. Inverted pyramid reflecting relative frequencies of neonatal resuscitation efforts for the newborn who does not have meconium-stained amniotic fluid. Note that a majority of newborns respond to simple measures. (Reproduced with permission. *Textbook of Pediatric Advanced Life Support,* **1994. Copyright American Heart Association.)**

    4. After brief and gentle stimulation, reassess respiration, heart rate, and color.

B. Oxygen

    1. All neonates receive 100% oxygen during resuscitation.

    2. Oxygen can be withdrawn slowly if the newborn has a heart rate greater than 100 and is pink. One rule of thumb is the following: Oxygen (flowing at 5 liter/minute) provides 80% at 0.5 inch from the nose/mouth, 60% at 1 inch, and 40% at 2 inch.

    3. After initiating oxygen therapy, reassess respiration, heart rate, and color.

C. Ventilation: bag-valve-mask (BVM) and endotracheal tube intubation (ETT)

    1. BVM ventilation

        a. Indications include apnea, gasping, or heart rate less than 100 bpm.

        b. Equipment is outlined in sec. **I.B.1.a.–c.** and in Table 6-1.

        c. Most newborns respond to brief BVM ventilation. Place the baby in the sniffing position and use an appropriately sized mask with a tight seal. Ventilate at 40–60 breaths/minute and observe the chest rise to deliver an estimated tidal volume of 6–8 cc/kg. Initial peak inspiratory pressures may require 20–40 cm of H_2O. Initial breaths should be slow with a relatively long inspiratory time.

        d. Common pitfalls include improper positioning of the newborn, incorrect mask size, a poor seal be-

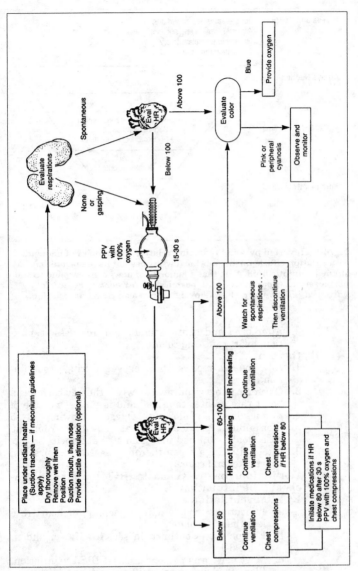

Fig. 6-2.   Overview of resuscitation. (Reproduced with permission. *Textbook of Neonatal Resuscitation*, 1987, 1990, 1994. Copyright American Heart Association.)

tween the mask and face, bag size greater than 500 ml, overly vigorous ventilation, and gastric distention.

    e. After initiating BVM ventilation, reassess respiration, heart rate, and color.

  2. ETT intubation

    a. Indications include poor response to BVM ventilation and ongoing need for PPV (e.g., severely depressed infants, small prematures with poor lung compliance). Candidates for primary intubation, with no BVM ventilation, are neonates with suspected or diagnosed diaphragmatic hernia or thick meconium at delivery (see sec. **V.B.2.**).

    b. Equipment is outlined in **I.B.1.e.** and in Table 6-1. Check the function of the laryngoscope prior to intubation. Stylets are optional but must not protrude beyond the end of the ETT.

    c. Preoxygenate and preventilate the baby who should be in the neutral, sniffing position. The assistant monitors respiration, heart rate, and color. Intubation attempts should not exceed 20 seconds. Place the ETT according to the "7-8-9" rule (see sec. **I.B.1.e.**). Observe chest rise. Listen over both hemithoraces and stomach. Secure the tube.

    d. Common pitfalls include poor positioning of the newborn, failure to visualize the glottis, esophageal intubation, incorrect depth of ETT placement, overly vigorous PPV, iatrogenic pneumothorax, and inadequate ETT securing/taping.

    e. After intubation and PPV, reassess respiration, heart rate, and color.

D. Chest compressions

  1. Indications are for heart rate <80 bpm.

  2. Either the two-finger or thumb compression technique is used at a rate of 120/minute.

  3. Depth of compression is ½ to ¾ of an inch. Compress just below the intermammary line, evenly and perpendicularly.

  4. Common pitfalls include compressing too slowly or too quickly, incorrect depth of compression, and iatrogenic trauma from incorrect finger placement, including fractures, pneumothorax, or hemorrhage.

  5. After initiating chest compressions, reassess respiration, heart rate, and color.

E. Medications (Table 6-3)

  1. Resuscitation drugs

    a. Indications for medication administration include heart rate <80 bpm despite 30 seconds of PPV and chest compressions.

    b. **Epinephrine** is the drug of choice. Administration can be repeated every 3 to 5 minutes. The dose is 0.01–0.03 mg/kg of the 1:10,000 solution.

    c. The use of **sodium bicarbonate** is controversial. Recommended dose is 2 mEq/kg, slowly infused over at least 2 minutes at a concentration of 0.5 mEq/ml (4.2% solution).

Table 6-3. Medications for neonatal resuscitation

Medication	Concentration to administer	Preparation	Dosage/Route*	Total dose/Infant			Rate/Precautions
Epinephrine	1:10 000	1 ml	0.1–0.3 ml/kg IV or ET	Weight (Kg) 1 2 3 4		Total ml 0.1–0.3 0.2–0.6 0.3–0.9 0.4–1.2	Give rapidly. May dilute with normal saline to 1–2 ml if giving ET.
Volume expanders	Whole blood 5% albumin-saline Normal saline Ringer's lactate	40 ml	10 ml/kg IV	Weight (Kg) 1 2 3 4		Total ml 10 20 30 40	Give over 5–10 minutes.
Sodium bicarbonate	0.5 mEq/ml (4.2% solution)	20 ml or two 10-ml prefilled syringes	2 mEq/kg IV	Weight (Kg) 1 2 3 4	Total Dose (mEq) 2 4 6 8	Total ml 4 8 12 16	Give slowly, over at least 2 minutes. Give only if infant is being effectively ventilated.
Naloxone hydrochloride	0.4 mg/ml	1 mL	0.1 mg/kg (0.25 ml/kg) IV, ET IM, SQ	Weight (Kg) 1 2 3 4	Total Dose (mEq) 0.1 0.2 0.3 0.4	Total ml 0.25 0.50 0.75 1.00	Give rapidly. IV, ET preferred. IM, SQ acceptable.
	1.0 mg/ml	1mL	0.1 ml/kg (0.1 ml/kg) IV, ET IM, SQ	1 2 3 4	0.1 0.2 0.3 0.4	0.1 0.2 0.3 0.4	
Dopamine	$\dfrac{\text{Weight (kg)} \times \text{Desired dose } (\mu g/kg/min)}{\text{Desired fluid (ml/h)}} = $ mg of dopamine per 100 ml of solution		Begin at 5 μg/kg/min (may increase to 20 μg/kg/min if necessary) IV	Weight (Kg) 1 2 3 4		Total μg/min 5–20 10–40 15–60 20–80	Give as a continuous infusion using an infusion pump. Monitor heart rate and blood pressure closely. Seek consultation.

Source: Reproduced with permission. *Textbook of Neonatal Resuscitation*, 1987, 1990, 1994. Copyright American Heart Association.

    d. Atropine and **calcium** are not indicated for delivery-related resuscitation.

    e. Naloxone can be used to reverse maternal-derived narcosis; however, acute withdrawal and seizures can be precipitated in neonates of narcotic-addicted mothers, and so naloxone is contraindicated for these infants.

    f. Epinephrine (and naloxone) can be administered intravenously or via the ETT. When administered endotracheally, epinephrine can be diluted 1:1 with normal saline (NS). Intravenous administration is preferable, but do not delay medications if an ETT is in place.

    g. After administering medication, reassess respiration, heart rate, and color.

  2. Volume expanders

    a. Volume expanders are indicated for evidence of blood loss with clinical signs of hypovolemia. Signs include persistent pallor, weak pulses with good heart rate, and poor response to resuscitation.

    b. Hypotension is a late sign of shock in neonates.

    c. Volume expanders include NS, Ringer's lactate (RL), 5% albumin, and whole blood.

    d. Dosage is 10 ml/kg over 5–10 minutes.

    e. After delivering a bolus of volume, reassess respiration, heart rate, and color.

IV. Umbilical venous access. During resuscitation, the preferred route of venous access is the umbilical vein (see Figs. 6-3 and 6-4).

  A. Preparation. The umbilical stump normally contains two muscular-walled arteries and one large flaccid vein. The vein is the easiest to cannulate. Commercial umbilical catheterization kits are available. These contain flexible sterile catheters, ties, clamps, lidocaine, saline, povidone-iodine, and a scalpel. Umbilical catheters are available in two sizes, 3.5 or 5.0 French. In a bind, any

Fig. 6-3. Umbilical line position. (Reproduced with permission. *Textbook of Neonatal Resuscitation,* 1987, 1990, 1994. Copyright American Heart Association.)

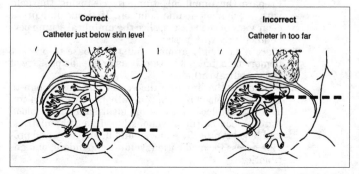

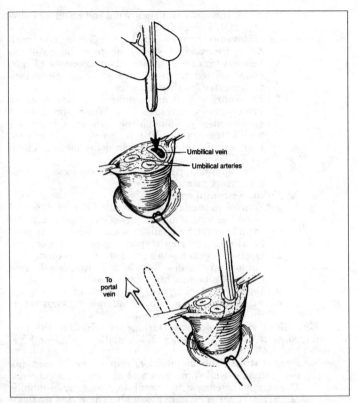

Umbilical vein

Umbilical arteries

To portal vein

Fig. 6-4.   Umbilical cross section. (From Fleisher G, Ludwig S. *Textbook of Pediatric Emergency Medicine* (3rd ed.). Baltimore: Williams & Wilkins, 1993.)

sterile flexible catheter, tube, or line of comparable size can be substituted.

B. Procedure of umbilical vein placement

1. Prepare the umbilical stump by cleansing the field with a povidone-iodine solution. If tissue impairs a clear view of the vessels, slice the umbilical stump perpendicularly with a scalpel.

2. Place a tie firmly around the stump base to prevent hemorrhage, but not so tightly as to impede passage of the umbilical catheter.

3. Cannulate the line into the vessel just far enough to get an easy blood return, generally no more than 4 cm. The initial blood draw is an ideal sample for blood count, blood cultures, venous blood gas, chemistries, and blood typing. The line should flush easily and provide access for medication, volume expanders, and antibiotics.

4. Do not remove the umbilical line until another definitive access site has been secured.
5. After placing the line, tighten the umbilical tie and secure the line.
6. Common pitfalls include incorrect depth of line placement with infusion into the liver and inadequate line securing with loss of venous access.

V. **Specific resuscitation situations.** Many different problems including prematurity, meconium aspiration, sepsis, hypovolemic shock, pneumothorax, diaphragmatic hernia, congenital heart disease, and others may require neonatal resuscitation. Prematurity and meconium aspiration, which are the most common problems, are discussed briefly here.

A. **Prematurity**
1. Prematurity is abnormal. An attempt should be made to ascertain the causes (e.g., chorioamnionitis, placental abruption or previa, trauma, or substance abuse). Knowing the etiology may facilitate the resuscitation and care of the neonate.
2. Attempt to determine the **estimated gestational age** (EGA). Ask about the mother's last menstrual period, ultrasounds, and estimated date of delivery. The EGA may help predict course and viability of the neonate.
3. Premature infants are at risk for several problems:
   a. Respiratory distress syndrome secondary to underdeveloped lungs and lack of surfactant.
   b. Central apnea due to brain stem immaturity.
   c. Sepsis/infection is a common cause of prematurity. Antibiotics (ampicillin and gentamicin) often are started presumptively.
   d. Hypoxic-ischemic encephalopathy and intraventricular hemorrhage.
   e. Thermal dysregulation due to evaporation from a large surface area of thin skin.
   f. Hypoglycemia due to low glycogen stores that are rapidly depleted with physiologic stress.

B. **Meconium aspiration.** Meconium excretion commonly occurs prior to birth and may be a sign of fetal distress.
1. Thin meconium usually is not a problem and does not require specific intervention.
2. Thick meconium must be removed from the airway prior to initiation of respiration to prevent aspiration of the material. **Meconium aspiration syndrome,** a common cause of persistent pulmonary hypertension of the neonate (PPHN), is associated with high morbidity and mortality. Therapy for PPHN includes **extra-corporal membrane oxygenation;** at present, many centers are studying the use of inhaled nitric oxide. Prevention of meconium aspiration is critical. If thick meconium is present, modify the standard resuscitative approach to "S-ABC", in which "S" stands for suctioning of the trachea and "ABC" stands for airway, breathing, and circulation.
   a. Once the head of the neonate has been delivered, suction the mouth and nose prior to delivery of the

body. Usually this is done by the obstetrician or the practitioner doing the delivery.

   b. If possible prior to commencement of breathing, the first step is intubation of the trachea with an ETT wall suction adapter.
   c. Suction pressure must be <100 mm Hg.
   d. Apply continuous suction while withdrawing the ETT. (Do not use suction catheters through the ETT. They are ineffective for thick meconium.)
   e. If particulate matter or thick meconium is found below the vocal cords, repeat the procedure as tolerated. PPV is required frequently after this event.
   f. After ETT suctioning for thick meconium, reassess respiration, heart rate, and color.

VI. Post-resuscitation care and disposition. Prior to transfer, all tubes and lines must be secured. ETT dislodgement occurs frequently in neonates and can be problematic. A warm, humidified isolation unit is recommended for transport. Once stabilized, all neonates should be transferred to a unit that can provide ongoing reassessment and therapy.

Bibliography

American Heart Association Emergency Cardiac Care Committee and Subcommittees. Guidelines for cardiopulmonary resuscitation and emergency cardiac care, VII: neonatal resuscitation. *JAMA.* 268:2276–2281, 1992.

Bloom RS, Cropley C, et al. *Textbook of Neonatal Resuscitation.* Dallas: American Heart Association, 1994.

Burchfield DJ, Berkowitz ID, Berg RA, Goldberg RN. Medications in neonatal resuscitation. *Ann Emerg Med.* 22:435–439, 1993.

Fleischer G, Ludwig S. *Textbook of Pediatric Emergency Medicine* (3rd ed.), Baltimore: Williams & Wilkins, 1993.

Wimmer, JE Jr: Neonatal resuscitation. *Pediatr Rev.* 15:255–265, 1994.

Pediatric Resuscitation

Daniel J. Scherzer and Daniel M. Cohen

CPR was developed for the treatment of sudden cardiac arrest in adults. Children progress slowly to cardiopulmonary arrest. In contrast to adults, ventricular dysrhythmias are uncommon in children with arrest. The usual presenting dysrhythmia is bradycardia or asystole in the context of severe trauma or illness. These preterminal rhythms are commonly due to hypoxia (90%). Survival with any degree of neurologic recovery for children presenting to the emergency department (ED) in cardiac arrest is dismal, at less than 7%. Therefore, prevention, early recognition, and intervention are critical for successful resuscitation. Accurate evaluation of airway patency, breathing, and circulation (ABCs) is contingent on recognizing compensatory mechanisms: increased heart and respiratory rates, use of accessory muscles of respiration, and decreased peripheral perfusion. Skilled, timely intervention, particularly for airway and breathing support, is vital.

Etiologies of childhood cardiopulmonary arrest are age-related. Medical problems such as respiratory illnesses, sudden infant death syndrome (SIDS), and congenital anomalies account for the majority of children under 1 year of age who require resuscitation. For children older than 1 year, trauma is the most common cause of death. Trauma accounts for 40% of all deaths in children 1–4 years old and for 50%–70% in children over the age of 5 years old. In some states, drowning is the leading cause of mortality and neurologic morbidity in young children. Nationally, the predominant causes of trauma are motor vehicle accidents and violence.

Emergency personnel must be prepared to provide pediatric life support for a wide range of ages and sizes. Preparation with medication charts or cards saves time and improves accuracy. One useful tool, the Broselow Pediatric Emergency Tape, details equipment size and medication dosages based on the patient's length. Two recommended courses, Pediatric Advanced Life Support (PALS) and Advanced Pediatric Lifesaving (APLS), provide training in pediatric resuscitation.

I. **Airway management** (see also Chap. 2, secs. **I.** and **IV.**)
   A. **Airway management with cervical spine immobilization.** In cases of known or suspected trauma or when the history is vague, maintain airway control with cervical spine immobilization. Vague histories may be associated with nonaccidental trauma, such as shaken and abused infants.
      1. Commercial pediatric cervical collars are available in different sizes.
      2. When these are unavailable or too large, towel rolls, sandbags, or foam rubber attachments can be taped to the backboard for immobilization. Tape the child's forehead to prevent excessive neck flexion or extension and to maintain the "sniffing" position.
   B. **Airway patency.** Quickly determine the patient's level of consciousness and airway patency. If the child is verbalizing or crying, the airway is patent.

1. If the patient has vomited or if there is debris in the mouth, logroll the patient to the side and suction the mouth.
2. If the patient is obtunded, stridorous, or exhibiting suprasternal retractions, perform a chin lift or jaw thrust maneuver. Look, listen, and feel for air movement.

C. **Airway adjuncts.** The most common airway impediment in obtunded children is hypotonia of the mandibular soft tissues. The chin lift or jaw thrust maneuver may provide insufficient relief.
   1. Oropharyngeal airways stent the airway and enhance ventilation. The method of insertion differs from that used in adult patients.
      a. Depress the tongue and insert the oropharyngeal airway directly into place.
      b. Do *not* insert the oropharyngeal airway upside-down and rotate; this may exacerbate tongue obstruction in children.
      c. Oropharyngeal airways should be used only in comatose patients. In the awake or semiconscious child they may induce vomiting.
   2. Nasopharyngeal airways can be used in semiconscious patients with no evidence of head injury or bleeding diathesis.
      a. In suspected head trauma, nasopharyngeal airways must be avoided because of the risk of penetrating the cribriform plate or of introducing infection through basilar skull fractures.
      b. Appropriate sizing is critical to avoid exacerbation of airway obstruction.
   3. Oro- and nasopharyngeal airway adjuncts are always used with 100% oxygen and ventilatory support as needed. The proper size is determined from the Broselow tape or by measuring the airway on the patient.

D. **Definitive airways.** A definitive airway is a tube in the trachea. Orotracheal intubation with direct laryngoscopy is preferred in children.
   1. Indications for securing a definitive airway include cardiopulmonary arrest, inability to adequately oxygenate or ventilate by other means, a closed head injury requiring hyperventilation, and preparation for transport of the patient at risk of losing his or her airway protective reflexes or CNS control of ventilation.
   2. Charts, formulas, and the Broselow tape aid in selecting endotracheal tubes, laryngoscope blades, and suction catheters. Always have a wide range of sizes available (Table 7-1).
   3. Intubation may be accomplished after preoxygenation and ventilation with a bag-valve-mask (BVM) device or by rapid sequence induction, if indicated.
   4. Pediatric airway pitfalls
      a. Difficulty passing the endotracheal tube (ETT) suggests that the tube is too large. The narrowest

Table 7-1.   Pediatric equipment table

Age	Weight (kg)	Suction nasogastric (Fr)	Endotracheal tube (mm)	Foley catheter (Fr)	Chest tube (Fr)
Newborn	3	8	3.5	5–8	12–18
6 mo	7	8	3.5–4.0	5–8	14–20
1 yr	10	10	4.0–4.5	8–10	14–24
2 yr	12	10	4.5–5.0	8–10	14–24
3 yr	14	12	4.5–5.0	10	14–24
4 yr	16	12	5.0–5.5	10–12	20–32
5 yr	18	12	5.0–5.5	10–12	20–32
6 yr	20	12–14	5.5–6.0	10–12	20–32
8 yr	25	12–14	6.0–6.5*	12	20–32
10 yr	25–30	14	7.0*	12–14	28–32
12 yr	30–35	14	7.0*	12–14	28–32
14 yr	40–50	14	7.0–8.0*	12–14	28–32

Laryngoscope blade: NB–3 yr: 1 straight
4–12 yr: 2 straight or curved
>12 yr: 3 straight or curved
* Cuffed endotracheal tube.
Note: These guidelines must be individualized.
Source: Children's Hospital, Columbus, OH.

part of a child's airway is the subglottic area, not the vocal cords. As a general guideline, use non-cuffed tubes in patients less than 8 years old.

b. If intubation has been accomplished but there is an audible air leak with inadequate chest rise, then reintubate with a tube 0.5 mm larger.

c. Poor or intermittent application of the Sellick maneuver during positive pressure ventilation may lead to gastric distention and cause emesis, aspiration, or inadequate ventilation.

d. Blind nasotracheal intubation is generally not recommended for pediatric patients. Esophageal obturator airways are contraindicated.

e. Needle cricothyrotomy is indicated in the rare circumstance of airway obstruction that is insurmountable by BVM ventilation or intubation. This may occur with severe facial or laryngeal injuries. Even in cases of critical croup or epiglottitis, BVM ventilation can provide adequate airway and ventilatory support. However, for these cases, the optimal site for definitive airway establishment is the operating room, with an anesthesiologist and surgeon in attendance. A child with severe airway obstruction or the possibility of progressive airway obstruction should have a secure airway prior to transport.

II. Breathing. After establishing and maintaining airway patency, ensure adequate ventilation and oxygenation (see Chap. 2, secs. **I.** and **IV.**).

   A. Minute volume ventilation assessment. Observe the patient's chest rise (tidal volume) and respiratory rate, which is age-dependent (Table 7-2). Auscultation assesses airway disease and time constants.

      1. The need to initiate positive pressure ventilation (PPV) is determined by the child's respiratory effort, rate of deterioration, and mechanism of illness or injury, not by blood gas results.

      2. If an ETT is in place, end-tidal CO_2 monitors or color indicators will be helpful. Other end-tidal CO_2 monitoring devices, such as transcutaneous or nasopharyngeal monitors, may be available.

      3. Obtain an arterial blood gas reading to confirm adequate ventilation. For children with suspected increased intracranial pressure, a PCO_2 of 28–33 mm Hg is targeted.

   B. Assisted ventilation

      1. Mouth-to-mouth breathing has been modified by the recommendation that a pocket mask be placed between the rescuer and the patient. In the ED a BVM device must be immediately available.

      2. Bag-valve ventilation can be accomplished with a mask or an ETT.

         a. The use of a mask requires more skill than is generally appreciated. The mask must be fitted to provide gentle yet leak-proof coverage from the bridge of the nose to the chin. With one hand, the resuscitator holds the mask firmly in position while maintaining chin lift and avoiding compression of the mandibular soft tissue. The resuscitator's other hand is used to compress the bag. Meanwhile, another person must administer cricoid pressure. Cricoid pressure protects against aspiration and gastric distention. Obtaining a good mask seal and providing adequate tidal volume sometimes may require one person to hold the mask and another to compress the bag.

         b. Self-inflating bags require less skill to operate

Table 7-2.   Normal pediatric vital signs

Age	Pulse	Respirations	Blood pressure*
Newborn	120–160	30–60	Systolic = 60–70
<1 yr	120–140	30–50	
1–2 yr	100–140	30–40	Systolic = 70 + (2 × age)
3–5 yr	100–120	20–30	Diastolic = 2/3 systolic
6–10 yr	80–100	16–20	

* Blood pressure is often an unreliable indicator of shock. Assess peripheral perfusion and pulses.
Source: Children's Hospital, Columbus, OH.

than anesthesia bags. They may have preset pressure pop-off valves (some can be occluded), O_2 reservoir attachments, and optional positive end-expiratory pressure (PEEP) adapters.

  c. Anesthesia bags are very effective at delivering a desired FIO_2, maintaining PEEP, and providing pressure support for spontaneous breaths. These are recommended only for resuscitators trained and skilled with this system.

3. **Mechanical ventilators** are used in the poststabilization phase for ongoing ventilation. Small infants require pressure ventilation, and older children are volume-ventilated depending on their respiratory pathophysiology.

C. **Oxygenation assessment.** Transcutaneous pulse-oximetry will adequately assess arterial oxygenation in most resuscitative circumstances. The most notable exception is severe shock.

D. **Oxygen delivery systems.** For spontaneously ventilating patients, there are several oxygen delivery systems. All oxygen delivery systems are run with humidified 100% O_2. The FIO_2 that is actually delivered to the patient will vary depending on the system.

1. **Nasal cannulas** are easy to use. The supplemental oxygen mixes with oropharyngeal air to provide an FIO_2 of 30%–40%. These are best suited for cooperative older children. Preschool children usually remove them. On infants, the prongs often fall out of place or irritate the nasal septum.

2. **Oxygen hoods** for infants are very well tolerated. They provide a local environment in which FIO_2, humidity, and temperature can be controlled.

3. **Oxygen tents,** occasionally used for young children, are falling out of vogue. They may invoke anxiety in the child and impair visualization and monitoring of the child.

4. **Oxygen masks** are available in a variety of sizes and offer the control of FIO_2.

  a. Simple face masks are lightweight and easy to use. A flow of 6 liter/min is required to flush out the dead space and prevent CO_2 rebreathing. It delivers an FIO_2 of 30%–60%.

  b. Partial rebreathing masks provide a wider range and more reliable FIO_2, but they require attachments.

  c. Nonrebreathing masks are combined with O_2 reservoir attachments. The nonrebreathing mask has one-way exhaust valves and can deliver nearly 100% oxygen to the patient. This is the device of choice for critically ill or injured children who are spontaneously breathing.

5. All children requiring (PPV) should initially receive 100% FIO_2.

III. **Circulation**

A. **Definition and recognition of shock.** Shock is a clinical syndrome in which the circulation of oxygenated blood to vital organs is not meeting metabolic demands. Florid shock is easy to recognize. The recognition of early circulatory compromise requires attention to the child's use of compensatory mechanisms.

1. In children who are in critical condition, the measurement of **blood pressure** is an insensitive method of assessing circulatory function. Children can lose over 40% of their blood volume and still maintain a normal blood pressure. In shock, a low blood pressure is a late indicator of decompensation.

2. In children the first cardiovascular compensatory mechanism is **tachycardia;** however, this is a fairly nonspecific response and must be interpreted in context.

3. Evidence of poor peripheral perfusion such as cool or **mottled skin,** weak distal pulses, and prolonged capillary refill (>2 seconds) is more indicative of cardiovascular compromise.

4. Combativeness, sleepiness, or **altered mental status** indicates that the most vital end-organ, the brain, is suffering from inadequate perfusion.

B. **Categories of shock.** The three most common types of shock in children are hypovolemic, distributive, and cardiogenic.

1. **Hypovolemic shock** occurs most commonly secondary to dehydration or hemorrhage. Gastroenteritis is a common cause of dehydration in young children. Worldwide, diarrhea is the leading cause of dehydration, shock, and death. Hemorrhage should be suspected in any patient in shock after a trauma.

2. **Distributive shock,** also known as relative hypovolemia, is caused by dysregulation of vascular tone. Inappropriate vasodilatation increases vascular capacitance to the point that the circulating volume becomes ineffective. Gram-negative toxemia, anaphylaxis, and disruption of the cervical spinal cord are examples of etiologies.

3. **Cardiogenic shock** refers to pump failure as seen with myocardial ischemia, myocarditis, or an ineffective rhythm.

   a. **Myocardial ischemia** in children is usually the result of respiratory failure or hypovolemic shock. Rarely, it is caused by an aberrant left coronary artery or other congenital anomaly.

   b. **Myocarditis** is uncommon and should be suspected in the child presenting with evidence of congestive heart failure after a prodromal upper respiratory tract infection (URI).

   c. The most common primary **ineffective rhythm** is symptomatic supraventricular tachycardia (SVT).

   d. A growing subset of children at risk for cardiogenic shock are survivors of **congenital heart disease**. The risk and degree of compromise depend on the child's underlying anatomy.

C. **Initial approach to shock.** The initial approach to the patient in shock is the same for all etiologies.

1. **ABCs.** Optimize ventilation and oxygenation. PPV is highly recommended in children in late shock even with no primary respiratory problem.
2. Obtain **vascular access.**
3. Identify and treat the **underlying cause**.

D. **Vascular access.** Vascular access is often difficult in small children with hemodynamic compromise (see Chap. 3, sec. **VI.**).

1. **Peripheral** IV lines are adequate for children requiring resuscitation. A supradiaphragmatic central line would be ideal; however, the procedure requires several minutes and may interfere with resuscitative efforts.
2. **Intraosseous (IO)** lines are indicated for the young child in critical condition when an IV line has not been established within 60 to 90 seconds. All fluids and resuscitative medications can be given by IO infusion. The greatest impediment to IO use is attitudinal (see Chap. 3 sec. **VI.C.**).
3. **Central lines.** When time permits and a peripheral IV line cannot be obtained, central venous access using the Seldinger technique is recommended. Femoral venous lines are most convenient in small children requiring resuscitation. A venous cutdown should be considered a last resort because it is time-consuming and provides only small, distal access (see Chap. 3 sec. **VI.B.**).
4. **Umbilical venous lines.** This may remain a viable route of access for as long as 2 weeks after delivery (see Chap. 6, sec. **IV.B.** for insertion technique).
5. **(ETT) drug instillation.** The ETT is an alternate, albeit unreliable, route of access to the circulation for delivery of resuscitative medications.
   a. Epinephrine is the most important and the most studied drug. Large doses and deep instillation are recommended. Use high-dose epinephrine (0.1 mg/kg) of 1:1000 diluted to a volume of 3–5 ml with normal saline (NS). Flush into the ETT with a catheter and follow by a few PPV breaths.
   b. Atropine, lidocaine, and naloxone can also be administered by ETT.

E. **Primary resuscitative medications** (Table 7-3)

1. **Oxygen** is the primary medication for children with circulatory failure. During resuscitation, all children should receive 100% O_2.
2. **Isotonic fluid boluses,** NS or lactated Ringers solution (LR), are the crystalloid solutions of initial choice. Glucose-containing solutions should be used only with documented hypoglycemia.
   a. Fluid boluses for children are 20 ml/kg. Children in septic shock may require large volumes of fluid: 60–100 ml/kg. Administer boluses as rapidly as possible. Repeat to restore effective circulating volume, reversing the metabolic acidosis secondary to poor perfusion.
   b. Large hemorrhagic losses are replaced by blood, preferably cross-matched when the patient's condition permits.

Table 7-3. Common pediatric medications

Drugs (how supplied)	Dose		Route*	Remarks
Adenosine (3 mg/ml)	0.1–0.2	mg/kg	IV	SVT, rapid push followed by saline flush
Albuterol	2.5	mg	Aerosol	Indicated for wheezing
Atropine (0.1 mg/ml)	0.02	mg/kg	IV, ET, IO	Minimum dose 0.1 mg
50% dextrose (0.5 g/ml)	1–2	ml/kg	IV, IO	Must dilute 50% 1:1 to ½ strength (25%)
Diazepam (Valium) (5 mg/ml)	0.2	mg/kg	IV, IO	Respiratory depressant, useful in seizures
	0.5	mg/kg	Rectal	Maximum dose 10 mg
1:10,000 epinephrine (0.1 mg/ml)	0.1	ml/kg	IV, IO	First dose for cardiac arrest
1:1000 epinephrine (1.0 mg/ml)	0.1	ml/kg	IV, IO, ET	Second and subsequent doses in arrest; all doses per ET route
1% lidocaine (10 mg/ml)	1.0	mg/kg	IV, IO, ET	Maximum dose 3 mg/kg
Midazolam (Versed) (1.0 mg/ml)	0.1	mg/kg	IV, IO	Useful for sedation
Naloxone (0.4 mg/ml)	0.1	mg/kg	IV, IO, ET	Indicated in OD and decreasing level of conscious (LOC)
Phenytoin (Dilantin) (50 mg/ml)	20	mg/kg	IV, IO	Give 1 mg/kg/min, maximum dose 50 mg/min
Phenobarbital (65 mg/ml)	15	mg/kg	IV, IO	Give over 15 min, respiratory depressant
8.4% bicarbonate (1 mEq/ml)	1	mEq/kg	IV, IO	Ventilation must be established, dilute 1:1 ½ strength for infants

* Route: IV = intravenous; ET = endotracheal; IO = intraosseous.
Source: Children's Hospital, Columbus, OH.

    c. Close attention to the volume administered and the response to therapy is critical.

    d. Never use hypotonic fluids for boluses.

  3. Epinephrine is the adrenergic agent of choice for pediatric resuscitation. Epinephrine is vasoconstrictive, inotropic, and chronotropic.

    a. The indications for epinephrine are cardiac arrest (asystole, fine ventricular fibrillation, pulseless electrical activity), symptomatic bradycardia unresponsive to ventilation and oxygenation, and hypotension unresponsive to fluid boluses (cardiogenic shock, distributive shock).

    b. Epinephrine is available in two dosage forms: standard dose or high dose. The standard dose is 1:10,000 or 0.1 mg/ml. The high dose is 10 times more concentrated, 1:1000 or 1 mg/ml.

    c. The dosing by volume stays the same. It is always 0.1–0.2 ml/kg; however, by changing to the concentrated solution, the dose/kg will be increased tenfold.

    d. The first dose of epinephrine is the standard dose. (ETT dosing is always high dose.)

    e. If subsequent doses are needed, use the high dose.

    f. These guidelines are based on animal studies and on one pediatric study. Outcome data from ongoing clinical trials are pending.

F. Secondary resuscitative medications (see Table 7-3)

  1. Adenosine is indicated for SVT and may be administered by IV or IO. Adenosine should be administered through an IV line situated proximally to the heart, preferably a left brachial line. Children with SVT who are in shock need synchronized cardioversion.

    a. Prior to and following administration of adenosine, 12-lead ECGs should be obtained. Critical information such as the presence of treatable bypass tracts may be obtained.

    b. The initial dose is 0.1 mg/kg rapid IVP followed by an immediate 5-ml NS flush. The dose may be doubled and then tripled if there is no response.

    c. The maximum dose is 12 mg.

  2. Atropine can be administered through IV line, IO line, or ETT.

    a. The dose is 0.02 mg/kg regardless of the route.

    b. The minimum dose is 0.1 mg, theoretically to prevent the paradoxical bradycardia associated with lower doses.

    c. The maximum dose is 1.0 mg.

    d. Atropine is commonly administered for rapid sequence induction because children are prone to a profound vagal response with laryngoscopy.

  3. Glucose should be used only with documented hypoglycemia.

    a. The dose is 0.5–1.0 g/kg; 2–4 ml of a 25% dextrose solution.

    b. If only 50% dextrose is available, dilute 1:1 with NS and administer 2–4 ml/kg.

    c. If the child simultaneously requires volume, a 20-ml/kg bolus of a 5% dextrose-containing isotonic solution (for example, D5-LR or D5-NS) will deliver 1 g/kg of glucose.

  4. **The sodium bicarbonate** dose is 1 mEq/kg.

    a. For older children, the dose is 1 ml/kg of 8.4% solution, the standard solution.

    b. In infants, a 4.2%, half-strength solution should be used to prevent damage from the hyperosmolarity.

  5. **Naloxone** can be administered through IV, IO, SQ, or ETT routes.

    a. The dose is 0.1 mg/kg. Repeat as needed.

    b. A common pitfall in pediatrics is underdosing of naloxone because of unfamiliarity with current dose recommendations.

  6. **Corticosteroids**

    a. There are several indications: upper and lower obstructive airway disease, meningitis, elevated intracranial pressure (ICP), spinal cord injury, adrenal insufficiency, and congenital adrenal hyperplasia.

    b. The choice of medication and dosing depends on the disease process.

    c. The role of steroids in gram-negative septic shock remains controversial.

  7. **Catecholamine drips** including epinephrine, dopamine, dobutamine can be administered IV or IO.

    a. Epinephrine drips are frequently used in the postresuscitative care of children.

    b. The dosing and titration are similar to those in adults (see Chap. 5 sec. **V.**).

G. **Cardiac compressions** (see Chap. 1 sec. **III.C.**)

  1. The indication for cardiac compressions is the absence of palpable pulses.

    a. The presence of an apical pulse is a poor indicator of perfusion to vital organs.

    b. Because of a child's thin chest wall and the heart's anterior location, ineffective cardiac activity may generate an apical pulse.

  2. Symptomatic bradycardia unresponsive to oxygenation and ventilation is also an indication. In children, symptomatic bradycardia is defined as a heart rate less than 60 bpm associated with hypotension and obtundation.

  3. Technique

    a. Compressions are applied over the midsternum. This position allows for the generation of adequate intrathoracic pressures with avoidance of rib fractures and liver laceration.

    b. The child's back should be against a firm surface, such as a backboard.

    c. Alternatively, in a newborn or small infant, the rescuer may encircle the patient's thorax with his or her hands, supporting the patient's back with his or her fingers and compressing the midsternum with the thumbs.

   d. Take care not to limit respiratory movements with this technique.

4. Compression rate and depth

	Infant	Child
Compressions/minute	100	80
Compression depth (in.)	$\frac{1}{2}$–1	1–$1\frac{1}{2}$

5. Common pitfalls include slow compression rates, shallow compression depths, and poorly located hand position.

IV. **Specific resuscitation situations**

A. **Trauma.** The principles of pediatric trauma resuscitation are essentially the same as those for adult patients, with a few notable exceptions listed below.

   1. All patients require oxygen and maintenance of their airway with cervical spine immobilization.

   2. Children with closed head injury are prone to apnea; poor airway management leads to morbidity and mortality.

   3. Blunt trauma associated with suboptimal oxygenation, obtundation, or a Pediatric Glasgow Coma Score of less than 8 or 9 is an indication for ventilatory support.

   4. Rib fractures in a child are pathognomonic for high impact injury.

      a. Because the pediatric rib cage is comparatively supple, a child can suffer enough impact to result in a pulmonary contusion or pneumothorax without any rib fracture.

      b. The presence of rib fractures indicates probable pulmonary injury or serious blunt trauma to other organ systems.

   5. Although a pediatric trauma victim may look good initially, a high index of suspicion for serious injury should be maintained. The vasoconstrictive capacity of children will often enable them to maintain a normal measurable blood pressure despite significant volume loss. Early surgical consultation is advisable.

   6. Head injury is not an explanation for vascular collapse; assume hypovolemic shock. Fluid resuscitation supersedes volume restriction in head injuries in the setting of shock.

   7. Maintain a high index of suspicion for nonaccidental trauma and multisystem trauma in cases of vague or unusual histories that fail to fit the clinical picture.

B. **Sudden infant death syndrome (SIDS)** is a unique problem in infancy.

   1. Victims of SIDS are typically less than 6 months old.

   2. Upon presenting to the ED, they are usually unresuscitatable, in terminal bradyarrhythmia or asystole.

   3. The diagnosis is based on history, physical examination, and autopsy.

   4. SIDS is a diagnosis of exclusion. The diagnosis is made when the death cannot be explained by sepsis, congenital heart disease, upper airway obstruction, trauma (abuse), or apnea due to respiratory syncytial virus, pertussis, or other discoverable cause.

5. Infant siblings of children who died of SIDS may be at increased risk of a life-threatening event. Referral and follow-up are advisable.

C. Apparent life-threatening event (ALTE)

1. This is occasionally mislabeled "near miss SIDS."
2. The diagnosis of an ALTE is based on a thorough history. This can be challenging considering that the historian may be distraught and may not have witnessed the entire event.
3. The differential diagnosis includes sepsis, airway obstruction, gastroesophageal reflux, seizure, abuse, periodic breathing, apnea of prematurity, and apnea of other etiologies.
4. All infants diagnosed with an ALTE should be admitted to an appropriate inpatient service.
   a. Inpatient investigations are guided as much as possible by the history and physical examination.
   b. The possibility of sepsis must be strongly considered, even in the absence of other signs or symptoms.
   c. Occasionally after hospitalization, an infant may be discharged with an apnea-bradycardia monitor. These monitors must be accompanied by counseling, training, and regularly scheduled follow-up.

D. Ductal-dependent lesions. A cardiovascular emergency unique to infants is congenital heart disease that is dependent on blood flow through a patent ductus arteriosus (see Chap. 28).

1. Typically, these infants present within 2 weeks of birth with respiratory distress and cyanosis, coinciding with closure of the ductus.
2. The initial approach is to apply the ABCs.
3. Arterial oxygen saturation (SaO_2) or PaO_2 that responds poorly to supplemental oxygen or PPV is a strong indicator of a cardiac right-to-left shunt, or incomplete communication of the pulmonary and systemic circulation.
4. Immediate pediatric cardiac consultation is recommended.
5. In the event of rapid deterioration, ventilatory support will be required and prostaglandin$_1$ may be warranted as a palliative measure to maintain ductal patency.
   a. The initial dose of prostaglandin$_1$ is 0.05 to 0.10 µg/kg/min.
   b. The dose is adjusted as necessary to maintain an acceptable baseline SaO_2 or PaO_2.
   c. The major side effects of prostaglandin infusion are apnea, bradycardia, fever, and hypotension. Newborns should be intubated prior to transport and should have two intravascular sites in case volume or pressor support is needed.

E. Near-drowning. Drowning accounts for approximately one-third of pediatric deaths in this country. Victims are typically toddlers or adolescents. The following points are especially applicable to infants and children.

1. In adolescents, the risk of substance abuse, cervical

spine injury, head injury, and other traumatic complications should be highly suspected.

2. Infants and toddlers are top-heavy and may fall head first.

3. Infants can drown in surprisingly small bodies of water such as that in buckets and toilets. Abuse and neglect must be suspected.

4. The following criteria defined by Orlowski predict poor outcome.
   a. Age less than 3 years.
   b. Submersion time greater than 5 minutes.
   c. No CPR at the scene for greater than 10 minutes.
   d. Initial pH less than 7.1.
   e. Coma upon presentation.

5. Brain injury and cardiovascular collapse with multisystem organ injury occur as a result of ischemia and reperfusion.

6. Pulmonary function may be further compromised by aspiration.
   a. Fresh water aspiration tends to disrupt surfactant and alveolar epithelium.
   b. Salt water aspiration creates an intra-alveolar osmotic gradient.

7. In both cases, gas exchange is impaired and intrapulmonary shunting occurs.

8. Cold water near-drowning events (specifically in icy water) have been associated with survival after rewarming, despite prolonged resuscitation.

9. All children with submersion injuries should be admitted for observation because their injuries can progress during the first several hours.

F. **Supraventricular tachycardia (SVT).** SVT is the most common type of significant pediatric dysrhythmia (see Chap. 5, sec. **II.C.** and Chap. 17, sec. **VI.**). SVT in infants and children differs somewhat from SVT in adults:

1. SVTs have a variety of etiologies and are characterized by a narrow-complex QRS with ventricular rates much greater than the maximum expected for age.

2. On presentation, the duration and etiology may be unknown.

3. Therapy is customized to the severity of the patient's signs and symptoms.

4. The first pitfall may be misdiagnosing sinus tachycardia as supraventricular tachycardia.
   a. In the context of fever, dehydration, fear, or other stressors, children may increase their sinus rhythm to the high 100s and infants can reach rates up to 220.
   b. These same stressors can trigger SVT.
   c. The ECG in sinus tachycardia demonstrates a narrow QRS with P waves of normal position and axis and undisturbed T waves. In this situation the underlying condition is treated.
   d. In SVT, the ECG demonstrates a very rapid, very regular narrow QRS. P waves look identical and may be anywhere or buried in the QRS complex.

5. Children with SVT who are in shock should be synchronously cardioverted with 0.5 watt/kg.
6. Stable SVT can be cardioverted with adenosine (see sec. **III.F.1.**).
7. Before and after cardioversion, ECGs should be obtained to evaluate for treatable bypass tracts.

V. Postresuscitation care. The key to postresuscitation care is recognizing that the hemodynamic stability that has been achieved is fragile. Hypoxic-ischemic injury has probably occurred with the initiation of multisystem organ failure. Transport, whether to another institution or to the pediatric intensive care unit within the same facility, should be arranged with a team prepared to manage rapid changes or deterioration. Invasive monitoring (e.g., Foley catheter, central venous line (CVL), Swan-Ganz catheter, arterial line) is often necessary.

For pediatric survivors of full arrest, delayed death is the most common outcome, followed by poor neurologic survival. The most common outcome of prehospital pediatric arrest is death. The following concepts will assist in the management of pediatric arrest victims.

1. Be prepared to manage the family.
2. Use family support resources and respect the family's wishes as much as possible.
3. Know your state's laws regarding coroner cases, autopsies, and organ donation.
4. Recognize the state laws and your duties regarding child abuse and neglect. Remember that other children may be at risk.

During resuscitation, transport, and postresuscitation phases, let the family be physically close to the child as frequently as possible.

Bibliography

American Heart Association Emergency Cardiac Care Committee and Subcommittees. Guidelines for cardiopulmonary resuscitation and emergency cardiac care, VII: neonatal resuscitation. *JAMA* 268:2276–2281, 1992.

Chameide L, Hazinski MF, et al. *Textbook of Pediatric Life Support.* Dallas: American Heart Association, 1994.

Fleisher G, Ludwig S. *Textbook of Pediatric Emergency Medicine* (3rd ed.). Baltimore: Williams & Wilkins, 1993.

Luten RC, et al. Length-based endotracheal tube and emergency equipment in pediatrics. *Ann Emerg Med* 21:900–904, 1992.

Zaritsky A. Pediatric resuscitation pharmacology. *Ann Emerg Med* 22:445–455, 1994.

8

Hemodynamic Monitoring

Michael Dick

The hemodynamic monitoring of patients allows for the detection of physiologic abnormalities not apparent through physical examination. Patients with acute cardiovascular decompensation often require therapy that can only be titrated with the information gained through advanced monitoring techniques. However, patient monitoring, whether invasive or noninvasive, is not therapeutic. Its value is determined only by the accuracy of the information and how the practitioner utilizes the data to modify therapy.

I. Arterial blood pressure monitoring

A. Automated noninvasive blood pressure monitoring. Most automated noninvasive blood pressure measuring devices use an oscillometric technique, where the cuff is inflated to a pressure above systolic pressure. The device then detects small oscillations in pressure during deflation. The initial oscillations, the point of maximal oscillations, and the rapid disappearance of the oscillations represent systolic, mean, and diastolic pressures, respectively. With these devices, the mean pressure is a direct measurement and is the most accurate of the three pressures. These devices are most appropriately utilized for frequent blood pressure determinations in relatively hemodynamically stable patients.

B. Invasive blood pressure monitoring

1. **Indications.** There are two primary indications for the placement of an arterial catheter: (1) continuous monitoring of blood pressure, and (2) frequent arterial blood sampling. Continuous monitoring of blood pressure is indicated in those patients who are hemodynamically unstable, either hypo- or hypertensive, those require high levels of respiratory support, and receive vasoactive or inotropic agents.
2. **Placement technique.** Table 8-1 lists the sites for arterial cannulation along with their advantages, disadvantages, and preferred catheter length. Arterial catheters may be placed using either a catheter over the needle technique or preferably a catheter over a guidewire (modified Seldinger technique). Twenty-gauge catheters provide adequate lumen size for monitoring and blood withdrawal with lower complication rates than with larger catheters. Placement of arterial catheters in hypotensive patients, obese patients, or those with significant edema may be difficult at best. Cannulation may be aided by locating the artery with a hand-held Doppler device. Catheters with Doppler probes in the stylet (Smart Needle™) and vascular ultrasound scanners are also available to locate arteries.

   Invasive blood pressure measurement always requires that the transducer be set at a reference point, and be "zeroed." The commonly used reference point is

Table 8-1. Arterial catheterization sites

Site	Advantages	Disadvantages	Catheter length (in.)
Radial	Accessible; good collaterals; easy to maintain	Difficult to cannulate in hypotensive patients	1.5–2.0
Ulnar	Same as radial	Tortuous at wrist	1.5–2.0
Brachial	Poor collaterals	Accessible	1.5–2.0
Axillary	Large lumen; good collaterals; proximal location	Less accessible	4–6
Temporal	Accessible; good collaterals	Tortuous; small diameter	1.5–2.0
Dorsalis pedis	Accessible	Prone to thrombosis; unreliable pressure except for mean	1.5–2.0

the mid-axillary line or right heart level. Zeroing compensates for differences in the transducer, tubing, and electronics. Arterial catheter systems display systolic, diastolic, and mean pressure. Mismatch of the catheter and tubing with the vessel, damping of the waveform due to air bubbles or thrombus, movement of the catheter in the vessel (catheter whip), and the distance of the catheter from the heart all contribute to discrepancies between measured systolic and diastolic blood pressure and true intraluminal blood pressure. Determining a return-to-flow blood pressure by inflating a manual blood pressure cuff until the arterial waveform disappears, then deflating the cuff until the first waveform pulsation occurs, allows confirmation of the pressure that most closely approximates intraluminal systolic pressure. Mean arterial pressure can be estimated by the systolic BP + 2 (diastolic BP) /3. The true mean pressure is determined by the area under the arterial pressure waveform. This calculation is performed automatically by most monitoring systems, and makes the mean pressure the most accurate pressure.

3. **Complications.** Complications of arterial catheterization include line sepsis, thrombosis, and embolization. Arterial catheters do not require routine changes. However, the site should be inspected daily, and the catheter should be changed at the first sign of erythema or drainage. The risks of distal ischemia are reduced by avoiding sites with poor collateral circulation (e.g., the brachial artery). Assessment of collateral circulation using the Allen test may be carried out prior to insertion of radial artery catheters. Flushing of catheters should be performed in a pulsatile manner to reduce the risk of retrograde flow and embolization.

II. **Central venous pressure (CVP) monitoring.** Measurement of central venous pressure can aid in the assessment of intravascular volume or preload. In patients without left or right heart failure, central venous pressure can be used as a rough estimate of left atrial pressure or left-side preload. However, there are often marked differences in right and left atrial pressures, which makes this means of volume assessment unreliable in critically ill patients.

The insertion of central venous catheters is described in Chapter 3. The addition of an electronic transducer provides a means of measuring central venous pressure. The pressure should always be measured at end expiration. In the spontaneously breathing patient, this will generally be the highest pressure. In the mechanically ventilated patient, central venous pressure will be the lowest pressure recorded.

Central venous pressure approximates right atrial pressure and therefore, right ventricular filling pressure or preload. In the absence of pulmonary hypertension, right ventricular preload provides an estimate of the adequacy of left ventricular filling pressures, or intravascular volume. In general a low CVP is always indicative of low intravascular volume and low ventricular filling pressures. Midrange or high central venous pressures may represent normal or increased intravascular volume. However, these pressures may also reflect pulmonary hypertension, cardiac tamponade, tension pneumothorax, high ventilatory pressures, or valvular heart disease. If there is any possibility that one of these states exist, or the patient's response to therapy guided by the central venous pressure is unexpected, the reliability of the measurement should be questioned.

III. **Pulmonary artery catheters**

    A. **Introduction.** The standard balloon tip flow-directed pulmonary artery catheter provides significantly more information than monitoring central venous pressure. The catheters used by Swan and Ganz in 1970 had a double lumen and measured pulmonary artery pressure and pulmonary artery occlusion pressure (wedge pressure). Subsequent catheter development included the addition of a right atrial port for measuring right atrial or central venous pressure and a thermistor on the distal tip to allow the determination of thermodilution cardiac output. The next major step in catheter development was the inclusion of fiberoptic bundles running to the distal end of the catheter. This allowed continuous monitoring of mixed venous oxygen saturation and, therefore, an assessment of oxygen delivery and consumption. Catheters are also available with additional infusion ports, lumens for placement of a right ventricular pacing wire, and rapid-response thermistors for measuring right ventricular ejection fraction. Continuous cardiac output catheters are the latest development for hemodynamic monitoring.

       In spite of the tremendous amount of information obtainable from pulmonary artery (PA) catheters, there have been no studies that demonstrate a difference in mortality in patients monitored with these devices. However, there remains general consensus that the information gained from these catheters, if interpreted and acted on correctly, is useful for diagnosis and management in certain clinical scenarios. The general indications for pulmonary artery catheterization are listed in Table 8-2.

    B. **Insertion technique.** Sites for insertion of a pulmonary artery catheter are those which provide access to the central venous circulation. The easiest sites in terms of catheter placement and flow are the right internal jugular, which offers a straight path to the right atrium, and the left subclavian, which provides a similar, gently curved path to the right atrium. The axillary vein is an alternative route for catheter placement. Once the introducer has been placed following standard techniques for placing central venous catheters, the pulmonary artery catheter is "floated." Prior to insertion of the catheter into the introducer, the pressure monitoring system must be set up and calibrated, the catheter lumens flushed, and the balloon integrity checked. In addition, catheters with oximetric capabilities must have the oximeter calibrated.

       Just prior to insertion, the catheter tip should be gently shaken to ensure a waveform is present on the monitor. The catheter should be positioned so that its natural curve approximately follows the intended path to the pulmonary

Table 8-2. Indications for pulmonary artery catheterization

Hypotension unresponsive to fluid resuscitation

Oliguria unresponsive to fluid resuscitation

Pulmonary edema of uncertain etiology

Congestive heart failure unresponsive to standard therapy

To define relation of intravascular volume to cardiac function

To assess effect of vasopressors, inotropes, and vasodilators

To assess effect of high ventilatory pressures on cardiac function

To assess and optimize oxygen transport

To diagnose pericardial tamponade

To guide fluid therapy in patients with myocardial infarction and hypotension

To guide fluid therapy in patients with severe burns

To guide therapy in any patient with contradictory management goals, (e.g., congestive heart failure and hypotension, head injury and hypotension)

artery. Pulmonary artery catheters are placed with continuous pressure monitoring and recognition of specific wave forms during insertion. Generally, fluoroscopic guidance is not required.

Once the catheter has been inserted 15–20 cm into the introducer, the balloon is inflated with 1.5 ml of air. The catheter is advanced steadily until the characteristic right ventricular pressure tracing is observed. From this point, the occlusion pressure ("wedge pressure") should be observed with less than 15 cm of further catheter advancement. The pulmonary artery pressure tracing is recognized by an increase in diastolic pressure from the right ventricle. The catheter is advanced farther until the balloon occludes the pulmonary artery branch, which results in a characteristic atrial tracing with smaller pressure excursions and a lower mean pressure. If the occlusion pressure is not observed within 15 cm of the right ventricle, the catheter should be withdrawn to the ventricle and advanced again. Once the occlusion pressure tracing has been obtained, the balloon should be deflated and the PA tracing should return. The catheter should be withdrawn in 1-cm increments with subsequent reinflation of the balloon and demonstration of the occlusion pressure. This ensures that the catheter is placed at the minimum distance that allows attainment of pulmonary artery occlusion pressure. The typical pressure tracings seen during catheter placement are illustrated in Fig. 8-1.

C. **Complications.** Complications during catheter insertion include ventricular arrhythmias and coiling of the catheter in the right ventricle (RV). Dysrhythmias are minimized by advancing the catheter quickly through the ventricle. Coiling of the catheter can be avoided by closely monitoring the length of the catheter inserted. As noted above, no more than 15 cm of catheter should be needed to obtain an

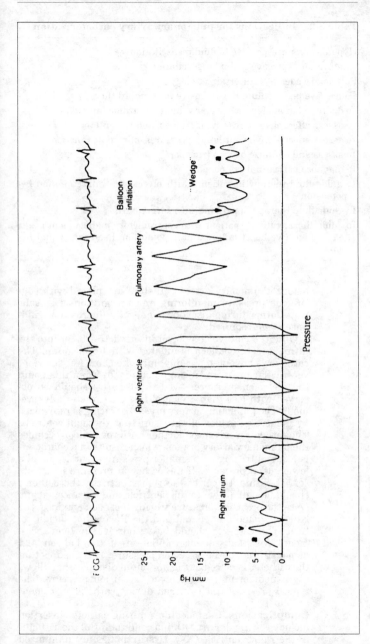

Fig. 8-1.   Pressure tracings seen during advancement of a pulmonary artery catheter. (From Kaur S, Heard SO. Airway management and endotracheal intubation. In Rippe JM, Irwin RS, Fink MP, Cerra FB (eds.), *Intensive Care Medicine* (3rd ed.). Boston: Little, Brown, 1996.)

**Table 8-3.   Approximate distance
from insertion site to PAOP**

Insertion site	Distance to PAOP (cm)
Internal jugular	40–55
Subclavian	35–45
Axillary	45–55
Femoral	55–70

occlusion pressure from the right ventricle. Approximate
catheter distances from routine insertion sites are listed in
Table 8-3. Additional complications of pulmonary artery
catheters are noted in Table 8-4.

D. **Pulmonary artery pressure measurements.** Normal
   pressure measurements are noted in Table 8-5. Elevated
   pulmonary artery pressures are seen in conditions with
   elevated pulmonary vascular resistance, such as pulmonary embolus, pulmonary hypertension, atelectasis or
   lobar collapse, and hypoxia. If pulmonary vascular resistance and left ventricular function are normal, diastolic
   pulmonary artery pressures will closely approximate pulmonary artery occlusion pressure (PAOP).

   When the catheter balloon is inflated, there is a continuous column of fluid from the catheter tip to the left atrium.
   Therefore, PAOP will approximate left atrial pressure. If
   the mitral valve is normal, left atrial pressure approximates left ventricular end diastolic pressure. If the compliance of the ventricle is normal, end diastolic pressure
   reflects end diastolic volume and therefore preload. PAOP
   then is used as an indicator of left ventricular preload.
   However, a disturbance in any of the above assumptions al-
   ters the ability of the PAOP to reflect preload accurately.

**Table 8-4.   Complications associated
with pulmonary artery catheters**

All usual complications associated with central venous cannulation
Complications associated with placement of catheter
   Atrial and ventricular dysrhythmias
   Right bundle-branch block
   Complete heart block (preexisting left bundle-branch block)
   Catheter knotting
   Cardiac perforation
Complications associated with indwelling catheter
   Catheter infection/sepsis
   Pulmonary infarction
   Pulmonary artery rupture

Table 8-5. Normal pulmonary pressure measurements

Location	Normal pressure (mm Hg)
CVP (right atrium)	2–8
Right ventricle	Systolic 20–30; diastolic 2–8
Pulmonary artery	Systolic 15–30; diastolic 5–12
Pulmonary artery occlusion pressure	2–12

Positive end expiratory pressure (PEEP) will increase measured PAOP to a variable degree. At levels of PEEP less than 10 cm H_2O there is little effect on PAOP. As with central venous pressure, PAOP should always be measured at end expiration in both spontaneously breathing and mechanically ventilated patients. The PAOP in various hypoperfused or shock states is shown in Table 8-6.

E. **Cardiac output.** Pulmonary artery catheters utilize the thermodilution method for determining cardiac output. A known quantity of solution with a known temperature that is cooler than blood (room temperature) is injected through the right atrial port. The resultant change in blood temperature is noted by the thermistor as blood flows by the distal tip of the catheter. The change in temperature over time is inversely proportional to blood flow. Monitoring systems calculate the flow based on the indicator dilution theory, providing a cardiac output in liter/minute. Three measurements within 15% of each other should be obtained at each cardiac output determination.

F. **Mixed venous oxygen saturation.** Pulmonary artery blood represents true mixed venous blood. The mixed ve-

Table 8-6. Hemodynamic characteristics of shock

Type	CO	PAOP	SVR	S$\bar{v}$O$_2$
Hypovolemic	⇓	⇓	⇑	⇓
Cardiogenic				
RV MI	⇓	nl–⇓	⇑	⇓
LV MI	⇓	⇑	⇑	⇓
Septic				
Early	nl–⇑ ⇓	⇓	nl–⇑ ⇓	nl–⇑ ⇓
Late	⇓	nl	⇑	⇓
Obstructive				
Tamponade	⇓	⇑	⇑	⇓
Pulmonary embolism	⇓	nl–⇓	⇑	⇓

Note: nl = normal; ⇑ = increasing level; ⇓ = decreasing level.

nous oxygen saturation ($S\bar{v}O_2$) can be obtained by co-oximetry analysis of a sample drawn from the distal port of the catheter. Alternatively, the $S\bar{v}O_2$ can be determined utilizing catheters containing fiberoptic bundles. Reflection spectrophotometry is used to provide a continuous measurement of $S\bar{v}O_2$.

The $S\bar{v}O_2$ is determined by the balance of oxygen supply and oxygen consumption. Oxygen supply is dependent on three variables: (1) cardiac output, (2) hemoglobin concentration, and (3) systemic arterial oxygen saturation. Oxygen consumption is dependent on the inherent metabolic rate as well as situations that either increase or decrease oxygen utilization, such as hyper- or hypothermia, increased work of breathing, and shivering. Normal $S\bar{v}O_2$ is 65%–75%. A sustained drop in the $S\bar{v}O_2$ below this level suggests a decrease in oxygen supply (an abnormality in one of the three transport variables) or an increase in oxygen demand. Increases in $S\bar{v}O_2$ are seen with sepsis and other scenarios that lead to shunting of oxygenated blood by tissues. Changes in the oxygen supply–demand ratio, which are reflected by changes in the $S\bar{v}O_2$, occur early in the decompensating patient, providing an opportunity for aggressive intervention. In addition, monitoring of the $S\bar{v}O_2$ provides a gauge of resuscitation beyond the attainment of "normal" vital signs.

IV. **Additional methods of hemodynamic assessment**
  A. **Echocardiography.** Transthoracic and transesophageal echocardiography provide additional means of assessing cardiovascular function. They are particularly useful in the diagnosis of dissecting aneurysms, infective endocarditis, valvular heart disease, and pericardial effusions or tamponade. In addition, echocardiography allows a detailed assessment of ventricular function including contractility, regional myocardial function, and estimation of ventricular filling or preload. This is particularly helpful when abnormal ventricular compliance makes the interpretation of PAOP difficult.
  B. **Noninvasive cardiac output.** Noninvasive methods that are used to determine cardiac output include **Doppler probes** positioned in the suprasternal notch, the esophagus, or the aorta. Currently this technology does not compare reliably with thermodilution techniques and is not routinely used. **Bioimpedance** methodology quantitates flow through the thoracic aorta by assessing changes in impedance when current is applied across the thorax. Currently bioimpedance determined cardiac output requires intermittent correlation with thermodilution methods and has not gained widespread acceptance.

Bibliography

Civetta JM, Taylor RW, Kirby RR (eds.), *Critical Care.* Philadelphia: Lippincott, 1992.

Ermakov S, Hoyt JW. Pulmonary artery catheterization. *Crit Care Clin* 8:773, 1992.

Hall JB, Schmidt GA, Wood LDH (eds.), *Principles of Critical Care*. New York: McGraw-Hill, 1992.

Society of Critical Care Medicine. *Fundamental Critical Care Support Course Syllabus*. Anaheim, CA: 1996.

Acute Myocardial Infarction

Diagnosis of Acute Myocardial Infarction

Gerard X. Brogan Jr.

I. **Etiology.** Occlusive thrombosis on a coronary artery atheromatous plaque is the most common cause of myocardial infarction. Rupture of the plaque is the most likely precipitating event. Vasospasm, resulting in part from the loss of endothelium-dependent dilator mechanism in atherosclerosis, may predispose to thrombus formation. Acute vasospasm also may induce plaque rupture.

Sudden complete occlusion of a coronary artery of duration less than 15–20 minutes (such as in unstable angina) results in impaired regional myocardial function due to myocardial ischemia. Although there is no irreversible injury, there is reversible impairment of ventricular function ("myocardial stunning"). Complete occlusion lasting longer than 20 minutes generally is associated with actual necrosis (myocardial infarction) even if flow is restored. Areas of myocardium adjacent to the necrotic area (infarct area) exhibit the stunning phenomena. Restoration of flow within 6 hours of occlusion onset is associated with substantial salvage of myocardium.

II. **Scope of the problem.** As many as 5 million patients present annually to emergency departments with a chief complaint of chest pain. Four million are admitted to the cardiac care unit (CCU) to "rule out" acute myocardial infarction (AMI), of which up to 70% eventually do "rule out." It is estimated that 2 to 3 billion dollars per year could be saved if this subset could be identified earlier and cared for in a less expensive hospital setting. Each year in the United States, coronary artery disease causes over 650,000 deaths and results in 1.3 million patients with nonfatal myocardial infarction. North American men have a 1-in-5 chance of experiencing acute myocardial infarction or sudden cardiac death before 65 years of age.

III. **Medicolegal considerations.** Up to 8% of patients presenting to the emergency department with acute myocardial infarction and chest pain are unintentionally released. This phenomenon accounts for 20% of malpractice dollar losses in emergency medicine and, more important, increased patient morbidity and mortality. The "missed" myocardial infarction patient tends to (1) be younger, (2) have a more atypical presentation, and (3) be evaluated by a less experienced clinician. Common issues in litigation of missed myocardial infarction focus on (1) poorly documented and incomplete history and physical examination, (2) ECG misinterpretation (emergency department ECG is diagnostic in only 55% of AMI patients), and (3) a reluctance by clinicians to admit patients with atypical or less than classic symptoms ("soft story").

IV. **Presentation.** The most widely accepted guidelines for the diagnosis of AMI are the World Health Organization's diagnostic criteria for AMI. These criteria utilize a triad of findings: (1) history and physical exam suggestive of acute coronary ischemia, (2) electrocardiographic changes compatible with AMI, and (3) a characteristic rise and fall of cardiac isoenzyme CK-MB. In essence, patients should meet two of the three criteria. However, a characteristic ECG evolution of infarction or a characteristic rise and fall of CK-MB is generally accepted as diagnostic as well.

A. **History.** The most accurate history is obtained by asking the patient whether or not he or she is having any type of **chest discomfort.** Patients, when asked if they are having any chest "pain," may not relate to the clinician a sensation of pressure or tightness that they do not consider as "pain." Chest discomfort is present in 80%–85% of patients with MI. The classic description of discomfort is a pressure or tightness in the substernal region or left chest. Patients may report similar but less intense prior episodes of discomfort. This type of chest discomfort, lasting 20 minutes or more, is most consistent with the discomfort of acute myocardial infarction. The **pain may radiate** to the left shoulder, neck, back, jaw, right shoulder, or epigastrium. Although pain radiating to the left arm is more common, studies have shown that radiation to the right arm or the jaw is more specific for AMI than other radiation patterns. Symptoms of radiation of pain to the back, although consistent with AMI, should also suggest the possibility of aortic aneurysm or dissection. Patients also may complain of **associated symptoms** of shortness of breath, nausea, and diaphoresis. Other accompanying symptoms may include vomiting, belching, a sense of "impending doom," and an urge to defecate.

Approximately 23% of myocardial infarctions go unrecognized because of the absence of symptoms or the absence of classic chest discomfort ("silent MI"). Patients with diabetes often fall into this category.

It is important to note that up to 20% of adults with acute myocardial infarction may present with **atypical symptoms.** Patients presenting with less than the classic symptoms of AMI may be undiagnosed. Studies have shown that up to 5% of patients presenting with AMI may report sharp or stabbing pain, and more than 20% of patients may describe their chest discomfort as burning or indigestion. In a group of patients diagnosed with MI, 13% complained of a chest ache and 5% described their pain as sharp and stabbing. In this same group of patients with myocardial infarction, 5% described their pain as partly pleuritic, whereas approximately 2% described their pain as fully positional. About 4%–5% of patients stated that their pain was fully reproduced by chest palpation.

Patients presenting with new onset of congestive heart failure or dysrhythmias may in fact be having acute myocardial infarction.

The classical symptoms of chest discomfort, vomiting, and diaphoresis are less common with advancing age. In patients presenting older than 85 years of age, shortness of breath is more common than chest discomfort. With increasing age, symptoms such as syncope, acute confusion, and stroke become even more common. The clinician should have a very low threshold for considering AMI in the differential in elderly patients presenting with these conditions. The clinician should never rule out myocardial infarction merely because of the presence of one atypical symptom in a patient's symptom complex (e.g., reproducible chest pain). Studies have noted that patients with atypical AMI presentations, on average, were ten years older, smoked less, and rarely described a prior history of angina, compared with patients with typical presentations.

B. Physical examination. The overall appearance of patients presenting with myocardial infarction can vary from no apparent clinical stress to obvious dyspnea, diaphoresis, and cyanosis. **Vital signs** may reveal a bradycardia, tachycardia, or irregular pulse. Up to 60% of patients with inferior wall myocardial infarction will manifest a bradycardia in the initial hours. Persistent sinus tachycardia beyond the initial 12–24 hours is predictive of a high mortality rate. Blood pressure is usually normal but may be increased secondary to anxiety or decreased from cardiac failure. Blood pressure also may be decreased as a result of severe bradycardia. Diaphoresis is common. Cyanosis, mottling, or pallor suggest a significant drop in cardiac output (cardiogenic shock). Pulmonary examination frequently reveals basilar rales. Cardiac failure diagnosed on the basis of mild pulmonary congestion occurs in 30%–40% of patients with otherwise uncomplicated myocardial infarction.

On **auscultation** the first and second heart sounds are often soft as a result of decreased contractility. The first heart sound may be diminished also because of a prolonged PR interval. If there is tachycardia, a short PR interval may result in a somewhat accentuated first heart sound. The second heart sound is usually normal; however, with extensive myocardial damage there may be a single second heart sound. A third heart sound is heard in probably only 15%–20% of patients with acute infarction. A fourth heart sound is often audible in patients with AMI. A pericardial friction rub, usually not heard until 48 to 72 hours after the onset of myocardial infarction, occurs in about 10% of patients and is more common in right ventricular and inferior infarcts. A new systolic murmur may indicate ischemic mitral regurgitation or a ventricular septal defect, particularly in the presence of heart failure or cardiogenic shock. Mitral regurgitation is most commonly due to ischemia of the posterior medial papillary muscle. Rales and an S3 gallop are associated with left ventricular failure, whereas jugular venous distention, a positive hepato-jugular reflex, and peripheral edema suggest right ventricular dysfunction. Isolated right heart failure suggests right ventricular infarction.

Clinical classification proposed by Killip provides some uniformity in terms of describing cardiac failure and provides approximate in-hospital mortality rates. Class I patients do not have any pulmonary rales or a third heart sound and have an in-hospital mortality rate less than

5%. Class II patients have rales to a mild-to-moderate degree, involving less than 50% of the lung fields, and may or may not have an S3 (10% mortality in-hospital). Class III patients have rales more than halfway up the lung fields and an S3 gallop (30% mortality). Class IV patients are those in cardiogenic shock (80%–90% in-hospital mortality). Studies have demonstrated that patients with evidence of myocardial dysfunction including third heart sound, fourth heart sound, or rales on arrival at the emergency department are at much greater risk for adverse cardiovascular events, including nonfatal AMI, stroke with deficit, life-threatening arrhythmia, the need for cardiac surgery, and death. Since acute ischemic coronary disease is a dynamic process, serial physical examinations should be performed.

C. **Cardiac risk factors.** Recognized risk factors for the development of atherosclerotic coronary heart disease include hypercholesterolemia (or a low HDL), family history, male gender, cigarette smoking, diabetes mellitus, and hypertension. Other cardiac risk factors include cocaine use, previous history of angina or MI, and peripheral vascular disease. The presence of risk factors for coronary artery disease may alert the clinician to the consideration of the diagnosis of acute ischemic coronary syndrome or AMI in younger patients or those presenting with atypical symptoms. Patients taking cardiovascular medications (antianginals, antiarrhythmics, antihypertensives, anticoagulants, or digitalis) should raise the clinician's suspicion that the pain may be of ischemic origin. In addition, the unsuccessful utilization of medications such as antacids, sulcrafate or H2 blockers by the patient for presumed symptoms of dyspepsia should alert the clinician to the possibility of a cardiac etiology of the patient's symptoms. Table 9-1 describes conditions that should be considered in a differential of a patient presenting with prolonged chest discomfort.

V. **Assessment.** In addition to the classic history, physical examination, and ECG criteria that patients present with, patients frequently may present with less than classic, subtle, or vague signs and symptoms of AMI. Of note, the initial ECG may be nondiagnostic in up to 55% of patients with documented AMI. Cardiac enzymes may never be elevated above the absolute threshold established at local laboratories. In fact, the ECG may be normal or show only nonspecific ST-T wave changes in 4% of patients presenting with acute myocardial infarction (normal in 1%, nonspecific ST-T wave changes in 3%).

A. **ECG criteria**
   1. **General comments.** The early ECG changes of T-wave inversion or ST-segment elevation/depression may reflect ischemia or infarction. ST-segment elevation is more specific for AMI and reflects the epicardial injury associated with total occlusion of an epicardial coronary artery. The hallmark of AMI is the development of abnormal Q-waves, which on average appear 8–12 hours from onset of symptoms but may not de-

Table 9-1. Causes of chest discomfort

Cardiac	Gastrointestinal
Acute myocardial infarction	Esophageal reflux/dysmotility
Unstable angina	Esophageal rupture
Angina	Gallbladder disease
Mitral valve prolapse	Peptic ulcer disease
Aortic stenosis	Pancreatitis
Hypertrophic cardiomyopathy	
Pericarditis	**Vascular**
	Thoracic aortic dissection/aneurysm
Pulmonary	
Pulmonary embolism	**Other**
Pneumonia	Musculoskeletal
Pneumothorax	Herpes zoster
Pleurisy	

velop for 24–48 hours. The classic diagnostic serial ECG changes consist of ST-segment elevation with the development of the T-wave inversion and then the evolution of abnormal Q waves. The appearance of abnormal Q waves is very specific for AMI; however, they are present in less than 50% of patients with documented AMI. Most of the other patients who have AMI will have ECG changes restricted to T-wave inversions and ST-segment depression, or no change at all. These patients represent a group with non-Q-wave infarction.

Right bundle-branch block does not mask ST-segment elevation, and the diagnosis of myocardial infarction is possible. Preexisting left bundle-branch block masks pathologic ST-segment and T-wave changes. Marked reduction of the QRS amplitude versus prior ECG, presence of any size Q wave in V5 and V6, or small Q waves in V1 or V2 may indicate AMI. A small percentage of patients will have left bundle-branch block that may mask the development of most abnormal Q waves. Serial ECGs increase the sensitivity of the electrocardiogram for the diagnosis of AMI.

The evolution of a Q-wave myocardial infarction can be separated electrocardiographically into four phases: (1) hyperacute, (2) acute, (3) subacute, and (4) chronic stabilized. In the hyperacute phase, which is usually the earliest ECG manifestation of an acute infarction, straightening of the normal upward concavity of the ST-T segment occurs. With further evolution (acute phase), the straightened ST-T segment becomes elevated. The ST-T segment usually slopes upward since the portion of the ST-T nearest the T wave is more

elevated than the proximal portion. The amplitude of
the T wave usually is increased also. The ST-T wave
depression in leads oriented towards the presumably
noninfarcting myocardium was traditionally termed a
reciprocal change. Recent data indicate that such
ST-T wave depressions usually reflect more extensive
infarction. In the subacute phase, the abnormal Q
wave representing myocardial necrosis begins to appear, but the T-wave vector still points toward the infarct zone. In the fully evolved phase, the ST-T segment
begins to diminish in amplitude and becomes coved or
convexed upward. The ST segment blends into the now
symmetrically inverted T waves. The abnormal Q
waves (greater than .03 seconds in duration and more
than 30% of the R wave amplitude) appear during this
stage. During the chronic phase, generally there is resolution of the ST-T wave changes, with the only residual change being the abnormal Q wave.

Reciprocal changes are defined as horizontal or down-
sloping ST-segment depressions in leads opposite to
ST-segment elevation in patients with AMI. The multiple causes of reciprocal changes include: (1) ECG phenomena caused by displacement of the injury current
vector away from the noninfarcted myocardium, (2) coexisting distant ischemia, or (3) manifestation of infarct
extension. Table 9-2 summarizes the ECG patterns for
acute myocardial infarction by location in the reflecting
leads.

The false positive rate for ST elevation that is greater
than or equal to 1 mm in the diagnosis of AMI on the
initial ECG is 12%–15%. There are other cardiac and
noncardiac conditions that may present with ST-
segment elevation and/or T-wave inversion. These entities are summarized in Table 9-3.

AMI patients may present 3%–4% of the time with
an ECG that is normal or has minimal nonspecific
changes. These patients had an associated mortality of
6%, versus 12% in patients with ECG evidence of AMI.
A study of 1900 patients with AMI revealed that 80%
of AMI patients demonstrated Q waves, new ST-
segment abnormalities, or T-wave inversion; 10% had

**Table 9-2. ECG patterns of various
myocardial infarction locations**

Location	Leads	ECG finding
Anterior	V1–4	ST elevation
Inferior	II, III, avf	ST elevation
Lateral	I, avl, V5–6	ST elevation
Posterior	V1–3	ST depression
	V8–9	ST elevation
Right ventricular	V4R	ST elevation

**Table 9-3. Causes of ST-segment deviation
and/or T-wave inversion**

Condition	Effect
Myocarditis	ST-segment and T-wave changes
Pericarditis	ST elevation
Hemorrhagic stroke	T-wave inversion
Ventricular aneurysm	ST-segment elevation
Pregnancy	Precordial T-wave inversion
Benign early repolarization	ST-segment elevation
Hyperkalemia	ST-segment elevation
Left bundle-branch block	ST-segment elevation
Hypothermia	ST-segment elevation

left bundle-branch block or a paced rhythm; and the final 10% had a normal ECG or only minimal nonspecific changes.

The initiating events in the pathogenesis of Q wave and non-Q-wave infarction are thought to be identical. There is evidence to indicate that in non-Q-wave infarction, early spontaneous reperfusion occurs. Table 9-4 summarizes differences between patients with Q-wave and non-Q-wave myocardial infarctions.

Determining the anatomical location of AMI requires an understanding of the location of the ECG electrodes in relation to the orientation of the heart. The anatomical location of an AMI can be used to estimate the amount of myocardium in the infarct zone. In general, patients with anterior MI have a greater amount of jeopardized myocardium than the patients

**Table 9-4. Comparison of Q-wave and
non-Q-wave myocardial infarction**

Characteristic	Q-wave MI	Non-Q-wave MI
Prevalence	47%	53%
ST-T segment elevation	80%	25%
ST-T segment depression	20%	75%
Postinfarction angina	15%–25%	30%–40%
Incidence of early reinfarction	5%–8%	15%–25%
Mortality		
1 month	10%–15%	3%–5%
2 years	30%	30%
Infarct size	Moderate to large	Small
Residual ischemia	10%–20%	40%–50%
Acute complications	Common	Uncommon

with inferior AMI. The greater the amount of myocardium at jeopardy, the higher the morbidity and mortality.

2. **Anterior wall myocardial infarction.** The left anterior descending artery supplies the anterior and anterior-lateral wall of the left ventricle and two-thirds of the intraventricular septum. Anterior wall myocardial infarction ECG diagnosis is made utilizing leads V1–4. When I, avl, V5, or V6 demonstrate ST-segment elevation, the infarct has extended to the lateral wall (anterior lateral wall myocardial infarction). Preexisting right bundle-branch block or left bundle-branch block may make the diagnosis of myocardial infarction more difficult. Figure 9-1 illustrates a 12-lead ECG diagnostic for acute anterior myocardial infarction. Reciprocal changes are found in 37% of patients with anterior AMI. The presence of reciprocal changes in anterior MI has been associated with more extensive myocardial necrosis, a higher incidence of multivessel disease, and lower ejection fractions.

3. **Lateral wall myocardial infarction.** The lateral wall is supplied by the left circumflex, LAD, or a branch of the right coronary artery (RCA). Isolated lateral wall infarctions are not as common as lateral wall infarction associated with anterior or inferior wall myocardial infarction (Fig. 9-2).

4. **Inferior wall myocardial infarction.** The right coronary artery supplies the inferior wall of the left ventricle and the atrioventricular (AV) node in 90% of patients. Inferior wall myocardial infarction is characterized by ST elevation in at least two of the inferior leads (II, III, and avf). Figure 9-2 illustrates the classic changes in inferior wall AMI.

Patients with inferior wall myocardial infarction associated with reciprocal changes in the anterior precordium, lateral wall extension (V5 and V6), or right ventricular infarction are at increased risk for high-degree AV block and have a 23%–29% in-hospital mortality rate. All patients with suspected inferior or lateral AMI should have lead VR4 included in their ECG to detect a right ventricular infarction (see Chap. 5). Reciprocal changes are most common in patients with inferior wall MIs and have been found in 72% of such patients. These patients generally have larger MIs, lower ventricular rejection fractions, and higher mortality rates than patients with inferior wall myocardial infarction without reciprocal changes.

Although only 8% of inferior wall myocardial infarctions will present with high-degree AV block in the emergency department, 66% will develop AV block within 24 hours of admission.

5. **Posterior wall myocardial infarction.** Posterior wall myocardial infarction occurs most commonly in association with inferior or lateral wall myocardial infarction. The ECG demonstrates an increase in voltage of the R waves in the right to mid-precordial leads

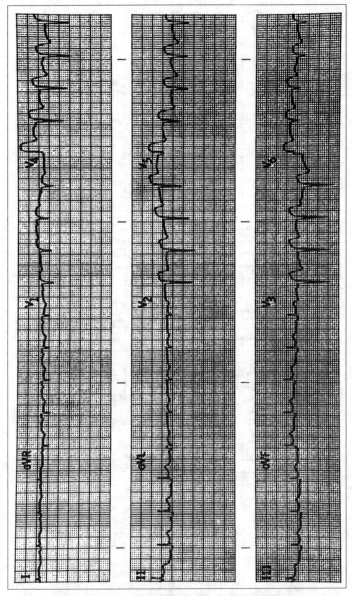

Fig. 9-1. Anterior wall myocardial infarction. Q waves in all precordial leads (V1–6) with ST-segment elevation and T wave inversion. (From Chung E. *Electrocardiography*. Norwalk, CT: Appleton & Lange, 1988.)

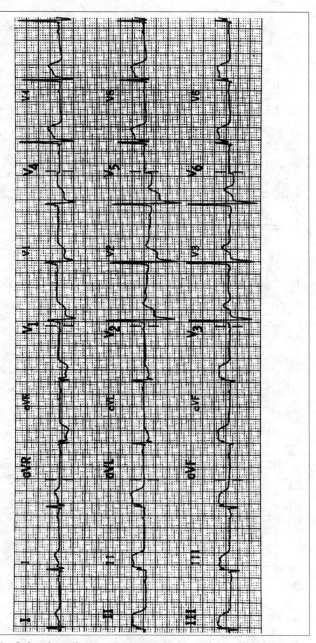

Fig. 9-2.   Infero-lateral-posterior myocardial infarction. ST-segment elevation in leads II, III, avf, and V4–6 indicate inferior and lateral wall involvement. The tall R wave in V1 with marked ST depression in leads V1 and V2 are indicative of posterior wall myocardial infarction. (From Chung E. *Electrocardiography.* **Norwalk, CT: Appleton & Lange, 1988.)**

with an R wave greater than or equal to 0.04 seconds in V1 and an RS ratio greater than or equal to 1 in V2. Horizontal ST-segment depression with upright precordial T waves in leads V1–3 are typical with posterior wall myocardial infarction (see Fig. 9-2). It has been suggested that ST elevation in V8 and V9 (see 12-lead ECG in Fig. 9-2) increases the sensitivity of the ECG for posterior wall myocardial infarction.

Posterior myocardial infarction occurs in the posterior left ventricular wall. Isolated true posterior infarction is quite uncommon. The ECG changes of a true posterior infarction are seen as mirror-image representations in leads V1–3. It is helpful to turn the ECG upside down and look at it from the back while holding it up to a strong light. The changes in leads V1 and V2, which might be overlooked at a quick glance, are seen as abnormal Q waves, ST elevation, and T-wave inversion when viewed from this perspective.

6. **Non-Q-wave myocardial infarction.** Symmetrical convex downward ST-segment depression or inverted or biphasic T waves are characteristically seen in a non-Q-wave infarction. There are significant prognostic differences between Q-wave and non-Q-wave myocardial infarctions (see Table 9-4). Other causes of T-wave inversion are juvenile T-wave patterns, left ventricular hypertrophy (LVH), acute myocarditis, Wolff-Parkinson-White (WPW) syndrome, acute pulmonary embolus, and cerebrovascular accident.

B. **ECG and historical risk stratification.** Studies have shown that patients admitted to "rule out" myocardial infarction with ECGs that demonstrate evidence of infarction, ischemia or strain, LVH, left bundle-branch block, or paced rhythm are at a higher risk for life-threatening complications (ventricular fibrillation, sustained ventricular tachycardia, heart block), compared to the same patients with normal ECGs (14% vs. 0.6%). The combination of three clinical variables—(1) sharp or stabbing pain, (2) no history of angina or myocardial infarction, and (3) pain that was reproduced by chest wall palpitation or that had a pleuritic or positional component—identified a low-risk group (0 out of 48 patients had a diagnosis of MI, unstable angina (UA), or angina (A)). Currently, the history, physical examination, and initial ECG can yield sensitivity of 95%–100% with an associated clinical specificity of 40%–50%.

C. **Novel ECG analyses**

1. **15-lead ECG.** Other diagnostic strategies have been investigated to improve clinical sensitivity and specificity for detecting acute ischemic coronary syndromes. Fifteen-lead ECGs have resulted in an 11.7% increase in sensitivity with no loss of specificity utilizing leads V4R, V8, and V9. Lead V4R was placed on the right anterior chest opposite to the corresponding left chest lead of V4. The posterior leads were placed at the level of the anterior fifth intercostal space, with lead V8 in the midscapular line and V9 at the medial border of the scapular. The 15-lead ECG may assist the clinician in more

accurately assessing acute inferior MIs by identifying posterior wall or right ventricular wall involvement. Utilization of the 15-lead ECG would be most appropriate when the standard 12-lead ECG demonstrates one of the following: (1) ST-segment depression in leads V1–3 or isoelectric segments in leads V1–3; (2) borderline ST-segment elevation in leads V5 and V6 or in leads 2, 3, and avf; (3) ST-segment elevation in leads 2, 3, and avf; or (4) isolated ST-segment elevation in V1 or ST-segment elevation in lead V1 greater than that seen in lead V2.

2. **22-lead ECG.** The 22-lead ECG utilizes ten additional leads in addition to those of the standard 12-lead ECG. These additional unipolar leads are distributed at specific locations on the anterior and posterior thorax and measure deviations in myocardial conduction velocity that may be associated with clinically significant coronary artery disease. Early studies evaluating 22-lead ECGs demonstrate a sensitivity for early AMI detection comparable to the sensitivity of the CK-MB sampling at three hours after presentation. When combined with clinical judgment, the 22-lead ECG could provide a 97.6% sensitivity for AMI diagnosis while possibly reducing unnecessary admissions for "rule-out" AMI by 69%. The negative predictive value of the 22-lead ECG was 89%, compared to 79% for the 12-lead ECG. Further study of this modality should elucidate the future role of 22-lead ECGs in the workup of acute myocardial infarction.

3. **Serial 12-lead ECG.** It has been demonstrated that serial ECGs at 0 hours and 3 hours after patient presentation increase the sensitivity of the ECG from 39% to 68%. Minor ECG changes indicative of ischemia may prompt the clinician to admit a patient with evolving AMI who otherwise would have been released.

4. **Continuous 12-lead ECG monitoring.** Transient elevation or depression of ST-segments without chest discomfort may identify high-risk patients who otherwise would have been released from the emergency department. This modality detects silent ischemia and identifies patient subgroups at risk for AMI, showing promise in the workup of patients who are in emergency departments for chest pain.

D. **Seriologic and biochemical markers of myocardial infarction**

1. **CK-MB.** A characteristic rise and fall of both total creatine kinase (CK) and its cardiac isoenzyme CK-MB is the standard enzymatic component for diagnosis of myocardial infarction. Within 4–8 hours of myocardial cell necrosis, CK-MB becomes elevated in the serum, peaks in 12–20 hours after the onset of cell necrosis, and returns to baseline in 36–48 hours. Initial determinations of CK-MB in patients presenting to the emergency department have a low sensitivity (30%–40%) for AMI. The use of a single or "spot" CK-MB to exclude pa-

tients having AMI is unreliable and discouraged. Initial determinations of CK-MB can neither reliably diagnose nor exclude AMI. Current immunochemical methods for measuring CK-MB require only ten minutes to perform, are automated, and are available to the emergency physician. Serial CK-MB sampling over a period of three hours in the emergency department can achieve sensitivities and specificities greater than 90% using this immunochemical methodology. A positive CK-MB in a patient with a nondiagnostic ECG may alert the clinician to the possibility that the patient is having a myocardial infarction and has been associated with a higher risk of complications during hospitalization.

Traditional sampling for CK-MB occurs at 0, 8, and 16 hours after patient presentation and may include a fourth specimen at 24 hours. False-positive elevations for CK-MB may occur in patients with muscular dystrophy, renal failure, rabdomyolosis, prostate surgery, or Cesarean section and after strenuous athletic activity. The criteria for positive CK-MB are summarized in Table 9-5.

2. **Myoglobin**. As a result of its relatively small molecular weight (17,000, compared to 82,000 for CK-MB), myoglobin is released earlier in the setting of myocardial necrosis. Myoglobin levels become elevated within 1–3 hours of symptom onset and peak within 4–6 hours after the onset of cell necrosis. As a result, myoglobin has a sensitivity of 45% (versus 15% for CK-MB) for AMI patients presenting within 3 hours of symptom onset. Because of the rapid rise and clearance of myoglobin, two myoglobin determinations, at the time of presentation and one hour later, improved sensitivity to 91% (versus 41% for CK-MB), with a specificity of 96% and a negative predictive value of 99% for AMI. This study defined a positive test as a single value greater than or equal to 110 ng/ml or a difference of greater than or equal to 40 ng/ml between hourly specimens. The use of several myoglobins may reduce the number of non-AMI rule-out admissions to the CCU. Rapid immunochemical technologies are available for

Table 9-5. Summary of criteria for a positive CK-MB in diagnosing acute myocardial infarction

Serial increase then decrease of CK-MB with a >25% change between any two values.

CK-MB >9–13 U/liter and >2–5% total CK activity (the actual cutoffs vary by institution).

Increase in CK-MB activity >50% between any two samples, separated by at least 4 hours.

If only a single sample available, CK-MB elevation greater than two-fold.

myoglobin with an assay turn-around time of seven minutes.

Carbonic anhydrase is an enzyme specific to skeletal muscle and is released in conjunction with myoglobin during skeletal muscle damage. Carbonic anhydrase III is not known to exist in detectable quantities in myocardial tissue. Simultaneous determination of myoglobin and carbonic anhydrase III levels results in a sensitivity of 45% for the myoglobin and carbonic anhydrase III combination (versus that of 15%–20% for CK-MB) within three hours of symptom onset with comparable specificity (98.9% for myoglobin plus carbonic anhydrase, compared with 100% for CK-MB). False-positive results with serum myoglobin may be found in patients with renal failure and skeletal muscle disease.

3. **Cardiac troponin T.** Troponin T has a molecular weight of 39,000 daltons and is one of three proteins found in the contractile apparatus of the myocardial cell. Cardiac troponin T becomes elevated in the serum within 6–8 hours, peaks at 12–18 hours, and remains elevated for 3–7 days. One study demonstrated the sensitivity of troponin T for AMI to be 99% at 12–24 hours, versus 87% for CK-MB. In this same study, the specificity of troponin T was 46%, versus 79% for CK-MB. In another study, 56% of patients with unstable angina had elevated cardiac troponin T. Other investigators found troponin T elevated in 39% of patients with unstable angina, and those patients with an elevated troponin T experienced a higher incidence of in-hospital complications.

4. **Cardiac troponin I.** Troponin I, with a molecular weight of 23,000 daltons, slightly precedes the release of CK-MB into the serum and remains elevated for 3–10 days. Troponin I has been demonstrated to have sensitivities at least equal to CK-MB and to be perhaps the most specific of all of the cardiac markers. Troponin I is not elevated in patients with skeletal muscle injury, chronic skeletal muscle disease, or chronic renal failure or in marathon runners. As a result of troponin I's high sensitivity and superior specificity to other cardiac markers, it has been shown to be useful in diagnosing intra- and perioperative acute myocardial infarction.

5. **CK-MB isoforms.** Two isoforms of CK-MB have been identified: CK-MB2 and CK-MB1. CK-MB is released from the myocardium in the form of CK-MB2 during myocardial cell necrosis. Upon appearance in the serum, a serum decarboxylase enzyme clears the terminal lysine from the MB2 molecule, creating a relatively more negative molecule that is identified electrophoretically as CK-MB1. CK-MB isoforms have a 92% sensitivity for AMI within 4–6 hours after symptom onset and 100% sensitivity for AMI within 6–8 hours of symptom onset.

6. **Myosin light chains.** Myosin light chains are released within 3 hours of myocardial cell necrosis, peak at 24–48 hours, and may remain elevated for 6–12 days. Recent studies have demonstrated that myosin light chains are more sensitive than CK-MB in the early hours of myocardial cell necrosis (within 0–4 hours after symptom onset) but lack the specificity of CK-MB.

E. **Echocardiogram.** Myocardial ischemia and infarction result in regional wall abnormalities that can be demonstrated by two-dimensional (2-D) echocardiography. Echocardiograms have a 94% sensitivity in detecting regional wall motion abnormalities in patients presenting to the coronary care unit within twelve hours after onset of symptoms for AMI. Two-dimensional echocardiography identifies regional wall motion abnormalities that characterize most transmural infarctions and some non-Q-wave infarctions. In one study patients without known coronary artery disease or infarct were evaluated by 2-D echocardiography. Two-dimensional echocardiography diagnosed acute myocardial ischemia with a sensitivity of 88% and specificity of 78%. Two-dimensional echocardiography is a useful tool for diagnosing acute myocardial ischemia among patients with nondiagnostic chest pain. The clinical utility of 2-D echocardiography is limited in patients with preexisting regional wall motion abnormalities. Echocardiography can detect left ventricular thrombi, which are present in up to 40% of patients with anterior wall MI. Echocardiography also can evaluate abnormalities of the valves, septum, ventricular walls, and the pericardium.

F. **Nuclear medicine studies.** The use of technetium 99m–labeled red blood cells for blood pool labeling is very helpful in assessing ejection fraction and regional wall motion abnormalities in both the left and right ventricles. Evaluation of ejection fraction and regional wall motion abnormalities is essential in establishing a prognosis for myocardial infarction patients. Thallium scintography both detects reperfusion defects in both the right and left ventricles and outlines the septum. Areas of decreased thallium uptake indicate ischemic or infarcted areas of the myocardium. Thallium scanning does not distinguish between new and old infarcts and is less accurate than serum enzyme analysis in detecting acute necrosis.

Technetium 99m sestamibi (Tc-99m hexakis 2-methoxy-2-isobutyl isonitril) shows considerable promise as an agent for estimating both area at risk and the actual necrotic zone in AMI patients. This agent is taken up by the myocardium in proportion to blood flow and demonstrates minimal redistribution. Technetium 99m sestamibi tomographic imaging currently is being evaluated in patients presenting to the emergency department with suspected acute ischemic coronary syndromes. Resting sestamibi scans appear promising as an adjunct in the emergency department diagnosis of chest pain patients.

G. **MRI.** MRI is being explored extensively for both assessment of infarct size and estimation of coronary blood flow in patients with myocardial infarction. It may be able to differentiate noninfarcted viable ischemic myocardium from the infarcted areas and ultimately assess myocardial perfusion. It also offers improvement over present techniques for assessing wall thickness and making overall estimates of chamber size. It remains to be seen what role, if any, MRI will play in the routine assessment of AMI patients.

H. Clinical algorithms. Computer algorithms with a sensitivity of 88% for AMI detection are essentially equal to the clinician's impression. However, specificity was signficantly better using the algorithm and would have reduced CCU admissions by 11.5% in patients without AMI (while admitting the same number of patients with AMI). Following the clinical algorithm, patients without enzymatic evidence of infarction or recurrent ischemic chest pain during the first 12 hours after admission experienced a 0.5% incidence of acute myocardial infarction. This clinical algorithm utilized clinical characteristics of each patient's history and physical examination in conjunction with enzymatic and ECG data. The investigators were able to identify a large subgroup of patients with whom a 12-hour period of observation was considered sufficient to exclude acute myocardial infarction.

I. Time-insensitive predicted instrument. Use of multivariate logistical regression analysis has been developed as a predictive instrument to give clinicians an estimate of a patient's likelihood of acute ischemia as well as myocardial infarction. Physicians' diagnostic specificity for acute ischemia increases when the probability value provided by this predictive instrument is available to them. Among patients with a final diagnosis of "not acute ischemia," the number of CCU admissions decreased by 30% without any increase in missed diagnosis of ischemia. The predictive instrument demonstrated a diagnostic sensitivity of 95% for acute ischemia and increased specificity from 73% to 78%. Diagnostic accuracy was therefore increased from 74% to 89% using the predictive instrument.

VI. Clinical pearls

A. A normal ECG does not rule out acute myocardial infarction. About 1% of AMI patients will present with a normal ECG, and 3% will present with ECGs manifesting only nonspecific ST or T wave changes.

B. An accurate and detailed history remains the most sensitive single means of detecting myocardial infarction.

C. Although negative serologic enzymes may reliably rule out myocardial necrosis in the appropriate time interval, other acute ischemic coronary syndromes such as unstable angina and angina are not ruled out by these negative enzymes.

D. Use of antacids, viscous lidocaine preparations, or similar agents should not be used as primary diagnostic aids in patients presenting with chest discomfort. Relief of symptoms after an antacid may represent either a causal relationship or coincidence.

Bibliography

Brogan GX Jr, Friedman S, McCuskey C, et al. Evaluation of a new rapid quantitative immunoassay for serum myoglobin versus CK-MB for ruling out AMI in the emergency department. *Ann Emerg Med* 24:665–671, 1994.

Gibler WB, Lewis LM, Erb RE, et al. Early detection of acute myocardial infarction in patients presenting with chest pain and nondiagnostic ECGs: serial CK-MB sampling in the emergency department. *Ann Emerg Med* 19:1359–1366, 1990.

Hedges JR, et al. Serial ECGs are less accurate than serial CK-MB results for the emergency department diagnosis of MI. *Ann Emerg Med* 21:1445–1450, 1992.

Hoekstra JW, Gibler WB, Levy RC, et al. Emergency department diagnosis of AMI and ischemia: a cost analysis of two diagnostic protocols. *Acad Emerg Med* 1:103–110, 1994.

Lee TH, Juarez G, Cook EF, et al. Ruling out acute myocardial infarction: a prospective multicenter validation of a 12-hour strategy for patients at low risk. *N Engl J Med* 324:1239–1246, 1991.

McCarthy B, Beshansky J, D'Agostino RB, et al. Missed diagnoses of AMI in the emergency department: results from a multicenter study. *Ann Emerg Med* 22:579–582, 1993.

Thrombolytic Therapy in Myocardial Infarction

Erica E. Remer

I. **Epidemiology.** Each year more than one million people in the United States suffer a myocardial infarction, and approximately 500,000 succumb. Over half of the deaths occur suddenly, within 1 hour of onset of the symptoms, and before the possibility of medical intervention. Although 60%–65% of patients with acute myocardial infarction (AMI) are eligible for thrombolytic therapy (TT), only 20%–40% currently receive it. Fewer than 10% are treated within the first hour, frequently because of patient delay in seeking medical attention.

Treatment of AMI has evolved significantly over the past 20 years. Initially, treatment was limited to bedrest and observation. Currently, the goal is to limit the extent of myocardial damage through reperfusion therapy and aggressive management of cardiovascular complications. Multiple studies have unequivocally demonstrated that early TT reduces mortality and morbidity.

II. **Pathophysiology.** Acute coronary artery occlusion is the etiology of almost 90% of AMIs. Typically, thrombus formation at the site of an atheromatous plaque occludes the lumen of the coronary artery. Platelets aggregate and the coagulation cascade is activated, converting fibrinogen to fibrin. The threatened muscle does not die immediately, but necrosis proceeds in progressive wavefronts from endocardium to epicardium over the following 4–6 hours. The mechanism of action of the commonly used thrombolytic agents is conversion of plasminogen to plasmin, which then lyses fibrin and circulating fibrinogen.

The "open artery hypothesis" is that rapid, total, and persistent recanalization produces maximal patient benefit by limiting infarct size and thereby reducing mortality. Reperfusion probably has a dual impact, depending on when therapy is begun in relation to the onset of occlusion. Thrombolytic therapy within 2 hours of symptoms results in myocardial salvage by reperfusion of affected and potentially threatened cardiac muscle. Later effects are related to improved healing, less adverse ventricular remodeling, reduced frequency of ventricular aneurysm, and improved electrophysiologic stability.

III. **Pharmacology.** Three thrombolytic agents are presently FDA-approved and commonly used in the United States. These are discussed below. Unapproved thrombolytics include urokinase, pro-urokinase (saruplase), and double-chain tissue plasminogen activator (duteplase). There are also experimental agents under investigation, such as vampire bat t-PA, novel recombinant-DNA-produced r-PAs like TNK-tPA, and staphylokinase, which may play a role in the future of TT.

   A. **Streptokinase (SK).** Streptokinase is produced by beta-hemolytic streptococci and combines in a 1:1 ratio with plasminogen to form a stable activator complex. It then functions as a catalyst to activate more plasminogen to plasmin. The activator complex has a plasma half-life of 30 minutes and is not specific for the fibrin-bound clot. This results in the depletion of systemic fibrinogen. The major advantage of SK is that it is relatively inexpensive. Disadvantages include lack of specificity, allergenicity, and occasional hypotension. Patients treated with SK are at risk for allergic reactions upon rechallenge with the drug in the future.

B. **Anisoylated plasminogen-SK activator complex (APSAC, anistreplase).** APSAC is an inactive combination of SK and lys-plasminogen. It was designed to be more thrombus-selective than SK. The active component is the same as in SK, but its half-life is 70–100 minutes, allowing bolus administration. It also reduces circulating fibrinogen. APSAC's principal advantages are speed and ease of administration. The cost is intermediary between that of SK and t-PA. Its disadvantages are similar to those of SK, including allergic reactions.

C. **Recombinant tissue plasminogen activator (r-TPA, t-PA, alteplase).** Recombinant tissue plasminogen activator is a DNA-recombinant form of a human protein plasminogen activator that shows an affinity for the plasminogen-fibrin complex. Although theoretically selective, in vivo fibrinogen levels still fall to 30%–40% of pretreatment levels. The half-life is 3–4 minutes. As an endogenous compound, it is not antigenic. It is therefore the drug of choice in the patient with remote reinfarction. Its drawbacks are a complicated dosing regimen, the need for concomitant heparin administration, and expense.

IV. **Conclusions from clinical trials**

A. **Which agent is best?** Many international clinical trials have demonstrated statistically significant reductions in mortality when TT is compared with placebo. However, there is no clear frontrunner thrombolytic agent. Accelerated t-PA dosing provides improved early patency, but SK and APSAC "catch up" within 2–3 hours and may be associated with less reocclusion of the infarct-related artery. There may be a slightly higher risk of hemorrhagic stroke with t-PA compared with SK, but the frequency of confirmed hemorrhagic cerebrovascular accident appears to be similar. Major bleeding complications are more common with SK (0.9% vs. 0.6% for t-PA), but this does not seem to increase mortality.

B. **Injury site.** Patients with elevated ST segments, which are consistent with transmural AMI, benefit from TT regardless of site of injury. The maximal advantage is seen in anterior infarctions (37 lives saved per 1000 patients treated), but inferior AMIs benefit as well (8 lives saved per 1000 patients treated). In patients with left bundle-branch blocks (LBBBs) where the likely site of infarction cannot be ascertained, the mortality rate is still much lower (49 lives saved per 1000 patients treated) in treated patients versus controls. This strongly suggests that patients with LBBBs should be considered candidates for thrombolysis.

C. **When should TT be administered?** Most myocardial damage occurs in the first 1–2 hours of symptoms, and maximal benefit is seen in this group presenting for early treatment. Patients presenting within the first hour of symptoms can be spared from most myocardial damage. Clear benefit from TT has been documented up to 12 hours after symptom onset in the EMERAS (Estudio Multicéntrico Estreptoquinas Repúblicas de América del Sur Collective Group) and LATE (Late Assessment of Thrombolytic Efficacy) studies. Administering TT beyond 12 hours may be beneficial in some patients with stuttering symptoms, but its use is controversial. There may be islands of viable tissue that can still be salvaged, and late reperfusion may also affect electrical stability. Dilatation of the left ventricle and aneurysm formation may be prevented. Finally, if a vessel is recanalized, it may provide collateral blood flow to areas that can become compromised in the future. Although the window of opportunity for the benefits of TT may be wider than once thought, the sooner TT is instituted, the better the results.

D. **Patient factors**
   1. **Gender.** Women with AMI tend to be treated less aggressively than men and are misdiagnosed more often. However, when treated with thrombolytics, the absolute effects on mortality are similar to those of men.
   2. **Age.** Historically, trials have excluded patients over 70–75 years of age. The elderly are more apt to have hypertension, diabetes, prior strokes, and the general physiologic effects of aging. These factors render them more likely to have bleeding complications, including intracerebral hemorrhage. The elderly also have an increased risk of dying from an AMI. The Fribrinolytic Therapy Trialists' (FTT) collaborative group evaluated data from multiple studies and found that the absolute mortality reductions were similar irrespective of age. The physician should not use age as the primary determinant of whether to use TT, but should consider physiologic factors on an individual basis.
   3. **Vital signs.** Cardiogenic shock is the major complication of AMI and imparts up to an 80% mortality without reperfusion. Current recommendations suggest that primary PTCA should be used in these patients; however, the FTT results suggest that TT may be effective when PTCA is not available. Patients with systolic BP under 100 mm Hg were at high risk of death, and these patients benefited significantly from TT (60 lives saved per 1000 patients). Patients with tachycardia also derived benefits from thrombolysis, and those with the combination of low blood pressure and heart rate greater than 100 demonstrated the maximal reduction in mortality (73 lives saved per 1000 patients treated).

   Controlled chronic hypertension is not automatically a contraindication to TT. In contrast, a persistent BP greater than 200/120 mm Hg is considered an absolute contraindication to TT. The approach should be to lower the elevated BP with appropriate medical management and then to treat the AMI patient with TT.

V. Indications for thrombolytic therapy (Fig. 10-1)
   A. Patient selection. The decision to administer TT is based on an individual assessment of the risk-benefit ratio. The absence of contraindications should be explored and clearly documented. Acute ischemia without an injury pattern on the ECG is not an indication for thrombolytics.
   B. Eligibility criteria (Table 10-1). Approximately half of patients are missed on ECG criteria because their initial

Fig. 10-1.   Thrombolytics in AMI algorithm.

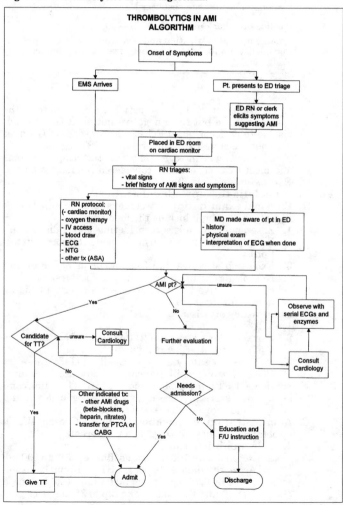

**Table 10-1.   Eligibility criteria
for thrombolytic therapy**

Clinical

Chest pain or equivalent consistent with AMI

  Lasting <20–30 min and ≤12 hr

  Unrelieved by nitroglycerin

with:

ECG (any of the following)

≥1-mm ST elevation in ≥ contiguous limb leads

≥2-mm ST elevation in ≥2 contiguous precordial leads

New bundle-branch block

Evidence of acute true posterior MI

Cardiogenic shock in AMI

Emergency catheterization and revascularization, if possible. Consider thrombolysis if catheterization not immediately available.

ECGs are negative. In those patients who seem to fit the clinical criteria but have negative initial ECGs, it is advisable to perform serial ECGs. The presence of Q waves does not preclude TT in the presence of ST-segment elevation. Patients who have prolonged or stuttering symptoms and meet ECG criteria are considered candidates for TT.

  C. **Exclusion criteria** (Table 10-2)

VI. **Thrombolytic therapy administration**

  A. **Physical examination.** Careful examination prior to administration should include the following:
    1. Assessment of pulses (considering aortic dissection).
    2. Blood pressure in both arms (considering aortic dissection).
    3. Exclusion of pericardial friction rub or new murmur.
    4. Neurologic examination to rule out focal lesion.
    5. Signs of active bleeding or recent surgery (including hemocculting stool).

  B. **Laboratory studies**
    1. ECG.
    2. Portable chest x-ray (CXR) (for signs of aortic dissection or congestive heart failure).
    3. Routine laboratory studies usually include those for CBC, electrolytes, BUN/creatinine, glucose, liver function, PT/PTT, myoglobin, and CK-MB. If bleeding complications are a concern, draw fibrinogen levels and type and screen (or cross, as indicated).

  C. **Administration of thrombolytic agent.** Consent should be obtained (in most settings it can be verbal).
    1. **t-PA administration**
      a. Reconstitute 100 mg with saline or D5W to 100 ml.
      b. Accelerated dose (as per GUSTO): 15-mg bolus followed by 0.75 mg/kg over 30 minutes (not to exceed 50 mg) and then 0.5 mg/kg (up to 35 mg) over next

Table 10-2. Exclusion criteria

Absolute contraindications

Altered consciousness

Aortic dissection, proven or suspected

Known bleeding disorder

Head trauma of recent onset

Hemorrhagic cardiovascular accident (CVA) in past

Active internal bleeding

Intracranial or intraspinal surgery within previous 2 months

Pregnancy

Spinal cord or cerebral arteriovenous malformation or tumor

Trauma or surgery within previous 2 weeks that could result in bleeding into a closed space

Uncontrolled hypertension of >200/120 mm Hg

Relative contraindications

Chronic, uncontrolled hypertension (diastolic BP >100 mm Hg), treated or untreated

CPR (prolonged or traumatic)

Any hemorrhagic retinopathy

Ischemic or embolic CVAs in past

Major trauma or surgery, >2 weeks and <2 months previously

Oral anticoagulation, therapeutic

Active peptic ulcer disease, or heme-positive stools

Acute pericarditis, infective endocarditis, intracardiac thrombus

Subclavian or internal jugular cannulation

Previous allergic reaction to SK or APSAC (or prior use within 1 yr)—should use t-PA

---

60 minutes. Maximal dosage is 100 mg for patients who weigh more than 65 kg.

2. **Streptokinase administration**
   a. May premedicate with hydrocortisone 100 mg IV and diphenhydramine 25–50 mg IV.
   b. Reconstitute 1.5 million units with bacteriostatic water. The vial should not be shaken because foaming denatures the drug. Dilute in 100–250 ml D5W.
   c. Infuse 1.5 million units over 60 minutes.

3. **APSAC administration**
   a. May premedicate as for streptokinase.
   b. Reconstitute 30 units with 5 ml bacteriostatic water. The vial should be gently rolled to avoid foaming. It must be used within 30 minutes of reconstitution.
   c. Inject 30 units over 2–5 minutes.

D. **General management** (Table 10-3)

E. **Conjunctive therapies**
   1. **Anticoagulation.** Intravenous heparin is important in maintaining patency following t-PA. A commonly

Table 10-3.   General management of patients receiving thrombolytics

Perform	Cautions
Continuous cardiac monitoring	No arterial punctures or excessive venipuncture unless absolutely necessary
Supplemental oxygen	
2 peripheral IV lines (18-gauge, if possible) in same arm	
3-way heplock in opposite arm for blood draws	Avoid central lines in noncompressible sites
Aspirin, unless allergic	Avoid intramuscular injections
Nitroglycerin, morphine, etc. as indicated	Avoid nasogastric or nasotracheal intubation
Monitor labs: CBC, CPKs, PTT, and, as needed, fibrinogen	Minimize patient handling
	Expect dysrhythmias (routine lidocaine drips are no longer used)
Repeat ECG after infusion is complete and every 6–8 hours	
Maintain pressure on all puncture sites for 20–30 min	

used dosage for anticoagulation is a 5000-unit bolus and 1000 U/hr for initial maintenance. It should be administered as the t-PA infusion is completed. The PTT should be monitored and the dosing appropriately adjusted. Heparin is not necessary in conjunction with streptokinase or APSAC, even though its use is common in this setting.

2. **Aspirin.** Multiple studies support the use of antiplatelet therapy with TT. Aspirin clearly reduces reocclusion of the infarct-related artery after successful thrombolysis. Administer 160–324 mg of aspirin prior to TT.

3. **Other medications.** Nitrates, morphine, beta-blockers, and other cardiac medications can be used in conjunction with thrombolytic agents as indicated (see Chap. 11).

VII. **Consequences of thrombolytic therapy**
   A. **Analysis of reperfusion**
      1. **Coronary artery catheterization.** One of the major problems of thrombolytic therapy is that there is no reliable bedside method for identifying the establishment of infarct-related artery patency and reperfusion. The gold standard is cardiac catheterization, which, because of its invasiveness, has inherent risks. Institutions with the capability to perform immediate angiography often bypass thrombolytics and perform emergent angioplasty on patients with impending or evolving AMI (see Chap. 12). Another drawback to angiography is that it is performed at a specific time point and cannot be used to monitor the dynamic process in the period following thrombolysis.
      2. **ECG.** The success of TT is usually measured by ECG ST-segment normalization and monitoring of serial car-

diac enzymes. The triad of rapid relief of pain, ST-segment normalization, and the appearance of an idioventricular rhythm is highly specific but not sensitive to detecting reperfusion. Continuous ST-segment monitoring with vector analysis is sensitive and specific. It may ultimately be the standard of care for following the patient's response and recuperation, but it is not yet widely available.

3. **Enzyme studies.** An early peak of CPK can be suggestive of reperfusion, but the time delay of laboratory results makes this sign less useful. Early peaking of myoglobin may prove helpful but is not universally available or effectively concurrent.

4. **Other studies.** Echocardiography may demonstrate hypokinesis and assist in the diagnosis of AMI, but resolution of wall motion abnormalities lags behind reperfusion.

   Some nuclear medicine studies (thallium, technetium) can demonstrate changes with reperfusion, but baseline imaging is necessitated and portable studies are not practical. MRI or MRA is promising but is not applicable in the coronary intensive care unit setting.

B. **Complications of TT**
   1. **Bleeding.** Most bleeding complications are at venous access sites and do not require transfusions. Gastrointestinal, genitourinary, and retroperitoneal bleeding can result in higher blood loss. Bleeding complications necessitating transfusion occur in 8%–11% of patients receiving TT.
   2. **Strokes.** AMI is complicated by stroke in 1%–3% of patients. TT has decreased the frequency of thrombotic and embolic events but has increased the number of intracranial hemorrhages. The incidence is approximately 1%. Risk factors include advanced age, low body weight, and hypertension. Prior cerebrovascular accidents also increase the risk, as does the use of oral anticoagulants.
   3. **Allergic reactions.** Approximately 5% of patients receiving streptokinase derivatives are prone to allergic reactions. Symptoms are usually mild, like pruritus, rash, or fever, and are easily managed with antihistamines and antipyretics. Anaphylaxis is rare, occurring in approximately 0.1% of treated patients. If there has been a recent culture-proven streptococcal infection or streptokinase therapy within the prior year, t-PA should be administered rather than SK or APSAC.
   4. **Hypotension.** This complication is seen in 10%–15% of patients receiving SK and is believed to be due to vasodilation. The infusion of thrombolytic should be slowed, and intravenous volume repletion can be accomplished with isotonic fluids.

VIII. **Impediments to TT**
   A. **Prehospital delays.** Many patients delay seeking treatment for AMI. The impact emergency physicians can have on prehospital delay is twofold. First, the public should be

educated on signs and symptoms of AMI and encouraged
to seek treatment early. Second, it is likely that prehospital diagnosis of AMI will be possible in the future. TT or
preparations for such treatment may then be started in
the field by emergency personnel.

B. Hospital delays

1. **"The four Ds."** The National Heart Attack Alert Program (NHAAP) coordinating committee identified four
   time points in the treatment of AMI. These times ("the
   four Ds") are patient arrival at the emergency department (door), ECG performance (data), the decision to
   administer TT (decision), and infusion of the medication (drug). These define the time intervals on which
   the hospital phase of treatment can be affected: door to
   data, data to decision, and decision to drug.

   a. **Time interval I—door to data.** Triage personnel
      need to be alert to the symptoms of AMI. They need
      to recognize atypical complaints and have a high
      index of suspicion. Patients who may be having an
      AMI must be brought back immediately and regis-
      tered in the emergency department (ED). If a
      stretcher is not available, the department needs to
      be rearranged to accommodate the patient.

      Another opportunity for improvement is in the
      prompt obtaining of an ECG. Most EDs have a pro-
      tocol that allows nursing personnel to order an
      ECG prior to physician contact. ECG capability
      should reside in the ED; the necessity for paging
      an ECG technician to the ED can greatly delay the
      workup.

   b. **Time interval II—data to decision.** The staff
      need to be aware that possible AMI patients are a
      top priority. The ECG analysis is of paramount im-
      portance. Computerized analysis or nursing educa-
      tion to recognize significant ECG patterns may be
      helpful in alerting the nursing personnel to notify
      the physician earlier. Access to previous ECGs is
      very helpful.

      The decision to administer thrombolytics should
      rest with the emergency physician. Requiring a
      cardiology consult on average adds 15 minutes to
      the process. A thrombolytic therapy protocol is very
      useful to expedite and facilitate the administration
      of TT. A checklist of contraindications should be in-
      cluded in the protocol packet.

   c. **Time interval III—decision to drug.** The facts
      that the patient needs in order to give informed
      consent should be available in the thrombolytic
      protocol so that consent may be readily obtained.
      TT should be performed in the ED; delay until the
      patient is transported to the critical care unit
      (CCU) is unacceptable.

      TT should not be delayed for other medications,
      although it is reasonable to try sublingual nitro-
      glycerin to ensure that the event is truly injury
      and not ischemia. The major delay at this time

point is in the preparation and receipt of the reconstituted medication. Having the thrombolytic present in the ED expedites its administration. This is especially important if the pharmacy is geographically distant from the ED.

2. **Continuous quality improvement (CQI).** TT is ideal for CQI monitoring. Barriers to prompt administration are identified, changes in the system are made, and objective time measurements are compared. Continuous process reevaluation should be done with the goal of shortening the "door-to-drug" time. The American Heart Association and the NHAAP recommend that this goal should be 30 minutes. Morbidity and mortality from myocardial infarction are clearly affected by TT; it is time that AMI patients are treated with the same sense of urgency as major trauma victims, but the time should be a "golden half-hour" instead of a "golden hour."

Bibliography

Dellborg M, Topol EJ, Swedberg K. Dynamic QRS complex and ST segment vector cardiographic monitoring can identify vessel patency in patients with acute myocardial infarction treated with reperfusion therapy. *Am Heart J* 122:943–948, 1991.

FTT Collaborative Group. Indications for fibrinolytic therapy in suspected acute myocardial infarction: collaborative overview of early mortality and major morbidity results from all randomised trials of more than 1000 patients. *Lancet* 343:311–322, 1994.

Granger CB, Califf RM, Topol EJ. Thrombolytic therapy for acute myocardial infarction. *Drugs* 44:293–325, 1992.

Grines CL. Thrombolytic, antiplatelet, and antithrombotic agents. *Am J Cardiol* 70:18I–25I, 1992.

NHAAPCC, Emergency Department. Rapid identification and treatment of patients with acute myocardial infarction. NIH Publication No. 93-3278, 1993.

Pharmacologic Therapy in Myocardial Infarction

David Reyes

Coronary artery disease is a major health problem in the United States. It is by far the leading cause of death. Even with current preventive efforts, 7 million Americans are diagnosed with coronary artery disease each year, and more than 450,000 persons will die annually from a complication of coronary artery disease. One bright note is the decline of the death rate due to coronary artery disease. Between 1980 and 1991 the age-adjusted death rate for heart disease declined 27% to 148.2 deaths per 100,000 population, continuing the downward trend of the 1970s. Since 1980, the age-adjusted death rate for heart disease declined 29% for white men, 25% for white women, and 17% to 18% for black men and black women. The decline is due, in part, to the pharmacotherapy of acute myocardial infarction (AMI).

This chapter includes a discussion of the nonthrombolytic therapy of AMI, including everything from oxygen to angiotensin converting enzyme (ACE) inhibitors. The typical history and physical findings in AMI, the differential diagnosis of AMI, the diagnostic methods used in patients with AMI, and thrombolytic therapy for AMI are discussed in Chaps. 9 and 10. Angioplasty and mechanical interventions for AMI are discussed in Chap. 12. Antiarrhythmic therapy and therapy for the treatment of complications of AMI are covered in Chaps. 14–19.

I. **AMI patient management.** The typical patient who presents to the emergency department with signs and symptoms that suggest AMI needs to be treated early, aggressively, and expectantly in order to avoid complications.

   A. **Initial evaluation.** Aggressive treatment of AMI begins with securing the airway, breathing, and circulation (ABCs). Ensuring an adequate airway is essential in patients with AMI. Cardiogenic shock and CHF can cause the patient to deteriorate rapidly, due to poor oxygenation, poor ventilation, and increased myocardial ischemia. If a need for intubation is indicated, it should be accomplished early. Oxygen should be administered empirically at a rate that ensures adequate oxygenation via pulse oximetry. Arterial blood gases should be avoided, if possible, until the decision not to give thrombolytic therapy is made.

      Intravenous access should be established early for drug administration. An isotonic solution is preferred in case fluid boluses are needed to maintain preload. Often two IV lines are needed to avoid mixing incompatible drugs.

      Continuous cardiac monitoring should be instituted early to watch for the development of arrhythmias.

   B. **Standard AMI drug therapy.** The patient with chest pain that suggests myocardial ischemia or AMI should receive certain standard therapy, by protocol if needed. This therapy includes:

1. **Oxygen,** 2–4 liter/min by nasal cannula. More is needed if congestive heart failure (CHF) is evident, if the patient is in shock, or if the patient has poor oxygenation by pulse oximetry.
2. **Aspirin,** 160 mg chewed, if the patient is not on aspirin already and is not allergic.
3. **Nitrate therapy,** either sublingual 1/150 g repeated every 5 minutes, topically as 1–2 in. of nitroglycerin paste, or intravenously at 5–100 μg/min titrated to pain or to keep the systolic blood pressure less than 120 mm Hg and greater than 100 mm Hg.
4. **Beta-blocker therapy,** typically with atenolol 5 mg IVP, repeated up to 15 mg, especially for patients with tachycardia or hypertension. Beta-blockers should be avoided in patients with bradycardia, CHF, or heart block.
5. **Symptomatic therapy,** with narcotic therapy for pain relief, anxiolytics for sedation, and antiemetics for nausea.
6. **Other therapies** including heparin, antiarrhythmic therapy, magnesium, ACE inhibitors, or calcium channel blockers should be instituted as indicated by the patient's condition (see discussion below).
7. **Thrombolytic therapy** (see Chap. 10).
8. **Therapy for complications of AMI** (see Chaps. 14–19).

II. **Pharmacotherapy for AMI.** What follows is a listing of the standard therapies available for the treatment of AMI. Each drug's indications, contraindications, therapeutic benefits, and potential complications in the setting of AMI are discussed.

A. **Oxygen**

1. **Indications.** Oxygen therapy is indicated for the treatment of all patients with suspected AMI. Hypoxemia is common in the setting of AMI, especially in patients with underlying lung disease or congestive heart failure. Patients with tachypnea, dyspnea, cyanosis, or shock are especially at risk for tissue hypoxia, and higher administration rates of oxygen are indicated in these patients. Adequate supplemental oxygen should be given to maintain oxygen saturation greater than 95% by pulse-oximetry or arterial blood gases. Administration of 100% oxygen by face mask is the best method to provide maximum hemoglobin saturation, but patients tend to tolerate nasal cannula administration of 2–4 liter/min better, as long as hemoglobin saturation is assured by pulse oximetry.

2. **Contraindications.** In general, there are no absolute or relative contraindications to using oxygen during AMI. However, it should be used with caution in patients with chronic lung disease and CO_2 retention.

3. **Therapeutic benefits.** The goal of pharmacological therapy for AMI is to preserve myocardial tissue. AMI is secondary to a decrease in the flow of oxygenated blood through the coronary arteries. Quite simply, by augmenting the oxygen content of the blood, myocardial ischemia decreases in areas of the myocardium

that are poorly perfused. In the setting of shock or cardiac arrest, peripheral tissue hypoxia occurs due to low blood flow. Administration of oxygen in these patients helps counteract the lactic acidosis produced by anaerobic metabolism.

4. **Complications.** Oxygen therapy can cause CO_2 retention and acidosis in patients with chronic lung disease or chronic obstructive pulmonary disease (COPD). These patients depend on hypoxia more than CO_2 to drive their ventilation. They may become acidotic and apneic if giving them oxygen causes them to lose their ventilatory drive. Administration of high-percentage oxygen for prolonged periods of time is associated with pulmonary fibrosis, but this is rarely a concern in the acute treatment of AMI.

B. Aspirin

1. **Indications.** Aspirin should be given immediately to all patients suspected of having an acute coronary ischemic syndrome. Therapeutic benefits have been documented in both unstable angina and AMI. The Second International Study of Infarct Survival (ISIS-II) recommends a dosage of 160 mg/d, administered immediately at presentation, and daily thereafter. Enteric-coated aspirin should be avoided, since its absorption is delayed. If possible, the aspirin should be chewed and then swallowed for maximal therapeutic benefit.

2. **Contraindications.** Aspirin is contraindicated in those patients with aspirin allergy or hypersensitivity. Because of its antiplatelet properties, any patient with preexisting bleeding disorders (hemophilia, Von Willebrand's, or other platelet dysfunction) or peptic ulcer disease may experience an increased risk of bleeding.

3. **Therapeutic benefits.** Aspirin exerts its action at the platelet level. It blocks thromboxane A_2, which aggregates platelets and constricts arterioles. By inhibiting platelet coagulation activity, aspirin decreases arterial thromboembolism production. In ISIS-II, aspirin alone, when started within 24 hours of the onset of symptoms, reduced by 23% the vascular mortality rate five weeks post AMI. This mortality benefit in AMI was independent of thrombolytic therapy.

   Aspirin also reduces by 49% the incidence of early recurrence of nonfatal reinfarction. A synergistic reaction occurs when aspirin is combined with a thrombolytic agent. In ISIS-II, there was a 42% reduction in mortality when aspirin was combined with streptokinase. Additionally, aspirin decreased the occurrence of nonfatal stroke by 46%.

4. **Complications.** Aspirin, like other anticoagulants, causes an increased risk of bleeding. Gastrointestinal hemorrhage is possible in patients with preexisting gastritis or peptic ulcer disease. Additionally, its irritative effects on the gastrointestinal system may result in simple pyrosis (heartburn), gastritis, or peptic ulcer disease.

C. Nitroglycerin

1. **Indications.** Nitroglycerin (NTG) is indicated in the treatment of suspected ischemic chest pain, unstable angina, or AMI. It can be administered sublingually, transdermally, or intravenously. For precise, minute-to-minute control, continuous IV infusion is preferable. NTG via any route is indicated for ischemic pain relief associated with AMI. Its coronary vasodilatory properties increase collateral blood flow to ischemic myocardium, reducing ischemia and ischemic pain. NTG is indicated for the treatment of pulmonary congestion due to congestive heart failure in the setting of an AMI. It causes venodilation in the pulmonary vessels, thereby reducing preload. NTG is also indicated for the treatment of hypertension associated with AMI. Its peripheral vasodilating properties facilitate afterload reduction.

2. **Contraindications.** Contraindications to NTG stem from its hypotensive effect. Hypotension and hypovolemia are clear contraindications. Once these conditions are reversed, usually with IV fluid boluses or inotropic therapy, NTG therapy can be reinstituted. Because of the NTG effect on preload, it should be used cautiously in patients with right ventricular infarction, which can accompany acute inferior infarction (see Chap. 18). NTG is contraindicated if angina is associated with idiopathic hypertrophic subaortic stenosis (IHSS) or hypertrophic cardiomyopathy (see Chap. 24). The vasodilatory effects of NTG cause a decrease in preload, which the IHSS heart needs to maintain an adequate stroke volume and cardiac output.

   NTG is contraindicated when head trauma is present or at any time when there is increased intracranial pressure; nitroglycerin's vasodilatory effects on the cerebral vessels can exacerbate intracranial hypertension.

3. **Therapeutic benefits.** Nitroglycerin has proven to be very useful in the therapy of AMI. The fundamental problem of poor perfusion to ischemic myocardium is alleviated by NTG in three ways: (1) NTG decreases coronary artery spasms and actually dilates collateral coronary artery vessels; (2) by lowering left ventricular preload, it increases myocardial perfusion pressure, thereby enhancing myocardial blood flow; and (3) because it decreases afterload, it decreases myocardial workload. Thus, not only is there more oxygenated blood available to the heart, but also the heart has to do less work and thus use less oxygen in order to get the oxygenated blood. Ischemia is therefore decreased, and infarct size may be limited. Previous clinical studies reported a 35% reduction in mortality from AMI with NTG use. The Third Gruppo Italiano per lo Studio della Sopravvivenza Nell' Infarcto Miocardico (GISSI-3) trial, however, demonstrated only a 17% decrease in mortality when nitrates were given

with angiotensin converting enzyme (ACE) inhibitors during AMI. Furthermore, in neither the Fourth International Study of Infarct Survival (ISIS-IV) nor GISSI-3 has there been shown an independent effect of NTG on mortality reduction in AMI. In these studies, nitroglycerin's major therapeutic benefits in AMI were shown to be symptom relief and a decrease in pulmonary congestion, not a decrease in mortality. It should be noted, however, that there was no increase in mortality or morbidity with NTG use, so no contraindication to the use of NTG was demonstrated.

4. **Complications.** As NTG dilates the peripheral vasculature, reflex tachycardia may occur, causing an increase in myocardial oxygen demand. This can usually be alleviated by proper volume loading. Transient bradycardia, which is a vagal response to NTG, has also been reported, and is especially common in inferior AMI. The vasodilatory effects of NTG have also caused hypotension, syncope, nausea, clammy skin, and dizziness. In addition, NTG's vasodilatory effects characteristically cause transient flushing of the face. Headache is also a common side effect.

   NTG-induced hypotension may exacerbate myocardial ischemia in the setting of AMI. Hypotension is most common with an inferior infarct with right ventricular involvement (see Chap. 18). These patients are very preload-dependent, and NTG reduces preload. The result is hypotension.

   Complications such as hypotension and myocardial depression are exacerbated with alcohol intoxication. Nitroglycerin may also aggravate hypoxemia by increasing ventilation-perfusion mismatch. If large quantities of NTG are given over a prolonged period of time, methemoglobinemia may occur.

D. **Beta-adrenergic blockers**
   1. **Indications.** Beta-adrenergic blockers are indicated as adjunctive therapy in the treatment of AMI. They are also indicated for treatment of many of the dysrhythmias associated with AMI. These include reflex tachycardia, ventricular tachycardia, recurrent ventricular fibrillation, supraventricular arrhythmia, atrial fibrillation, and atrial flutter. Beta-adrenergic blockers are also indicated following a completed MI. According to the Metroprolol in Acute Myocardial Infarction (MIAMI) study, mortality reduction was greatest in a high-risk subgroup with three or more of the following: (1) history of previous MI, (2) history of previous angina, (3) congestive heart failure, (4) diabetes mellitus, (5) diuretic intake, and (6) digitalis intake.

   2. **Contraindications.** Beta-adrenergic blockers have both absolute and relative contraindications. Beta-blockers should not be used on patients who have bradycardia (<60 bpm), heart block, hypotension (systolic BP < 100 mm Hg), congestive heart failure, or bronchospasm due to COPD or asthma. Given its myo-

cardial depressant properties, it should not be used in patients with low cardiac output, left ventricular dysfunction, or right ventricular failure secondary to pulmonary hypertension. Beta-blockers are contraindicated in patients with AV conduction abnormalities such as first-degree heart block with a PR greater than 0.22, type I and type II second-degree AV block, or complete heart block.

Relative contraindications include a history of asthma, current use of beta-blockers, current use of calcium channel blockers, severe peripheral vascular disease, or brittle insulin-dependent diabetes mellitus.

3. **Therapeutic benefits.** Beta-blockers consistently have demonstrated beneficial effects for patients suffering from AMI. The effects include a decrease in recurrent ischemic chest pain associated with AMI. Beta-blockers, like NTG, decrease myocardial oxygen demand. This is done by reducing the effects of excessive catecholamines on the myocardium. Thus, the heart rate and negative inotropic effects decrease. The long-term effects include a lowered incidence of recurrent ischemic events, cardiac rupture, and nonfatal reinfarction. Its effects on reduction of ventricular dysrhythmias are controversial.

Many studies support beta-blocker benefits. According to the Timolol en Infarcto, Republica, Argentina (TIARA) study, timolol maleate exerts an antiarrhythmic effect by increasing the ventricular fibrillation threshold. Other studies have not confirmed this antiarrhythmic effect. ISIS-I evaluated the effects of atenolol on vascular mortality at one week in patients with transmural AMI. It demonstrated a decreased mortality in patients treated with beta-blockers compared to controls. There was a marked reduction in cardiac rupture, thought secondary to a beta-blocker–induced reduction in myocardial wall stress. The Second Thrombolysis in Myocardial Infarction (TIMI-2) trial investigated the effect of metoprolol on mortality, recurrent ischemia, and reinfarction. Patients treated with IV metoprolol on day 1 had a decrease in recurrent ischemia and reinfarction when compared to patients who received treatment on day 6. Also, if treatment was initiated within 2 hours of AMI, mortality and recurrent MI rates were both decreased. These findings corroborate those of the MIAMI study, which demonstrated a reduction in mortality in patients treated with metoprolol.

4. **Complications.** Cardiac complications from beta-blockers include bradycardia, hypotension, and AV block. Most significantly, beta-blockers decrease myocardial contractility, which potentially can lead to the exacerbation of congestive heart failure. Pulmonary complications include COPD/asthma exacerbation, and bronchoconstriction.

Effects of beta-blockers on the gastrointestinal system may include nausea/vomiting and diarrhea.

Patients have also reported dizziness and fatigue, as well as fluid retention.

E. **Analgesics, antiemetics, and anxiolytics**
  1. **Narcotics**
     a. **Indications.** Morphine is indicated for pain relief in the treatment of AMI. The typical dose is 2–4 mg intravenously titrated to pain relief. Its analgesic and sedative effects provide relief in patients experiencing ischemic chest pain. Moreover, morphine's vasodilator effects have made it an adjunctive therapy for associated pulmonary edema, which may complicate AMI. Meperidine hydrochloride (Demerol) 12.5–50 mg IVP may be more useful than morphine in acute inferior wall myocardial infarction since it has vagolytic effects.
     b. **Contraindications.** Hypersensitivity to morphine sulfate is a contraindication. In the setting of hypovolemia, morphine may cause hypotension secondary to its vasodilatory properties. It should be used with caution or avoided in patients with hypotension. The use of morphine or any narcotics should be avoided in patients with altered mental status. In addition, in patients who are being treated with nitrates, the pain relief response to therapy may be difficult to discern in patients who have been given narcotics. Since morphine is metabolized by the liver, it should be avoided in patients with hepatic failure. Its dose should be reduced in renal failure.
     c. **Therapeutic benefits.** Morphine has many properties that are beneficial to a patient suffering with an AMI. First, morphine acts at the vascular level. By blocking the sympathetic efferent discharge at the CNS level, both preload and afterload decrease. Thus, morphine is a venodilator and arterial dilator. Furthermore, it decreases the patient's pain and anxiety. This leads to decreased catecholamine levels and diminished myocardial oxygen demand. Both vascular and CNS actions decrease the work on the heart and subsequently reduce ischemia and infarct extension.
     d. **Complications.** In patients with respiratory distress due to CHF or lung disease, narcotics may lead to respiratory depression and sedation. In patients who are hypovolemic, morphine administration may result in hypotension.

       Complications may arise from morphine's effect on the gastrointestinal system. Morphine decreases bowel motility and increases intrabiliary pressure. Nausea and vomiting have been frequent complications of morphine use.

       After administration of morphine, histamine release may occur. Patients may complain of pruritis, urticaria, bronchospasm, or hypotension.

       Merperidine use in combination with monoamine oxidase (MAO) inhibitors can precipitate a catecholamine crisis.

2. **Anxiolytics**

   a. **Indications.** Benzodiazepines are indicated in the treatment of AMI to reduce anxiety. They should be used sparingly, and only as an adjunct to other therapeutics such as nitrates or narcotics. Diazepam 2.5–10.0 mg IVP or lorazepam 1–4 mg IVP are typical first-line drugs.

   b. **Contraindications.** Contraindications to benzodiazepines include altered mental status or delirium. In addition, benzodiazepines cause peripheral vasodilatation, making their use contraindicated in patients with shock or hypovolemia. They are contraindicated in patients with concomitant alcohol or sedative use. Doses should be reduced in patients with hepatic or renal insufficiency.

   c. **Therapeutic benefits.** Anxiolytics cause sedation and relaxation, which theoretically result in decreased catecholamine levels in the anxious patient. The result is lowering of myocardial workload. This is especially effective in patients who are undergoing benzodiazepine or alcohol withdrawal.

   d. **Complications.** In hypotensive or hypovolemic patients, benzodiazepines can cause lowering of arterial blood pressure. The effect is usually treatable with volume infusion. With overzealous use, respiratory depression can occur. Allergic reactions are rare, but possible. Altered mental status, agitation, and confusion are common side effects, especially in elderly patients.

3. **Antiemetics**

   a. **Indications.** Promethazine hydrochloride, prochlorperazine, and other antiemetics are indicated for treatment of nausea and vomiting associated with AMI or narcotic use in the treatment of AMI. They should be used sparingly and not empirically. A typical dose of promethazine hydrochloride is 12.5–25.0 mg IVP; of prochlorperazine, 2.5–5.0 mg IVP.

   b. **Contraindications.** Antiemetics should be avoided in patients with altered mental status, because they can cause sedation. This is particularly noticeable in patients who have been treated with sedatives, narcotics, or narcotic analgesics. In addition, use in patients with hypotension or hypovolemia should be avoided because antiemetics cause mild degrees of hypotension as a result of peripheral alpha receptor blocking properties. Dosage should be reduced in hepatic insufficiency, and use should be avoided in allergic patients.

   c. **Therapeutic benefits.** Patient comfort is enhanced with antiemetics, theoretically leading to lower catecholamine levels and lower myocardial workload.

    d. Complications. Complications from antiemetic use include sedation, especially in patients who use concomitant sedative or narcotic drugs. Common anticholinergic effects include dry mouth, blurred vision, dry skin, and urinary retention. Tachycardia and hypotension can be detrimental to myocardial oxygen metabolism in the setting of AMI. Dystonic reactions and oculogyric crises can also occur.

F. Angiotensin converting enzyme (ACE) inhibitors

  1. Indications. ACE inhibitors have been advocated for the treatment of patients after AMI. Administration should begin once the patient is hemodynamically stable. Recent studies suggest that ACE inhibitors are beneficial at the time of presentation with the acute infarct. The patients having the clearest benefit are those who have heart failure associated with ventricular systolic dysfunction or hypertension in the setting of AMI.

  2. Contraindications. Contraindications to ACE inhibitors include bilateral renal artery stenosis or hyperkalemia. ACE therapy is not beneficial in the patient with renal artery stenosis, and ACE therapy has been shown to exacerbate hyperkalemia. In addition, since ACE therapy causes afterload reduction and subsequent systolic blood pressure reduction, it should be avoided in patients with hypotension or cardiogenic shock.

  3. Therapeutic benefits. ACE inhibitors increase survival from AMI. During and after an AMI, activation of the renin-angiotensin-converting enzyme causes an increase in systolic and coronary vascular resistance, myocardial oxygen requirements, and ventricular wall stress. The combination of these forces can lead to an infarct expansion and ventricular wall remodeling with ventricular aneurysm formation. ACE inhibitor therapy counteracts these forces.

    In GISSI-3, lisinopril therapy, given over a 6-week period post MI, decreased mortality by 11% and decreased ventricular dysfunction. Additionally, lisinopril, when given in combination with nitrates at the time of presentation in acute MI, decreases mortality by 17%. ACE inhibitors decrease left ventricular enlargement and slow the progression to congestive heart failure. In Acute Infarction Ramipril Efficacy Study (AIRE), heart failure patients who received ramipril had a 27% reduction in mortality and cardiovascular events. In Studies of Left Ventricular Dysfunction (SOLVD), enalapril decreased mortality in those patients with ejection fractions less than 35%.

    Captopril also has been shown to decrease mortality following myocardial infarction. It decreases ventricular arrhythmia and reinfarction. According to the Survival and Ventricular Enlargement (SAVE) study, early and continued administration of captopril to patients with asymptomatic left ventricular dysfunction post MI reduced mortality by 19%, reduced cardiac events 21%, and reduced reinfarction. These results were corroborated by ISIS-IV, in which PO captopril, given early in AMI, increased survival.

In contrast, the Second Cooperative New Scandinavian Enalapril Survival Study (CONSESUS-II) demonstrated no benefit and, in fact, possible harm from IV enalapril given within 24 hours of presentation with AMI. There was an increase in cardiogenic shock with IV enalapril use early in AMI.

To summarize, ACE inhibitors improve mortality from AMI. They should be given as soon as possible in the course of AMI, but should be given orally, not intravenously. Benefits are greatest in those patients most prone to infarct expansion and remodeling (e.g., large MI, anterior MI, clinical LV dysfunction, and hypertension).

4. **Complications.** Complications include hypotension or cardiogenic shock secondary to afterload reduction. Other complications of ACE inhibitors include hyperkalemia, increased creatinine, angioedema, and a persistent, nonproductive cough.

G. Calcium channel blockers

1. **Indications.** The role of calcium channel blockers in the treatment of AMI is limited. Routine use is not recommended. Calcium channel blockers are indicated for unstable or postinfarction angina. Diltiazem is a calcium channel blocker that provides limited benefits (secondary prevention and prophylactic against recurrent ischemia) in patients with non-Q-wave infarction. For the spastic effects of Printzmetal's angina, calcium channel blockers are advantageous. They are also indicated for persistent chest pain when no relief from nitrates is apparent.

   Calcium channel blockers with significant AV nodal blocking effects (e.g., verapamil, diltiazem) may be helpful for atrial fibrillation or atrial flutter with rapid ventricular response complicating acute MI (see Chap. 16). For severe hypertension, calcium channel blockers may be helpful in rapidly decreasing blood pressure (see Chap. 45).

2. **Contraindications.** Calcium channel blockers are contraindicated in patients who have depressed left ventricular function, ventricular tachycardia, and atrial fibrillation with wide QRS associated with Wolff-Parkinson-White (WPW) syndrome.

   Furthermore, calcium channel blockers should not be used with patients who are experiencing hypotension (systolic BP < 90 mm Hg), high-degree AV block, pulmonary edema, sick sinus syndrome or a heart rate less than 60 bpm.

3. **Therapeutic benefits.** The therapeutic benefits of calcium channel blockers include dilatation of the coronary arteries with secondary augmentation of blood flow to ischemic areas of the myocardium. Afterload and contractility are also decreased, thus

decreasing the work placed on the heart. The oxygen demand of cardiac tissue is reduced by lowering both blood pressure and heart rate.

At the nodal level, calcium channel blockers are therapeutic because there is a reduction in AV node conduction as well as in the sinoatrial (SA) node rate. The result is a slowing of the heart rate, especially in patients with atrial fibrillation or flutter.

One advantage of calcium channel blockers over beta-blockers is that they do not cause bronchoconstriction. Experimental evidence suggests that calcium channel blockers may prevent myocardial stunning in AMI. However, the data suggest that patients need to be given the medication before the AMI occurs.

4. **Complications.** Complications experienced with calcium channel blockers include a decrease in afterload, which causes hypotension and a reflex tachycardia. This is seen most often with dihydropyridines (e.g., nifedipine). An increase in heart rate creates a paradoxical increase in oxygen demand. The effect of calcium channel blockers on slowing the atrial nodes may also lead to a total SA and AV block with subsequent bradycardia and shock. Negative inotropic effects may worsen congestive heart failure. Diltiazem is potentially harmful in patients with Q-wave MI and LV dysfunction.

H. Magnesium

1. **Indications.** Magnesium is indicated in the treatment of refractory ventricular fibrillation as well as torsades de pointes associated with AMI. Most recently, it has been used as a prophylactic antiarrhythmic medication in AMI or AMI with associated hypomagnesemia. The typical dosage is 1–2 g IV for 5–30 minutes, depending on the severity of the clinical situation. Its empiric use for AMI is controversial, however, and cannot be recommended at this time.

2. **Contraindications.** Multiple studies including ISIS-IV reveal that magnesium is safe if used correctly in the treatment of AMI. Magnesium, however, is contraindicated in those patients experiencing shock, persistent severe hypotension, or complete heart block. It should be used with caution in patients with a history of renal failure.

3. **Therapeutic benefits.** Like NTG and calcium channel blockers, magnesium has systemic and coronary vasodilatory effects. The subsequent reduction in peripheral vascular resistance causes a decrease in myocardial workload and oxygen demand. The size of an MI and the incidence of recurrent ischemia can be limited by the fact that magnesium decreases platelet aggregation. Magnesium's antiarrhythmic effects are beneficial in the treatment of torsades de pointes as well as postinfarction ventricular arrhythmias. Magnesium has been shown to provide protection against catecholamine-induced myocardial necrosis. According

to the Second Leicester Intravenous Magnesium Intervention (LIMIT-2), there was a 24% decrease in mortality among patients treated with magnesium compared to patients treated with placebo during AMI. However, ISIS-IV, which was a much larger study than LIMIT-2, convincingly demonstrated no survival benefit from routine magnesium use. Its empiric use in AMI is not supported at this time.

4. **Complications.** Complications of magnesium include shock, respiratory arrest, and asystole. If it is given rapidly (2 g/5 sec), it is associated with ventricular fibrillation and hypotension. Other complications include sedation, diaphoresis, and renal failure as well as respiratory and skeletal muscle depression.

I. Heparin

1. **Indications.** Anticoagulant therapy (heparin) is used most often as an adjunctive therapy with thrombolytics. Its use is indicated following rTPA, and its use following streptokinase is common. Atrial fibrillation in the setting of AMI is also an indication to initiate anticoagulant therapy, to avoid systemic emboli from the left ventricle or left atrium. Large anterior apical infarcts, which tend to cause mural thrombi, are an indication for anticoagulant therapy. Inferior and non-Q infarcts rarely produce mural thrombus. Other indications include poor ejection fraction, unstable angina, and dilated cardiomyopathy.

   Typical dosing of heparin is 5,000–10,000 units IVP, followed by a continuous infusion of 700–1,200 U/hr to maintain a partial thromboplastin time (PTT) in the 50- to 70-second range.

2. **Contraindications.** Heparin use is contraindicated in those patients who are at risk for excessive bleeding. These include patients with peptic ulcer disease, recent GI or GU hemorrhage, recent major surgery, concomitant anticoagulant use, or bleeding diatheses. Recent intracerebral hemorrhage or intracerebral/intraspinal surgery are also contraindications.

   Anticoagulants are also contraindicated in patients with a history of heparin hypersensitivity–type reaction. Hypertension and hepatic or renal disease are relative contraindications.

3. **Therapeutic benefits.** At the molecular level, heparin binds antithrombin III, which leads to factor V inhibition and factor VIII induction by circulating thrombin. Clinically, heparin prevents arterial emboli. It decreases the incidences of reocclusion and reinfarction after thrombolytic use. It diminishes the incidence of left ventricular thrombus, reducing the chances of ischemic stroke after AMI. Furthermore, there is a diminished incidence of deep venous thrombosis and pulmonary emboli with heparin therapy.

   Heparin is used most often as an adjunctive therapy to thrombolytic use. No survival benefit has been shown with heparin following either streptokinase or TPA, but angiographic data have shown a reduction in reocclusion of the infarct-related artery with heparin use after TPA. Following both TPA and streptokinase, the incidence of hemorrhagic stroke is increased with heparin use. Heparin use following TPA continues as the standard of care, with close monitoring to keep the patient's PTTs in the 55- to 85-second range. Use of heparin following streptokinase cannot be recommended.

4. **Complications.** Hemorrhage, especially intracerebral hemorrhage, is the most common complication from anticoagulants. According to GISSI-2, subcutaneously heparin and aspirin are associated with increased frequency of noncerebral and cerebral hemorrhage. Thrombocytopenia (associated with arterial thrombus known as "white clot" syndrome) is another complication. Hypersensitivity to anticoagulants results in chills, fever, urticaria, and anaphylaxis.

J. **Lidocaine**
1. **Indications.** Lidocaine therapy is indicated for therapy of frequent PVCs (>6/min), multifocal PVCs, bigeminy, trigeminy, and paroxysmal ventricular tachycardia in the setting of AMI. Furthermore, lidocaine is indicated for closely coupled (R-on-T phenomena) premature ventricular contractions (PVCs). Additionally, lidocaine is indicated for the treatment of ventricular tachycardia, ventricular fibrillation, and wide-complex tachycardia in the setting of AMI (see Chap. 17). A typical dosage is 1 mg/kg IVP repeated at 5 to 10 minutes, followed by a continuous infusion of 2–4 mg/min.

   Routine use, however, for prophylaxis against ventricular arrhythmias in AMI is associated with increased mortality and is not indicated.
2. **Contraindications.** Lidocaine use should be avoided in patients with junctional idioventricular rhythms, especially accelerated idioventricular rhythm associated with reperfusion. Lidocaine can precipitate ventricular standstill in these patients. In patients with cardiogenic shock or low cardiac output, lidocaine can exacerbate the myocardial depression. Lidocaine use necessitates a decrease dosage with those patients who are more than 70 years of age, patients with hepatic failure, and those undergoing CPR.
3. **Therapeutic benefits.** The therapeutic benefits of lidocaine include a decrease in ventricular dysrhythmias by increasing ventricular fibrillation threshold. Another benefit of lidocaine is that it decreases reentrant arrhythmia in ischemic muscle. Nevertheless, there is no positive overall effect on mortality, and there may be even a possible detrimental effect. Lidocaine should therefore be limited to only those patients who are very early (<6 hours) into their AMI with evidence of complex ventricular ectopy.
4. **Complications.** Complications of lidocaine include CNS and cardiac toxicity. Extreme examples of CNS toxicity include seizures or coma. Patients may com-

plain of tremors, blurred vision, lightheadedness, or decreased hearing. On examination, physicians may note slurred speech, tremors, or muscle twitching. Close monitoring of lidocaine levels can alleviate some of this problem.

Cardiac toxicity secondary to lidocaine includes bradycardia, heart block, myocardial depression, hypotension, asystole, decreased automaticity, and decreased conduction velocity. Overall, class I antiarrhythmics demonstrate a statistically significant increased risk of death in those patients treated prophylactically post MI.

Bibliography

Cody RJ: Comparing angiotensin-converting enzyme inhibitor trial results in patients with AMI. *Arch Intern Med* 154:2029–2035, 1994.

The GISSI Investigators. Effects of lisinopril and transdermal glyceryl trinitrate singly and together on 6-week mortality and ventricular function after AMI. *Lancet* 343:1115–1121, 1994.

Gunnar RM, et al. Guidelines for the early management of patients with AMI. *J Am Coll Cardiol* 16:249–292, 1994.

Heesch C, et al. Magnesium in AMI. *Ann Emerg Med* 24:1154–1160, 1994.

The ISIS Study Investigators. A randomised comparison of streptokinase vs TPA vs anistreplase and of aspirin plus heparin vs aspirin alone among 41,299 cases of suspected AMI. *Lancet* 339:753–766, 1992.

Mitchell JM, et al. The golden hours of the myocardial infarction: nonthrombolytic interventions. *Ann Emerg Med* 20:540–548, 1990.

National Center for Health Statistics. *Health, United States 1993*. Hyattsville, MD: Public Health Service, 1994.

Teo K, et al. Effects of prophylactic antiarrhythmic drug therapy in AMI: an overview of results from randomized controlled trials. *JAMA* 270:1589–1594, 1993.

Angioplasty in Acute Myocardial Infarction

Aaron L. Bender

I. **Coronary artery occlusion and myocardial infarction.**
Coronary artery disease remains the leading cause of death in residents of the United States. Approximately 1.3 millon people per year in the United States experience a myocardial infarction (MI). It is extremely important that the emergency physician have an understanding of the pathophysiology, the treatment goals and modalities, and the management of patients with acute myocardial infarction (AMI).

It has been shown by angiography that approximately 97% of patients with transmural AMI have greater than 95% stenosis of the infarct-related artery at 4 hours (Fig. 12-1). The major thrust of therapy for AMI over the past two decades has been to establish timely reperfusion in the infarct-related artery, thereby reestablishing blood flow to the ischemic myocardium and reversing the wavefront of necrosis that occurs after coronary artery occlusion. It has been shown that in patients suffering AMI, in-hospital mortality of those with occluded infarct arteries is approximately three times as high as that of those who have patent infarct arteries. It is also well documented that complications of MI such as congestive heart failure (CHF) or ventricular arrhythmias are less common in those patients who have patent infarct artery (Table 12-1). Therefore, it is of utmost importance that initial therapy of AMI be directed in establishing reperfusion, either pharmacologically, or through mechanical means such as coronary artery angioplasty (PTCA) or coronary artery bypass surgery (CABG).

II. **The technique of coronary artery angioplasty.** Coronary angioplasty was first performed intraoperatively in 1977 by Gruntzig in Switzerland. Since that time the technique of PTCA has been modified and perfected, and it is now a relatively safe and effective means of treating coronary insufficiency. When performing PTCA, arterial access is obtained via the femoral or brachial artery. A guiding catheter is fed retrograde to the aorta and placed at the coronary ostium. Angiography is then performed to delineate the area of occlusion. The dilating catheter is fed through the guide and placed into the appropriate coronary artery. The balloon is directed across the area of stenosis and is inflated to 3–5 atmospheres of pressure or until the balloon contour is fully distended on fluoroscopy. In doing this, the area of atherosclerotic plaque is fractured and pushed into the wall of the coronary artery, thus reducing the area of original stenosis. During the procedure, heparin is used to prevent thrombogenesis, and often intracoronary nitroglycerine (NTG) is used to stimulate intracoronary vasodilation. Postdilation angiography is performed to define the residual stenosis.

The indications, contraindications, and timing of PTCA vary with the patient's clinical condition. Acute PTCA may oc-

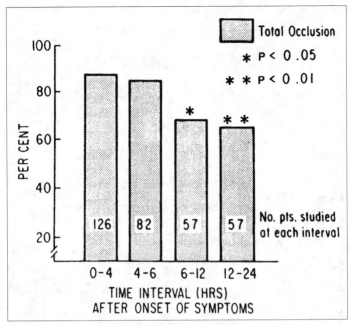

Fig. 12-1. Percentage of coronary occlusion after myocardial infarction. (Reprinted by permission of *The New England Journal of Medicine,* Dewood MA, Prevalence of total coronary artery occlusion during early hours of acute myocardial infarction. *New Engl J Med* 303:899. Copyright 1980, Massachusetts Medical Society.)

cur with thrombolytic therapy (TT), after unsuccessful thrombolytic therapy, or instead of thrombolytic therapy. In stable patients post AMI without ongoing ischemia, it may be deferred until days after the AMI to reduce complication rates. These options, indications, and contraindications are outlined below.

III. **Angioplasty in conjunction with thrombolytic therapy.**
With the advent of thrombolytic therapy and its documented efficacy treatment of AMI, the role of PTCA in those patients with MI who have already received thrombolytic therapy is controversial. It is intuitive that in those patients who have successfully reperfused with thrombolytic therapy but still may have residual coronary stenosis documented by angiography, immediate PTCA to reduce the stenosis would likely prevent or decrease hospital mortality or recurrent ischemic events. Three large clinical trials (TIMI-2, TAMI-1, and ECSG) were designed to evaluate the appropriate timing of angioplasty after TT. The conclusion of these three trials was that immediate or even somewhat deferred PTCA within 18–48 hours after TT did not reduce in-hospital mortality or improve left ventricular function and actually led to increased complication rates. In TIMI-2, it was discovered that a more conservative approach, in which PTCA was used for coronary

Table 12-1. Comparison of those patients with reperfusion (group 1) versus those without reperfusion (group 2)

	Group 1 (n = 64) Perfusion grades 2,3	Group 2 (n = 115) Perfusion grades 0,1	p value
Age (yr)	46 ± 9	47 ± 10	NS*
No. men (%)	44 (69)	88 (77)	NS
No. of days from MI* to catheterization	25 ± 30	28 ± 26	NS
Risk factors for ASCVD* (%)			
Hypertension	26 (41)	56 (49)	NS
Cigarette smoking	50 (78)	94 (82)	NS
Diabetes mellitus	16 (25)	23 (20)	NS
Serum cholesterol >270 mg/dl	8 (13)	16 (14)	NS
Duration of follow-up (mo)	46 ± 29	48 ± 28	NS
Medications after MI (%)			
Calcium antagonists	32 (50)	50 (43)	NS
Beta-blockers	27 (42)	47 (41)	NS
Long-acting nitrates	32 (50)	64 (56)	NS
Aspirin	35 (55)	40 (35)	NS
Antiarrhythmics	9 (14)	23 (20)	NS
Left ventricular volumes			
End-diastolic volume (ml/m^2)	67 ± 17	72 ± 21	NS
End-systolic volume (ml/m^2)	33 ± 14	36 ± 18	NS
Ejection fraction	0.52 ± 0.14	0.52 ± 0.11	NS
Morbid events (%)			
Unstable angina	6 (9)	29 (25)	0.012
Subsequent MI	3 (5)	14 (12)	NS
Congestive heart failure	4 (6)	20 (17)	0.031
Mortality (%)	0 (0)	21 (18)	<0.001

*ASCVD = atherosclerotic cardiovascular disease; MI = myocardial infarction; NS = not significant.
Source: Cigarroa R. Prognosis after acute myocardial infarction in patients with and without anterograde coronary blood flow.
Am J Cardiol, 1989;64:156. Reprinted with permission from *American Journal of Cardiology.*

stenosis in only those patients who had evidence of recurrent ischemia, either spontaneous or provocable, resulted in equally low in-hospital and one-year mortality and reinfarction rates, while avoiding the complications encountered using immediate post-thrombolytic PTCA (Fig. 12-2). As such, a more conservative approach to PTCA following thrombolytic therapy is now advocated.

A. **Indications for PTCA following thrombolytic therapy**
   1. Evidence of continued ischemia (rescue PTCA, see sec. **III**).
      a. Persistent chest pain unresponsive to pharmacologic therapy
      b. Persistent ST-segment elevation on ECG
   2. Hemodynamic instability (cardiogenic shock)
B. **Contraindications to PTCA following thrombolytic therapy**
   1. Successful reperfusion of infarct artery
   2. Severe left main coronary stenosis
   3. Triple vessel disease
   4. Large thrombus in the infarct artery (too long for angioplasty)
   5. Stenosis associated with large area of myocardium at risk (relative contraindication)
C. **Complications**
   1. Emergent CABG (approximately 1%)
   2. Coronary artery dissection
   3. Abrupt reocclusion and infarct extension
   4. Bleeding at catheterization site requiring transfusion
D. **Morbidity and mortality**
   1. One-year mortality
      a. 6.9% invasive strategy (emergent PTCA)
      b. 7.4% conservative strategy (delayed PTCA)
   2. One-year reinfarction rates (Fig. 12-3)
      a. 9.4% invasive strategy
      b. 9.8% conservative strategy
IV. **Rescue angioplasty after unsuccessful thrombolytic therapy.** Of the current topics involving the role of angioplasty in treatment of AMI, by far the most controversial is the role of rescue or salvage angioplasty after apparent thrombolytic therapy failure. One of the most challenging aspects of managing AMI is the recognition of thrombolytic therapy failure and the decision to attempt emergency rescue angioplasty.

Prior to salvage angioplasty, the physician must be able to adequately recognize those patients who have had unsuccessful thrombolysis. The current method of recognizing thrombolytic success hinges on the resolution of chest pain, return of ST segments to near baseline, the appearance of reperfusion arrhythmias, or return of hemodynamic stability. The most specific of the above measures is reduction in ST-segment elevation (50% reduction in elevation predicting 97% successful reperfusion); however, only 40% of those patients with patent infarct arteries meet this criterion. Reperfusion remains difficult to document, but fortunately, with new modalities under investigation such as vector cardiography,

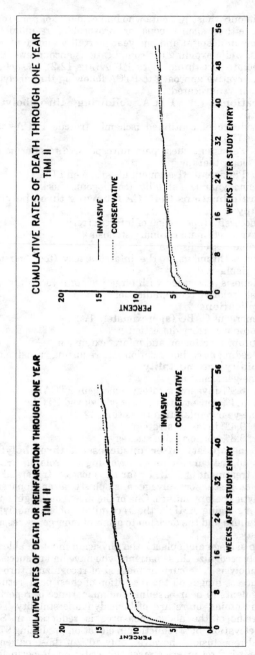

Fig. 12-2.   Event rates after immediate post-thrombolytic angioplasty versus conservative elective angioplasty. (From Williams D. One-year results of the Thrombolysis in Myocardial Infarction Investigation (TIMI) phase II trial. *Circulation* 1992;85:537–538. Reproduced with permission. *Circulation.* Copyright 1992 American Heart Association.)

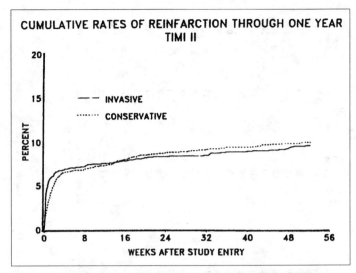

Fig. 12-3.   Reinfarction after immediate post-thrombolytic PTCA
versus conservative elective PTCA after thrombolysis. (From Williams
D. One-year results of the Thrombolysis in Myocardial Infarction
Investigation (TIMI) phase II trial. *Circulation* 1992;85:537–538. Reproduced with permission. *Circulation*. Copyright 1992 American Heart Association.)

serum enzyme levels, and nuclear medicine studies, more
sensitive and specific methods of defining reperfusion after
TT are sure to develop.

There have been few randomized studies to date evaluating
the merits of rescue angioplasty (Table 12-2). The largest trial
to date, the RESCUE study, randomized patients with failed
thrombolysis to receive either rescue angioplasty or medical
therapy only. The trial revealed a trend in mortality reduction
from 10% to 5% and a reduction in the combined incidence of
death or congestive heart failure from 17% to 10% in those patients who received rescue angioplasty. It must be noted that
the patients enrolled in this study were those who had the
most myocardium at risk (i.e., those with anterior infarctions). It also must be noted that while other trials have revealed similar promising mortality reductions in patients
with successful angioplasty, the mortality in patients with
unsuccessful rescue angioplasty has been as high as 39%.

A. **Patient selection.** Current recommendations on the timing and value of rescue angioplasty include certain situations and types of patients who would benefit from acute
catheterization and angioplasty (if anatomy permits) immediately after thrombolytic therapy. Given that unsuccessful rescue angioplasty may be associated with high
mortality, this procedure should be reserved for those patients who are at high risk and have the most to gain from

Table 12-2. Pooled results of randomized rescue angioplasty trials

First author	No. of pts	Thrombolytic regimen	Success (%)	Reocclusion (%)	ΔEF	Mortality (%)
Topol	86	rt-PA	73	29	−1	10.4
Califf	15	rt-PA	87	15	+1	NR
	25	UK	84	12	+1	NR
	12	rt-PA + UK	92	0	+2	NR
Belenkie	16	SK	81	NR	+2	6.7
Fung	13	SK	92	16	+10	7.6
Topol	22	rt-PA + UK	86	3	+5	0.0
Grines	12	rt-PA + SK	100	8	NR	NR
Holmes	34	SK	71	NR	−11	11.0
Grines	10	rt-PA + SK	90	12	+5	10.0
O'Connor	90	SK	89	14	−1	17.0
Baim	37	rt-PA	92	26	NR	5.4
Whitlow	26	rt-PA	81	29	−2	NR
	18	UK	89	25	+1	NR
Ellis	109	rt-PA	79	20	+1	10.1
	5	rt-PA + UK	80	20	+2	20.0
	59	SK	76	18	+4	10.2
Pooled SK, UK or combination	308*		260/308 (84%)†	31/223 (14%)	−1	11.2
Pooled rt-PA only	252‡		191/252 (76%)†	38/157 (24%)	−1	9.5
Total	560*‡		451/560 (80%)	69/380 (18%)	−1	10.6

* Five patients included in both series of Topol.
† p = 0.01
‡ 21 patients included in both series of Califf.
Source: Reprinted with permission from the American College of Cardiology (*Journal of the American College of Cardiology*, 1992, 19, p. 684.)

the procedure. The criteria below should guide patient selection.

B. Inclusion criteria for rescue PTCA
  1. History
     a. Persistent chest pain after TT
     b. History of limited systolic function (e.g., CHF)
     c. Previous myocardial infarction (limited myocardium)
  2. Physical findings
     a. Evidence of CHF
     b. ECG criteria
        (1) Anterolateral infarction
        (2) Large increases in ST-segment elevation
        (3) ST-segment elevation in multiple leads
        (4) Inferoposterior infarction
        (5) Persistent ST elevation after TT
     c. Hemodynamic instability (cardiogenic shock)

  After the administration of TT, patients with both persistent chest pain for more than 90 minutes, not controlled with nitroglycerin or heparin, and any number of the above risk factors should be considered candidates for rescue PTCA. Consultation with a cardiologist is imperative to make the decision regarding emergent PTCA. Transfer to a facility that has PTCA available should proceed as soon as possible. This is especially true for patients with CHF or cardiogenic shock who would benefit the most from an attempted mechanical revascularization procedure, whether salvage PTCA or emergent CABG.

V. Primary angioplasty 0–6 hours after AMI onset. One of the most exciting and ever-changing aspects of angioplasty in acute myocardial infarction is that of primary PTCA. Coronary angioplasty has evolved over the past 15 years into a viable and possibly superior therapeutic option to TT in AMI. Although clinical trials of primary angioplasty are relatively small compared to randomized trials of TT, primary angioplasty has been associated with very low in-hospital mortality rates, ranging from 3% in the Primary Angioplasty Registry to 8% in the Myocardial Infarction Triage and Intervention (MITI) Registry (Table 12-3). Infarct-related artery patency in these studies has been shown to be higher than patency achieved with thrombolytic therapy, to levels over 90%. When looking at randomized studies comparing primary angioplasty to TT, it is evident that PTCA is a viable treatment option in AMI. The two largest of these trials, the Netherlands trial and the Primary Angioplasty in Myocardial Infarction (PAMI) study, both demonstrated a statistically lower combined endpoint of in-hospital mortality and reinfarction compared to TT.

A. Indications for primary PTCA
  1. Symptoms consistent with AMI (see TT indications, Chap. 10, sec. **V.**).
     a. Chest pain of more than 30 minutes not relieved with NTG
     b. ST elevation of 1 mm in 2 contiguous leads
  2. Access to catheterization lab with experienced cardiologist

**Table 12-3.   Primary angioplasty
in myocardial infarction trial results**

Event	PTCA (n=185)	t-PA (n=200)	p value
Reinfarction	2.6%	6.5%	0.06
Death overall	2.6%	6.5%	0.06
Low risk*	3.1%	2.2%	0.69
Not low risk*	2.0%	10.4%	0.01
Nonfatal reinfarction or death	5.1%	12.0%	0.02

* Patients defined as being at "low risk" had no high-risk factors. Those in the "not low risk" category were older than 70, had an anterior infarction, or had a heart rate of more than 100 bpm on admission.
Source: Kleiman N, Primary angioplasty for acute myocardial infarction: current status, *Clinical Challenges in Acute Myocardial Infarction,* 4(2):6.

    3. Ability to perform PTCA within 90 minutes of presentation
    4. Patients with the following clinical characteristics:
        a. Contraindication to thrombolytics
        b. Cardiogenic shock
        c. Diagnostic uncertainty
B. Contraindications to primary PTCA
    1. Inability to gain timely access to PTCA
    2. Poor vascular access
    3. Left main coronary artery disease with infarct artery in the left anterior descending (LAD) or circumflex artery
    4. Severe triple vessel disease
    5. Large intracoronary thrombus
C. Complications of primary PTCA
    1. Infarct extension
    2. Emergent CABG (approximately 1.4%)
    3. Coronary artery dissection
    4. Cardiac arrhythmias—more often with right coronary artery
    5. Hemorrhage requiring blood transfusions (as high as 18%)

Primary PTCA is a very attractive and effective option in the therapy of AMI, and one additional benefit it ensures is the actual assessment of the coronary anatomy and the severity of disease. In doing this, one can direct therapy more appropriately for each patient. This is a benefit that is not realized after acute thrombolytic therapy. Conversely, one must be aware that immediate angioplasty in the patient with acute myocardial infarction is an option not available at most centers. Angioplasty capability is currently available at approximately 12% of the hospitals across the United States. Coronary bypass backup should be available as well, given that the emergent CABG rate is approximately 1.5% post PTCA.

Whether PTCA can be performed at centers without CABG capabilities is now being evaluated. In a study performed in

Seattle, it was shown that PTCA performed in centers without surgical backup did not affect the overall patient mortality rate, compared to those centers with emergent CABG capability. Although these results are promising, more data must be generated before this strategy can become a viable option.

VI. **Primary PTCA 6–24 hours after AMI onset.** Initial studies of reperfusion therapy demonstrated that myocardial salvage is negligible 4–6 hours after symptom onset. More recent studies, however, including the Late Assessment of Thrombolytic Efficacy (LATE) and Estudio Multicéntrico Estreptoquinas Repúblicas de América del Sur Collective Group (EMERAS) trials, have demonstrated mortality benefits of TT in the 6- to 12-hour window. In the ISIS-II trial, there was a reduction mortality in patients receiving therapy as late as 24 hours after the onset of symptoms. It has been suggested that reperfusion of the infarct artery patency decreases myocardial remodeling after AMI. In so doing, myocardial infarct expansion is limited, the injured myocardium is electrically stabilized, and it is therefore less susceptible to malignant post-MI arrhythmias and congestive heart failure.

Studies performed on late PTCA in AMI are limited in patient numbers. Subpopulations of the PAMI study who received PTCA after 6 hours of symptoms did very well, with mortality rates less than those treated with TT and reperfusion rates greater than 90%. In a recent study performed at the University of Michigan, late direct PTCA, when successful, was associated with a low in-hospital mortality rate of 5.5%. When PTCA was unsuccessful, which occurred in 30 of 139 patients (22%), in-hospital mortality was 43% (13 of 30). Although the overall mortality rate was similar to patients presenting late in MI who were treated with conventional therapy (13.7% vs. 13.9%), patients in the angioplasty trial were on profile a much higher risk group (14% vs. 2% cardiogenic shock, and 25% vs. 15% with previous MI). Given this increased risk profile and similar mortality rates achieved, it is reasonable to assume that certain patients should not be denied a trial of angioplasty on the premise of presenting after 6 hours. In patients of relatively young age (<65 years) who are suffering from hemodynamic compromise or continued ischemia, a trial of mechanical reperfusion late in the course of myocardial infarction appears to be indicated.

VII. **PTCA in patients with contraindications to TT.** Given the extensive list of contraindications to thrombolytic therapy, it is not surprising that in patients presenting with AMI, as many as 25%–30% have contraindications to TT (Fig. 12-4). Although the inclusion criteria for TT have been relaxed significantly over the past 5 years, still many patients will be denied thrombolysis. It is in these patients that angioplasty plays a significant role in the therapy of AMI. A recent study by Himbert examining patients with contraindications to TT demonstrated very promising results. An initial patency rate of 93% was achieved with an in-hospital mortality rate of 9% and a predischarge infarct patency rate of 97%. Given that conventionally treated patients with contraindications to TT have an in-hospital mortality from 17% to 29%, this

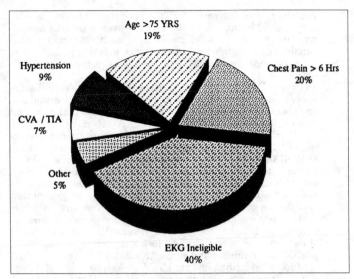

Fig. 12-4.   Exclusion criteria for thrombolytic therapy. (From Feldman T, et al. Direct percutaneous transluminal coronary angioplasty for patients with exclusions from thrombolysis. *Am Heart J* 1994;5:122).

represents a significant clinical improvement. Although this study was limited in patient numbers, it supports the use of PTCA as a viable treatment option for the patient with contraindications to TT and PTCA. See Chap. 10 for TT contraindications.

VIII. **PTCA in patients with cardiogenic shock.** Cardiogenic shock is the leading cause of death in patients who are admitted to the hospital with AMI. Cardiogenic shock can be defined as (1) a systolic blood pressure less than 80 without inotropic or aortic balloon pump support, (2) a systolic blood pressure less than 90 with inotropic or balloon pump support, or (3) no evidence of hypovolemia (see Chap. 14). Cardiogenic shock is associated with large MIs that involve at least 40% of the myocardium. The mortality rate associated with cardiogenic shock in patients treated with conventional therapy is approximately 80%. Unfortunately, the significant benefits associated with the use of TT in AMI have not translated to patients with cardiogenic shock. This is most likely the result of low (<40%) recanalization rates of the infarct-related artery in patients with cardiogenic shock.

One of the most exciting and beneficial uses of angioplasty in AMI is its use in patients with cardiogenic shock. Similar to the treatment of AMI without shock, the most essential aspect of therapy in AMI with cardiogenic shock is achieving infarct artery patency. In fourteen studies examining the performance of PTCA in patients with cardiogenic shock, the mortality benefits with reperfusion were striking. In patients with successful recanalization of the infarct artery, mortality was 30%, compared to 80% in those with unsuccessful angio-

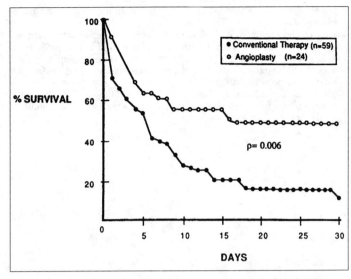

Fig. 12-5. Survival using PTCA versus conventional therapy in cardiogenic shock. (From Lee L, et al. Percutaneous transluminal coronary angioplasty improves survival in acute myocardial infarction complicated by cardiogenic shock. *Circulation* **1988;78:1348. Reproduced with permission.** *Circulation.* **Copyright 1988 American Heart Association.)**

plasty. The overall success rate was 73%, with an overall mortality of 44% in patients presenting with cardiogenic shock treated with PTCA. This represents a 50% reduction in mortality in patients presenting with cardiogenic shock (Fig. 12-5).

Although the benefits of angioplasty in patients with cardiogenic shock are significant, PTCA capability is available at only 12% of hospitals. At centers without angioplasty availability, transfer to a hospital that can perform PTCA is indicated. Whether thrombolytic therapy in those without contraindications should be administered before transfer is a decision that should be made in concert with the accepting cardiologist.

Bibliography

Cigarroa G, Lange R, Hillis D. Prognosis after acute myocardial infarction in patients with and without residual anterograde coronary blood flow. *Am J Cardiol* 64:155–160, 1989.

Eisenhauer AC, Matthews RV, Moore L. Late direct angioplasty in patients with myocardial infarction and fluctuating chest pain. *Am Heart J* 123:553–559, 1992.

Himbert D, Jean-Michel J, Steg G, et al. Primary coronary angioplasty for acute myocardial infarction with contraindication to thrombolysis. *Am J Cardiol* 71:377–381, 1993.

Kurz H, Krone R. Which MI patients are candidates for rescue angioplasty? *J Crit Illness* 9:753–768, 1994.

Landau C, Glamann B, Willard J, et al. Coronary angioplasty in the patient with acute myocardial infarction. *Am J Med* 96:536–543, 1994.

Lee L, Erbel R, Brown T, et al. Multicenter registry of angioplasty therapy of cardiogenic shock: initial and long-term survival. *J Am Coll Cardiol* 17:599–603, 1991.

Williams D, Braunwald E, Knatterud G, et al. One-year results of the thrombolysis in myocardial infarction investigation (TIMI) phase II trial. *Circulation* 85:533–542, 1992.

13

Prehospital Diagnosis and Treatment of Acute Myocardial Infarction

Diane L. Gorgas

Chest pain is one of the most frequent chief complaints registered by Emergency Medical Service (EMS) systems. Although most of the calls for assistance do not represent acute myocardial infarctions (AMIs), cardiac ischemia in all degrees of severity makes up a sizable percentage of these calls.

The literature clearly shows that therapy—especially thrombolytic therapy—should be instituted as early as possible in AMI. Several collaborative clinical studies have demonstrated improved left ventricular function, lower peak creatinine and CK-MB levels, smaller infarct size, and reduced mortality in AMI when thrombolytic therapy is instituted in the early stages of infarction (<2 hours) than when treatment is delayed (>4 hours). Obviously early diagnosis of AMI in the prehospital arena is also desirable.

I. **Phases in delay of treatment.** Unfortunately, only a small percentage of AMI patients are given definitive treatment or clot lysis within the 60- to 90-minute period after AMI. The cause for delay in definitive therapy can be divided into two phases.

  A. **Phase I.** The first phase consists of time from symptom onset to emergency department (ED) arrival. Most of the time delay within phase I is associated with the patient's own decision to seek medical care and activate EMS. The remainder of the delay in phase I is associated with EMS response, stabilization, diagnosis, and transport of the patient.

  B. **Phase II.** Phase II begins with the patient's arrival in the ED. Time-consuming activities during the initial evaluation include gathering demographic data, establishing IV access if this was not already accomplished in the prehospital setting, recording and interpreting the initial ECG, sending laboratory samples, beginning mainstay medical therapy such as aspirin, nitrates, or morphine, and in some institutions awaiting cardiology approval before initiating thrombolytic therapy. Phase II delays commonly take 60–90 minutes as based on US studies. This puts the vast majority of thrombolytic candidates out of "the golden hour" before definitive therapy can be given.

II. **Limiting the time to therapy.** Appropriately, efforts have been made to analyze delays and improve the time to definitive treatment in phases I and II. This discussion focuses on phase I, the prehospital phase.

  A. **Patient and bystander delays.** The delay in patient activation of EMS can be substantial. As many as 50% of patients with chest pain wait more than 4 hours before seeking medical care. Of the patients who do present to the ED or to a local physician's office, only 30%–40% acti-

vate EMS at all. The remainder in most studies are transported by private vehicle. Improvement in this delay is
the most difficult to achieve. Public awareness programs
have the potential for reaching the largest number of
high-risk individuals in the general population. Also important is education of high-risk individuals by primary
physicians and cardiologists. All potential patients should
be urged to call 911 when they experience chest pain.
B. **EMS delays.** Once EMS has been activated, typical delays occur in the scene response time (the time from dis-
patch to patient arrival), in obtaining histories and
physical examinations in the field, in placing the patient
on a cardiac monitor, in obtaining IV access, in beginning
initial therapy, in readying for transport, and in the transport time incurred en route to the nearest medical center.
European-based studies have explored the possibility of
placing physicians or "mobile ICUs" in the field to more
rapidly administer thrombolytic therapy. Prehospital
ECGs are obtained and interpreted in the field by on-site
physicians. Indications and contraindications for thrombolytic therapy are reviewed on scene and treatment is begun before transport.

In the United States, however, physicians are traditionally hospital-based. Therefore, efforts have focused on
EMS activation and communication via telemetry to
hospital-based physicians, who make the ultimate decision regarding thrombolytic therapy administration.
III. **Prehospital EMS systems.** The success of prehospital
thrombolytic therapy depends heavily on the EMS system.
Some important concepts to understand in evaluating the feasibility of prehospital thrombolytics are on-line versus off-line
medical control, first-response systems, and paramedic capabilities (see also Chap. 4).
A. **On-line versus off-line medical control.** Medical control can be established in any system via standing protocols (off-line) or by radio or phone communication with a
control physician (on-line). The most common system in
urban areas in the United States is a combination of the
two. Chief complaints generate a set protocol of evaluation and therapy. The on-line arm of the system is used after initial protocol is begun. Telemetry of rhythm strips or
12-lead ECGs occurs during the on-line communication
and is interpreted by the medical control physician. Therapy is further determined by medical control based on
transmitted findings.

On-line medical control is a crucial feature of a prehospital ECG and/or thrombolytic program. Because correlation between computer interpretation of ECGs and
physician readings has not yet been adequately established, on-line communication is necessary before the initiation of prehospital thrombolytic therapy. The most
commonly used portable 12-lead ECG recorders have
ECG cellular phone transmission that is fully automated. After electrodes are placed and patient information is logged into the ECG machine, the collection and
transmission of the ECG by phone takes approximately 30

seconds. Virtually error-free transmission can be achieved. A study by Grim et al. showed good correlation between the field copy of the ECG obtained by paramedics, the ECG transmitted from the field, and the ECG obtained upon ED admission with respect to PR interval, QRS duration, QT interval, R and T axis, and morphologic characteristics.

Special training is recommended for medical control physicians when a prehospital ECG program is initiated. It is essential that physicians check potential false-positive ECGs for AMI. They should be familiar with EMS standing orders, field protocol, and ECG labeling and identification. A crucial part of medical control quality assurance is the testing of physicians for their ability to interpret ECGs.

B. **Tiered systems.** EMS activation itself can take many different forms, each of which can influence the success of out-of-hospital thrombolytic therapy. In general, paramedic units are a much-valued resource. There are fewer advanced life support (ALS) units per capita than basic life support (BLS) units, and therefore response times are, on average, longer. Some systems have compensated for longer ALS response times by establishing a **two-tiered response system** (see Chap. 4). For life-threatening chief complaints, including chest pain and unresponsiveness, a BLS unit is dispatched simultaneously with an ALS unit. When BLS units arrive first at the scene, they operate under standing protocols in taking vital signs and beginning initial assessment. This helps free ALS units to begin administering therapy and establishing on-line medical control more quickly.

Another facet of EMS activation that should be considered before evaluating the potential success of any prehospital thrombolytic therapy program is the **mode of activation.** Although "911" is becoming much more common throughout the United States, many communities, especially in rural settings, have yet to establish this access system.

C. **Paramedic capabilities.** Other features that must be considered in assessing the feasibility of prehospital thrombolytic therapy are paramedic capability and the strength and direction of medical control. Typically, paramedics undergo over 1000 hours of a **training program** before certification. Systems that already have prehospital ECG capabilities have found that an additional 5- to 7-hour training period is necessary for paramedic education. Trials examining the potential for prehospital thrombolytic therapy have quoted at least three to four times this period for adequate training in thrombolytic therapy administration.

Paramedics who obtain prehospital ECGs should be educated in the pathophysiology of AMI and cardiac ischemia, in appropriate patient selection, in correct ECG lead placement, and in correctly identifying transmitted ECGs with the base physician. A review of the management of complications associated with AMI and thrombolytic therapy is another necessary part of training. Paramedics must also understand the benefits of prehospital ECGs and thrombolytic therapy in reducing hospital delays and the definitive time to treatment versus the risk of prolonged scene times.

New policies, protocols, and procedures will be associated with either a prehospital ECG program or with the use of prehospital thrombolytics. One of the most important indicators of success is the frequency with which these new protocols and procedures are used. **Quality assurance** in such a program is a major concern, and the feasibility of a program often depends on the skills of the paramedics. Frequent practice is therefore needed, along with periodic testing of skills.

D. **Equipment requirements.** The physical equipment necessary for prehospital ECGs has advanced rapidly since field 12-lead ECG telemetry capabilities were first introduced in 1986. Current models have standard cardiac monitors, defibrillators, and 12-lead ECG capabilities in a single unit that is no larger than a typical "Life-Pac" unit. Most ECGs are transmitted via cellular phone, but land-line transmission is possible through any touch-tone phone jack. Transmission can be to a centralized base station, to an alternate base station as determined by the geographic location of the transmitting squad, or to the receiving hospital.

E. **Prehospital thrombolytic therapy.** If thrombolytic therapy is to be initiated in the field, patient selection will be one obstacle. The paramedic's ability to perform an accurate physical examination is therefore essential. Screening questions should be read from a list that the paramedic must understand in detail should any questions arise. An example of such a list is provided in Table 13-1.

Thrombolytic administration protocols need to be set up well in advance. The thrombolytic or protocol of choice may depend on patient characteristics, cost, or physician preference. European and U.S. studies have demonstrated that streptokinase, urokinase, anisoylated plasminogen-SK activator complex (APSAC), and tissue plasminogen activator (t-PA) can be used safely in prehospital settings. The "front-loaded" protocol for the use of t-PA is advantageous in the prehospital use of thrombolytics because no infusion pump is required and only a fraction of the dose is needed before arrival at the hospital.

IV. **Feasibility of prehospital ECGs.** Prehospital diagnosis and treatment of AMI will not become an accepted practice overnight, nor should it be. Limitations to its use are clear. A Milwaukee study demonstrated that in the initial stages of starting a prehospital ECG program, approximately 33% of all attempted ECG transmissions were received and reviewed "adequately." After 6 months, the success rate had significantly increased. Reasons for failed transmissions were most commonly cellular "dead space," interfering structures (for instance, attempted transmission from a basement), busy cellular airways, and operator error. Land-line use can decrease the percentage of unsuccessful transmissions to 5%–7%. Hu-

Table 13-1. Screening questions for potential prehospital thrombolytic therapy patients

Inclusion criteria

Y	N	Typical chest pain?
Y	N	Age <75 years?
Y	N	Pain duration <6 hours?
Y	N	Pain persists despite sublingual nitroglycerin?
Y	N	Systolic BP between 90 and 180?
Y	N	Diastolic BP <110?
Y	N	Systolic BP R arm vs L arm <20?
Y	N	12-lead ECG successfully sent to base physician and interpreted?
Y	N	Patient is oriented and can give consent for therapy?

Exclusion criteria

Y	**N**	History of myocardial infarction?
Y	**N**	History of trauma, arterial lines, central lines in past 2 months?
Y	**N**	History of surgery in last 2 months?
Y	**N**	Stroke, seizure, brain surgery?
Y	**N**	Brain tumor, aneurysm, arteriovenous malformation?
Y	**N**	Takes warfarin (Coumadin; "blood thinner")?
Y	**N**	History of Crohn disease, colitis, or GI bleed in last 12 months?
Y	**N**	Cancer, kidney, liver problems, diabetes?
Y	**N**	Hematuria in last 12 months?
Y	**N**	Suspected or known aortic problems?
Y	**N**	Pregnancy or currently menstruating female?
Y	N	Patient meets criteria on checklist?

man error, however, can never be eliminated from the system even with a successful transmission. Concerns have arisen regarding orders that were based on the wrong ECG when two were being received simultaneously at the base station. Detailed documentation and double-checking of ECG labels are therefore necessary, both in the field and at the base station.

Regardless of the success of transmission, obtaining field ECGs does represent a delay in patient transport, albeit small compared to hospital delays in obtaining ECGs. In some situations, any delay should be seen as unwarranted. Hemodynamic instability or electrical cardiac instability must be written into protocol as contraindications for field ECGs or prehospital thrombolytic therapy. Suggested criteria for patients in whom prehospital ECGs should be obtained are listed in Table 13-2.

Studies have been completed within the U.S. system to verify the feasibility of prehospital ECGs. Some of the work done by Aufderheide et al. in Milwaukee demonstrated a threefold reduction in time to the obtainment of ECGs by paramedics in

Table 13-2.   Patients for whom prehospital ECGs may be obtained

Patients with hemodynamic stability
  Systolic BP >90 and <200
  Heart rate >50 and <140
Patients with absence of dysrhythmias (ventricular tachycardia, ventricular fibrillation, second- or third-degree heart block)
Adults >18 years and <75 years
Patients with nontraumatic cause of chest pain
Patients who meet above criteria and whose transport will not be significantly delayed by obtaining the ECG

the prehospital environment versus in the ED (8.4 ± 5.1 minutes by prehospital providers versus 24.2 ± 21.6 minutes after the patient entered the ED). On-scene time increased by an average of 5.2 minutes when compared with retrospective response times for chest pain. Furthermore, the study demonstrated a 99.2% specificity and a positive predictive value of 92.8% with 54.2% of all AMI patients having diagnostic ECGs. The second phase of the Milwaukee Prehospital Chest Pain Project looked at the feasibility of prehospital thrombolytic therapy, but again focused on prehospital ECG collection and its reliability. This phase of the project again verified the feasibility of prehospital ECG collection with high specificity (99.7%) and acceptable sensitivity (42%). A review of U.S. studies done to analyze the accuracy of prehospital ECGs is given in Table 13-3.
V. **Feasibility of prehospital thrombolytic therapy.** The feasibility and safety of obtaining prehospital ECGs is much less of an issue than the feasibility and safety of giving prehospital thrombolytic therapy. Because any errors encountered with prehospital ECGs may be multiplied when prehospital thrombolytic therapy is given, the administration of thrombolytics in the prehospital setting has its own set of risks. The number of patients who qualified for prehospital thrombolytic therapy in a number of U.S. studies has been very low. It is often unclear whether uniformity and expertise in administration can be achieved when a procedure is used

Table 13-3.   Time delays in obtaining prehospital ECGs and reliability

Study	Scene time to obtain ECG (min)	Specificity of +ECG (%)	Sensitivity of +ECG (%)
Aufderheide	5.2	99.2	54.2
Milwaukee Prehospital Chest Pain Project	4.0	99.7	48.0
Grim	1.0	—	—

only sporadically. Whether it is cost-effective or even realistic to thoroughly train paramedics in administering thrombolytic therapy when the protocol is so infrequently used remains a valid question. How much more of a delay is involved when thrombolytic therapy is begun in the field, and is this delay justified only when the distance to the nearest medical facility is excessive? If so, this would almost guarantee that patients in more remote locations would be the only ones for whom prehospital initiation of thrombolytic therapy could be justified. But this would present a dilemma, since rural medics would naturally have the lowest volume of patients and therefore the least experience.

The question regarding the number of potential cases that would benefit from thrombolytic therapy in the prehospital setting has been addressed by several studies. Most of these studies have assessed the candidacy of patients for prehospital thrombolytic therapy without actually administering thrombolytics. In most of these studies, the paramedics obtained a prehospital ECG, transmitted it to the base hospital, and administered a checklist to the patient of thrombolytic indications and contraindications. **The real utility of these studies was in demonstrating the amount of time saved from ED presentation to definitive therapy when a prehospital ECG had been obtained.** This information is given in Table 13-4.

The Milwaukee Prehospital Chest Pain Project found, as did later studies, that the number of patients who met criteria for field thrombolytic administration was disappointingly low (12 out of 439, or 2.7%). None of these studies has been able to document a thrombolytic therapy candicacy rate greater than 10%. This again emphasizes the difficulty in time commitment and financial expenditure of establishing a program that would be used only occasionally. The Myocardial Infarction Triage Intervention (MITI) trial in Seattle, Washington, has suggested screening criteria for the likeli-

Table 13-4. Feasibility of prehospital thrombolytic therapy

Study	Estimated time savings (min) from ED presentation to therapy	% of all patients with chest pain eligible for prehospital thrombolytic therapy
Milwaukee Prehospital Chest Pain Project	—	2.7
PAST-MI	20	4.2
O'Rourke	60–90*	4.3
Gibler (Nashville study)	—	8.2
Keriakes (Cincinnati study)	20	4.2
Weaver (MITI study)	40	4.1

* Prehospital thrombolytic therapy actually administered—no estimated time saved after ED presentation.

hood of cardiac disease and the presence of AMI. Prehospital ECGs were completed on 1973 patients who met the following criteria: age less than 75 years, duration of pain less than 6 hours, the absence of uncontrolled systolic or diastolic hypertension, recent surgery, syncope, stroke, or known kidney or liver disease. This study's potential inclusion rate for prehospital thrombolytic therapy was then raised to 360 out of 1973 (18%). This percentage clearly stands above projections from other studies, suggesting that screening criteria administered before prehospital ECGs are obtained may make prehospital thrombolytic therapy an attainable goal.

In summary, the acquisition of prehospital ECGs in select patients has proved to be both safe and effective in decreasing the time to definitive treatment in AMI in the urban and suburban setting. The feasibility of prehospital thrombolytic therapy has yet to be fully assessed. Preliminary work shows a low utilization rate and costly expenditures in additional EMS personnel training. Logically, preliminary efforts should be focused on establishing reliable prehospital ECG capabilities throughout the EMS system. Expansion to a prehospital thrombolytic therapy program may be undertaken once safety and efficacy have been proven.

Bibliography

Aufderheide TP, Keelan MH, Hendley GE, et al. Milwaukee Prehospital Chest Pain Project—phase I: feasibility and accuracy of prehospital thrombolytic candidate selection. *Am J Cardiol* 69:991, 1992.

Gibler WB, Aufderheide TP. *Emergency Cardiac Care.* St. Louis: Mosby, 1994.

Grim P, Feldman T, Martin M, et al. Cellular telephone transmission of 12-lead electrocardiograms from ambulance to hospital. *Am J Cardiol* 60:715, 1987.

Keriakes DJ, Weaver WD, Anderson JL, et al. Time delays in the diagnosis and treatment of acute myocardial infarction: a tale of eight cities. Report from the Prehospital Study Group and Cincinnati Heart Project. *Am Heart J* 120:773, 1990.

Weaver WD, Cerqueira M, Hallstrom AP, et al. Prehospital-initiated versus hospital-initiated thrombolytic therapy: the myocardial infarction triage and intervention trial. *JAMA* 270:1211, 1993.

Complications of Acute Myocardial Infarction

Acute Heart Failure and Cardiogenic Shock

Steven C. Carleton

I. **Significance.** Of the 1.5 million annual hospital admissions for acute myocardial infarction (AMI) in the United States, 15% to 20% manifest some degree of cardiac pump failure at the time of initial presentation, and 4% to 7% present in frank circulatory shock. Overall, cardiac pump failure complicates the hospital course of 40% and 60% of all admissions for AMI, and cardiogenic shock and congestive heart failure comprise the leading sources of postinfarction, in-hospital mortality. In the absence of emergent coronary revascularization, mortalities from refractory congestive heart failure and cardiogenic shock exceed 80%. Invasive hemodynamic monitoring, aggressive pharmacotherapy, and mechanical circulatory support have had little influence. However, coupling of these therapeutic modalities with early reperfusion can substantially improve survivorship. Percutaneous transluminal coronary angioplasty (PTCA), in particular, appears to hold promise as the therapy of choice for maximal salvage of patients with severe hemodynamic instability after AMI. Optimal care of the patient with postinfarction circulatory collapse requires an expedient, physiologically-based, directed strategy, which involves appropriate application of fluid and oxygen therapy, mechanical ventilation, pharmacologic support, mechanical circulatory assistance, and reperfusion techniques. Definitive care for such patients must necessarily be delivered in a referral center with the ready availability of personnel and facilities for coronary angiography, angioplasty, and cardiothoracic surgery.

II. **Etiology. Ventricular dysfunction** after AMI reflects the aggregate effects of acute, irreversible myocardial necrosis and reversible myocardial "stunning," myocardial scarring from remote infarctions, unfavorable ventricular loading conditions, and various mechanical complications of AMI. Regardless of the mix of contributing factors, the result is a reduction of ventricular performance to the point where stroke volume (SV) and cardiac output (CO) are compromised. The clinical status of the patient with ventricular power failure is a reflection of the volume of involved myocardium. With ischemic dysfunction of 20% to 25% of the left ventricular (LV) myocardium, signs and symptoms of acute **congestive heart failure** (CHF) occur. The clinical definition of CHF requires the presence of **pulmonary congestion.** The hemodynamic definition requires LV filling pressures to be pathologically elevated, with the pulmonary capillary wedge pressure (PCWP) exceeding 18 mm Hg. With involvement of greater than 35% to 40% of the LV myocardium, cardiac performance is depressed to the point where physiologic compensatory mechanisms are insufficient to maintain coronary, renal, cerebral and peripheral perfusion, and **cardiogenic shock** (CS) ensues. The clinical definition of CS includes a systolic blood pressure less than 90 mm Hg, or a 30% decline in systolic pressure in patients with known hypertension, accompanied by evidence of renal, cerebral, or peripheral hypoperfusion. Hypoperfusion may be reflected as altered mental status, cool, clammy skin, or reduced urine output (< 20 ml/hr). The definition assumes the correction of hypovolemia, hypoxia or dysrhythmia as contributing factors. CS is defined hemodynamically as an intra-arterial systolic blood pressure less than 90 mm Hg, with a cardiac index (CI) of less than 1.8 to 2.0 liter/minute/m^2. Hypoperfusion is generally not clinically evident until CI is less than 2.2 liter/min/m^2. Hypoperfusion may be subclinical in a range of CI from 2.2 to 2.7 liter/min/m^2. It is important to recognize that in the absence of frank hypovolemia, the majority of patients in CS will also manifest some degree of pulmonary congestion.

III. **Pathophysiology.** Experimental studies, autopsy data, and clinical observations suggest that myocardial ischemia progresses over time as a wavefront of necrosis and stunning. The progressive nature of injury accounts for the observed time course of the development of CHF and CS after AMI; the majority of patients do not manifest evidence of ventricular power failure at the time of initial presentation, but develop this complication over a period of hours. When pump failure is evident at the time of initial presentation, or becomes evident during the patient's early hospital course, the natural history is one of rapid worsening toward circulatory collapse. As a critical mass of myocardium becomes involved, signs and symptoms of pump failure develop, and a vicious cycle is established—ischemic injury leading to reduced coronary perfusion that results in further ischemic injury. Interruption of this cycle is central to the successful management of the hemodynamically compromised patient. It is of paramount importance that the consequences of various therapeutic interventions on myocardial energetics are understood. Situations that worsen the myocardial oxygen supply and demand balance, and increase the potential for infarct extension, must be avoided. It is also of critical importance that the concepts describing the response of the myocardium to altered loading conditions are understood. It is through these concepts that the physiologic rationale for therapy is formed.

A. **Preload.** The Frank-Starling relationship states that the developed tension of an individual myocardial fiber increases in direct proportion to the initial fiber length or stretch. The degree of initial fiber stretch is defined as **preload.** In the intact heart, preload is equivalent to the end-diastolic volume (EDV) of the ventricle. EDV relates directly to end-diastolic pressure (EDP) in a nonlinear fashion that is determined by the diastolic compliance of the ventricle. LVEDP can be estimated by PCWP, whereas developed tension roughly corresponds to CI. As such, the Frank-Starling relationship can be reformulated to relate CI to PCWP, allowing the contruction of a **ventricular function curve** (Fig. 14-1). This relationship predicts brisk increases in CI as ventricular filling pressures rise over the range describing the steep portion of the curve. Over the flat portion of the curve, successive incremental

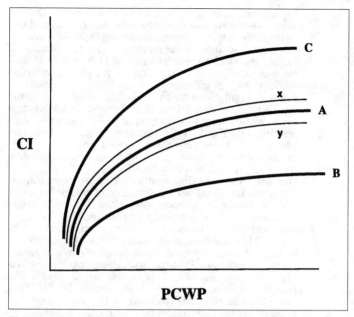

Fig. 14-1. A family of ventricular function curves showing the relationship between PCWP and CI at (A) baseline, (B) in the setting of LV failure, and (C) with augmented LV contractility. Note that loss of contractility is reflected by shift of the curve downward and to the right (A to B), whereas increased contractility results in a shift of the curve upward and to the left (A to C). The x and y curves represent parallel shifts of the ventricular function curve with reduced (x) and increased (y) afterload. At any given level of preload and contractile state, reduction of afterload results in increased ventricular emptying, whereas increased afterload causes a reduction in ventricular emptying.

increases in PCWP result in only modest gains in CI. There is a peak in the curve beyond which further increases in PCWP result in no further improvement in cardiac performance. Depression of contractility is reflected graphically as flattening and shifting of the curve downward and to the right (A to B). This predicts a lower CI for any given filling pressure and a reduced gain in CI for any given increase in PCWP. Augmentation of contractility results in steepening of the curve and a shift upward and to the left (A to C). With increased contractility, CI is greater for any given level of filling pressure, and incremental elevations of PCWP result in greater increases in cardiac performance than in the basal state.

B. Afterload. The velocity of shortening of a myocardial fiber varies inversely with the load imposed on the fiber during contraction. The load imposed on the myocardium during contraction is defined as **afterload** and represents ventricular wall stress during systole. The determinants of afterload for the intact heart are multifactorial but can be approximated by mean aortic pressure for the LV. Velocity of shortening directly relates to CI. At a fixed inotropic state, a fall in afterload augments systolic ventricular emptying, thereby increasing CI. As the fraction of ejected ventricular volume increases, LVEDP falls. Reductions in afterload thus can improve peripheral perfusion while reducing pulmonary congestion. The effects of changes in afterload on the Frank-Starling relationship are reflected as parallel shifts in the ventricular function curve without any attendant change in ventricular contractility (see Fig. 14-1). Integrating the effects of contractility, preload, and afterload permits prediction of the results of volume loading, diuretics, inotropes, vasodilators, and pressors on pump function.

C. **Diastolic dysfunction and ventricular compliance.** Although the principal determinant of pump failure in AMI is systolic dysfunction, alterations in diastolic relaxation contribute significantly to pathologic elevations of ventricular filling pressure. Myocardial infarction and ischemia alter the visco-elastic properties of the ventricular wall, producing stiffening and reduced diastolic distensibility. Ischemia also leads to incomplete ventricular relaxation during diastole. This reduction in myocardial compliance yields large increases in ventricular EDP for a given increment in EDV relative to the basal state. Decreased ventricular compliance limits the beneficial effects of increasing preload on CI that are achievable through the Frank-Starling mechanism. In the setting of a noncompliant ventricle, unacceptable levels of LV filling pressure with resultant pulmonary congestion may occur before CI can be significantly improved by volume loading.

D. **Myocardial energetics.** The determinants of myocardial oxygen consumption include heart rate, myocardial contractility, and ventricular wall tension. In AMI with hemodynamic compromise, physiologic compensation for reduced cardiac output increases myocardial oxygen requirements through reflex tachycardia and stimulation of contractility. Neurohumeral compensation after AMI also increases systemic vascular resistance and afterload, elevating LV filling pressures. Elevated filling pressures and reduced myocardial compliance increase ventricular wall tension through the Laplace's law, further increasing myocardial oxygen demand. The myocardium is unable to increase oxygen extraction in the face of ischemia, depending instead on coronary vasodilation to increase oxygen delivery in the face of rising metabolic demand. With fixed proximal stenoses, the coronary circulation is unable to increase oxygen delivery through this mechanism. With superimposed reduction of mean coronary perfusion pressure to less than 60 to 70 mm Hg, coronary autoregulation fails and coronary flow cannot be maintained in response to further decreases in aortic root pressure.

Myocardial oxygen supply may be further compromised by reduced atrial oxygen content. Hypoxemia is encountered in 80% of patients after AMI. With moderate congestive failure, the mean value of PaO_2 is 71 mm Hg. The mean PaO_2 in patients with frank alveolar edema or shock is less than 60 mm Hg. Hypoxemia after AMI principally occurs as a consequence of ventilation-perfusion mismatching and shunting within the pulmonary circulation. As pulmonary congestion progresses and closing volume exceeds functional residual capacity, small airways collapse, ventilation of distal alveoli is decreased, hypoxic pulmonary vasoconstriction occurs, intrapulmonary shunts develop, ventilation-perfusion mismatching becomes prominent, and hypoxemia worsens. The already unfavorable myocardial energetics encountered in AMI are enhanced. Ischemia progresses, and in the absence of effective intervention, progression toward circulatory collapse is unchecked.

IV. **The clinical syndrome of congestive heart failure in AMI**

   A. **Presentation.** The clinical presentation of AMI complicated by CHF or CS is generally distinctive and characteristic. The diagnosis usually can be established quickly by history, physical findings, electrocardiography, and chest film. Often, initial therapeutic interventions must precede definitive diagnosis.

   1. **History.** In the setting of hemodynamically complicated AMI, the history is most useful as a means of establishing a connection between the observed findings of acute congestive failure or shock and the inciting event of myocardial injury. Historical findings commonly will reveal classic cardiac risk factors or an established history of ischemic disease. Although AMI with hemodynamic compromise may occur as the initial manifestation of atherosclerotic coronary artery disease, it more commonly represents the superimposition of a new infarction on a previously damaged heart. Classically, the patient will complain of typical cardiac chest pain, generally of acute onset and greater than 10-minutes duration (see Chap. 9). Complaints of dyspnea should alert the clinician to the potential for significant pulmonary congestion in any patient presenting with an ischemic history. The inability of the patient to supply a cogent history should alert the physician to the possibility of inadequate cerebral perfusion pressure or advanced hypoxia. Alternative sources of historical information, including family, pre-hospital personnel, and the medical record should be sought aggressively in this circumstance.

   2. **Physical examination.** Physical findings in CS and acute CHF reflect the peripheral and end-organ effects of low cardiac output, the results of elevated ventricular filling pressures on the pulmonary and systemic venous circulations, and the changes in cardiac mechanisms imposed by ventricular dilatation, segmental wall motion abnormalities, and altered valvular function.

      a. **Inspection.** Physical findings on inspection that suggest pulmonary congestion include tachypnea, nasal flaring, use of accessory respiratory muscles, chest retractions, and expiratory grunting. A cough may be present, and in severe pulmonary edema it will produce pink, frothy sputum. The patient in congestive failure may be observed to prefer a seated or standing posture. Elevated central venous pressures may present as jugular venous distension. Findings suggestive of peripheral hypoperfusion include pallor, diaphoresis, and altered mental status. Changes in mental status accompanying CS or hypoxia secondary to severe CHF may include anxiety, agitation, obtundation, lethargy, or complete unresponsiveness. Inspection of the chest wall may reveal a hyperdynamic precordium.

b. **Palpation.** Cool, clammy skin reflects peripheral vasoconstriction and sympathetic overactivity in response to reduced CI. Palpation of the precordium may reveal thrills secondary to valvular dysfunction and precordial heaves or the downward and lateral displacement of the point of maximal impulse indicating chamber enlargement or ventricular dyskinesia.

c. **Auscultation.** Rales are considered to be the defining physical finding of **pulmonary congestion.** Rales generally begin in the dependent lung fields but progress to involve all lung fields as pulmonary edema becomes generalized. Auscultation also may reveal expiratory wheezing that results from bronchospasm or peribronchiolar edema. It should be recognized, however, that significant elevations of LV filling pressure may occur without any accompanying auscultatory findings. Rales are only audible with the advent of alveolar edema and are absent in even severe interstitial edema. Because the signs and symptoms of pulmonary congestion overlap those of obstructive airway disease to a considerable extent, a chest x-ray may be required to assist in differentiation.

Auscultation **of the precordium** may reveal a soft or inaudible first heart sound (S_1), suggesting decreased ventricular contractility, and accentuation of the pulmonic component of the second heart sound (P_2), indicating pulmonary hypertension. The presence of a third (S_3) or fourth (S_4) heart sound reflects ventricular noncompliance during rapid ventricular filling and atrial systole. The presence of a new holosystolic murmur at the apex or left lower sternal border suggests acute mitral regurgitation or ventricular septal defect.

B. **Assessment**

1. **Laboratory studies.** Laboratory evaluation is generally of little importance in the evaluation and management of hemodynamic instability accompanying AMI. As an exception, arterial blood gases can be extremely useful in identifying hypoxia as an indication of subclinical pulmonary congestion or acidemia as an indication of subclinical peripheral hypoperfusion. In-

terpretation of any acidemia discovered on blood gas analysis would be assisted by a renal panel. Although of little value in the acute management of the patient, a complete blood count, coagulation profile, and cardiac enzyme series should be sent for to establish pretreatment base lines. Anticipation of the need for thrombolysis or invasive interventions mandates collection of blood for type and crossmatch.

2. **Electrocardiography.** Electrocardiography is essential in establishing the diagnosis of AMI in patients presenting with acute pump failure. Generally, infarctions resulting in CS and severe CHF are large and transmural. Anterior MIs are more commonly represented than inferior MIs in the population of patients with hemodynamic instability because of the larger volume of LV myocardium at risk with thrombotic occlusion of the left anterior descending coronary artery. Occasionally, the ECG may be nondiagnostic in this setting. Electrocardiography also permits rapid recognition of rhythm disturbances that may contribute to compromised cardiac performance.

3. **Chest x-ray.** Radiographic findings of pulmonary congestion occur in an orderly progression as LV filling pressures increase. At mildly elevated pressures, there is redistribution of pulmonary blood flow to the upper lobe vasculature. The appearance of this redistribution pattern on the chest film is considered to be the earliest reliable clinical sign of LV failure. As LV filling pressures continue to rise, there is transudation of intravascular fluid into the interstitial spaces of the lung, resulting in perivascular and peribronchial cuffing, Kerley septal lines, visible fluid in the fissures, or a diffuse reticular pattern in the lung fields. Further elevation of LV filling pressures leads to alveolar edema. Alveolar edema has a variety of radiographic manifestations, including perihilar "batwing" densities, or diffuse densities that may be uniformly distributed, patchy, or confined to the dependent lung fields. Because the development of auscultatory or radiographic pulmonary congestion may lag behind measured increases in PCWP by many hours, the absence of physical or radiographic findings of congestion should not be interpreted as evidence of normal filling pressures in the patient with subjective complaints or objective findings of respiratory compromise.

4. **Echocardiography.** Echocardiography can rapidly confirm the presence of global or regional LV wall motion abnormalities and valvular regurgitation, define the adequacy of RV and septal function, and ascertain the existence of various mechanical complications of AMI when the etiology of shock or congestive failure is uncertain.

5. **Swan-Ganz catheterization.** Pulmonary artery catheterization represents the "gold standard" for the assessment of hemodynamic status and provides a

means for monitoring the response to therapy in real time. Typically, the patient with LV dysfunction will exhibit an elevation in PCWP, and decreased CI. Invasive hemodynamic monitoring offers the only method for tailoring therapy to the specific pathophysiology of the patient. The pulmonary artery catheter allows for the direct measurement of right atrial pressure, right ventricular systolic and diastolic pressures, pulmonary artery systolic and diastolic pressures, pulmonary artery occlusive (or capillary wedge) pressure, and cardiac output. Pulmonary artery catheterization allows for the calculation of SV, stroke work, pulmonary and systemic vascular resistance, coronary perfusion pressure, and indices of peripheral oxygen transport and utilization (see Chap. 8, sec. **III**). In the setting of AMI with hemodynamic instability, the pulmonary artery catheter is utilized most appropriately as a means of optimizing filling pressures and gauging physiologic response to therapeutic interventions. Use of the pulmonary artery catheter clearly is indicated in any patient suffering CS or CHF who fails to respond to initial, empiric pharmacotherapy.

6. **Arterial pressure monitoring.** Because auscultated cuff blood pressures are notoriously inaccurate in the setting of hemodynamic instability, direct measurement of arterial pressures via an intra-arterial catheter should be considered in any patient with hypotension or hypoperfusion after AMI. In addition to allowing accurate, serial determinations of blood pressure, the arterial line allows for serial blood gas determinations that may be critical in determining the course of respiratory therapy offered to the patient.

C. **Patient classification.** Patients may be classified by clinical or hemodynamic status after AMI. Classification schemes are useful in mortality prediction and for stratification of patients into physiologically distinct subsets that can be utilized to direct therapy. Several different classifications have been developed, each with its own utility.

1. **Killip classification.** The original Killip classification (Table 14-1) segregates patients into four functional categories based on presenting clinical findings. It is predictive of mortality but does not relate clinical and hemodynamic status within patient groups. Modifications of the Killip classification relate the four functional categories to parallel measurements of hemodynamic parameters (Table 14-2).

2. **Forrester classification.** The Forrester classification (Table 14-3) segregates patients based on the presence or absence of clinical pulmonary congestion and peripheral hypoperfusion and relates these clinical findings to specific hemodynamic states. In developing this classification it was demonstrated that the presence of clinical pulmonary congestion accurately predicted a PCWP of greater than 18 mm Hg, whereas the presence of clinical hypoperfusion accurately predicted a CI of less than 2.2 liter/min/m^2. By the For-

Table 14-1.   Killip classification of patients with acute myocardial infarction

	Definition	Patients with acute myocardial infarction admitted to CCU in this category (%)	Approximate mortality (%)
Class I	Absence of rales over the lung fields and absence of S_3	30–40	8
Class II	Rales over 50% or less of the lung fields or the presence of an S_3	30–50	30
Class III	Rales over more than 50% of the lung fields (frequently pulmonary edema)	5–10	44
Class IV	Shock	10	80–100

Source: Pasternak RC, Brauwald E, Sobel BE. Acute myocardial infarction. In Brauwald E, (ed.), *Heart Disease: A Textbook of Cardiovascular Medicine* (3rd ed.). Philadelphia: Saunders, 1988:1237. Also from Killip T. Treatment of myocardial infarction in a coronary care unit. *Am J Cardiol* 1967;20:459. Adapted with permission from *American Journal of Cardiology.*

rester classification, all patients in subsets IV and many in subset III are in CS, whereas patients in subsets II and IV have significant CHF. Subset I represents patients with uncomplicated MI. The most common predictive error of this classification scheme is its failure to recognize significant but subclinical reductions in CI in up to 44% of patients classified in subset II. As such, there should be considerable suspicion of depressed CI in any patient who lacks physical findings of hypoperfusion but demonstrates clinical pulmonary congestion. Although the Forrester classification also misses approximately 15% of significant elevations in PCWP, these occur almost exclusively in subset I and are not characterized by any mortality difference from patients in subset I who do not have elevated PCWP. Like the Killip classification, Forrester subset classification predicts mortality. The mortality rates in subsets I, II, III, and IV are 2.2%, 10.1%, 22.4%, and 55.5%, respectively. Mortality in subset II is limited to those patients with subclinical depression of CI. By allowing the prediction of hemodynamic status based on clinical findings, subset classification allows for the initiation of therapy based on physiologic principles when invasive monitoring is unavailable and defines specific therapeutic goals for patients classified to each subset. This latter feature renders the

Table 14-2.   Classification of left ventricular failure after acute myocardial infarction

	Class I	Class II	Class III	Class IV
Clinical				
Consciousness	Normal	Worried	Anxious	Restless, subcomatose
Skin	Warm, dry	Tepid	Cool, dry	Cold, moist, cyanosis
Pulse	Normal	Normal	Weak	Very weak, absent
Heart sounds	Normal	Normal	Soft	Very soft
Gallops	No S_3	No S_3	S_3, S_4	S_3, S_4
Moist rales <	None	Bases	10–15 cm	Pulmonary edema
Chest roentgenogram	Normal	Dilatation of upper lobar veins	Interstitial edema	Alveolar edema
Hemodynamic				
HR (min^{-1})	70–85	85–100	90–110	>100
BP (mm Hg)	>90	80–90	60–80	<60
PAP (mm Hg)	<12	12–14	14–18	>18
CI (liters·min^{-1}·m^{-2})	>3.0	2.5–3.0	2.0–2.5	<2.0
LVW (liter·mm Hg·min^{-1}·m^{-2})	>270	200–270	120–200	<120
SWI (ml·mm Hg·m^{-2})	>3000	2000–3000	1200–2000	<1200
Urine (ml·hr^{-1})	>50	40–50	20–40	<20

BP = mean arterial pressure; CI = cardiac index; HR = heart rate; LVW = left ventricular work; SWI = stroke work index; Urine = urine production.
Source: Hagemeijer F. Effectiveness of intraaortic balloon pumping without cardiac surgery for patients with severe heart failure secondary to a recent myocardial infarction. *Am J Cardiol* 1977;40:952. Reprinted with permission from *American Journal of Cardiology.*

Table 14-3. The Forrester classification of hemodynamic status after AMI defining four clinical subsets and providing hemodynamic correlates to each subset

Subset	CI	PCP
I. No pulmonary congestion or peripheral hypoperfusion	2.7 ± 0.5	12 ± 7
II. Isolated pulmonary congestion	2.3 ± 0.4	23 ± 5
III. Isolated peripheral hypoperfusion	1.9 ± 0.4	12 ± 5
IV. Both pulmonary congestion and hypoperfusion	1.6 ± 0.6	27 ± 8

Source: Forrester A. Correlative classification of clinical and hemodynamic function after acute myocardial infarction. *Am J Cardiol* 1977;39:137. Reprinted with permission from *American Journal of Cardiology.*

Forrester classification useful even when hemodynamic monitoring is available. It cannot be overemphasized that the accurate assessment of CI, PCWP, and arterial pressure is essential to formulating a rational, physiologically-based treatment plan.

D. Management. Management of AMI with pump failure is directed at restoring and maintaining adequate cardiac output, reducing pulmonary congestion, optimizing peripheral oxygen delivery, and salvaging ischemic myocardium. Attainment of the first three of these four goals must be balanced against the potential for precipitating increased myocardial oxygen demand or reduced coronary perfusion pressure as a consequence of therapeutic interventions. Interventions that increase ventricular wall tension, heart rate, and myocardial contractility, or reduce systemic vascular resistance and aortic root pressure should be applied cautiously and monitored closely.

1. **Supportive care**
   a. **Oxygenation and ventilation.** Any patient who exhibits altered mental status or is unable to protect the airway should be immediately intubated. Patients who are alert and making adequate respiratory effort should be placed on supplemental O_2 with a goal of maintaining a PaO_2 of greater than 60 to 70 mm Hg, or an arterial oxygen saturation (SaO_2) greater than 90%. If there is any clinical evidence of pulmonary congestion, O_2 should be administered by face mask at 10 to 15 liter/minute. Arterial blood gases should be obtained on initial presentation and periodically thereafter to monitor the efficacy of therapy. Continuous pulse oximetry can be used for the early detection of hypoxemia. End-tidal CO_2 monitoring can be used for the early detection of hypoventilation. If the patient with a stable airway is observed to tire, or if oxygenation or ventilation become inadequate, the patient should be intubated or given a trial continuous positive airway pressure (CPAP) by face mask. In

the intubated patient, reductions in preload should be anticipated if high levels of positive end-expiratory pressure (PEEP) are required to maintain oxygenation.

b. **Positioning.** If blood pressure permits, the patient with pulmonary congestion should be placed in the seated position with dangling legs. This position can significantly reduce venous return and LV filling pressures, thereby increasing vital capacity, decreasing the work of breathing, and reducing pulmonary congestion. If the patient is hypotensive and must be placed supine or in reverse Trendelenburg position, reductions in vital capacity and functional residual capacity should be anticipated.

c. **Heart rate and rhythm.** Primary ventricular **dysrhythmias** and supraventricular **tachycardias** of nonsinus origin may precipitate hemodynamic deterioration and unfavorable myocardial energetics and should be aggressively treated (see Chaps. 16 and 17). **Bradycardia** is poorly tolerated in patients with depressed stroke volume, and should be promptly reversed with atropine or pacing if hypotension is present. If pacing is required, sequential atrioventricular pacing may offer hemodynamic advantages over ventricular demand pacing by preserving the salutary effects of atrial systole on ventricular filling. A heart rate of 90–100 bpm should be the therapeutic goal in treating symptomatic bradycardia.

Sinus tachycardia after AMI may represent a necessary compensatory adjustment for reduced CO but can limit diastolic filling, reduce SV and exacerbate myocardial ischemia when rates are excessive (>120 bpm). Noncompensatory sinus tachycardia may occur as a result of pain or anxiety. **Morphine sulfate** administered in intravenous doses of 4 to 10 mg may be useful in treating noncompensatory sinus tachycardia, and offers the potential benefit of improved myocardial O_2 delivery mediated through a reduction of coronary vascular resistance and reduced pulmonary congestion mediated through a reduction in pulmonary vascular resistance. However, because morphine can cause generalized dilation of capacitance and resistance vessels, it should be used cautiously to avoid precipitation of hypotension. Although beta-adrenergic blocking agents are useful for the treatment of noncompensatory sinus tachycardia after AMI, these agents have not proven useful in the treatment of CS or postinfarction CHF and are, in fact, contraindicated in the setting of pump failure due to their negative inotropic effects.

d. **Fluid therapy.** Patients presenting with hypotension or other evidence of hypoperfusion should have intravenous access established with two large-bore IV lines. A trial of volume expansion is indicated as long as evidence of clinical or hemodynamic pulmonary congestion is absent. In approximately 20% of patients with AMI and shock, hemodynamic monitoring demonstrates frank hypovolemia at the time of presentation. In this significant minority the signs and symptoms of shock may be reversed solely by volume expansion. Appropriate fluids for volume expansion include isotonic crystalloid, hydroxyethyl starch solutions, and high-molecular-weight dextran solutions. There are no compelling advantages to the use of colloid solutions in preference to crystalloid for resuscitation from shock, and normal saline or lactated Ringer's solution may be used with confidence.

If invasive hemodynamic monitoring is not available, fluid should be administered in small volumes (100 ml) over 5- to 10-minute intervals with careful reassessment of blood pressure, heart rate, peripheral perfusion, and breath sounds between successive administrations. If invasive hemodynamic monitoring is available, volume should be administered until a PCWP of 18 mm Hg is attained. Volume loading to this level of LV filling pressure will maximize SV by the Frank-Starling mechanism without precipitating significant pulmonary congestion. Volume loading beyond this level is unlikely to further augment cardiac output and may result in alveolar edema and compromised gas exchange. Even when volume loading is unsuccessful in reversing hypotension and hypoperfusion, optimization of LV filling pressures by volume administration will permit maximal benefit from the subsequent use of inotropic agents.

2. **Specific pharmacotherapy**

   a. **Diuretics.** Diuretics are used to reduce intravascular volume, thereby relieving the signs and symptoms of elevated LV filling pressure. The agents of choice for acute pulmonary congestion are loop diuretics. Although extremely useful for the treatment of pulmonary congestion, loop diuretics should be used with caution in patients with significant ventricular dysfunction. As a group, these agents induce a potent natriuretic diuresis within minutes of administration. Diuresis may induce delayed hemodynamic deterioration through excessive reduction of preload if overzealously applied. Hypokalemia is also a potential danger. The prototypic agent for the treatment of pulmonary congestion is intravenous furosemide. Bumetanide and ethacrynate sodium, although effective as loop diuretics, offer no compelling advantages in comparison to furosemide.

      (1) **Furosemide.** Furosemide induces a diuresis with onset at 5 minutes. Peak effect occurs at

30 to 60 minutes. Furosemide also has direct hemodynamic effects that precede the onset of diuresis, inducing dilation of capacitance vessels and reduction of preload within minutes after administration. The acute hemodynamic effects of furosemide are maximized at a dose of 20 mg IV. The diuretic effects increase linearly with dose. In patients with acute pulmonary edema, the starting dose of furosemide is generally 40 mg IV. This may be repeated or doubled at 20-minute intervals if initial therapeutic response is inadequate. In patients with antecedent chronic renal insufficiency, initial doses of 80–160 mg may be required for the production of significant diuresis.

(2) **Bumetanide.** Bumetanide is administered in doses of 0.5–1.0 mg IV. Onset of diuretic effect can be anticipated to begin within minutes, with peak effect at 15 to 30 minutes after administration.

(3) **Ethacrynate sodium.** This sodium salt of ethacrynic acid is administered in doses of 0.5–1.0 mg/kg, or 50 mg IV. Onset of diuretic action is within 5 minutes of administration, with peak effects and duration of action following a similar time course as for furosemide.

b. **Vasodilators.** Vasodilators are useful for the reduction of both preload and afterload; predominant hemodynamic effects vary with the principal site of action of the agent selected. Preload reduction is accomplished by dilation of venous capacitance vessels. The signs and symptoms of pulmonary congestion are relieved as central blood volume is redistributed to the periphery and ventricular filling pressures fall. Afterload reduction is accomplished through dilation of resistance vessels. This augments cardiac output by allowing more complete systolic emptying of the ventricle.

Afterload reduction can reduce filling pressures through this mechanism, as well. **Nitroglycerine (NTG)** is primarily a venodilator, though arteriolar dilation and afterload reduction occur in higher dose ranges. **Sodium nitroprusside (NP)** is a balanced vasodilator, affecting both arteriolar and venous tone at conventional doses. **Captopril,** an angiotensin converting enzyme ACE-inhibitor, and **phentolamine,** an alpha-adrenergic antagonist, act principally as afterload reducers.

(1) **Nitroglycerine.** Because of proven efficacy, safety, and ease of use, NTG has emerged as the drug of choice for acute ischemic pulmonary congestion. At conventional doses NTG reduces PCWP by 29% to 50% with little change in blood pressure or heart rate. CI is generally preserved or even increased. NTG dilates coronary conductance vessels and collat-

eral channels, increasing blood flow to areas of ischemic myocardium and protecting watershed areas. The hemodynamic effects of NTG also reduce ventricular wall stress, thereby decreasing myocardial O_2 demand. Infarct expansion is limited as long as critical reductions in coronary perfusion pressure are avoided. NTG should be administered cautiously in patients with a systolic blood pressure less than 110 mm Hg, and strictly avoided when systolic pressure is less than 90 mm Hg. Maxmal benefit is obtained when mean arterial pressure is maintained above 80 mm Hg, and benefit is lost when mean pressure falls below 70 mm Hg.

End points for therapy with NTG are a 10% decline in mean arterial pressure without lowering systolic pressure below 90 mm Hg, an increase in heart rate not exceeding 20 bpm, a decrease of 30% in PCWP, or a maximum dosage of 200 µg/min. When pretreatment blood pressure is borderline, NTG can be coadministered with dobutamine to permit safe exploitation of its desirable effects on hemodynamics and myocardial O_2 supply/demand balance.

NTG may be administered in sublingual, topical, and intravenous formulations. Sublingual and topical NTG are useful primarily as a bridge until IV therapy can be started. Sublingual administration is initiated with 0.4–1.2 mg, which may be repeated at 5- to 10-minute intervals. Onset of action is 2 minutes, with peak effect at 8 to 10 minutes and a duration of action of approximately 20 minutes. NTG is applied topically as ½ to 2 inches of 2% ointment. The onset of hemodynamic effects of topical NTG are delayed approximately 30 minutes and can persist from 3 to 6 hours. IV administration of NTG is initiated by continuous infusion at 10–20 µg/min and is titrated upward at increments of 10 µg/min at 3- to 5-minute intervals until therapeutic end-points are achieved. Venodilatation and preload reduction predominate at dosages less than 50 µg/min. Infusion rates of 20–100 µg/min are commonly encountered.

(2) **Sodium nitroprusside.** NP is a balanced vasodilator, having nearly equivalent effects on resistance and capacitance vessels. It is useful principally as an afterload reducer and can dramatically improve SV and CO in the failing heart, particularly in the setting of arterial hypertension complicating CHF. NP is not as effective as NTG at reducing LV filling pressure, but can achieve 25% reductions of PCWP in patients with severe LV failure and markedly elevated filling pressures.

The hemodynamic effects of NP and intravenous NTG in AMI are comparable, but available evidence suggests that NP has significant disadvantages when applied in the setting of acute myocardial ischemia. Although NP decreases myocardial O_2 requirements by reducing afterload, preload, and ventricular wall stress, it may extend ischemic damage by redistributing coronary blood flow away from zones of ischemic myocardium and through induction of reflex tachycardia and inadequate coronary perfusion pressure.

NP is administered by continuous IV infusion. Therapy is generally initiated at 10 μg/min and titrated upward in increments of 5 to 10 μg/min at 5-minute intervals until therapeutic end points or dose-limiting hypotension is achieved. NP is particularly effective in reducing the regurgitant fraction and improving CO in severe mitral insufficiency, and is probably most appropriately reserved for this purpose and for pump failure complicated by severe hypertension.

(3) Captopril. Captopril has not been studied in a controlled fashion for the treatment of CS or acute ischemic CHF, but has shown utility for this indication in small case-series and anecdotal reports. Inhibition of the peripheral conversion of angiotensin-I to angiotensin-II reduces afterload, increasing CI and urine output while reducing PCWP. Captopril also may inhibit deleterious effects of angiotensin-II on coronary blood flow, improving myocardial O_2 supply; administration of captopril to patients with acute ischemia reduces anginal symptoms and ST-segment depression. Use of captopril for acute ventricular power failure is inhibited by inconvenient dosing and unfavorable pharmacokinetics.

Captopril can be administered intravenously as a 1 mg/min infusion to a total of 25 mg every 6 hours or by sublingual, oral, and nasogastric routes. It has a protracted half-life compared with NP or NTG, and is therefore less titratable than these standard agents.

(4) Phentolamine. Phentolamine is an arteriolar vasodilator. It reduces afterload and improves SV and cardiac output in the setting of acute ischemic pump failure. Therapy is initiated by IV infusion at 0.1 mg/min and increased in increments of 0.1 mg/min at 5-minute intervals to a maximum dose of 2.0 mg/min. Phentolamine is hampered by its effects on myocardial oxygen consumption. It commonly induces reflex tachycardia and may directly precipitate nodal tachycardia by causing release of cardiac norepinephrine. It is less titratable than either

NP or NTG, and has no compelling advantages to support its use over these agents in the treatment of AMI complicated by pump failure.

c. **Inotropes and pressors.** Inotropic therapy for acute pump failure is directed at the fundamental pathophysiologic consequence of myocardial ischemia and necrosis—loss of contractility. Pressors are utilized to maintain perfusion pressure in the range supporting autoregulation in the vascular beds of critical organs. Several classes of inotropic agents have been applied as initial therapy for acute pump failure after AMI, including adrenoreceptor agonists, cardiac glycosides, and phosphodiesterase inhibitors. Two agents, dopamine (DA) and dobutamine (DB), have emerged as the inotropes of choice. DA, in addition to its utility as an inotrope, can be utilized for pressure support in the hypotensive patient with adequate ventricular systolic function.

(1) **Dopamine.** DA is a naturally occurring metabolic precursor to norepinephrine (NE). It is administered by continuous IV infusion, and has well-characterized hemodynamic effects that vary in a predictable manner with increasing doses. DA acts by interacting directly with adrenoreceptors and releasing endogenous myocardial and vascular NE.

At dosages less than 2.5 µg/kg/min, the predominant action of DA is mediated through specific dopaminergic receptors (DA_1-receptors) in the renal, splanchnic, and coronary vasculature. Stimulation of these receptors causes vasodilation and increased organ blood flow. Systemic vascular resistance falls by up to 20%. Interaction with myocardial $beta_1$ receptors at dosages from 2.5 to 5 µg/kg/min stimulates heart rate and contractility. Stroke volume and cardiac output increase with little change in peripheral vascular tone. At dosages from 5 to 10 µg/kg/min, $alpha_1$-adrenergic effects are superimposed on $beta_1$ effects. Mean arterial pressure and systemic vascular resistance increase, and PCWP rises by approximately one-third. Perfusion of the viscera and skin are reduced. Gains in CO induced by $beta_1$ stimulation are largely preserved. Heart rate increases between 10% and 20%. At dosages in excess of 10 µg/kg/min, alpha effects completely dominate and SV falls in the face of excessive afterload. As infusion rates approach 20 µg/kg/min the hemodynamic effects of DA parallel those of NE.

DA has significant arrhythmogenic potential at doses that increase heart rate and increases all of the determinants of myocardial O_2 consumption. As such, there are potential dangers inherent to its use as an inotrope. Although DA is extremely useful as a pressor, infusion rates that produce significant alpha-effects tend to offset improvements in coronary perfusion pressure with disadvantageous increases in coronary vascular resistance.

(2) **Dobutamine.** DB acts principally as an agonist at myocardial beta$_1$ receptors. Weak beta$_2$ and alpha effects exist, but balance over the clinically useful dosage range. DB does not release endogenous NE. It is administered by continuous infusion at an initial rate of 2.5 μg/kg/min, and is titrated to effect in increments of 2–3 μg/kg/min at 10- to 30-minute intervals. Desired effects are commonly obtained at dosages from 7.5 to 15 μg/kg/min. Arrhythmogenic, positive chronotropic, and peripheral vasodilatory effects limit use at higher doses. At conventional infusion rates, DB produces dose-dependent increases in SV with little chronotropic effect. PCWP is reduced secondary to improved systolic emptying and mild venodilation. Systemic vascular resistance falls in response to weak beta$_2$ effects and the stimulation of carotid baroreceptors by forceful systolic ejection, but reductions in mean arterial pressure are prevented by augmentation of cardiac output. Increases in mean arterial pressure of up to 25% have been observed after administration of DB, though reduced or static blood pressures are more commonly noted. DB is not a clinically important pressor, and can cause hypotension when administered at dosages of 20 μg/kg/min.

DB has complex effects on myocardial energetics. While myocardial O_2 consumption is increased in concert with increased contractility, O_2 requirements are reduced as filling pressures and ventricular wall stress decline. The effects of wall stress reduction appear to predominate in the setting of LV failure. As long as increases in heart rate of greater than 10% or reductions in mean arterial pressure (MAP) to less than 70 mm Hg are avoided, the aggregate effects of DB on myocardial energetics appear to be neutral or even mildly beneficial.

In comparison to DA, DB produces significantly greater increases in CI. MAP improves significantly with DA, but changes little with DB. DA significantly increases PCWP, whereas DB causes slight reductions. DA has greater positive chronotropic and arrhythmogenic effects. The choice of one agent over the other is dependent on the pretreatment hemodynamic status of the patient. When there is peripheral hypoperfusion and significant hypotension, DA is preferred for its ability to increase MAP and restore adequate coronary, cerebral, and renal perfusion. In the patient with significant pulmonary congestion and only mild hypotension, DB is preferable. Coadministration of both agents at the modest infusion rate of 7.5 µg/kg/min in patients with hypoperfusion, hypotension, and pulmonary congestion minimizes the disadvantageous effects of the individual drugs while exploiting the salutary effects of both.

(3) **Norepinephrine.** NE is a beta$_1$- and alpha-adrenergic agonist across its dosage range. NE augments contractility, but this effect is offset by potent peripheral vasoconstrictive effects. Gains in cardiac output are of lesser magnitude than those achievable with DA and DB, while CI actually decreases when systolic blood pressure is elevated above 90 mm Hg. Other undesirable effects on renal and coronary blood flow, ventricular filling pressures, and myocardial energetics limit the efficacy of NE as an inotrope. Its principal utility is as a pressor that preserves CO to a greater extent than pure alpha-agents. In the setting of AMI, NE is best utilized to maintain MAP between 70 and 80 mm Hg in patients who fail to respond to DA. Therapy with NE is initiated at an infusion rate of 8–12 µg/kg/min then adjusted upward or downward as indicated by clinical response.

(4) **Digitalis glycosides.** Cardiac glycosides are useful inotropes for the treatment of chronic CHF but have significant disadvantages for the emergent management of acute pump failure. Digoxin is not titratable to effect, having a serum half-life of greater than 30 hours and a delayed onset of hemodynamic effect. It is a significantly less-potent inotrope than DB, producing less than one-third of the improvement in CO seen with the latter agent. It has no beneficial effect on ventricular filling pressures or wall stress, and may worsen myocardial energetics as contractility improves.

(5) **Phosphodiesterase-III (PDE-III) inhibitors.** The effects of beta-adrenergic agonists are mediated at the cellular level by increases in intracellular cyclic adenosine monophosphate (cAMP). Inhibition of PDE-III similarly can increase intracellular cAMP, causing changes in ventricular contractility and vascular smooth muscle tone identical to changes seen after administration of beta agonists. PDE-III inhibitors have been applied in the treatment of acute congestive failure and CS but have not been investigated in a controlled manner for this indication. **Amrinone,** the parent drug of this class, increases CI by 50% while reducing PCWP and SVR by 25% to 30%

when administered to patients with CHF. Amrinone generally reduces MAP and is unsuitable for use in the hypotensive patient. Amrinone improves myocardial energetics by reducing oxygen demand in the absence of ischemia, but is associated with infarct extension in the setting of acute coronary occlusion.

Therapy with amrinone is initiated by bolus injection of 0.75–1.50 mg/kg, followed by continuous infusion at 5 to 40 µg/kg/min. Vasodilator effects predominate at lower infusion rates. Serum half-life is greater than 2 hours. As such, amrinone is less titratable than DA or DB. It has similar arrhythmogenic potential to the catecholamines. Other PDE-IIIs such as **milrinone** and **enoximone** have comparable hemodynamic properties to amrinone, but are more potent. Amrinone has been demonstrated to have additive salutary effects on CI and PCWP when used in combination with DB, and enoximone compares favorably to therapy with diuretics, nitrates, and beta agonists for the treatment of acute pulmonary edema. When used in CS, enoximone yields increases of 60% in CI, 9% reductions in PCWP, and insignificant changes in MAP. Still, there is no convincing evidence to suggest that any of the PDE-III inhibitors should displace DB as the first-line intervention for acute ventricular power failure. The chief utility of these compounds appears to be for supplementation of DB in patients with inadequate response to catecholamines due to down-regulation of beta receptors.

3. **Pharmacotherapy by Forrester subset**
   a. **Subset II: Isolated pulmonary congestion.** Patients in subset II represent a heterogeneous population. They may have high, normal, or borderline blood pressure, severe, moderate, or mild pulmonary congestion, and normal or subclinically depressed CI. Therapy is directed at the reduction of LV filling pressures, but this reduction must not be so great as to precipitate relative hypovolemia. The failing LV operates optimally at a filling pressure of 18 mm Hg. Rapid reduction of PCWP to less than this value may precipitate reflex tachycardia, increased myocardial O_2 demand, and infarct extension. It may also reduce preload to the point where subclinical hypoperfusion becomes manifest.

   Assuming normal blood pressure and cardiac output, therapy for pulmonary congestion in the setting of ongoing ischemia should be initiated with **NTG**. Administration by continuous IV infusion is preferred since it offers the greatest precision in titration to desired end-points. End points of NTG therapy include clinical improvement and reclassification of the patient to subset I, a fall in systolic pressure to less than 90 mm Hg, a 10% decline in MAP, a 10% increase in heart rate, a reduction in CI to less than 2.2 liter/min/m^2, or a reduction in PCWP to less than 18 mm Hg. Patients who develop borderline blood pressure or inadequate peripheral perfusion should have the dosage reduced. Failure to respond to reduced dosing may require the addition of sympathomimetic amines.

Patients in subset II will benefit from simultaneous administration of **diuretics.** The goal of diuretic therapy is maintenance of a urine output greater than 50 ml/hr.

Severely hypertensive patients classified in subset II may benefit from initial vasodilator therapy with NP. NP is a superior to NTG for the reduction of systemic vascular resistance and arterial blood pressure. It is less effective than NTG for the reduction of PCWP but is still capable of lowering LV filling pressures by 25%. Precipitation of marked increases in heart rate or reductions in MAP to less than 70 mm Hg are potential hazards associated with the use of NP and should be avoided.

Patients classified to subset II with borderline blood pressures or subclinical hypoperfusion may require support of cardiac output with **inotropes** in order to exploit the salutary effects of vasodilators. Administration of DB in this setting can augment CI and increase systolic blood pressure to an extent that permits the initiation of vasodilator therapy with NTG. DA is less effective than DB in this setting due to its potential for causing alpha-mediated increases in afterload and LV filling pressures.

b. **Subset III: Isolated hypoperfusion.** Isolated hypoperfusion is uncommon after AMI, occurring in only 20% of patients with CS. In approximately one-third of patients classified in subset III, PCWP will be less than 18 mm Hg, and hypoperfusion can be reversed with volume administration. Relative hypovolemia in this group results from peripheral venous pooling, shift of intravascular volume to the interstitium, and right ventricular failure. In a smaller minority, hypoperfusion occurs with normal or elevated blood pressure as a result of excessive systemic vascular resistance. These patients may respond to vasodilator therapy once filling pressures have been brought into the optimal range by **volume expansion.** The majority of patients in subset III will be hypotensive, and will require support with **inotropes** and pressors in addition to volume expansion to restore adequate CI and mean arterial pressure. Both DA and DB are capable of augmenting CO in patients with isolated hypoperfusion. When blood pressure is adequate, DB is the preferred agent. DB is less likely to worsen myocardial energetics or precipitate pulmonary congestion than is DA, and it is more effective in improving CI. However, when MAP is less than 70 mm Hg, the pressor effects of DA are required to maintain adequate coronary perfusion pressure.

  c. **Subset IV: Hypoperfusion with pulmonary congestion.** Subset IV presents the classic picture of CS. Controversy exists regarding whether vasodilators, inotropes or pressors represent the most appropriate initial therapy for this group. The issue is one of priorities; although both pulmonary congestion and hypoperfusion are independently associated with increased mortality after AMI, the critical factor for avoiding irreversible circulatory collapse is prevention of infarct extension and rescue of stunned myocardium. The strategy employed in accomplishing this goal depends on the pretreatment blood pressure. In the most common situation mean arterial pressure is inadequate, and the therapeutic priority must be the restoration and maintenance of an adequate coronary perfusion pressure. The beneficial effects of vasodilator therapy on CO, filling pressures, and myocardial energetics cannot be exploited while the overriding consideration of inadequate perfusion pressure remains.

  In the patient with frank hypotension, therapy is best initiated by **inotrope** therapy with DA at 5 µg/kg/min. Should hypotension and hypoperfusion resist titration to a dosage of 20 µg/kg/min, DA should be abandoned in favor of NE. Failure to promptly restore adequate arterial pressure while maintaining peripheral perfusion with NE requires the initiation of mechanical circulatory assistance. Should DA succeed in elevating MAP to adequate levels, DB may be added to augment cardiac output and allow weaning of DA to levels that do not produce unacceptable side effects. Addition of DB may allow DA to be weaned to the point where only splachnic vasodilatory effects persist, thereby improving renal perfusion, urine output, and pulmonary congestion. Beneficial effects on myocardial O_2 balance will be realized whenever DB is substituted for DA as long as coronary perfusion pressure is maintained. NTG or NP might also be added to DA to augment SV and reduce filling pressures once systolic blood pressure has been stabilized at greater than 90 mm Hg. In practice, this combination differs little in hemodynamic effect from DB when administered by itself.

  When the patient in subset IV has an initial systolic pressure of 90 to 100 mm Hg, DB should be used as first-line therapy at 4–8 μg/kg/min. If blood pressure improves, vasodilators can be added to further increase cardiac output and reduce filling pressures. Should mean arterial pressure fall, DA may be added, with further interventions to follow in the pattern outlined above.

A minority of patients in Subset IV will have an initial systolic pressure of greater than 100 mm Hg. In this subgroup, therapy is most appropriately initiated with vasodilators. Although NTG is generally preferred over NP in the setting of ongoing myocardial ischemia, NP is the favored agent when hypoperfusion results from an inappropriately high SVR or from hemodynamically significant mitral regurgitation. Because of the potential for disastrous reductions in mean arterial pressure with the vasodilators, strict end-points must be used to guide therapy. NP should be initiated in this group when SVR exceeds 1,200 dyne×sec×cm^{-5}. Therapeutic end-points include reduction of SVR to 700 to 800 dyne×sec×cm^{-5}, an increase in heart rate of no more than 10%, and maintenance of a systolic pressure greater than 90 mm Hg. If vasodilator therapy is poorly tolerated, DB should be added and NP weaned until an adequate perfusion pressure is restored.

The treatment of pulmonary congestion necessarily takes a back seat to the correction of inadequate perfusion pressure in the majority of patients with CS. Once arterial pressure is stabilized, measures to reduce filling pressures with nitrates and diuretics can be attempted. Exacerbation of ischemia will be minimized during this phase of therapy if marked increases in heart rate are avoided.

4. **Mechanical circulatory support.** The vast majority of patients classified in subset III or IV will die in the absence of heroic measures if respiratory care and pharmacotherapy are unsuccessful in promptly reversing hemodynamic instability. Although mechanical circulatory support in and of itself does not significantly influence mortality from CS or refractory CHF, it is capable of stabilizing the majority of patients in whom it is applied and plays a critical role in the preservation of adequate organ perfusion until myocardial salvage can be accomplished. Mechanical circulatory assistance is appropriately utilized only as a bridging therapy pending coronary revascularization by angioplasty, thrombolysis, or coronary artery bypass grafting (CABG). It does not represent a definitive therapy in the absence of revascularization efforts. Any patient who remains in CS or refractory CHF despite optimization of ventricular filling pressures and 30 to 60 minutes of maximal pharmacotherapy should be considered a candidate for mechanical assistance. The inadequacy of maximal fluid and

pharmacologic support will be reflected by the following measured or derived hemodynamic indices: (1) a CI less than 1.8 liter/min/m^2 and systolic blood pressure of less than 90 mm Hg in patients with a PCWP greater than 20 mm Hg, (2) a right atrial pressure of less than 15 mm Hg, and (3) a systemic vascular resistance of greater than 2,000 dyne×sec×cm^{-5}. Severe right ventricular failure, in which LV filling pressure remains low despite a central venous pressure exceeding 20 mm Hg, is a further indication for mechanical support. Three principal techniques are available: (1) intra-aortic balloon counterpulsation (IACP), (2) percutaneous cardiopulmonary bypass (CPB), and (3) the transvalvular, intraventricular, rotary, axial screw pump [Hemopump™ (HP)]. IACP is the most widely applied and available of the three methods, and should be the first modality considered in patients who fail less invasive therapies. Until experience and familiarity with CPB and HP increase, these methods should be reserved for patients who fail an initial trial of IACP and are at, or near, a facility where the technology is available. Regardless of the method chosen, the salutary effects of mechanical assistance include augmentation of myocardial oxygen supply through improvement of coronary perfusion pressure, reduction of myocardial oxygen demand through unloading of the left ventricle, and improvement in cardiac output.

a. **Intra-aortic balloon counterpulsation.** IACP has been used in the treatment of AMI complicated by CS or refractory CHF for over three decades, and remains the most widely applied mechanical circulatory assist device. IACP provides phased inflation of an intra-aortic balloon placed in the descending thoracic aorta just distal to the take-off of the left subclavian artery. The balloon is placed percutaneously, generally through the femoral artery. Improvements in catheter technology have resulted in reduction of the size of the insertion sheath to 8.5 French, limiting vascular and thromboembolic complications associated with prolonged use. Inflation and deflation are linked to the ECG or arterial pressure tracing to provide systolic relaxation and diastolic inflation of the balloon. This results in systolic unloading of the LV and augmentation of runoff during diastole. Systolic blood pressure is generally reduced and diastolic pressure increased without significant changes in mean arterial pressure. When applied in CS, IACP is capable of increasing cardiac output by 500–800 ml/min. Urine output is improved and metabolic acidosis reduced, reflecting improved peripheral perfusion. PCWP is reduced by approximately 25%, reflecting improved systolic emptying. Myocardial energetics improve as reflected by a reduction in coronary sinus lactate levels during balloon use. Myocardial pressure work and oxygen consumption fall secondary to reductions in afterload and ventricular wall tension during systole. IACP also may improve myocardial oxygen supply by augmenting aortic root pressure and increasing coronary collateral flow during diastole. In approximately 80% of patients in whom it is applied, IACP will result in temporary resolution of pulmonary congestion and shock. Use of IACP also reduces the rate of coronary reocclusion following PTCA and may increase the efficacy of thrombolysis in CS. Commonly encountered complications of IACP include local vascular trauma with bleeding, thromboembolism and limb ischemia, infection, hemolysis, and thrombocytopenia. Although complication rates increase with the duration of use, IACP has been used safely for weeks without the development of limiting complications. Use of IACP for a period of several days is fairly routine.

b. **Cardiopulmonary bypass.** Percutaneous CPB has been applied principally for mechanical circulatory assistance during complicated PTCA. Its application in CS or refractory CHF outside this setting has not been examined in a controlled fashion. CPB is not widely available, but this technique has tremendous potential as a means of preserving patient viability pending attempts at reperfusion. Insertion of the perfusion ports and initiation of bypass can be accomplished in as little as 5 to 10 minutes. Unlike IACP, which depends on some degree of intrinsic cardiac activity, CPB remains effective in maintaining cardiac output even in the absence of effective ventricular contraction or a stable cardiac rhythm. This represents a significant advantage over IACP when intrinsic cardiac activity can be rapidly reestablished but is disastrous when myocardial salvage fails and the patient becomes completely dependent on bypass. Flow rates of 3.5–6.0 liter/min and mean aortic root pressures of 70–110 mm Hg are attainable. LV filling pressures under bypass commonly normalize to less than 10 mm Hg. Myocardial O_2 demand is decreased, coronary blood flow is increased, and infarct size may be reduced. Peripheral perfusion can improve to the point where mixed venous O_2 saturations indicate supranormal peripheral O_2 delivery. Usage of portable CPB is limited by the complications of hemolysis, thrombocytopenia, and thromboembolism with limb ischemia. CPB use is not recommended for more than 8 hours duration.

c. **Hemopump (HP).** HP utilizes a rotating, nonpulsatile, Archimedes screw pump that is inserted transfemorally by surgical cutdown or percutaneous technique, then advanced transvalvularly into the LV cavity under fluoroscopic control. The pump is capable of producing flow rates of up to 3.5 liter/min. When applied in patients in subset IV,

HP can support up to 80% of LV work, increase CI by 50% to 120%, boost mean arterial pressure to greater than 85 mm Hg, and lower PCWP into the optimal range. Use of HP reduces myocardial O_2 consumption while favorably redistributing coronary blood flow. The support functions of the pump have been sufficient to allow weaning of all cardiotonic agents while in operation. Insertion can be accomplished by surgical femoral arterotomy or by percutaneous technique. Insertion time is approximately 20 minutes by experienced hands. Complications of HP are similar to those of CPB. In addition, HP can precipitate ventricular dysrhythmias through direct irritation of the endocardial surface of the LV. Because of the size of the insertion sheath (21 French), HP cannot be placed in patients with significant aortic stenosis or atherosclerotic narrowing of the descending aorta, iliac, or femoral vessels. Application of this device is currently limited to investigational use at a few health centers. HP has not been studied in a controlled fashion as a means of stabilizing or maintaining patients with CS or severe CHF following AMI, but has been extremely successful in stabilizing postcardiotomy patients with shock.

5. **Revascularization.** Reperfusion strategies are applied with the rationale of salvaging myocardium that is reversibly ischemic, or "stunned." Clear survival benefits have been realized with revascularization of ischemic myocardium after AMI uncomplicated by shock or congestive failure. Although the benefits of coronary reperfusion are less well established in patients with CS or severe CHF, a wealth of data indicate that the pivotal factor influencing survival from hemodynamic instability after AMI is the restoration and maintenance of patency in the infarct-related artery. Available techniques for emergent reperfusion include administration of thrombolytic agents, PTCA, and CABG.

   a. **Thrombolysis.** The data on thrombolysis in AMI complicated by hemodynamic instability are limited. Among the 325 patients classified as Killip Class IV in the GISSI and Society for Coronary Angiography trials, there was no difference in mortality between the control group and the groups receiving intravenous or intracoronary streptokinase. Coronary angiograms of patients who received thrombolytic agents demonstrated that recanalization of the infarct-related artery occurs much less often in shock patients (45%) than in nonshock patients (71%). However, successful reperfusion of the infarct-related artery is associated with a 50% reduction of in-hospital mortality in the subset of patients with shock. As such, although successful thrombolysis is less likely to occur in the setting of CS, it is of significant benefit when it does. The available evidence—although scant—suggests that thrombolytic agents should be administered in patients with CS or severe CHF if PTCA is unavailable, or will be delayed. Administration of thrombolytic agents does not preclude subsequent PTCA and may contribute to a reduction in the rate of early reocclusion in comparison to patients undergoing angioplasty without antecedent thrombolytic therapy.

b. **Angioplasty.** PTCA has emerged as the therapy of choice for emergent coronary revascularization in the hemodynamic unstable patient. The rates of reperfusion and survival are greater in both shock and nonshock patients than the rates achievable with thrombolytic therapy. Successful recanalization of the infarct-related artery occurs in 60% to 88% of patients with CS. When patency of the infarct-related artery is attained, mortality drops dramatically. Reviews of case-series demonstrate survival rates of 40% to 100% after successful PTCA in AMI patients with CS or refractory CHF. Survival of such patients when angioplasty is unsuccessful, when no revascularization procedure is attempted, or when thrombolytic therapy fails, declines to the historical rate of 0% to 33%. Although of tremendous benefit in reducing both the morbidity and mortality of complicated AMI, PTCA is not useful when coronary disease is diffuse or when discrete disease affects the proximal left main coronary artery. Salvage in such patients is most appropriately attempted by thrombolytic therapy, or surgery.

c. **Coronary artery bypass grafting.** Surgical revascularization for AMI complicated by hemodynamic instability has not been studied in a controlled manner, but case-series have documented substantial gains in in-hospital survival when CABG is applied within 16 hours of symptom onset. Survival rates approximating two-thirds have been reported in several small series, compared to 10%–20% in historical controls. Survivorship is even more impressive when surgical revascularization can be accomplished within four hours of symptom onset, or when stability can be achieved preoperatively with IACP. Unfortunately, expeditious application of surgical revascularization in patients with CS or CHF is hampered by logistical issues, and emergent CABG is generally reserved for those who fail PTCA or have diffuse, multivessel stenoses.

E. **Disposition and consultation.** Maximal salvage of patients with hemodynamic instability after AMI requires resources that are available in only a minority of U.S. hospitals. Optimal management should begin in the field, with triage of patients to centers capable of providing emergent cardiac catheterization, PTCA, mechanical circulatory support, and cardiothoracic surgical backup. When complicated AMI is encountered in the emergency department or inpatient service of a community hospital lacking these services, emergent consultation with a cardiologist at a facility capable of delivering definitive care should be obtained. Transfer by the most expeditious means available should be arranged and, where possible, accomplished with a nurse and physician in attendance. If transfer is expected to be delayed or protracted, thrombolytic therapy should be strongly considered. Pending transfer, stabilizing care should be delivered in a manner consistent with the hemodynamic status of the patient as based on clinical classification to a Forrester subset, or direct measurement with a pulmonary artery catheter. When AMI with hemodynamic compromise is encountered at a tertiary referral center with appropriate and available resources for definitive care, the equipment and personnel necessary to the delivery of that care must be immediately mobilized if patient salvage is to be maximized.

Bibliography

Belskii NE, Pilipenko VA, Roshchin ST, et al. Use of nitroglycerine in the treatment of acute heart failure and cardiogenic shock in patients with myocardial infarction. *Cor Vasa* 29:89–97, 1987.

DeWood MA, Notske RN, Hensley GR, et al. Intraaortic balloon counterpulsation with and without reperfusion for myocardial infarction shock. *Circulation* 61:1105–1112, 1980.

Forrester JS, Diamond G, Chatterjee K, et al. Medical therapy of acute myocardial infarction by application of hemodynamic subsets. I. *New Engl J Med* 295:1356–1362, 1976.

Forrester JS, Diamond G, Chatterjee K, et al. Medical therapy of acute myocardial infarction by application of hemodynamic subsets. II. *New Engl J Med* 295:1404–1413, 1976.

Francis GS, Sharma B, Hodges M. Comparative hemodynamic effects of dopamine and dobutamine in patients with acute cardiogenic circulatory collapse. *Am Heart J* 103:995–1000, 1982.

Hibbard MD, Holmes DR, Bailey KR, et al. Percutaneous transluminal coronary angioplasty in patients with cardiogenic shock. *J Am Coll Cardiol* 19:639–646, 1992.

Mundth ED. Mechanical and surgical interventions for the reduction of myocardial ischemia. *Circulation* (Suppl. I):I-176–I-190, 1976.

Bradycardia and Conduction Block

Steve Marso, William J. Brady Jr., and
Andrew T. Guertler

I. **Etiology.** Bradyarrhythmias arising in the setting of myocardial infarction (MI) occur in 25% to 30% of patients with MI and result from abnormalities of either impulse formation (e.g., automaticity) or impulse conduction. In the majority of cases, these abnormalities are due to myocardial ischemia or infarction with necrosis of the cardiac pacemaker sites and/or conduction system. Other factors responsible for these bradyarrhythmias include altered autonomic influence, systemic hypoxia, electrolyte disturbances, acid-bases disorders, and complications of various medical therapies.

II. **The heart blocks.** The rhythm disturbances that complicate MI include the bradycardias and the conduction blocks of both the atrioventricular (AV) and the intraventicular systems. Sinus bradycardia (SB) is the most frequently encountered bradyarrhythmia in the setting of MI, whereas junctional (nodal) and idioventricular rhythms are encountered less often. Atrioventricular conduction disturbances are classified into first-degree AV block, second-degree (types I and II) AV block, and third-degree (complete) AV block (CHB). Left anterior fascicular block (LAFB, also known as left anterior hemiblock), left posterior fascicular block (LPFB, also known as left posterior hemiblock), left bundle-branch block (LBBB), right bundle-branch block (RBBB), and the nonspecific intraventricular conduction delay (NSIVCD) complete the list of disorders of intraventricular conduction seen in MI patients. Unifascicular block is described when a single branch of the trifascicular intraventricular conduction system is compromised, such as isolated LAFB, LPFB, or RBBB. Bifascicular blocks are composed of combinations of two intraventricular conduction disturbances. For example, LBBB is considered a bifas-cicular block in that both branches, or fascicles, of the left bundle are affected. Right bundle-branch block with either an LAFB or LPFB is considered the other form of bifascicular block. Trifascicular block, electrical dysfunction of the right bundle branch and both fascicles of the left bundle branch, results in a complete heart block (CHB), which is described as distal with a different electrophysiologic behavior compared to the proximal form of CHB seen in patients with atrioventricular node disease.

III. **Incidence of heart block in MI.** The incidence of the various **bradyarrhythmias** in the setting of MI, including both bradycardia and conduction block, is reported to be 25% to 30%. Of the rhythm disturbances, SB is found in approximately 25% of patients with myocardial infarction and is the most frequently encountered bradyarrhythmia in patients with MI. Junctional rhythm is noted in 20% of patients, and idioventricular rhythm occurs in 15% of such cases. Both junctional and idioventricular rhythms occur with failure of higher pacemaker site function or as escape rhythms in the setting of AV or intraventricular conduction block. Of the AV blocks, first- and second-degree type I AV blocks are found in 15% and 12% of patients with MI, respectively. Complete heart block (third-degree AV block) complicates 8% of infarctions. Second-degree type II AV block is rare. Of the intraventricular blocks, RBBB is noted in 6% to 8%, LAFB in 8%, and LBBB in 5% of patients with MI. Left posterior fascicular block is rare, occurring in less than 1% of such patients.

In the realm of **unstable bradyarrhythmias** complicating MI, complete heart block is most often encountered with an incidence of 40%. Sinus bradycardia (24%) and junctional rhythm (20%) are the next most frequently encountered hemodynamically compromising bradycardic rhythms in MI patients. Table 15-1 lists the incidence of the bradyarrhythmias occurring in the setting of MI. Table 15-2 reports the incidence of these rhythm disturbances in unstable patients experiencing acute myocardial infarction.

IV. **Anatomy of the conduction system.** The anatomy of the conduction system (Fig. 15-1) includes the sinotrial node (SAN), the interatrial conduction pathways, atrioventricular node (AVN), bundle of His, and the ventricular bundle branches. The SAN is found at the junction of the superior vena cava and the right atrium. The blood supply of the SAN, the sinus node artery, originates from the proximal portion of the right coronary artery (RCA) in 55% of patients, the circumflex artery (CXA) in 35%, and a dual supply from both arteries in 10%. The SAN is richly innervated by both the sympathetic and parasympathetic nervous systems. The interatrial conduction pathways, connecting the SAN to the AVN, are poorly defined anatomically. The vascular supply of these tracts includes both the sinus node artery and the AV nodal artery.

The AVN is located in the posteromedial portion of the right atrium immediately anterior to the coronary sinus. The vas-

Table 15-1.   The incidence of bradyarrhythmia in the setting of MI

Rhythm	Incidence (%)
Sinus bradycardia	25
Junctional	20
Idioventricular	15
First-degree AV block	15
Second-degree, type I AV block	12
Second-degree, type II AV block	4
Third-degree AV block	15
Right bundle-branch block	6–8
Left bundle-branch block	5
Left anterior fascicular block	8
Left posterior fascicular block	0.5

Table 15-2. The incidence of unstable bradyarrhythmia in the setting of MI

Rhythm	Incidence (%)
Sinus bradycardia	25
Junctional	20
Idioventricular	0
First-degree AV block	10
Second-degree, type I AV	4
Second-degree, type II AV block	1
Third-degree AV block	40

culature responsible for the AVN is the AV nodal artery, which is a branch of the posterior descending artery (PDA) in 80% of patients and of the CXA in 10%. The AV nodal artery arises from a dual supply of the PDA and CXA structures in the remainder of patients. The left anterior descending artery (LAD) also supplies collateral circulation to the AVN in most patients. The AVN is innervated by both divisions of the autonomic nervous system. Recall that the PDA is a branching continuation of the RCA.

Fig. 15-1. A diagrammatic representation of the myocardial conducting system and its blood supply. (From De Guzman MD, Rahimtoola MD. Controversies in coronary artery disease: What is the role of pacemakers in patients with coronary artery disease and conduction abnormalities? *Cardiovasc Clin* **13:192, 1983.)**

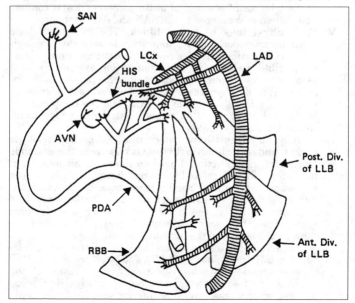

The AVN connects to the bundle of His, which enters the fibrous skeleton of the heart, courses through the membranous septum, passes adjacent to the noncoronary cusp of the aortic valve, and runs along the left side of the interventricular septum. The blood supply includes both the AV nodal artery and septal perforating branches of the LAD.

The bundle of His separates into two major divisions, the right and left bundle branches. The right bundle branch runs within the interventricular septum at the level of the subendocardium toward the base of the anterior papillary muscle of the right ventricle, receiving its vascular supply from both the AV nodal artery and septal perforating branches of the LAD.

The left bundle branch, a less well defined anatomical structure compared to the right bundle branch, further subdivides in the area of the aortic valve into the anterior and the posterior fascicles, spreading out in a fan-like distribution from the left side of the interventricular septum. The anterior fascicle, the smaller of the two branches of the left bundle, passes along the left ventricular outflow tract toward the anterior papillary muscle of the left ventricle. The posterior fascicle moves from the area of the aortic valve in a posteroinferior direction along the interventricular septum toward the posterior papillary muscle of the left ventricle. Considerable variation among individuals is found in the structure of the left bundle branch and its subdivisions. The vascular supply to the left bundle branch includes septal perforating branches of the LAD to the anterior fascicle and a combination of both LAD- and PDA-derived branches is responsible for perfusion of the posterior fascicle. This dual perfusion of the left posterior fascicle explains the relatively infrequent occurrence of LAFB in the settting of acute MI. Autonomic influence is minimal in the intraventricular conduction system as compared to the SAN and AVN systems.

V. **Pathophysiology of heart block.** The pathophysiologic mechanisms underlying the majority of bradyarrhythmic episodes in MI patients involve reversible ischemic injury to and irreversible necrosis of the conduction system as well as altered autonomic function. Additional mechanisms include myocardial hyperkalemia, local increases in adenosine, metabolic acidosis, systemic hypoxia, and the complications of medical therapy, in particular both beta- and calcium channel–blocking agents.

Many authorities have categorized the pathophysiologic background of the bradyarrhythmias relative to the anatomic location of the infarction. Based on the anatomic location of the infarction and related pathophysiology, the clinician is able to predict the likelihood in many cases of bradyarrhythmia development, the expected time course for the onset of arrhythmic difficulty, the associated risk of hemodynamic compromise, the response to acute therapy, the need for long-term treatments, and the ultimate prognosis.

A. **Inferior and inferoposterior infarctions.** Acute inferior (IMI), inferolateral (ILMI), and inferoposterior (IPMI) myocardial infarctions resulting from occlusion of the RCA are frequently complicated by bradyarrhythmias. The common association of inferior wall ischemic events and compromising bradyarrhythmias may be due to increased **parasympathetic influence,** especially early in the time course of the infarction. Such patients tend to abruptly develop compromising rhythm disturbances including second- and third-degree AV blocks **within six hours** after the onset of infarction, have relatively slow ventricular escape rates, and respond rapidly to atropine and/or isoproterenol therapy. Patients who develop bradyarrhythmia **after six hours** of infarction usually do so in a gradual progression with an equally slow return to normal sinus rhythm. The escape rhythm is usually of ventricular origin with a relatively high rate and poor response to medical therapy. These patients most likely are experiencing the rhythm disturbance due to **reversible ischemia** of the conduction system. Necrosis (irreversible damage) of the AVN is rare due to the presence of both extensive collateral circulation (RCA and LAD contributions in the most patients) as well as a relatively low metabolic rate with high glycogen reserves of such myocardial conducting tissue.

CHB in patients with IMI are said to develop a **"proximal" third-degree AV block** due to ischemic damage to the AVN and/or increased parasympathetic influence. In contrast, patients with anterior wall infarctions suffer **"distal" third-degree AV block** as a result of dysfunction of the trifascicular intraventricular conduction system. Patients with IMI and its anatomic variants who develop compromising bradyarrhythmias have a higher in-hospital mortality approaching 20% compared to patients without arrhythmic complications. This increased mortality does not result from the bradycardia or block themselves, but rather from a generally larger-sized myocardial infarction.

Patients with RCA-related infarctions also are at risk of developing **sinus node dysfunction,** manifested primarily by SB and sinus arrest. Sinus bradycardia is the most frequent bradyarrhythmia encountered in MI patients, particularly in patients with inferior wall involvement. In cases of sinus arrest, the escape rhythm originates from either the AVN, producing the narrow-complex junctional rhythm with ventricular rates of 45–60 bpm, or from the intraventricular conduction system, resulting in the wide QRS complex idioventricular rhythm with rates of 30–45 bpm. In many cases, patients have either a prior history of sick sinus syndrome or are using cardioactive medications such as beta-blocking agent, calcium antagonists, and cardiac glycosides that suppress SAN function. With the acute ischemic syndrome, either ischemic injury to the SAN and/or heightened parasympathetic tone are responsible for the clinical expression of the bradyarrhythmia.

B. **Anterior and anteroseptal MI.** Patients with anterior and anteroseptal (ASMI) infarctions most often have occlusion of the left main coronary artery, the proximal LAD, and the LAD-derived branches. Intraventricular and AV blocks that develop in this setting respond poorly to therapy, and these patients have a poor prognosis. Autopsy studies show extensive septal necrosis often accompanied by irreversible **malfunction of the bundle of His** and the bundle branches. Interesting in these cases, the AVN is often normal without evidence of necrosis, indicating the distal nature of the complete AV block in these patients. Patients with intraventricular conduction disorders have a very high early mortality. Patients with a pre-existing intraventricular conduction block are at slightly lower risk compared to patients with new-onset bundle-branch block. Patients with conduction disturbances occurring in the setting of AMI most often do not respond to medical therapy such as atropine or isoproterenol. Perfusion actually may be further impaired by the vasodilating effects of isoproterenol without an accompanying increase in the escape rhythm rate. Ventricular pacing by the transcutaneous or transvenous routes is required in compromised patients. The prophylactic presence of a ventricular pacer is encouraged in these patients who are hemodynamically stable on presentation.

VI. **Risk of complete heart block.** A considerable body of literature has grown around the issue of the risk of progression to CHB in patients with MI. It is felt that in patients with a high risk for CHB, **prophylactic ventricular pacing** can be made ready and employed rapidly with the development of third-degree AV block. Other patients, at lower risk for such a conduction abnormality, may be observed safely in the appropriate critical care setting with the institution of such resuscitation if the need arises. A useful method to predict the potential for such progression considers the electrocardiographic presence of the following **risk factors** including first-degree AV block, second-degree (types I and II) AV block, RBBB, LBBB, LAFB, and LPFB. Each risk factor, when noted on the 12-lead ECG, receives a score of 1. The total score is summed, giving the clinician the risk of progression to CHB in patients with MI. A score of 0 carries a 1.2% risk of CHB development whereas a score of 3 or more is associated with a significant possibility of CHB (36.4%). The total scores and the risk of third-degree AV block are listed in Table 15-3.

VII. **Bradycardia**

A. **ECG recognition. Sinus bradycardia** (Fig. 15-2) is noted on the 12-lead ECG when the ventricular rate is less than 60 bpm, the QRS complex is narrow, the rhythm is regular, and each P wave is associated with a QRS com-

Table 15-3. Risk of progression to complete heart block (CHB) in patients with MI based on the risk score

CHB total score	Predicted risk (%)
0	1.2
1	7.8
2	25.0
>2	36.4

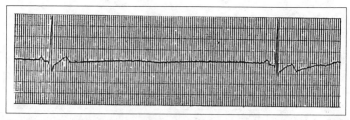

**Fig. 15-2.   Profound sinus bradycardia
in a 42-year-old man with acute MI.**

plex. Further, the P-wave morphology and the PR interval
are normal and consistent.

   Sinus arrest or exit block may be complete or incomplete. In complete sinus arrest, no P waves are found on
the ECG. Most often, a lower pacemaker assumes control.
The focus of the escape rhythm usually is the AVN and
produces a **junctional rhythm** (Fig. 15-3) with a narrow-
QRS complex and rates of 45–60 bpm. An **idioventricular rhythm** (Fig. 15-4) is noted if the focus of the escape
rhythm is found in the His bundle–branch system; the
QRS complex is wide with a rate of 30–45 bpm. Rarely, if
no pacemaker site is able to assume control, then complete ventricular asystole results. With incomplete sinus
arrest, an occasional P wave is dropped from the normal
electrical PQRST cycle.

B. Clinical presentation. Patients with SB and MI may
   not be adversely effected by the bradyarrhythmia and
   maintain adequate systemic perfusion. Alternatively, in
   approximately 25% of patients with hemodynamically
   compromising block or bradycardia occurring in the setting of MI, SB is responsible for the hypoperfusion, which
   is manifested by extreme fatigue, syncope, altered mental
   status, pulmonary edema, or systemic hypotension with
   systolic blood pressure less than 90 mm Hg. Since SB frequently occurs in the setting of IMI, the clinician also
   must consider right ventricular infarction with diminished preload as a cause of the hypoperfusion (see Chap.
   18). Sinus arrest, if compensated by an adequate escape
   rhythm, also may be asymptomatic. If the escape rhythm

**Fig. 15-3.   Junctional rhythm found
in lead II in the setting of AMI.**

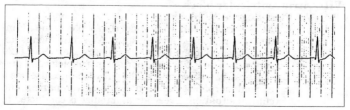

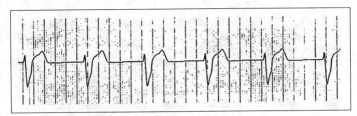

Fig. 15-4.   Idioventricular rhythm.

is inadequate, however, then systemic hypoperfusion will be noted as in SB.

   C. **Specific therapy**

     1. **Atropine.** Patients who present with SB or sinus arrest with an adequate escape rhythm should be observed with ECG monitoring. Patients with systemic hypoperfusion should receive intravenous atropine at conventional doses. When using atropine, the clinician is encouraged to use the full vagolytic dose, which is 0.04 mg/kg. For such bradyarrhythmias with systemic hypoperfusion, 0.6–1.0 mg IV should be used with repeat bolusing as needed up to the vagolytic dose. In cases of unstable SB in which atropine is ultimately successful in normalizing the vital signs, the first dose of atropine is likely to restore adequate perfusion. Subsequent doses are less likely to produce positive change, though the complete vagolytic dose is recommended. Additionally, extreme bradycardia is a risk factor for the development of frequent ventricular extrasystoles, ventricular tachycardia, and ventricular fibrillation. The use of atropine in this setting may abolish the ventricular irritability.

     2. **Isoproterenol.** If atropine is unsuccessful, isoproterenol is the next agent and should be used as a "medical bridge" to ventricular pacing via either the transcutaneous or transvenous routes. Isoproterenol infusion is started at 1 mg/min and titrated upward to achieve an adequate heart rate and blood pressure. Titrating isoproterenol in the setting of cardiac ischemia must be done with great care. Beta-adrenergic stimulation increases myocardial oxygen demand and can lead to malignant ventricular arrhythmias. Overshooting a target heart rate can lead to increased myocardial oxygen demand and further ischemia.

VIII. Atrioventricular block

   A. **First-degree AV block**

     1. **ECG recognition.** In first-degree AV block, the PR interval is prolonged and constant. AV conduction is delayed such that the PR interval is **greater than 0.20 seconds.** The P wave has normal morphology and precedes every QRS complex. The QRS complex also has a normal morphology and axis for the given patient and clinical situation. Every atrial impulse is conducted to

the ventricles. First-degree AV block may be associated with other conduction abnormalities as well.

2. **Clinical presentation.** Patients with first-degree AV block and concurrent acute myocardial infarction often exhibit a softened S1 on physical examination. The AV block is due to either increased vagal tone, AV nodal ischemia, or rarely, extensive necrosis of the His bundle–branch system. The majority of these patients have had an inferior infarction, causing increased vagal tone or AV nodal ischemia. A minority of patients have suffered an anterior infarction with necrosis of the intraventricular conduction system. First-degree AV block is usually a benign rhythm. However, patients with anterior infarctions and first-degree block are at an increased risk of developing high-grade AV block.

3. **Specific therapy.** First-degree AV block in the setting of MI is usually a benign rhythm, and the vast majority of patients are asymptomatic and require no specific intervention. There is an overall 13% risk of progression to higher-grade AV block in these patients. Given the relatively low risk of progression to high-grade AV block and the effectiveness of external pacers, prophylactic temporary transvenous pacing is not indicated in first-degree AV block unless other conduction abnormalities are present. Therefore, it is necessary only to monitor the patient closely for development of other conduction disturbances and hemodynamic compromise.

B. **Mobitz type I second-degree AV block (Wenkebach)**

1. **ECG recognition.** In Mobitz type I block (Fig. 15-5), there must be P waves and QRS complexes. The P waves and QRS complexes have normal morphology and axis for a given patient. The QRS complex is usually narrow (less than 0.12 seconds duration). In Mobitz type I block, there is a pattern to the P wave–QRS complex relationship. The PR interval is often normal in the first beat of the series. There is progressive PR interval lengthening with subsequent beats until an impulse is unable to reach the ventricles, resulting in a nonconducted P wave. After the dropped beat, the PR interval returns to normal and the cycle repeats itself. There is also a pattern to the RR interval in Wenkebach. As the PR lengthens with subsequent

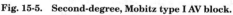

Fig. 15-5. Second-degree, Mobitz type I AV block.

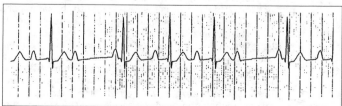

beats, the RR interval becomes shorter. Following the dropped beat, the RR interval in the subsequent beats tends to shorten. In fact, the RR interval containing the dropped beat is shorter than two of the shorter cycles. One also will notice on the rhythm strip a grouping of beats that is especially noticeable with tachycardia. Such a finding is referred to as **grouped beating of Wenkebach.** Evidence for Mobitz type I AV block includes the following:

a. Progressive lengthening of the PR interval, then dropped beat.

b. Progressive shortening of the RR interval.

c. The RR length of the dropped beat is less than twice the shortest cycle.

d. Grouped beating.

2. **Clinical presentation.** Patients with Mobitz type I AV block and acute myocardial infarction will exhibit an irregularly irregular pulse and beat-to-beat variability in the first heart sound, best appreciated at the apex. As the PR progressively lengthens, S1 will become so much softer that the loudest S1 is heard immediately following the dropped beat. The intensity of S2 remains constant throughout the cycle. Mobitz type I block is secondary either to increase vagal tone, to AV nodal ischemia, or rarely, to intraventricular conduction system ischemia. The site of the block is usually at or above the AV node; these patients usually have sustained an **inferior infarction.** Typically the QRS is narrow and the rate is sufficient to maintain adequate perfusion. Further, these patients tend to be hemodynamically stable. Type I second-degree AV block tends to occur within 72 hours of infarction and rarely lasts longer than 7 days. The presence of type I block does not increase mortality in patients with acute coronary syndromes. Patients with anterior infarction rarely will exhibit type I second-degree AV block. These patients have suffered extensive necrosis to the His bundle–branch system. In contrast to patients with inferior wall infarctions, these patients tend to have a wide QRS complex and may suddenly develop high-grade AV block with hemodynamic collapse.

3. **Specific therapy (inferior infarction).** Second-degree type I block in the setting of an inferior infarction and narrow QRS complex is usually a benign rhythm and requires only cardiac monitoring to identify the minority of patients who become symptomatic or progress to higher-grade AV block. In the occasional patient, this block is associated with hypotension, heart failure, or frequent ectopic beats. **Atropine** in these situations is the drug of choice. Atropine should be given in 0.5- to 1-mg boluses repeated every 5 minutes, not to exceed a total dose of 0.04 mg/kg. Atropine and other sympathomimetic drugs are more likely to be effective if AV block develops within 6 hours of the first signs of infarction. When effective, atropine will either abolish the block or accelerate the ventricular

rhythm. In a significant minority of patients, atropine seems to be ineffective. Recently it has been shown that adenosine may mediate some of the brady-arrhythmias and AV blocks during MI, possibly explaining atropine's lack of efficacy in certain clinical situations. **Methylxanthines,** such as aminophylline and theophylline, are competitive antagonists of adenosine and may be effective at abolishing AV block when atropine is not effective. If pharmacotherapy is ineffective, then a temporary **transvenous pacemaker** can be inserted. During placement of the transvenous pacer, a transcutaneous pacemaker can be placed if the patient is hemodynamically unstable.

4. **Specific therapy (anterior infarction).** The management of patients with anterior infarction complicated by type I AV block is controversial. These patients have sustained significant injury to the His bundle–branch system and are at increased risk of progression to higher-grade AV block. Atropine is rarely efficacious in this setting since the mechanism for AV block is extensive intraventricular conduction system ischemia rather than increased vagal tone. Some cardiologists favor prophylactic placement of a **transvenous pacemaker.** An acceptable alternative would be to place a transcutaneous pacemaker and proceed to a transvenous pacer only if the patient becomes unstable or develops high-grade block.

C. **Mobitz type II second-degree AV block**
   1. **ECG recognition.** The PR interval in type II second-degree AV block (Fig. 15-6) is constant. There must be P waves and QRS complexes with normal morphology and axis. The QRS complex is widened in most instances of type II second-degree AV block. The PR interval may be either normal or prolonged, but it is always constant without progressive PR interval lengthening from beat to beat. If there are three P waves for two QRS complexes, then it is a 3:2 block.

      Distinguishing type I from type II block is relatively straightforward unless there is 2:1 conduction. In this situation, there is no way to compare the PR intervals for the conducted beats. The physician must "assume the worst" in situations of 2:1 conduction, meaning that the block is Mobitz type II unless proven other-

Fig. 15-6. Second-degree, Mobitz type II AV block with a narrow QRS complex. (From Milwaukee County Paramedic System, Milwaukee, WI.)

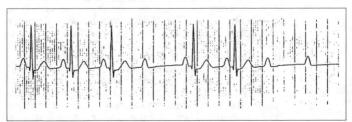

wise due to the relatively benign nature of type I block compared to the malignant course of type II AV block. *High-grade AV block* occurs when two or more P waves are not conducted. This implies advanced conduction disease and high risk for sudden development of complete heart block.

2. **Clinical presentation.** Patients with type II block will have a regularly irregular pulse. The heart sounds will be normal. The site of block in Mobitz type II is usually infranodal. These patients tend to have both widened QRS complexes with ventricular rates between 20 and 40 bpm and a higher risk of progression to CHB, most commonly in patients with extensive **anterior infarction.** Often these patients are hemodynamically unstable at the time of presentation. In contrast, patients who present with block at the level of the AV node tend to have narrow QRS complexes, are at less risk for progression to a high-grade AV block, and typically are experiencing an IPMI. These patients often are hemodynamically stable at the time of assessment in the emergency department. There is an increased mortality in patients with Mobitz type II and anterior AMI as compared to patients with inferior infarctions. Although the width of the QRS complex in Mobitz type II block can give the clinician information as to the level of block, it is not entirely predictable. For instance, type II block often is associated with preexisting ventricular conduction defects in patients with acute coronary syndromes. Therefore, the site of block may be within the AV node yet have a widened QRS complex.

3. **Specific therapy.** Patients with type II second-degree AV block may be unstable at the time of assessment or may develop third-degree block suddenly. If so, **transvenous pacing** should be instituted immediately. Patients can be supported with isoproterenol or transcutaneous pacing while the transvenous pacing wire is positioned. In patients with anterior MI with type II block, the risk of progression to complete block is quite high. A transvenous pacing wire often is placed for prophylactic measures in these patients. Patients with inferior infarcts and type II block often have ventricular rates greater than 40 and are hemodynamically stable. It would be appropriate to place transcutaneous pacers on these patients and transvenously pace them only if progression of block or hemodynamic compromise occurs. Atropine is rarely, if ever, the drug of choice for Mobitz type II block. Atropine may increase the sinus rate but not affect AV conduction, thus enhancing the degree of AV block.

D. **Third-degree AV block (complete heart block)**
1. **ECG recognition.** In complete heart block, no atrial impulses reach the ventricle through the AV conduction system. Therefore, the atria and ventricle are controlled by different pacemaker sites and function independently. The atrial pacemaker can be either si-

nus or ectopic (e.g., normal rate, bradycardic, tachy-cardic, flutter, or fibrillation). The ventricular escape rhythm also can have varying pacemaker sites, result-ing in differing rates. Rarely will there be no ventricu-lar escape rhythm, the patient presenting in asystolic arrest. More often the site of escape will be just below the level of the block. When the ventricular escape rhythm is located near the bundle of His, the rate ex-ceeds 40 bpm and the QRS complexes tend to be nar-row (Fig. 15-7). When the site of escape is distal to the bundle of His, the rate tends to be less than 40 bpm and the QRS complexes tend to be wide (Fig. 15-8). When examining the ECG for complete heart block, there will be no meaningful relationship between the P waves and the QRS complex. The P waves will ap-pear in a regular rhythm and will "march" through the rhythm strip at a specific atrial rate. As stated above, the ventricular rate will depend on the site of block. However, the QRS complexes should appear in a regu-lar fashion and will also "march" through the rhythm strip.

2. **Clinical presentation.** Patients with complete heart block will have beat-to-beat variation in the intensity of S1 best appreciated at the apex. S2 will be normal. Cannon A waves may be present when examining the jugular venous pulse on a minority of beats. Cannon A waves are a result of the right atria contracting against a closed tricuspid valve. About 60% of patients with complete heart block have had an **inferoposterior MI.** Most of these patients develop third-degree block after progression through first- and second-degree blocks. These patients tend to have narrow QRS complexes, escape rhythm with rates between 40 and 60 bpm, and hemodynamic stability. Complete heart block in this setting usually resolves in 3 to 7 days. Infrequently, a patient will remain in third-degree block for 2 weeks or more. In contrast to pa-tients with complete heart block and inferoposterior in-farcts, third-degree AV block in the setting of **anterior MI** carries a much higher in-hospital mortality and fre-quently leads to hemodynamic compromise. These pa-tients tend to have sudden onset of complete heart block (usually after Mobitz type II block), widened QRS complexes, and escape rates of less than 40 bpm.

Fig. 15-7. Complete heart block with narrow QRS-complex escape.

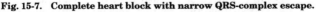

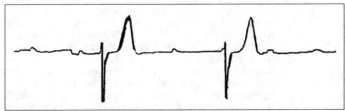

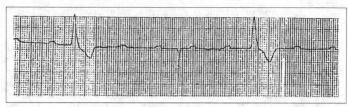

Fig. 15-8. Complete heart block with wide QRS-complex escape.

Despite aggressive medical management and transvenous pacing, these patients have a high in-hospital mortality because of extensive myocardial necrosis.

3. **Specific therapy.** Patients with third-degree heart block and **anterior MI** likely will be hemodynamically unstable at the initial assessment or will develop hemodynamic embarrassment suddenly. These patients should have a **transvenous pacemaker** placed urgently. Many of these patients will require permanent pacemakers. If the patient is unstable, atropine, isoproterenol, or transcutaneous pacing therapy can be instituted while placing the transvenous wire. In patients with **inferior MI,** the ventricular rate tends to be adequate to maintain cardiac output. If the ventricular rate is greater than 40 bpm and the patient is stable, one may elect to place a transvenous pacer only if the clinical situation deteriorates. If the patient develops hypotension, heart failure, oliguria, or ventricular arrhythmia, then atropine, isoproterenol, or transvenous pacing should be initiated. Patients with anterior infarctions and third-degree block should be treated aggressively for cardiogenic shock as it develops (see Chap. 14).

IX. **Intraventricular conduction defects**
  A. **Left bundle-branch block**
    1. **ECG recognition.** Interruption of the left bundle results in activation of the ventricles in a right-to-left direction (rather than the normal activation of left-to-right), inferiorly, and anteriorly more often than posteriorly. In complete LBBB, the QRS is prolonged measuring 0.12–0.18 seconds. A large QS or RS pattern is noted in lead V1, depending on whether the initial activation is directed anteriorly or posteriorly. A large, slurred or notched R wave is found in leads I and V6, reflecting the right-to-left activation in LBBB (Fig. 15-9). The QRS axis can be either normal or leftward (−30 to −90 degrees), each having equal prevalence. The direction of the ST segment and T wave is opposite that of the QRS vector. As the QRS complex in leads V1, V2, and V3 is directed downward, the expected ST segments will be elevated and the T wave will be upright. In leads I and V6, the QRS complex is upright; the ST segments are depressed and the T waves are inverted. Several attempts at establishing

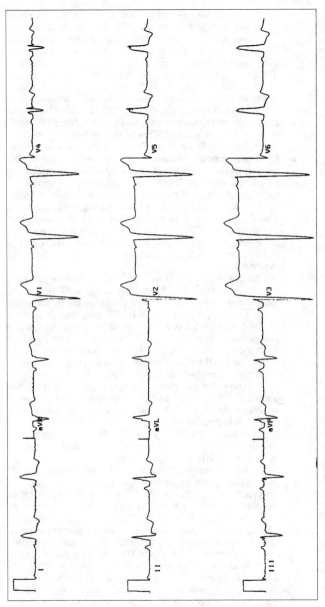

Fig. 15-9.   Left bundle-branch block.

ECG criteria for myocardial infarction in the presence of LBBB have proven unreliable. As a general rule, diagnosing ischemia and infarction in the presence of LBBB should be approached with caution. Occasionally, one will encounter a patient with ST-segment and T-wave changes directed in the same direction as the QRS complex. Such ECG findings are not the anticipated electrophysiologic result of LBBB and are highly suggestive of acute MI (Fig. 15-10). It should be stated that primary T-wave changes in the setting of LBBB are not always a reliable indicator of myocardial ischemia. See Table 15-4 for the ECG features of LBBB.

2. **Clinical presentation.** Patients with LBBB will have a paradoxically split S2. **Paradoxical splitting of S2** occurs when there is activation of the ventricles in a right-to-left direction causing a delay in aortic valve closure and splitting of S2 during expiration. A2 and P2 close simultaneously during inspiration. During expiration P2 actually closes before A2. Paradoxical splitting of S2 occurs in patients with LBBB and in patients with a transvenous pacemaker in the right ventricle.

   The presence of a new LBBB in patients with myocardial infarction has been associated with increased cardiovascular mortality and progression to complete heart block. The presence of LBBB and first-degree AV block carries an even higher risk of progression to complete AV block (up to 40% in some series). Patients with a new LBBB and MI likely are undergoing a large **anterior wall infarction** or experiencing ischemia in multiple vascular territories. Patients with LBBB tend to be older and more frequently are women. Transient LBBB also carries the same risk for progression to complete AV block and mortality as persistent LBBB. **Diagnosis of MI or ischemia in the setting of preexisting LBBB is difficult.** The exception is the demonstration of new ST-T wave changes in the setting of LBBB (see Fig. 15-10).

3. **Specific therapy.** Patients with new-onset LBBB most often have sustained extensive necrosis of the anterior wall and septum. They are at high risk to develop pump failure and an 11% risk to develop complete AV block. Some cardiologists would choose prophylactically to place a **transvenous pacemaker** in this group. A reasonable alternative would be to place a transcutaneous pacer and proceed to a transvenous wire if the clinical situation deteriorates. Patients with MI, LBBB, and first-degree AV block are at a much higher risk to progress to complete AV block. Therefore, prophylactic transvenous pacing is indicated in this group. If the patient becomes hemodynamically unstable and develops AV block, the use of atropine, isoproterenol, or transcutaneous pacing may be used as a temporizing measure until a transvenous pacemaker wire is placed.

   Many patients with MI and new LBBB will be

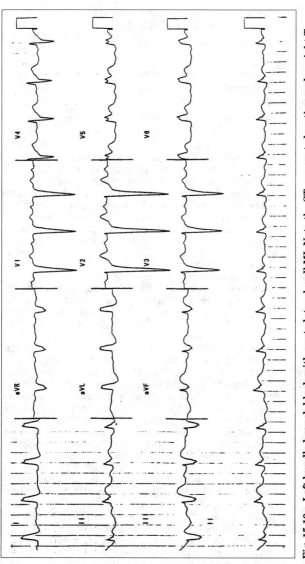

Fig. 15-10. Left bundle-branch block with acute lateral wall MI. Note the ST-segment elevation and upright T waves in the leads demonstrating acute infarction. Such findings are not the expected electrophysiologic result of LBBB. The ECG diagnosis of acute MI in patients with left bundle-branch block is difficult in most cases; this example is the rare patient in which AMI can be reliably diagnosed based on the ECG findings.

Table 15-4.   Electrocardiographic features of LBBB and RBBB

ECG finding	LBBB	RBBB
QRS axis	Normal/leftward	Normal
QRS duration	>0.12 sec	>0.12 sec
Lead V1	QS, rS	RSR′
Leads I and V6	Slurred R wave	Normal

hemodynamically unstable and require invasive hemodynamic monitoring. These patients are dependent on their right bundle. Placement of a Swan-Ganz catheter may interrupt the right bundle resulting in complete heart block. It would be appropriate to place a transvenous wire in patients who are hemodynamically tenuous prior to placing the right-heart catheter. In patients who are more stable, it would be appropriate to place transcutaneous pacer while placing the Swan-Ganz catheter.

B. **Right bundle-branch block**
   1. **ECG recognition.** In RBBB, the septum and left ventricle are activated normally in a left-to-right direction; however, right ventricular activation is delayed in a left-to-right, anterior, and superior direction. The characteristic pattern of RBBB (Fig. 15-11) is recorded in lead V1 as RSR′. The initial R wave reflects the normal septal activation, and the S wave reflects left ventricular activation. The R′ represents the delayed activation of the right ventricle from a left-to-right and anterior vector. The depth of the S wave in V1 can vary depending on whether left ventricular activation is directed anteriorly or posteriorly. The QRS axis in RBBB usually is normal but can be leftward or rightward. Left or right axis deviation usually signifies concomitant block of either the anterior or posterior fascicle of the left bundle. The T wave is inverted usually in V1 and sometimes in V2, and it is upright in the remaining precordial leads. Since septal and left ventricular activation is directed normally in RBBB, ECG diagnosis of myocardial ischemia is possible (Fig. 15-12). See Table 15-4 for ECG features of RBBB.
   2. **Clinical presentation.** Patients with RBBB have a widely fixed split S2 on examination. Patients with RBBB and MI usually are older and more often are women. They usually have sustained a large infarction of the anterior wall and septum, myocardium supplied by the LAD. In a minority of patients, the right coronary artery supplies the proximal portion of the right bundle; therefore, inferior ischemia can lead to RBBB. In patients with new RBBB and MI there is increased in-hospital mortality compared to patients without RBBB. Death is due usually to pump failure or malignant ventricular arrhythmias.

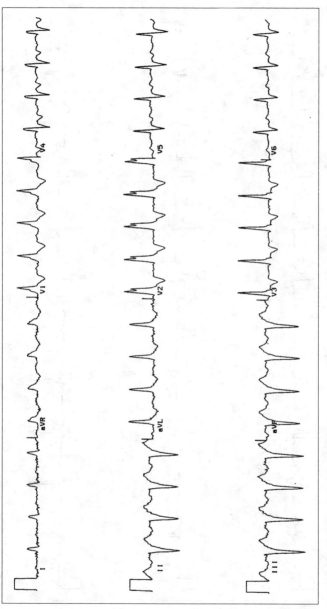

Fig. 15-11. Right bundle-branch block.

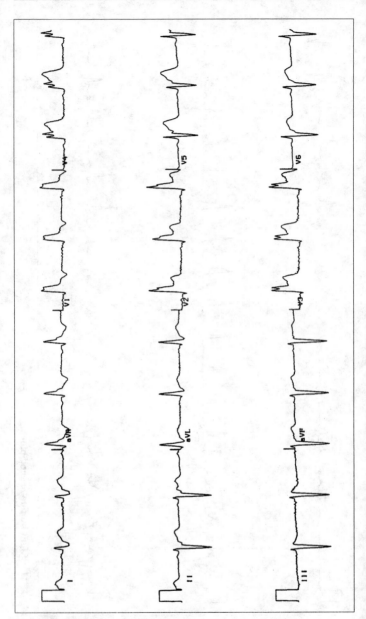

Fig. 15-12.   Right bundle-branch block with acute anterior
wall MI. The diagnosis of acute MI in patients with right bundle-
branch block is possible. (From Aufderheide TP, Gibler WR.
Emergency Cardiac Care. St. Louis: Mosby–Year Book, 1994:181.)

Table 15-5. Electrocardiographic features for the fascicular and bifascicular blocks

ECG finding	LAFB	LPFB	RBBB and LAFB	RBBB and LPFB
QRS axis	>−45	+90 to +120	−60 to −120	>+120
QRS duration	Normal	Normal	>0.12 sec	>0.12 sec
Leads I and avl	qR	rS	qR	rS
Leads II, III, and avf	rS	qR	rS	qR
Leads V1 and V2	–	–	RSR′	RSR′
Leads V5 and V6	S	No Qs	–	–

3. **Specific therapy.** Prophylactic pacing in patients with new RBBB is controversial. Recently published American Heart Association (AHA) guidelines do not recommend prophylactic pacing of patients with new RBBB. There is a definite risk to progression to complete heart block, and these patients should be closely monitored. A transvenous wire should be placed if bifascicular, complete heart block, or progressive AV block develops.

C. **Left anterior fascicular block**
   1. **ECG recognition.** In LAFB (Fig. 15-13), the septum is initially activated in an inferior, anterior, and rightward direction. This activation is followed by the inferior and apical portions of the left ventricle. The anterolateral and posterobasal segments are the last to be activated. The QRS is less than 0.12 seconds. The QRS axis is leftward and greater than −45 degrees. As the initial vector is directed inferiorly, there will be a small R wave followed by a deep S wave in leads II, III, and avf, indicating activation of the anterolateral and posterobasal segments of the left ventricle. Leads I and avl record a dominant R wave with or without small Q waves. Often there are persistent S waves in leads V5 and V6. There also may be small initial Q waves in the midprecordial leads, which can be mistaken for a septal infarct. The T waves are normally upright (except in avr).
   2. **Clinical presentation.** LAFB is the most common ventricular conduction defect in patients with MI, occurring in approximately 8% of patients. Patients with LAFB in the setting of MI are likely undergoing anterior and septal ischemia. These patients are only at a small risk of progression to complete AV block.
   3. **Specific therapy.** Most patients with LAFB and MI are unlikely to progress to complete AV block. Prophylactic pacing in these patients is not indicated. These patients should be closely observed and treated as indicated by the clinical situation.

D. **Left posterior fascicular block**
   1. **ECG recognition.** In LPFB, the mid-septum is

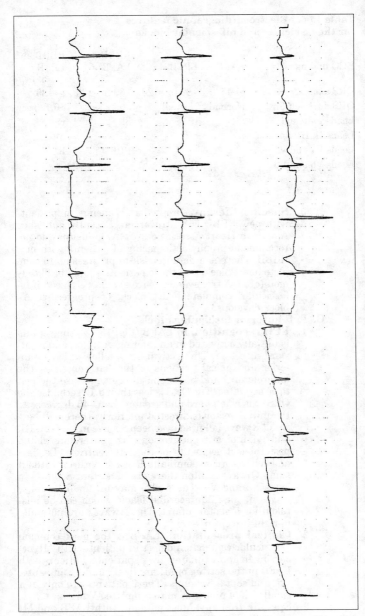

Fig. 15-13.   Left anterior fascicular block.

activated initially, followed by the anterior and anterolateral walls of the left ventricle in an anterior and
leftward direction. The inferior and posterior walls are
the last to be activated in an inferior, posterior, and
rightward direction. The QRS duration is less than
0.12 seconds, and the QRS axis is usually between +90
and +120 degrees. There is an RS pattern in leads I
and avl, and a qR pattern in leads II, III, and avf. To
meet ECG criteria for LPFB, there should be no electrocardiographic or clinical evidence for right ventricular hypertrophy (RVH), since RVH can produce the
same pattern as LPFB in the limb leads.

2. **Clinical presentation.** The presence of LPFB is rare
and almost always associated with RBBB. The posterior fascicle of the left bundle is the least vulnerable
because of dual blood supply. When affected, usually
the left anterior fascicle or right bundle is involved as
well. Increased cardiovascular morbidity and mortality in patients with isolated LPFB and AMI is found.
However, progression to high-grade AV block is not increased in isolated LPFB.

3. **Specific therapy.** Prophylactic transvenous pacing in
patients with isolated LPFB in the setting of MI is not
indicated. Like patients with LAFB, close observation
and treatment as indicated by the clinical situation is
appropriate.

E. **Right bundle-branch block and fascicular blocks
(bifascicular block)**

1. **ECG recognition.** In patients with RBBB, the diagnosis of LAFB also should be considered when the
QRS axis is markedly leftward between –60 and –120
degrees (Fig. 15-14). As in lone LAFB, there may be a
qR pattern in I and avl, and an Rs pattern in II, III,
and avf. Likewise, the diagnosis of RBBB and LPFB
should be considered when the QRS axis is markedly
rightward greater than +120 degrees (provided there
is no RVH). Further evidence would include a qR pattern in II, III, and avf, and an rS pattern in I and avl.

2. **Clinical presentation.** Patients with bifascicular
block and MI are at increased risk of sudden progression to complete AV block. In fact, 80% of patients with
RBBB and LPFB have concomitant AV conduction disturbances. About 25% of patients with bifascicular
block progress to complete AV block. The combination
of RBBB and LAFB is much more common than RBBB
and LPFB. Patients with new bifascicular block in the
setting of MI likely have extensive ischemia to the anteroseptal area. These patients are at increased risk of
sudden progression to **complete heart block** and development of **left ventricular failure.** They also
have an increased risk of in-hospital cardiovascular
mortality.

3. **Specific therapy.** Patients with a new bifascicular
block in the setting of MI are at increased risk of progression to sudden heart block. Recent AHA guidelines

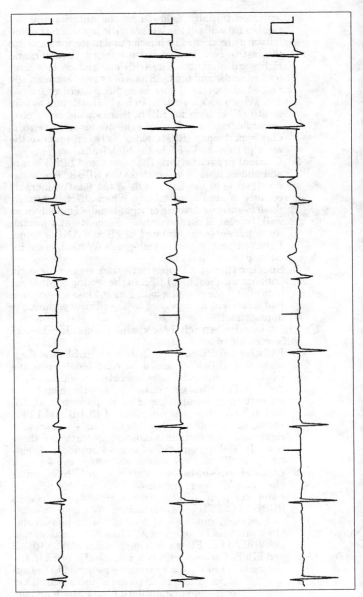

Fig. 15-14.   Left anterior fascicular block and incomplete right bundle-branch block, a bifascicular block.

recommend prophylactic transvenous pacemaker placement in these patients.

X. **General management and specific therapy for heart block**

A. **Approach to patient care.** Heart block and ongoing myocardial ischemia are medical emergencies and require immediate assessment, diagnosis, and initiation of treatment. As in all medical emergencies, the first priority is in assessing the airway, breathing, and circulation (ABC's). All patients should have IV access, receive supplemental oxygen, and undergo ECG monitoring. Although all patients with myocardial ischemia and conduction disturbances need a complete history and physical examination, the risk of hemodynamic compromise necessitates the need for a cursory history and physical. Initial assessment should include measurement of heart rate, blood pressure, respiratory rate, and oxygen saturation. The cardiovascular and pulmonary systems should be examined in detail, including peripheral pulses and jugular venous wave form. Diagnosing AV and intraventricular conduction defects in the setting of MI requires a detailed analysis of the 12-lead ECG and rhythm strip. However, the evaluation of QRS width and ST-segment motion should always be done in multiple leads on the electrocardiogram. Management of pain during myocardial infarction and administration of antithrombotic, antiplatelet, and thrombolytic agents also should have a high priority.

B. **Pharmacological therapy of bradycardia and heart block**

1. **Atropine.** Atropine increases the sinus rate and enhances atrioventricular conduction by blocking the effects of acetylcholine. The initial dose of atropine is 0.5–1.0 mg IV q5min if needed for a total dose, not to exceed 0.04 mg/kg, the amount to produce complete vagal blockade. The recommended indications for atropine therapy include but are not limited to the following:

   - Sinus bradycardia with hypotension, heart failure, or frequent ventricular premature contractions
   - Symptomatic type I second-degree AV block in the setting of acute IMI
   - Bradycardia and hypotension after administration of nitroglycerin
   - Nausea and vomiting after morphine administration
   - Asystole
   - Complete heart block at or above the level of the AVN

   Atropine is rarely the drug of choice in patients with infranodal AV block (e.g., type II second-degree AV block and complete heart block with a wide QRS complex). Adverse effects of atropine include the following.

   - Rarely can it cause paradoxical effect (i.e., worsening of bradycardia and depression of AV conduction).

- It can induce atrial fibrillation and rarely ventricular tachycardia and fibrillation during acute myocardial infarction.
- Other effects include dry mouth, cycloplegia, mydriasis, hyperpyrexia, urinary retention, confusion, and hallucinations.

2. **Isoproterenol.** Isoproterenol is a potent nonspecific beta-adrenergic agonist. There is negligble effect on alpha receptors at dosages that are used clinically. Stimulation of beta$_1$ receptors causes marked increase in heart rate, contractility, and conduction velocity. Stimulation of beta$_2$ receptors causes smooth muscle relaxation and bronchodilation. The combined stimulation of beta receptors results in an increase in cardiac output, systolic blood pressure, pulse pressure, contractility, and a decrease in systemic vascular resistance, pulmonary vascular resistance, and diastolic blood pressure. There is likely no net change in mean arterial pressure. As a result of increased heart rate and contractility, myocardial oxygen demand is increased. There is also a decrease in coronary perfusion pressure as diastolic blood pressure is decreased.

   Isoproterenol is rarely the drug of choice during acute myocardial infarction due to the increase in myocardial oxygen demand. However, isoproterenol can be administered as a temporizing measure to treat hemodynamically significant bradycardia and AV block in the setting of MI. Isoproterenol infusion should be administered to patients refractory to atropine while the transvenous pacemaker is placed. Isoproterenol infusion can be started at 1.0 mg/min and titrated to desired hemodynamic effects with a maximum of 4 mg/min. Isoproterenol has a half-life of 2 minutes and is rapidly cleared by the liver. Adverse drug effects include tachyarrhythmias, palpitations, headache, flushing, nausea, tremor, and dizziness.

3. **Aminophylline.** Aminophylline is a methylxanthine and a competitive antagonist of adenosine. Recently it has been shown that adenosine may mediate some of the conduction abnormalities during MI. Adenosine is likely released endogenously by ischemic cells and prolongs AV nodal conduction leading to AV block. In recent studies in animal and human models, the effects of adenosine-induced bradycardias and AV block can be inhibited by administration of aminophylline but not atropine. The dose is 5 mg/kg infused over 5 minutes.

C. **Transcutaneous and transvenous pacing in AMI**
   1. **Transcutaneous pacing.** Transcutaneous pacing is a rapid, minimally invasive, highly effective means of treating compromising bradyarrhythmias. Transcutaneous pacing electrodes are applied to the skin of the anterior and posterior chest walls; pacing is initiated with a portable pulse generator. In an urgent or emergent situation, compared to other methods of cardiac

pacing, such a pacing technique is easily and rapidly accomplished. The transcutaneous pacing apparatus is sufficiently portable such that its use in the emergency department and out-of-hospital settings is possible. In fact, a number of current-generation portable transcutaneous pacers are incorporated into defibrillation units.

Recommended **indications** for transcutaneous pacemaker use include both the prophylactic placement of pacer electrodes (i.e., without active pacing) and the active pacing mode. In patients with relatively lower-risk conduction block and acute coronary ischemic syndromes, the placement of transcutaneous electrodes on the patient provides immediate means of pacing should clinical deterioration occur while the transvenous approach is secured. Patients in any hemodynamically compromising bradyarrhythmia (e.g., intact though compromised circulation), asystole, and bradyarrhythmic cardiopulmonary arrest are all candidates for active transcutaneous pacing. In patients with unstable bradycardia or conduction block associated with MI who have not responded to atropine, transcutaneous pacers have proven to be useful in both the out-of-hospital and emergency department settings. Such pacing therapy is strictly temporary, however, and is intended as a therapeutic bridge to transvenous pacing. Animal studies and anecdotal human reports suggest that the use of transcutaneous pacing is safe for up to 1 hour without myocardial or other tissue damage. Longer periods of such pacing have not been fully investigated and cannot be recommended except in extreme cases.

Patients in cardiac arrest without spontaneous circulation frequently do not benefit from such therapy unless initiated very early in the course of resuscitation.

a. **Transcutaneous pacemaker placement technique.** Two sets of patient electrodes are required, one set for patient monitoring and the other for actual pacing. Standard ECG electrodes are used for cardiac monitoring purposes while larger electrodes with an 8-centimeter conducting surface are employed for pacing. One pacing electrode is placed over the mid-dorsal spine along the left paravertebral line, serving as the "ground," and the other is positioned over the left anterior chest (Fig. 15-15A). An alternative anterior placement method is described in Fig. 15-15B.

After application of the pacing electrodes, the unit is activated. In patients with compromising bradycardia or conduction block with intact though compromised circulation, the current output should be increased slowly from the minimal setting until electrical capture is observed on the filtered ECG (Fig. 15-16). Mechanical capture is

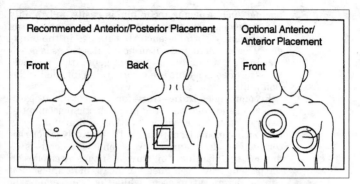

Fig. 15-15.   (Left) Proper positioning of transcutaneous pacer pads.
(Right) Alternative positioning of transcutaneous pacer pads. (From
ZOLL Medical Corporation, Burlington, MA.)

assessed by determining the presence of a palpable
pulse corresponding to the paced rhythm on the
cardiac monitor and/or through blood pressure
monitoring. The pacing rate is then adjusted according to the particular clinical situation. Current
output is minimized at a level immediately above
the threshold of electrical capture so as to limit patient discomfort.

Conscious patients or those patients who regain
consciousness during pacing must receive medication to limit pain and anxiety. Reasonable agents
include narcotic pain medications with or without
benzodiazepines. In patients with cardiac arrest,
the current output is maximized with subsequent
reduction if successful pacing is accomplished.

b. **Complications.** Complications associated with
transcutaneous pacing include pain, induction of
arrhythmia, tissue damage, and failure to recognize underlying rhythm changes such as ventricular fibrillation (VF). The risk of electrical shock
to health care personnel from patients who are
actively pacing via the transcutaneous mode is

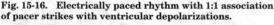

Fig. 15-16.   Electrically paced rhythm with 1:1 association
of pacer strikes with ventricular depolarizations.

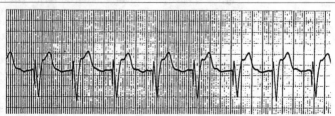

minimal; the power delivered is less than 1/1000 of that delivered in defibrillation. Chest compressions may be administered directly over the electrodes while pacing since inadvertent contact results in only a mild shock.

3. **Transvenous pacing.** Although there are no convincing data to show that temporary transvenous pacing during acute myocardial infarction reduces mortality, there are accepted indications for transvenous pacing and a general conception that some patients are salvaged. The vast majority of patients with progressive heart block have extensive myocardial damage, depressed left ventricular function, and an associated increased cardiovascular mortality. These patients often can be resuscitated and stabilized with a single ventricular lead with placement of a permanent, dual-chamber pacer at a later time.

   a. **Recommended indications** for temporary transvenous pacemaker insertion include:

      • Asystole
      • Complete heart block
      • Right bundle-branch block with left anterior or left posterior hemiblock developing in acute myocardial infarction
      • New left bundle-branch block with acute infarction (some authors would require a first-degree AV block in addition to the LBBB)
      • Type II second-degree AV block
      • Symptomatic bradycardia unresponsive to atropine
      • Type I second-degree AV block with hypotension unresponsive to atropine
      • Sinus bradycardia with hypotension unresponsive to atropine
      • Recurrent sinus pauses unresponsive to atropine
      • Atrial or ventricular overdrive pacing for incessant ventricular tachycardia

   b. **Venous access.** Transvenous pacing can be achieved through the femoral, subclavian, or internal jugular vein. The right subclavian vein has become the standard route of venous access for transvenous pacing for several reasons: 1) the subclavian vein is usually easily accessible; 2) further, the temporary pacing wire rests on the flat surface of the vein under the clavicle, allowing increased stability and easy maintenance in this position; and 3) a right-sided venous approach leaves the left side clear for a permanent pacer implant, if indicated. Venous access also can be obtained through the internal jugular vein if necessary. These sites should be avoided if the patient has a coagulopathy or recently received thrombolytic therapy since these veins are not easily compressible.

   c. **Insertion of ventricular leads.** Occasionally a patient will present in extremis and a transvenous pacemaker will need to be placed emergently. In these instances, the physician does not have the luxury of placing the pacemaker wire using fluoroscopic guidance. Placement of the pacemaker can be done either under electrocardiographic guidance or blindly, using a balloon-tipped flotation catheter. **Placement under electrocardiographic guidance** requires that the patient be connected to the limb leads of a grounded ECG machine. The distal end of the pacing wire is connected to the V lead of the ECG machine. The pacing electrode is advanced through the central venous line into the right ventricle while the V lead is monitored. As the electrode enters the superior vena cava, the P wave and QRS complex will be negative. When the catheter tip enters the high right atrium, both the P wave and QRS complex will be negative; the P wave will be larger than the QRS complex. As the catheter tip travels through the right atrium, the P wave becomes smaller and upright. As the catheter travels through the tricuspid valve, the P wave becomes smaller and the QRS larger. Once in the right ventricle, the tip is advanced until the contact is made with the endocardium, indicated by marked ST-segment elevation. Ideally the tip is located at the apex of the right ventricle. If a balloon-tipped flotation catheter is used, the balloon should be deflated once in the right ventricle.

Occasionally, in the absence of an ECG monitor, the pacemaker must be placed blindly. Once the pacemaker wire is in the vein of choice, the wire is connected to the pacing generator. The output should be set to an amperage that is unlikely to achieve capture (i.e., usually less than 0.2 mA). The unit is turned on and set to the "sense" mode, and the wire then is advanced. Upon entering the right ventricle, the electrode will sense ventricular depolarization. The amperage can be then increased to 4–5 mA and the wire advanced; the "pace" mode then is used. Electrical capture of the ventricle should occur after advancing the pacemaker wire approximately 10 cm. If not, the wire should be pulled back to its original position and advanced again.

In patients with asystolic arrest or complete heart block with malignant ventricular arrhythmia, blind placement of the transvenous wire must be performed in the pace mode. In this situation, connect the wire to the power source, turn the output to a maximum setting, and select the asynchronous mode. The catheter then is inserted blindly with the hope that the pacemaker lead will enter and subsequently capture the right ventricle.

If available, **fluoroscopy** is extremely useful in the placement of transvenous pacing wires. Advance the pacing wire through the sheath of the appropriate venous access until it lies in the right atrium. Rotate the wire, using the index finger and thumb, until the wire points down and to the patient's left. It is often easier to rotate the wire while advancing it forward. Ideally, the wire will pass through the tricuspid valve and slide along the floor of the right ventricle to the apex. If it is difficult to pass the tricuspid valve, then adjust the angle of the tip of the electrode. If difficulty is still encountered, try looping the wire in the right atrium with the tip facing the tricuspid valve. Advance the wire while applying either counterclockwise or clockwise torque force such that the tip is directed through the tricuspid valve. Once the wire is beyond the valve, direct the wire into the apex of the right ventricle (down and to the left) until minimal resistance is felt and a small bend in the wire is noted (Fig. 15-17).

Regardless of the technique used for insertion, adequate positioning can also be confirmed by activating the pacer. The ECG will demonstrate pacer spikes associated with ventricular depolarizations (see Fig. 15-16) when the wire is correctly positioned. Always remember to **obtain a chest radiograph** after placing a temporary pacing wire

Fig. 15-17.   Transvenous pacemaker insertion through the left subclavian vein. (From Benjamin G. Emergency transvenous cardiac pacing. In Roberts J, Hedges J (eds.) *Clinical Procedures in Emergency Medicine* (2nd ed.). Philadelphia: Saunders, 1991:189.)

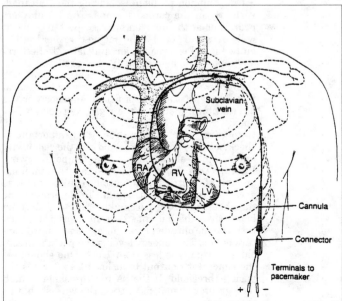

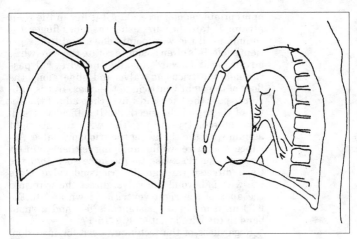

Fig. 15-18. Schematic of proper positioning of transvenous pacemaker wire on posteroanterior and lateral chest radiographs. (From Goldberger E. *Treatment of Cardiac Emergencies* (4th ed.). St. Louis: Mosby, 1985:277.)

to determine adequate placement and rule out an iatrogenic pneumothorax. See Fig. 15-18 for a schematic representation confirming adequate positioning on the chest radiograph of a transvenous pacing wire inserted through the subclavian vein.

One common problem is placing the lead inadvertently in the coronary sinus. The tip may appear to be at the apex on fluoroscopy, but either it will not capture or else the pacing threshold will be quite high. Posteroanterior and lateral chest radiographs will help identify this problem. If the coronary sinus has been inadvertently cannulated, then the wire will project posteriorly on the lateral film. The wire is always projected anteriorly on the lateral film if placed at the right ventricular (RV) apex.

d. Inspecting the pacemaker. It is important to check both the pacing threshold and the sensitivity immediately after placing the temporary wire. **Pacing threshold** is defined as the minimal amount of electrical stimulation required to cause a cardiac muscle contraction. To determine the threshold, turn the pacemaker rate to 5–10 bpm faster than the patient's current heart rate; then turn the amplitude of the voltage down until capture is lost. This energy level is the pacing threshold and usually is less than 1 mA. One should set the generator's output to at least 2 to 3 times the pacing threshold. If the pacing threshold is high (i.e., greater than 1 mA), then the wire should be repositioned.

Sensing is defined as the ability of the pacemaker to recognize and respond to electrical activity of the heart, usually by inhibiting pacemaker firing. To check the sensitivity function, turn the pacemaker rate to 10–20 bpm less than the patient's heart rate. If the pacemaker is sensing, there should be no pacemaker spikes noted on the rhythm strip. If the pacemaker was placed for prophylactic reasons, then the sensitivity should be at maximum pacing only when there is not an adequate intrinsic heart rate.

e. **Complications.** Complications associated with transvenous pacing include infection, phlebitis, venous thrombosis, perforation of the right ventricle, carotid artery perforation, hemothorax, pneumothorax, and induction of arrhythmias.

Bibliography

Aufderheide TP, Brady WJ. In Gibler B, Aufderheide TP (eds.). *Emergency Cardiac Care.* St Louis: Mosby, 1994.

Goldberger E. *Treatment of Cardiovascular Emergencies.* St Louis: Mosby, 1985.

Roberts J, Hedges J (eds.). *Clinical Procedures in Emergency Medicine.* Philadelphia: Saunders, 1991.

Atrial Tachydysrhythmias

Alan Gora

Supraventricular tachydysrhythmias can be a common complication of acute myocardial infarction (AMI) (Table 16-1). AMI-associated supraventricular dysrhythmias include sinus tachycardia, paroxysmal atrial tachycardia, atrial fibrillation, atrial flutter, and junctional tachycardia. In addition to the classic signs and symptoms associated with AMI, patients with atrial tachydysrhythmias can present with a spectrum of symptoms from simple palpitations to syncope and cardiovascular collapse. In the setting of an AMI, many of these atrial tachydysrhythmias can be detrimental. They cause relatively rapid heart rates, which decrease cardiac output and increase myocardial oxygen demand. These patients require aggressive management to control their dysrhythmias and to treat the underlying causes. Consequently, physicians working in emergent care settings should be familiar with the diagnosis and treatment of atrial tachydysrhythmias associated with AMI.

This chapter also discusses the diagnosis and treatment of a number of atrial tachydysrhythmias that are not classically associated with AMI. These include preexcitation syndromes, sick sinus syndrome, and multifocal atrial tachycardia.

I. **Atrial dysrhythmias in myocardial infarction**
   A. **Premature atrial contractions (PACs).** Premature atrial contractions occur relatively commonly after AMI (15%–40%). Although they occur in normal individuals as well, most PACs are found in patients with heart disease. PACs tend to be benign, except that they can initiate a more serious dysrhythmia like paroxysmal supraventricular tachycardia (PSVT), atrial flutter, or atrial fibrillation. In themselves, PACs are not associated with a higher mortality in the setting of an AMI.
      1. **Assessment.** The assessment of the patient with myocardial ischemia and PACs should include close cardiac monitoring. Special attention should be paid to the potential for the development of other atrial arrhythmias that may be triggered by a PAC. The ECG characteristics of PACs include the following (Figure 16-1):
         a. A premature P wave is present and usually of different morphology, although it may be buried under a QRS complex or a T wave.
         b. The PR interval is usually longer but may be the same or shorter.
         c. The QRS that follows the P wave is usually unchanged from conducted sinus beats.
         d. The postextrasystolic cycle is usually less than compensatory.
      2. **Management.** Treatment of PACs is generally not required. If another more severe dysrhythmia is triggered, then treatment is directed at that secondary dysrhythmia.

Table 16-1. Incidence of supraventricular dysrhythmias in AMI

Dysrhythmia	Incidence (%)
Sinus tachycardia	30–40
Premature atrial contractions (PACs)	15–40
Paroxysmal atrial tachycardia (PAT)	2–10
Atrial fibrillation	10
Atrial flutter	5
Junctional tachycardia (JT)	5
Paroxysmal junctional tachycardia	1–2

B. Sinus tachycardia. Up to one third of patients with AMI will develop sinus tachycardia at some point within the first 72 hours of presentation. The general causes of sinus tachycardia are diverse and are listed in Table 16-2. In the patient with AMI, the most likely etiologies are anxiety, pain, hypovolemia, and left ventricular dysfunction. Because sinus tachycardia causes an increase in myocardial oxygen demand and a decrease in end-diastolic filling time, it can be detrimental to the patient with AMI. In the setting of poor left ventricular (LV) function, however, stroke volumes are relatively fixed and a more rapid heart rate is required to maintain or increase cardiac output. Consequently, a sinus tachycardia may be a necessary physiologic response under these circumstances. Even in patients with poor LV function or hypovolemia, however, too rapid a heart rate can result in a decrease in cardiac output.

    1. Assessment. In the assessment of the patient with AMI and sinus tachycardia, attention should be given to identifying whether the tachycardia is a compensatory mechanism to increase cardiac output. Specific etiologies such as heart failure, fever, hypoxia, hypovolemia, or pericarditis should be identified and treated aggressively. The ECG characteristics of sinus tachycardia are as follows (Fig. 16-2):

Fig. 16-1. Premature atrial contractions. (From Weiderhold R. *Electrocardiography: The Monitoring Lead.* Philadelphia: Saunders, 1988:58.)

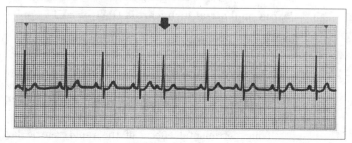

Table 16-2.   Causes of sinus tachycardia

Fever	Hypoxemia
Anxiety	Pulmonary embolus
Pain	Congestive heart failure (CHF)
Sepsis	Hyperthyroidism
Hypovolemia	Ethanol withdrawal
Anemia	Pericardial tamponade
Pericarditis	Hypotension
Medications	Sinoatrial (SA) node reentry

   a. The heart rate is between 100 and 160.
   b. The P-wave is normal (upright in II and down in avr).
   c. There is a P wave before each QRS with a normal PR interval unless a block is present.
   d. There may be a small variation in the P-to-P interval.

2. **Management.** Management of the patient with AMI and sinus tachycardia should focus on treating the ischemic event. If there is no evidence of heart failure (rales, S3, pulmonary congestion on chest x-ray), the patient does not appear hypovolemic or hypoxic, and the tachycardia is *not* felt to be a compensatory mechanism to maintain cardiac output, treatment with beta blockade can be instituted (Table 16-3). The dose of beta-blockers can be titrated to effect.

   In those patients with significant LV dysfunction or hypovolemia, beta blockade can be detrimental and can result in cardiogenic shock or pulmonary edema. In patients who appear to be clinically dehydrated, IV fluid boluses can be given prior to beta blockade to reduce the tachycardia. If there is no response, beta-blockers can be given cautiously. Patients with LV dysfunction can be treated as outlined in Chap. 14. Other potential etiologies of the tachycardia should be sought and treated. For example, analgesics for pain, anxiolytics for anxiety, and antipyretics for fever can reduce tachycardia when indicated. Swan-Ganz catheter monitoring can be extremely helpful in guiding fluid and beta-blocker management in the AMI patient.

C. **Paroxysmal atrial tachycardia (PAT or SVT).** Paroxysmal atrial tachycardia occurs in 2%–10% of patients following AMI. It may involve the sinoatrial (SA) node or an ectopic atrial focus. These dysrhythmias tend to be significant in the setting of myocardial ischemia because of the rapid ventricular rate, the increase in myocardial oxygen demand, and the decrease in cardiac output that they cause. Consequently, they are associated with a higher mortality in the context of AMI.

1. **Assessment.** Assessment of PAT should focus on identifying detrimental effects of the rapid ventricular

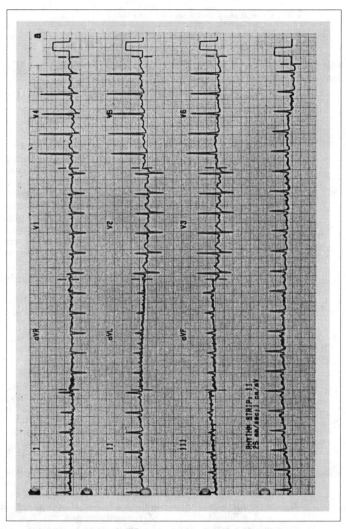

Fig. 16-2. Sinus tachycardia. (From Paine R. *Generation and Interpretation of the Electrocardiogram.* Philadelphia: Lea & Febiger, 1988.)

Table 16-3.   Commonly used beta-blockers

Drug	Dosage	Half-life
Propranolol	1–3 mg IVP	3–4 hr
Metoprolol, atenolol	5 mg IVP q5min, max 15 mg	3–4 hr
Esmolol	500 µg/kg/min bolus, 50 µg/kg/min infusion	9–10 min

response, such as worsening angina or significant decreases in cardiac output with hypotension or pulmonary edema. If the tachycardia is wide complex, an attempt should be made to differentiate between PAT with an aberrant conduction pathway versus ventricular tachycardia. In the setting of myocardial ischemia, however, wide-complex tachycardia is most likely to be ventricular in origin and should be treated as such (see Chap. 17). In narrow-complex tachycardia, the ECG should be examined to differentiate PAT from sinus tachycardia as a diagnosis. The following clues can be used to differentiate between sinus tachycardia and PAT (Fig. 16-3).

   a. Rate. Sinus tachycardia is usually <140 bpm, whereas PAT is usually >150 bpm. Both have a regular RR interval.

   b. Vagal maneuvers. These usually will slow a sinus tachycardia but not a PAT. They may convert a PAT to sinus rhythm.

   c. Onset. Sinus tachycardia usually has a gradual onset, whereas PAT usually begins and ends abruptly. In those patients receiving digitalis, PAT with block may be a manifestation of digitalis toxicity, necessitating withdrawal of the drug (see Chap. 30).

2. **Management.** Management should focus on controlling the ventricular rate and cardioversion to normal sinus rhythm (NSR). In the setting of myocardial ischemia, treatment should be rapid to terminate the high myocardial oxygen demand that results from a rapid ventricular rate. If the patient shows evidence of cardiogenic shock or worsening angina, the most rapid and efficient method of restoring sinus rhythm involves synchronized DC cardioversion beginning at 50 joules. Given the invasive nature of this intervention, pharmacologic interventions are often attempted first, time permitting. These include the following:

   a. Vagal maneuvers. Carotid sinus massage is usually the most effective of the vagal maneuvers. It should begin on the right side. If the tachycardia persists, massage of the left carotid sinus can be done after several minutes. Bilateral carotid massage should never be performed. A history of cardiovascular accidents (CVAs), advanced age, or diffuse atherosclerosis are contraindications to carotid sinus massage. The Valsalva maneuver is another

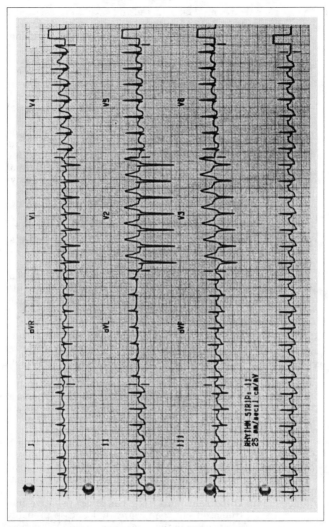

Fig. 16-3.   Atrial tachycardia. (From Paine R. *Generation and Interpretation of the Electrocardiogram.* Philadelphia: Lea & Febiger, 1988.)

effective method of increasing vagal tone, especially in older patients or patients with cerebrovascular disease. Other vagal maneuvers include squatting, inflation of MAST pants, rectal examination, or submersion of the patient's face in ice water.

b. Adenosine. Adenosine is highly effective at blocking the atrioventricular (AV) node and can convert 90% or more of PAT in adults. Because of its extremely short half-life (<10 seconds), its potential side effects are short-lived.

   (1) Dosage. The dose is 6 mg rapid IV push as close to the IV insertion site as possible. This should be followed rapidly by a normal saline flush. If 6 mg is not effective, a second dose of 12 mg can be used and repeated if the tachycardia persists.

   (2) Adverse effects. These include flushing, lightheadedness, chest pain, dyspnea, bradycardia, and sinus pause. The patient should be warned about these bothersome side effects. Adenosine may be less effective in patients receiving theophylline.

c. Calcium channel blockers. This class of drugs is highly effective at controlling the ventricular rate and converting PAT to sinus rhythm. Vagal maneuvers can be repeated after administration of a calcium channel blocker because the effect of the maneuvers will be enhanced. The administration of calcium (e.g., 1 g calcium gluconate or chloride) prior to the use of calcium channel blockers has been advocated as a way to reduce side effects.

   (1) Verapamil. This is usually quite effective but needs to be used cautiously because it can cause hypotension, worsen congestive heart failure (CHF), or produce bradycardia, especially in the face of concomitant beta-blocker therapy.

      (a) Dosage. The dose is 5 to 10 mg IV over 2 minutes. One may repeat up to 20 mg in 20–30 minutes.

      (b) Adverse effects. These include hypotension, CHF, bradycardia, and AV block.

   (2) Diltiazem. This drug has fewer negative inotropic effects than verapamil and is probably safer to use in the case of decreased LV function.

      (a) Dosage. The dose is 0.25 mg/kg over 2 minutes followed by 0.35 mg/kg over 5 minutes if necessary. This can be followed with a continuous infusion of 5–15 mg/hr.

      (b) Adverse effects. These include hypotension, CHF, bradycardia, and AV block.

d. Beta-blockers. This group of medications can also be effective in converting episodes of PAT to NSR. The commonly used beta-blockers are listed in Table 16-3 along with their respective doses.

   Adverse effects. These include exacerbation of asthma or chronic obstructive pulmonary disease

(COPD) worsening LV or sinus node dysfunction, and AV block.

e. **Digoxin.** Digoxin slows the ventricular rate by slowing AV node conduction time. It is used less often than adenosine or calcium channel blockers in the setting of PAT because of its slow onset of action. Its effects are additive to beta-blockers or calcium channel blockers, but it can be used simultaneously with both.

   (1) **Dosage.** The initial dose is 0.25–0.50 mg IV, with 0.25 mg given 30–60 minutes later. A total loading dose of 1 mg over the first 24 hours is needed to maintain effect. Serum levels can help guide loading doses.

   (2) **Adverse effects.** These include heart block, ventricular dysrhythmias, nausea, vomiting, and yellow-green visual halos.

f. **Overdrive pacing.** Overdrive pacing using a transvenous pacemaker has also been shown to be effective in converting refractory PAT.

g. **Vasopressors.** Medications such as phenylephrine can convert PAT by increasing arterial pressure and activating carotid baroreceptors. However, this could be extremely detrimental to the patient with AMI and should be avoided in this setting.

D. **Atrial flutter.** Atrial flutter occurs in less than 5% of patients following AMI. Its presence in the setting of myocardial ischemia is associated with a higher mortality. It is less common, but also less stable, than atrial fibrillation. It tends to be episodic but may be chronic in patients with underlying heart disease.

1. **Assessment.** Unlike in atrial fibrillation (see sec. **I.E.**), some semblance of the AV conduction sequence is maintained in atrial flutter. Rapid ventricular response to atrial flutter is common and can easily result in decreased filling time, low stroke volume, and hemodynamic compromise requiring rapid treatment.

   In atrial flutter, the atrial rate usually varies between 250 and 300 bpm. It most commonly appears as 2:1 block with a ventricular rate of approximately 150 bpm. The next most common presentation is 4:1 block, and 3:1 block is relatively rare. The salient ECG characteristics of atrial flutter are as follows (Fig. 16-4):

   a. "Sawtooth" pattern of flutter waves that may be difficult to see with faster ventricular rtates.

   b. The rhythm is regular unless variable block is present.

2. **Management.** Management of atrial flutter usually centers on cardioversion to normal sinus rhythm or slowing of the ventricular rate. Since this arrhythmia is often difficult to convert pharmacologically, synchronized DC cardioversion is commonly the initial treatment of choice, especially in the setting of AMI. Cardioversion is usually successful at energy levels as low as 10 joules, but 25 joules is the initial recommended energy level. In atrial flutter the atria

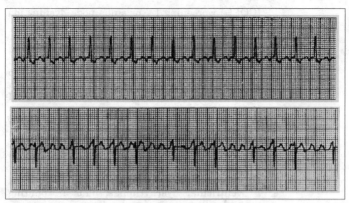

Fig. 16-4.   Examples of atrial flutter. (From Patel JM, McGowan SG, Moody LA. *Arrhythmias: Detection, Treatment, and Cardiac Drugs.* Philadelphia: Saunders, 1989.)

contract, resulting in fewer atrial thrombi. Therefore, anticoagulation is not usually necessary before attempted cardioversion to normal sinus rhythm. (It should be noted that many atrial flutter patients convert back and forth from atrial flutter to atrial fibrillation spontaneously, making generalizations regarding atrial thrombi difficult.)

If the situation permits, the ventricular rate can be controlled using calcium channel blockers, beta-blockers, or digoxin as described previously for the treatment of PAT. In the setting of transmural AMI, beta-blockers are probably preferred over calcium channel blockers to control ventricular rate because of beta-blockers' beneficial effects demonstrated in ISIS-I. Since spontaneous conversion to NSR frequently occurs in patients with new-onset atrial flutter, slowing the ventricular rate may be all that is needed to stabilize the patient prior to monitoring for spontaneous cardioversion to NSR.

E. **Atrial fibrillation.** Atrial fibrillation occurs in approximately 10% of patients with AMI. It is most often a result of atrial ischemia. It is frequently poorly tolerated in this setting and is therefore associated with a higher mortality. Other causes of atrial fibrillation are hypertension, rheumatic heart disease, cardiomyopathy, pericarditis, hyperthyroidism, congestive heart failure, and pulmonary disease (Table 16-4).

Like atrial flutter, atrial fibrillation tends to be episodic. Unlike in atrial flutter, however, no semblance of the AV contraction sequence is maintained in atrial fibrillation, and the atrial contribution to cardiac output is lost. This loss of the atrial contraction along with the rapid ventricular rate can result in significant reductions in cardiac output.

1. **Assessment.** Assessment of the patient with atrial fibrillation should include examination for hemody-

Table 16-4. Causes of atrial fibrillation

Acute myocardial infarction (AMI)	Hyperthyroidism
Pericarditis	Cardiomyopathy
Valvular disease	Pulmonary embolus
Congestive heart failure (CHF)	Sick sinus syndrome
Cardiac surgery	Idiopathic
Preexcitation syndrome	Myocardial contusion
Holiday heart syndrome	Catecholamines
(acute ethanol intoxication)	

namic instability and associated diseases that may be a contributing etiology for the dysrhythmia. Atrial fibrillation is usually readily identifiable by its irregularly irregular pulse and characteristic ECG. However, multifocal atrial tachycardia (see sec. **III.A.**) or NSR with PACs may be mistaken for atrial fibrillation. The salient ECG features of atrial fibrillation are as follows (Fig. 16-5):

  a. Irregularly irregular pattern of QRS complexes.
  b. Absence of P waves and the presence of fibrillatory or F waves that are usually best seen in lead V1.

  2. Management. The management of atrial fibrillation should involve addressing the underlying cause (e.g., ischemia, hypoxia, CHF), controlling the ventricular rate, cardioversion to normal sinus rhythm, and prevention of embolic phenomena.

  a. Treating the etiology. The causes of atrial fibrillation are diverse, and treating the precipitating factor may result in spontaneous cardioversion to NSR. Hypoxia and myocardial ischemia are perhaps the most easily reversible causes and should be aggressively treated. The specific treatments of these and other etiologies are covered elsewhere in this book.

  b. Controlling the ventricular rate. Several options are available, as discussed in the PAT section (see sec. **I.C.2**.). **Calcium channel blockers** (e.g., verapamil and diltiazem) are usually effective and

Fig. 16-5. Atrial fibrillation. (From Davis D. *Differential Diagnosis of Arrhythmias.* Philadelphia: Saunders, 1992.)

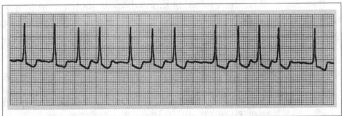

act quite rapidly. However, they should be avoided in those patients with wide-complex atrial fibrillation if there is any possibility of an accessory pathway. If calcium channel blockers are used in this group of patients, ventricular fibrillation may occur. If time permits, oral diltiazem (90–120 mg) is an effective alternative to the IV route and usually takes effect in approximately 30 minutes. **Beta-blockers** are another alternative (see Table 16-3) but should be avoided in those patients with poor LV function. Esmolol is probably the safest of the options in this class because of its relatively short half-life (<8 minutes), but it can be difficult to administer. It still takes approximately 30–40 minutes for its effects to completely disappear. **Digoxin** is also useful for controlling the ventricular rate in atrial fibrillation. However, it does not lead to conversion of NSR in itself. It takes longer to act than most of the above-stated therapeutic options (approximately 30–45 minutes), and its peak effect does not occur for several hours. **Clonidine** has been shown to be effective in this setting as well. Its mechanism of action is through decreasing sympathetic tone. The usual initial dose is 0.075 mg PO, and this dose may be repeated in 2 hours if no significant reduction in heart rate has occurred.

c. **Cardioversion to NSR.** How quickly a patient needs to be cardioverted to NSR depends on patient stability, duration of fibrillation, and etiology of the dysrhythmia. In those patients with hemodynamic instability from loss of atrial contraction and a rapid ventricular rate, synchronized *electrical cardioversion* is the treatment of choice. It should begin at 100 joules. Intravenous diltiazem may be used to rapidly slow the ventricular rate in an effort to increase cardiac output and stabilize the patient prior to cardioversion. Caution should be used, however, because calcium channel blockers may worsen hypotension.

Maintenance of NSR following cardioversion usually involves either single or combination antidysrhythmic therapy with quinidine, beta-blockers, and/or digitalis.

Quinidine and procainamide are the best-studied pharmacologic modalities for chemical cardioversion, but amiodarone, sotalol, and propafenone have also been studied in this regard. Prior to chemical cardioversion with quinidine or procainamide, the ventricular rate should be slowed using digitalis or calcium channel blockers to at least 100–110 bpm to prevent a paradoxical increase in ventricular rate when pharmacologic cardioversion is attempted. Once the ventricular rate is slowed, chemical cardioversion can be attempted as shown in Table 16-5.

Table 16-5. Pharmacologic cardioversion of atrial fibrillation

Drug	Dosage	Adverse effects
Intravenous procainamide	20–30 mg/min to a total of 17 mg/kg or until conversion occurs	Hypotension, prolongation of Q-T interval
Oral quinidine sulfate	300 mg PO q3hr for 4 doses or until side effects occur	Torsade, SLE, hypersensitivity reactions

Amiodarone has been investigated for its possible role in converting atrial fibrillation to NSR. It has numerous side effects, including interstitial pneumonitis, tremors, and ataxia. Currently more investigation is required to elucidate its role in converting atrial fibrillation and maintaining NSR.

Sotalol is a nonselective beta-blocker that also possesses some class III antidysrhythmic properties. Consequently, it can slow the ventricular response and has been shown to result in conversion in about 30% of cases. Its side effects are similar to those of other beta-blockers (e.g., CHF, bronchospasm). It also prolongs the QT interval, resulting in proarrhythmic effects as well.

Propafenone, an IC antidysrhythmic drug, has been shown to convert approximately 40% of patients from atrial fibrillation to NSR. It is also effective in slowing the ventricular response in those patients who do not convert.

d. **Prevention of embolic phenomena.** The potential for embolic events is a significant concern in atrial fibrillation. The risk is five to seven times that of patients without atrial fibrillation and may be even higher in those patients with concomitant mitral stenosis or mitral valve prolapse. In general, thrombi can form in the atria within 72 hours of the onset of atrial fibrillation. Consequently, patients presenting beyond this time frame should be anticoagulated prior to restoration of normal sinus rhythm. In general, patients with atrial fibrillation of less than 72 hours duration can safely undergo cardioversion.

II. **Junctional arrhythmias in myocardial infarction.** Junctional arrhythmias occur more commonly in patients following inferior wall myocardial infarctions. They may also result from CHF, myocarditis, electrolyte abnormalities, and digoxin toxicity.

A. **Premature junctional contractions (PJCs).** Premature junctional contractions, like PACs, tend to be benign except that they may trigger a more serious dysrhythmia. They are rarely symptomatic and are not associated with a higher mortality in the setting of AMI.

1. **Assessment.** A PJC can activate the atria before, during, or after ventricular depolarization. Consequently, the ECG can appear in one of three ways. An inverted P wave appears before, is buried within, or occurs after the QRS, depending on when atrial depolarization occurs. After the PJC, there is a less than compensatory pause before the next sinus beat occurs. (Fig. 16-6).
2. **Management.** Generally, treatment of PJCs is not required unless they begin to trigger other, more serious dysrhythmias. Treatment can then be directed at that specific dysrhythmia.

B. **Junctional tachycardia (JT).** Junctional tachycardia occurs in 5%–10% of patients with AMI and is more commonly seen following acute inferior wall infarction. It tends to occur transiently and will frequently resolve spontaneously. Two forms, paroxysmal and nonparoxysmal, have been described.

1. **Nonparoxysmal JT.** This dysrhythmia is also known as accelerated junctional rhythm. The rate is usually between 70 and 130 bpm, and the rhythm is usually regular. Unlike the paroxysmal form, nonparoxysmal junctional tachycardia has a gradual onset. Its mechanism is probably enhanced automaticity of a junctional focus. It can occur with digitalis toxicity, at which time the rhythm may be irregular secondary to a varying degree of block.

   a. **Assessment.** This dysrhythmia is usually well tolerated. If the rate is relatively rapid, signs or symptoms of instability may be evident. Potential or contributing etiologies such as digoxin toxicity or electrolyte abnormalities should be addressed. The ECG usually shows a normal QRS complex with absent P waves or the presence of inverted P

Fig. 16-6.   Examples of premature junctional contractions. (From Patel JM, McGowan SG, Moody LA. *Arrhythmias: Detection, Treatment, and Cardiac Drugs.* Philadelphia: Saunders, 1989.)

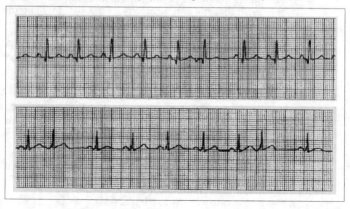

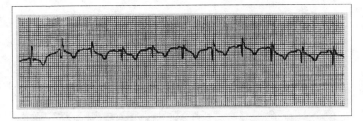

Fig. 16-7. Nonparoxysmal junctional tachycardia (lead III). (From Patel JM, McGowan SG, Moody LA. *Arrhythmias: Detection, Treatment, and Cardiac Drugs.* Philadelphia: Saunders, 1989. Used with permission.)

waves before or after the QRS complex (Fig. 16-7). The QRS morphology is unchanged from NSR.

b. **Treatment.** Treatment is generally not required except for treatment of the underlying cause (e.g., ischemia or digitalis toxicity). If the rate is rapid and there are no contraindications to their use, beta-blockers or calcium channel blockers can be used to slow the ventricular rate.

2. **Paroxysmal JT.** This tachydysrhythmia usually results in more rapid ventricular rates (140–250 bpm) and therefore tends to be more hemodynamically significant. Unlike the nonparoxysmal form, paroxysmal JT has an abrupt onset and abrupt termination. Its mechanism most likely involves an AV nodal reentry circuit. The rapid ventricular rates lead to increased myocardial oxygen consumption and can compromise LV function. The loss of AV contraction sequence may further contribute to hemodynamic instability. It can be difficult to distinguish it from PAT using routine eletrocardiography (Fig. 16-8). Fortunately, the emergent treatment is similar to that of PAT.

a. **Assessment.** Assessment of these patients should involve looking for serious signs or symptoms related to the rapid ventricular rates (e.g., worsening angina, hypotension, or CHF). The ECG should be studied in an attempt to differentiate JT from other possible tachycardias (PAT, sinus tachycardia) and for any evidence of an accessory pathway (wide QRS complex). This can be very difficult to do using the surface ECG alone. Figure 16-9 illustrates the morphologies of the P waves and their relationship to the QRS complexes as seen in the varying types of narrow-complex tachycardias.

b. **Treatment.** Treatment should progress as for PAT. Adenosine, calcium channel blockers, beta-blockers, or cardioversion can be used, depending on the clinical situation.

III. **Atrial dysrhythmias not associated with AMI**

A. **Multifocal atrial tachycardia (MAT).** Multifocal atrial tachycardia, also known as chaotic atrial tachycardia,

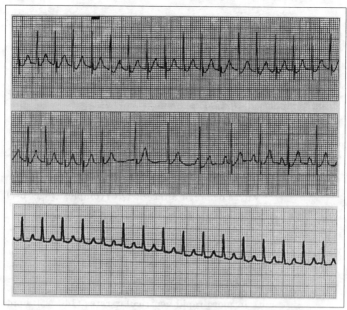

Fig. 16-8.   Paroxysmal junctional tachycardia and a continuous strip showing conversion to normal sinus rhythm. (From Patel JM, McGowan SG, Moody LA. *Arrhythmias: Detection, Treatment, and Cardiac Drugs*. Philadelphia: Saunders, 1989.)

Fig. 16-9.   Location and morphology of P waves in various causes of regular, narrow-complex tachycardias. (From Marriott HJL. *Practical Electrocardiography* (8th ed.). Baltimore: Williams & Wilkins, 1988.)

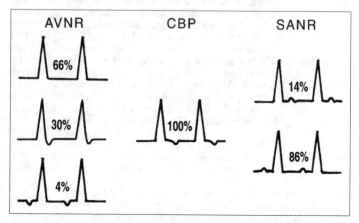

occurs most commonly in patients with chronic obstructive pulmonary disease or CHF. Less common causes of this dysrhythmia are digoxin toxicity and electrolyte abnormalities. It can be sustained or it can degenerate into atrial fibrillation or flutter. The in-hospital mortality of patients with MAT is relatively high, probably because of their underlying disease.

1. **Presentation.** Since MAT does not occur without significant heart or lung pathology, patients will most commonly present with worsening of some underlying condition like COPD or CHF. MAT is usually associated with relatively high ventricular rates, which may cause a deterioration of the patient's condition by increasing myocardial oxygen demand and decreasing cardiac output.

2. **Assessment.** This dysrhythmia is usually well tolerated. Assessment of the patient with MAT should attempt to define an etiology for the dysrhythmia. The patient should remain on a monitor to identify conversion to NSR or deterioration into atrial fibrillation or flutter. As always, a stat ECG should be obtained to define the cardiac rhythm. The classic ECG characteristics of MAT are as follows (Fig. 16-10):

   a. The ventricular rate is usually 100–150 bpm, but may be faster.

   b. There may be slight variations in the R-R intervals.

   c. At least three different P-wave morphologies exist.

   d. The QRS complexes are usually normal.

3. **Management.** Treatment usually involves correcting or treating the underlying disorder (e.g., exacerbation of COPD, CHF, or electrolyte abnormalities). Electrical cardioversion is rarely required. **Calcium channel blockers** are usually effective in controlling the ventricular rate, but digoxin is usually not effective and may worsen the condition. Consequently, digoxin should be avoided in the acute treatment of MAT. For those patients who are on digoxin chronically, the possibility of toxicity should be entertained as an etiology for the MAT and subsequent doses of digoxin should be avoided. **Beta-blockers** may be effective in controlling rapid ventricular rates but are contraindicated in patients with bronchospastic disease or CHF. Consequently, their role in the treatment of MAT is often limited. **Magnesium** given as 1–2 g IV may also potentially be helpful in the treatment of MAT.

4. **Disposition.** Most patients with MAT will require admission to a monitored bed because of the severity of the illness associated with this dysrhythmia. Furthermore, because of the potential of MAT to degenerate into atrial fibrillation or flutter, cardiac monitoring is appropriate. If the ventricular rate is well controlled and the dysrhythmia is well tolerated or chronic, the patient may be discharged with follow-up as indicated by their underlying clinical condition.

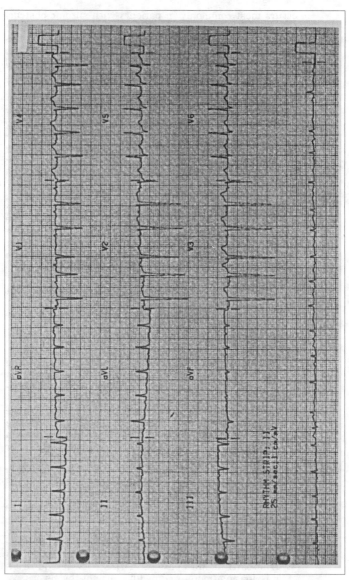

Fig. 16-10.   Multifocal atrial tachycardia. (From Paine R. *Generation and Interpretation of the Electrocardiogram.* Philadelphia: Lea & Febiger, 1988.)

B. **Preexcitation syndromes.** Preexcitation implies ventricular activation by an atrial impulse that occurs sooner than would be expected if the impulse used the normal AV conduction system. The impulse travels by way of an accessory pathway that allows the AV node to be bypassed. The tachycardia is usually sustained by reentry of an impulse through a circuit that uses the accessory pathway as one limb and the AV node as another. Wolff-Parkinson-White syndrome (WPW) is the most common of the preexcitation syndromes. The accessory pathway in WPW is referred to as the Kent bundle. Other preexcitation syndromes exist (e.g., Lown-Ganong-Levine syndrome), but they are rare and their emergent evaluation and treatment parallel that of WPW.

WPW is present in 0.1–0.3% of the population, but less than 50% of these patients are symptomatic. Males are affected twice as often as females, and a large majority of WPW patients have no associated underlying heart disease. The risk for sudden death exists, but it is exceedingly low and the prognosis of WPW generally is excellent.

Tachycardia in patients with WPW is usually triggered by a PAC or PJC. Reentry through the circuit can then occur in one of two ways. If conduction proceeds through the AV node and retrograde conduction occurs by way of the accessory pathway, a narrow QRS tachycardia usually results. This is referred to as **orthodromic conduction,** which is the most common mechanism for tachycardias in WPW. If conduction is reversed and initially travels through the accessory pathway and then retrograde to the atria by way of the AV node, then a wide-complex tachycardia occurs. This is referred to as **antidromic conduction.** It is more rare than orthodromic conduction. It also has a poorer prognosis because these patients are more likely to develop ventricular fibrillation.

Evidence of an accessory pathway can sometimes be appreciated on surface ECG because under normal conditions part of the ventricle is depolarized by the accessory pathway. In the case of WPW, the slurring of the upstroke of the QRS complex results from partial activation of the ventricle through the accessory pathway. This slurring of the QRS is referred to as the **delta wave.** Other ECG characteristics of WPW are a shortened PR interval and a QRS duration greater than 0.10 second (Fig. 16-11). Most patients with WPW will be missing one or more of the classic ECG characteristics. Any patient with PAT and a ventricular rate greater than 200 bpm should raise the suspicion for an accessory pathway.

1. **Assessment.** Assessment of patients with tachycardia and a preexcitation syndrome involves watching for signs or symptoms of instability. The duration of the QRS should also be noted because treatment will vary depending on the width of the QRS.

2. **Management.** Regardless of the duration of the QRS complex, if signs or symptoms of instability exist (e.g., hypotension and evidence of end-organ dysfunction), immediate synchronized cardioversion with 50–100

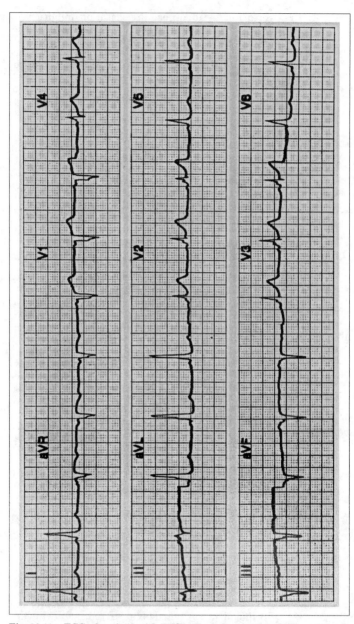

Fig. 16-11.   ECG of patient with WPW. (From Patel JM, McGowan SG, Moody LA. *Arrhythmias: Detection, Treatment, and Cardiac Drugs.* Philadelphia: Saunders, 1989.)

joules should be employed. In the stable patient, more time can be spent evaluating the clinical situation. Treatment of the stable patient varies, depending on the duration of the QRS complex.

    a. Narrow-complex WPW tachycardia. With orthodromic conduction or narrow-complex WPW tachycardia, treatment centers on prolonging conduction time through the AV node. Consequently, **vagal maneuvers** and/or **adenosine** can be used as described with PAT. Adenosine will convert a large majority of these tachycardias to normal sinus rhythm. **Calcium channel blockers** (verapamil, diltiazem) are also very effective, but beta-blockers are usually ineffective, and digitalis should probably be avoided in these patients. **Procainamide** is another pharmacologic option that is usually effective.

    b. Wide-complex WPW tachycardia. Treatment of antidromic or wide-complex WPW tachycardia differs from that of narrow-complex tachycardia. Many of the agents used in the treatment of narrow-complex tachycardia produce their effect through their action on the AV node and have little effect on conduction time through the accessory pathway. Consequently, using these agents in wide-complex tachycardia can result in preferential conduction down the accessory pathway, which can lead to ventricular fibrillation. Therefore, calcium channel blockers and beta-blockers should be avoided in this setting. Instead, **procainamide,** which slows conduction through the AV node as well as through the accessory pathway, is the treatment of choice for all antidromic WPW tachycardias. Patients with atrial fibrillation and WPW (Fig. 16-12) should not receive calcium channel blockers or digitalis either, because these medications can potentiate conduction through the accessory pathway and lead to ventricular fibrillation. Consequently, procainamide is the drug of choice for irregular WPW tachycardias.

3. Disposition. All patients who require electrical cardioversion or show signs of instability prior to chemi-

Fig. 16-12. WPW with atrial fibrillation.
(From Davis D. _Differential Diagnosis of_
Arrhythmias. Philadelphia: Saunders, 1992.)

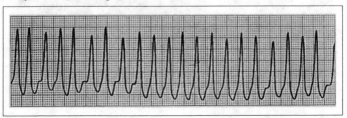

cal cardioversion should be admitted for observation. Patients who tolerate the tachycardia well and convert either spontaneously or with vagal or pharmacologic therapy can be referred for further outpatient evaluation. Preventing recurrences can be challenging pharmacologically because it is difficult to predict which medications will be effective. Furthermore, certain drugs may actually worsen the tachydysrhythmias. Two medications, quinidine and propranolol, can be used to effect conduction through both the AV node and the accessory pathway. The possibility of surgical ablation exists, and patients should be offered referral for electrophysiologic studies and possible ablation.

C. **Sick sinus syndrome.** The sick sinus syndrome is a term used to describe a variety of clinical conditions manifested by supraventricular tachydysrhythmias and/or bradydysrhythmias. Its causes are diverse, but it most commonly occurs as a result of myocardial infarction. Other potential etiologies include cardiomyopathies, pericarditis, electrolyte abnormalities, rheumatic heart disease, and connective tissue disorders. Medications in themselves do not cause sick sinus syndrome but may worsen the underlying dysrhythmias.

1. **Presentation.** The clinical manifestations of sick sinus syndrome are diverse and may result from either bradycardia or tachycardia. Patients most commonly present with palpitations, syncope, near syncope, angina, or transient mental status changes.

2. **Assessment.** Since several clinical conditions can occur in the context of sick sinus syndrome, the ECG characteristics of the syndrome are diverse. Severe or persistent bradycardia (Fig. 16-13) is the most frequent early presentation of sick sinus syndrome. Atrial fibrillation refractory to cardioversion or with extremely slow ventricular rates (Fig. 16-14) is the most common dysrhythmia seen in long-standing sick sinus syndrome. A bradycardia-tachycardia syndrome is also relatively common late in the course of this disease.

Fig. 16-13.   Severe bradycardia. (From Wiederhold R. *Electrocardiography: The Monitoring Lead.* Philadelphia: Saunders, 1988:296.)

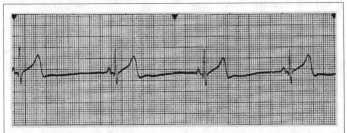

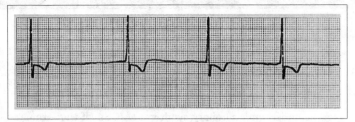

Fig. 16-14. Atrial fibrillation with slow ventricular rate. (From Davis D. *Differential Diagnosis of Arrhythmias*. Philadelphia: Saunders, 1992.)

Prolonged monitoring is usually required to identify the sick sinus syndrome, since many of the dysrhythmias are transient and are difficult to demonstrate on routine ECG. Therefore, ambulatory or in-hospital monitoring is usually necessary to make the diagnosis.
3. **Management.** Management of patients with sick sinus syndrome can be difficult but usually involves permanent pacing to combat the bradydysrhythmias with or without concomitant pharmacologic therapy for the tachydysrhythmias. Tachydysrhythmia medications, used alone in this syndrome to treat the tachydysrhythmias, can worsen the bradydysrhythmias without an indwelling pacemaker. They should not be used as a single treatment modality in the treatment of bradycardia-tachycardia syndromes.
4. **Disposition.** If sick sinus syndrome is suspected and the patient is symptomatic, has hemodynamic compromise, or has had a syncopal episode, admission to a monitored bed for definitive treatment is indicated. In those patients who present with symptoms suggestive of sick sinus syndrome but who are clinically stable, ambulatory monitoring should be arranged.

Bibliography

Braunwald E (ed.). *A Textbook of Cardiovascular Medicine*. Philadelphia: Saunders, 1992.

Goldberger E (ed.). *Treatment of Cardiac Emergencies*. St Louis: Mosby, 1990.

Jewitt D, Bacon R, Raftery E, et al. Incidence and management of supraventricular arrhythmias after AMI. *Lancet* 2:734–738, 1967.

Keefe D, Miura D, Somberg J. Supraventricular tachyarrhythmias: their evaluation and therapy. *Progress in Cardiology: Am Heart J* 111:1150–1161, 1986.

Wathen M, Klein G, Yee R, et al. Classification and terminology of supraventricular tachycardia. *Cardiol Clin* 11, 1993.

Ventricular Arrhythmias

Joseph J. Moellman and W. Brian Gibler

I. **Significance of ventricular arrhythmias.** Despite advancement in the rapid recognition and treatment of acute myocardial infarction (AMI), ventricular arrhythmias still remain one of the leading causes of death associated with the acute ischemic coronary syndrome (AICS). Of the estimated 300,000 to 500,000 sudden cardiac deaths (SCD) annually, nearly 25% occur in the setting of AMI. An additional 25% occur during transient ischemic episodes.

II. **Pathogenesis.** The pathogenesis of cardiac arrhythmias can be classified in terms of two major mechanisms: 1) automaticity and 2) reentry. Although it is a normal property of various cardiac tissues [e.g., sinus nodal, atrioventricular (AV) junctional, and His-Purkinje tissues], **automaticity** or simple spontaneous electrical activity can occur pathologically. Triggered activity is one example of pathologic automaticity where the induction of spontaneous electrical activity results from an impulse emanating from a remote site, which results in abnormal impulse formation.

   Reentry represents a disorder of impulse conduction in which an electrical impulse proceeds in a circuit. The components of the reentry mechanism include a dual conduction pathway that is characterized by both slow conduction and unidirectional conduction block (Fig. 17-1). As an impulse travels down the Purkinje fibers, it is blocked in one branch and travels slowly down the other. Since only a unidirectional block is present in the one branch, the impulse is conducted retrograde, which creates a circuit.

   In the setting of AMI, both of these mechanisms have been found to be responsible for the development of ventricular arrhythmias. It is well established that ventricular arrhythmias, in particular ventricular fibrillation (VF), are 15 times greater in the first 4 hours of AMI as compared to the subsequent 20 hours during the first day. Studies have shown that in this early phase, ventricular arrhythmias are usually the result of reentry arising from the ischemic zone. After conduction through the ischemic zone progressively worsens as the myocardium deteriorates, such early phase reentrant arrhythmias subside. In the later phase of AMI (8 to 72 hours), arrhythmias may arise from the development of abnormal automaticity from surviving Purkinje cells adjacent to necrotic myocardium. It is the reentrant, early phase arrhythmias that are the likely cause of the majority of sudden cardiac deaths accompanying AMI.

III. **Warning arrhythmias and sudden death.** As a result of emphasis placed on rapid recognition and treatment of AMI, medical personnel have been sensitized to the early phase arrhythmias of AMI. With an increased understanding of the basic pathogenesis underlying the development of such arrhythmias, the current major goal of investigators is to determine which ventricular arrhythmias pose the greatest threats to patients.

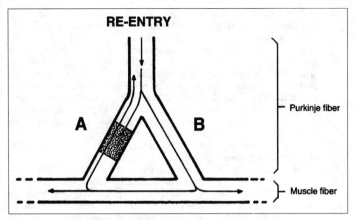

RE-ENTRY

Fig. 17-1. **Mechanism of reentry. (Reproduced with permission.** *Textbook of Advanced Cardiac Life Support,* **1994. Copyright American Heart Association.)**

The recognition of such **warning arrhythmias** in AMI has been well studied, yet remains controversial. Animal studies have confirmed the presence of ventricular ectopy occurring as soon as 30 minutes after occlusion of blood supply to myocardium. However, the type of ectopy ranged from simple premature ventricular contractions (PVCs) to VF. In an attempt to predict the degree of ectopy which would most likely indicate VF, Lown and Wolf proposed a grading system for ventricular ectopy (Table 17-1). They proposed that complex and frequent ectopy is associated with VF and SCD, and low grade ectopy is more benign in nature. Lown and Wolf recommended the prophylactic treatment of high grades of ectopy. Recent investigations have found that in up to 80% of patients with VF, such warning arrhythmias did not exist, thereby suggesting that ventricular ectopy is neither sensitive nor specific in predicting VF and SCD.

Table 17-1. Lown's grading system of ventricular ectopy

Grade	Description of ventricular extrasystoles
0	None
1	<30/hr
2	≥30/hr
3	Multiform
4A	Two consecutive
4B	≥3 consecutive
5	R-on-T

Source: Marriott H. *Practical Electrocardiography* (8th ed.). Baltimore: Williams & Wilkins, 1988.

Basic fundamental principles are associated with the management of ventricular arrhythmia in the setting of AMI. The clinician must be able to recognize rapidly the type of ventricular arrhythmia present, to assess efficiently the patient, and be flexible in critical actions and therapeutic strategies required to stabilize and treat the patient. Finally, the clinician must be familiar with appropriate in-hospital disposition and consultation. This chapter outlines an approach to ventricular arrhythmias accompanying AMI that is practical and systematic. The diagnosis and treatment of the patient with wide-complex tachycardia is also emphasized.

IV. **General therapy for ventricular arrhythmias post MI**
   A. **Patient presentation**
      1. **History.** Ventricular arrhythmias occurring in patients with AMI are a significant underlying concern in the management of these patients. Historic findings focus on symptom presentation for AMI. The time of onset of chest pain, dyspnea, nausea and vomiting, syncope, and diaphoresis should be ascertained to anticipate the risk of ventricular arrhythmia based on the likelihood of evolving AMI. Pertinent risk factors for coronary artery disease such as smoking, hypertension, diabetes mellitus, familial history, hypercholesterolemia, and cocaine abuse increase suspicion that the particular patient has ventricular arrhythmias due to myocardial injury.

      The patient's past medical history is essential and should focus on previous myocardial infarction (MI)—particularly recent MI—and a history of past arrhythmias. The patient's medications are equally relevant since many drugs, including antiarrhythmics and antidepressants, may be responsible for precipitating ventricular arrhythmias.

      One of the most important although often neglected historic features is the pre-hospital record. Frequently, rhythm strips from the field may delineate a specific arrhythmia. In some cases, the pre-hospital care providers will be the sole resource for these key historic data.

      2. **Physical examination.** The physical examination should focus on findings that suggest an etiology to the arrhythmia as well as consequences of the arrhythmia. Vital signs may indicate irregularities in the pulse rate and force as well as the blood pressure. The patient's general appearance, such as decreased mentation, may indicate evidence of hypoperfusion. Respiratory changes and skin color may also depict hemodynamic instability. A thorough cardiovascular examination should be performed to assess for evidence of pump failure. The venous system should be assessed for jugular venous distention and abnormal pulsations. Pulses should likewise be assessed for character in all extremities including rate, regularity, and form as well as for bruits. Auscultation of the lungs may detect rales that suggest left heart failure. Finally, examination of the heart should include

palpation for heaves, thrust, and thrills as well as auscultation for murmurs, gallops, or rubs. In some cases,
the stability of the patient will dictate the extent of the
physical exam. These physical findings should be
sought, if possible, in order to adequately assess the
patient.

B. **Patient assessment.** The assessment of the patient with
ventricular arrhythmias complicating AMI is dictated by
the stability of the patient. Obviously, in situations where
the patient is unstable, rapid treatment of the arrhythmia
must be undertaken without delay. Once stabilized, ancillary data should be gathered.

1. **ECG and rhythm strip.** In addition to key historic
information and specific physical findings, immediate
recognition of an abnormal cardiac rhythm strip is essential for the early diagnosis and treatment of the patient with ventricular arrhythmias. The patient with
AMI may present with or develop a number of different ventricular arrhythmias during the course of diagnosis and therapy. These specific arrhythmias and
their treatments will be discussed below.

   Rapid procurement of a **12-lead ECG** should be performed in order to confirm the suspicion of AMI or to
aid in the determination of the underlying rhythm
when the initial rhythm strip is inconclusive. Crucial
findings that must be addressed on the 12-lead ECG
include intervals such as R-R and Q-T, and signs of
electrolyte disturbances including U waves that may
contribute to the arrhythmias.

2. **Laboratory studies.** Serum electrolytes should be
evaluated, in particular potassium, magnesium, and
calcium. Hypomagnesemia and hypokalemia are perhaps the most common electrolyte abnormalities found
in such patients. Other laboratory studies should include levels of significant medications including digoxin, procainamide, and quinidine as well as cardiac
enzymes. Coagulation profiles and a complete blood
count should also be sent as a routine emergency department (ED) evaluation. **Oxygen saturation** in the
blood should be assessed to determine the patient's oxygenation and respiratory status.

3. **Chest x-ray.** A **chest x-ray** should be performed in
order to assess for the presence of congestive heart
failure, as well as to search for other contributing
causes for the arrhythmia such as pneumonia, pulmonary emboli, or aortic dissection.

4. **Echocardiogram.** Although not immediately indicated and not available in all emergency settings, an
echocardiogram can provide useful information. Assessment of wall motion abnormalities, ejection fraction, and valvular disorders can provide important
prognostic information as described below.

C. **General management.** The management of the patient
with ventricular arrhythmias complicating AMI is dependent on the stability of the patient, the time course after
infarction, and the particular arrhythmia present. The

basic tenets of cardiorespiratory resuscitation must prevail, including appropriate equipment and ancillary staff. The patient should be connected to a monitor, preferably one with a defibrillator, oxygen should be administered by nasal cannulae, and at least one large-bore IV line should be established. The monitor should be in sight at all times since frequently the patient may display a wide variety of arrhythmias, providing a harbinger for those arrhythmias requiring immediate action. Continuous reassessment of the airway, breathing, and circulation (ABCs) must be performed because the patient's condition may rapidly deteriorate. Management of specific arrhythmias is discussed below.

D. **Patient disposition.** Once the patient has been stabilized and the arrhythmia treated, immediate consultation with a cardiologist should be obtained. In those patients manifesting refractory ventricular arrhythmias, earlier consultation is recommended. Prognosis and long-term definitive care options are governed by the type of ventricular arrhythmia present (see below).

V. **Specific therapy for ventricular arrhythmias post MI.**
A. **Premature ventricular complexes (PVCs).** The incidence of PVCs in patients with AMI varies from 60% to 100%. The frequency increases for the first 6 hours post MI, with nearly 90% of patients experiencing PVCs during the first 4 hours. The persistence of frequent and complex PVCs seems to correlate with the size of the infarction, yet as previously discussed the significance of such warning arrhythmias typically does not correlate with the development of more malignant arrhythmias such as ventricular tachycardia (VT) and VF.

1. **Recognition.** PVCs are one of the most frequently encountered ventricular arrhythmias associated with AMI. Such complexes represent a premature depolarization of either ventricle producing a wide (>0.12 second), bizarre QRS complex on the ECG (Fig. 17-2). The ST segment and T wave are opposite from the QRS complex and if similar throughout the ECG are termed **unifocal PVCs** or simple focus PVCs. **Multifocal PVCs,** in contrast, have differing QRST configurations and represent different regions of the depolariz-

Fig. 17-2. Premature ventricular complex. (Reproduced with permission. *Textbook of Advanced Cardiac Life Support,* 1994. Copyright American Heart Association.)

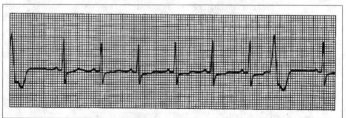

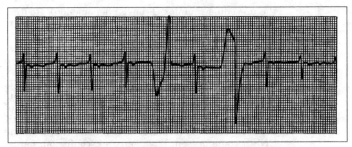

Fig. 17-3. Multiformed premature ventricular complex. (Reproduced with permission. *Textbook of Advanced Cardiac Life Support,* **1994. Copyright American Heart Association.)**

ing ventricle (Fig. 17-3). Whereas the complex interval that is the interval between previous normal beat and PVC is nearly constant with unifocal PVCs, it varies in the presence of multifocal PVCs. There is usually a full compensatory pause following the PVC. A PVC may be sufficiently premature in that it occurs at the apex of the T wave from the previous QRS. This is described as the **R-on-T phenomenon** (Fig. 17-4). PVCs may also occur in various frequencies such as in bigeminy where every other QRS is a PVC, in trigeminy where every third QRS is a PVC, and so forth. Two consecutive PVCs represent a couplet; three or more are considered VT.

2. **Treatment.** Perhaps one of the greatest controversies in antiarrhythmic therapy revolves around the treatment of PVCs accompanying AMI. Treatment of underlying electrolyte abnormalities, drug toxicity, or hypoxemia should take precedence. Although antiarrhythmics have been shown to decrease PVCs in the first 48 hours post infarction, controversy persists regarding its prevention of primary VF. Despite such controversy, the standard of care determined by the American Heart Association (AHA) is prophylactic treatment of warning arrhythmias. This includes more than 6 PVCs a minute, multifocal PVCs, coupled PVCs or runs of V-tach, and PVCs that fall on the T wave of

Fig. 17-4. R-on-T phenomenon. (Reproduced with permission. *Textbook of Advanced Cardiac Life Support,* **1994. Copyright American Heart Association.)**

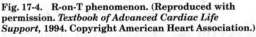
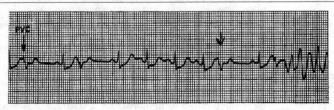

the preceding complex (R-on-T phenomenon). Routine use of prophylactic lidocaine without these findings is not indicated and may be harmful.

Antiarrhythmic drug therapy for PVCs has been extensively investigated regarding indications, precautions, dosages, and efficacy. **Lidocaine** is the most frequently used agent for treatment of PVCs and is considered the drug of choice. An initial 1 mg/kg bolus should be employed followed by an additional bolus of 0.5–0.75 mg/kg (maximum total dose ≤3 mg/kg) until the arrhythmia is terminated or if toxic effects on the CNS become present (e.g., seizures, confusion, paresthesias, or conduction disturbances such as AV block). The AHA recommends decreasing the dose by 50% in the presence of AMI, acute pulmonary edema, or shock and in those patients over the age of 70, due to the reduced volume of distribution.

Procainamide may be used as a second-line drug in patients refractory to lidocaine. A dose of 100 mg every 5 minutes or 20 mg/min is used until a total dose of 1.0 g is given or the arrhythmia is terminated. Other end-points include hypotension or widening of the QRS by 50% of its original width. An infusion of 1–4 mg/min may prevent recurrence. Due to the negative inotropic effects and ganglionic blockade of procainamide, hypotension and heart block may ensue.

Another second-line agent that may be useful in the suppression of PVCs is **bretylium**. An initial dose of 5 mg/kg IV over 5 to 10 minutes can be given followed by a repeat dose of 10 mg/kg IV over 10 to 20 minutes after 1 to 2 hours. If effective, an infusion of 1–4 mg/min may be employed to prevent recurrence. End-points of therapy include hypotension that is usually postural, or a total bolus of 25–30 mg/kg. In some cases, the hypotension is marked and may be refractory to norepinephrine and epinephrine. Awake patients may experience nausea and vomiting after rapid infusion. The only relative contraindication for the use of bretylium is in the instance of digitalis toxicity because catecholamine excess exacerbates the toxicity. A summary of the above agents can be found in Table 17-2 and Fig. 17-5.

3. **Prognosis and chronic therapy.** In the setting of AMI, the prognostic implication of complex PVCs depends on the time course. Although more common early after infarct (<48 hours), the early presence of complex PVCs does not appear to have prognostic implications. However, patients experiencing sustained ectopy after 72 hours appear to have an increased mortality. Furthermore, the presence of complex PVCs beyond 6 months after MI is associated with increased mortality.

Many clinical trials employing antiarrhythmic therapy have been conducted that attempt to suppress such ectopy and decrease mortality. Unfortunately, most have failed to demonstrate a treatment benefit.

Table 17-2. Drug treatment: premature ventricular contractions

First-line drug
Lidocaine

Initial dose	1 mg/kg initial bolus (75–100 mg)
Repeat dose	Additional bolus every 5 min (0.5–0.75 mg/kg) to maximum total dose ≤3 mg/kg
	Infusion may be given at 2–4 mg/min to prevent recurrence.
End-points	Arrhythmia terminated
	Toxic effects such as seizures, CNS changes, AV heart block
	Maximum IV bolus dose ≤3 mg/kg

Second-line drugs
Bretylium

Initial dose	5 mg/kg IV over 5–10 minutes
Repeat dose	10 mg/kg IV over 10–20 minutes; may repeat once
	If arrhythmia terminated, may give infusion at 2 mg/min
End-points	Arrhythmia terminated
	Postural hypotension
	Nausea, vomiting
	Maximum bolus dose ≤25 mg/kg

Procainamide

Initial dose	20 mg/min until arrhythmia terminated
Repeat dose	Infusion of 1–4 mg/min to prevent recurrence
End-points	QRS duration increased by 50% of original width
	Hypotension
	Total dose 1 g
	Arrhythmia terminated

Source: Gibler WB. Antiarrhythmics. In Barsan WG, Jastremski MS, Syverud SA (eds.), *Emergency Drug Therapy*. Philadelphia: Saunders, 1991.

Moreover, the highly publicized Cardiac Arrhythmia Suppression Trial (CAST) has demonstrated an increased risk of death in patients treated with the potent antiarrhythmics encainide and flecainide.

B. Ventricular tachycardia (VT). VT is another rhythm that may occur in the setting of AMI. The reported incidence of monomorphic VT in patients with AMI varies between 6% and 40%. Episodes of sustained VT are unusual within the first 24 hours. More commonly, acute ischemia is associated with multiple form VT or polymorphic ventricular tachycardia (see below).

1. **Recognition.** ECG findings that suggest VT include three or more consecutive beats of ventricular origin at a rate usually between 140 and 200 bpm (Fig. 17-6).

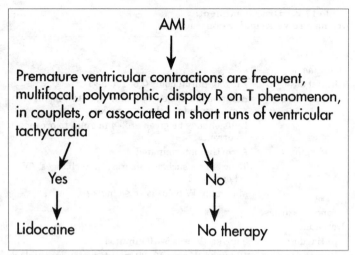

Fig. 17-5.   Treatment algorithm for PVCs. (From Aufderheide TP, Gibler WR. *Emergency Cardiac Care*. St. Louis: Mosby–Year Book, 1994.)

The rhythm is usually regular. VT is sustained if it lasts longer than 30 seconds or nonsustained if the rhythm ceases in less than 30 seconds. If the form of the QRS complex in each beat of sustained VT is constant, it is called **monomorphic ventricular tachycardia**. One of the most challenging situations for the clinician is distinguishing monomorphic VT from supraventricular tachycardia (SVT) with aberrancy (see sec. **VI.**).

2. **Treatment.** The treatment of sustained VT with a pulse is governed by the stability of the patient (Fig. 17-7). As depicted in the algorithm, for those patients

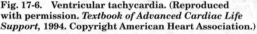

Fig. 17-6.   Ventricular tachycardia. (Reproduced with permission. *Textbook of Advanced Cardiac Life Support*, 1994. Copyright American Heart Association.)

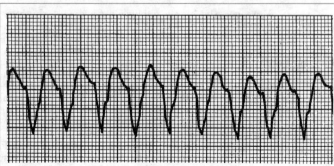

deemed **unstable** who are experiencing chest pain, dyspnea, hypotension, congestive heart failure (CHF), ischemia or evolving infarction, electrical cardioversion is the treatment of choice starting with 50 joules in the unsynchronized mode. In more stable patients, synchronized cardioversion with a short-acting anesthetic may be employed. If recurrent, lidocaine should be administered (1 mg/kg IV) and cardioversion attempted at the previously successful level. Procainamide and bretylium may be administered if lidocaine is unsuccessful.

In the **stable** patient with sustained VT, a trial of pharmacologic agents may be employed (see Fig. 17-7). Lidocaine is the agent of choice with procainamide and bretylium as second-line drugs. Dosages, end-points, and precautions are similar to the treatment of PVCs

Fig. 17-7.   Treatment algorithm for sustained ventricular tachycardia with a pulse. (From Aufderheide TP, Gibler WB. *Emergency Cardiac Care*. St. Louis: Mosby–Year Book, 1994.)

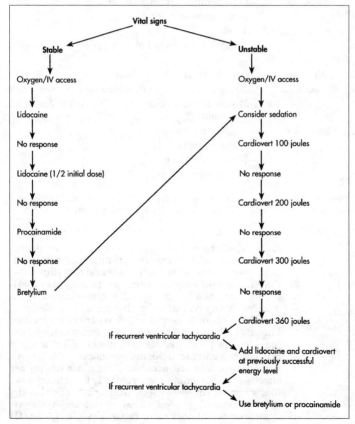

Table 17-3.   Drug treatment: ventricular tachycardia

First-line drug
Lidocaine
Initial dose	1 mg/kg initial bolus (75–100 mg)
Repeat dose	Additional bolus every 5 min (0.5–0.75 mg/kg) to maximum total dose ≤3 mg/kg
	Infusion may be given at 2–4 mg/min to prevent recurrence.
End-points	Arrhythmia terminated
	Toxic effects such as seizures, CNS changes, AV heart block
	Maximum IV bolus dose ≤3 mg/kg

Second-line drugs
Procainamide
Initial dose	20 mg/min until arrhythmia converted
Repeat dose	Infusion of 1–4 mg/min to prevent recurrence
End-points	QRS duration increased by 50% of original width
	Hypotension develops
	Total dose 1 g
	Arrhythmia terminated

Bretylium
Initial dose	5 mg/kg IV over 5–10 minutes
Repeat dose	10 mg/kg IV over 10–20 minutes; may repeat once
	If arrhythmia terminated, may give infusion at 2 mg/min
End-points	Arrhythmia terminated
	Postural hypotension
	Nausea, vomiting
	Maximum bolus dose ≤25 mg/kg

Source: Gibler WB. Antiarrhythmics. In Barsan WG, Jastremski MS, Syverud SA (eds.), *Emergency Drug Therapy*. Philadelphia: Saunders, 1991.

(Table 17-3). Electrical cardioversion, however, is usually recommended if the arrhythmia does not terminate after the use of procainamide and bretylium.

3. **Prognosis and chronic therapy.** In patients experiencing sustained VT during AMI, prognosis is dependent on many variables including age, underlying structural heart disease, and left ventricular function. Like PVCs, the occurrence of this arrhythmia in the convalescent phase of AMI (>72 hours) offers a worse prognosis including a higher incidence of SCD. Although myocardial revascularization alone has proved effective in controlling recurrent VT, few patients actually benefit. In most cases, antiarrhythmic therapy is administered, guided either by electrophysiologic studies or ambulatory monitoring. The use of Class III

antiarrhythmics such as amiodarone and sotolol has recently shown promise. Side effects limit their effectiveness.

C. **Torsades de pointes.** Although much confusion exists in the medical literature regarding its classification, most now recognize torsades de pointes as a subtype of **polymorphic ventricular tachycardia,** in which there is prolongation of the Q-T interval. Polymorphic VT with a normal Q-T interval usually develops during acute episodes of myocardial ischemia secondary to coronary artery occlusion or more classically coronary artery spasm (Prinzmetal's angina). It also occurs in patients taking antiarrhythmics such as quinidine or other medications that prolong the Q-T interval. Its association with AMI is rare, occurring in approximately 1% to 2% of patients. It tends to occur in individuals with extensive anterior AMI. Under this circumstance, polymorphic VT has the propensity to degenerate into monomorphic VT and VF. More recently, investigators have suggested that polymorphic VT is a more common dysrhythmia than previously recognized, especially in cases of SCD.

1. **Recognition.** Unlike monomorphic VT that has only one unchanging QRS complex, polymorphic VT is a tachyarrhythmia characterized by wide QRS complexes of varying amplitude and polarity. One form of polymorphic VT is torsades de pointes or "twisting of the points," first described by Dessertene. QRS complexes in torsades de pointes appear to twist around the isoelectric baseline of the ECG tracing (Fig. 17-8).

2. **Treatment.** Torsades de pointes often will terminate spontaneously. In cases of recurrent or sustained torsades de pointes, aggressive steps must be taken to prevent degeneration of this rhythm into VF. Treatment must include correction of hypomagnesemia, hypokalemia, and hypocalcemia if present. Agents responsible for prolonging the Q-T interval such as Class I-A antiarrhythmics, including procainamide and quinidine, should be avoided. Although this discussion is focused on torsades accompanying AMI, other etiologies must be excluded, including the presence of psychotropic agents that can cause this tachyarrhyth-

Fig. 17-8. Torsades de pointes. (Reproduced with permission. *Textbook of Advanced Cardiac Life Support*, 1994. Copyright American Heart Association.)

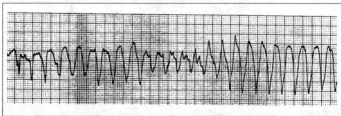

mia such as lithium, tricyclic antidepressants, and
thioridazine. In such cases, removal of the agent may
be facilitated by gut decontamination.

After such intervention has been completed or if the
patient is unstable, further management must proceed as outlined in Fig. 17-9. The **unstable patient**
must be rapidly **cardioverted** electrically starting
with 50 joules and proceeding as indicated.

In more **stable patients,** pharmacologic intervention can be attempted. Torsades requires different
pharmacologic intervention than monomorphic VT.

Magnesium sulfate, as an initial dose of 2 g IV
over 10 to 20 minutes followed by an infusion of 1
g/hour if successful, has recently been demonstrated
efficacious and is currently considered first-line drug
therapy. Magnesium is indicated prior to the use of isoproterenol, especially in the setting of AMI. As a cofactor of adenosine triphosphatase (ATPase) magnesium
transports potassium into the cell that has been postulated to promote electrical stabilization. The phar-

**Fig. 17-9.   Treatment algorithm for torsades de
pointes. (From Aufderheide TP, Gibler WB. *Emergency Cardiac Care.* St. Louis: Mosby–Year Book, 1994.)**

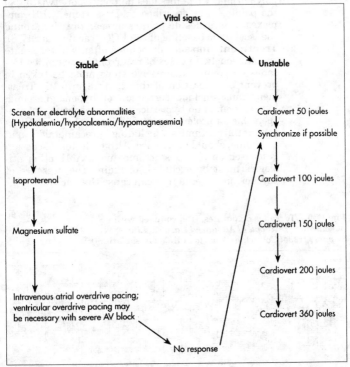

Table 17-4. Drug treatment: torsades de pointes

Magnesium sulfate

Initial dose	2 g IV over 10–20 minutes
Repeat dose	Infusion of 1 mg/min if successful; maintain serum K$^+$ level >4 mEq/liter
End-points	Arrhythmia terminated

Isoproterenol

Initial dose	1 mg is added to 500 ml D$_5$W; this gives a concentration of 1 µg/min to increase heart rate to 100–120 bpm and shorten QT interval
Repeat dose	Tirate to desired heart rate
End-points	Infusion rate of 20 µg/min without desired change in heart rate
	Hypotension
	Development of cardiac arrhythmias

Source: Gibler WB. Antiarrhythmics. In Barsan WG, Jastremski MS, Syverud SA (eds.), *Emergency Drug Therapy*. Philadelphia: Saunders, 1991.

macologic therapy for torsades de pointes is summarized in Table 17-4.

Isoproterenol, a sympathomimetic amine, is often recommended as a first-line drug in the treatment of torsades de pointes. At an infusion of 2–20 µg/minute, isoproterenol accelerates AV conduction and decreases the Q-T interval by decreasing temporal dispersion of repolarization. The infusion may be titrated to a heart rate of 100–120 bpm. Unfortunately, **isoproterenol is relatively contraindicated in the setting of AMI** and ischemia because it increases myocardial oxygen demand.

Transcutaneous overdrive pacing should be attempted if magnesium is unsuccessful. Although more invasive, atrial pacing can also be used. Overdrive pacing should be employed at a rate up to 120 bpm until the Q-T interval normalizes. Cardioversion should be a last resort in the stable patient because the rhythm will likely recur or degenerate to VF.

3. **Prognosis and chronic therapy.** Torsades de pointes in the setting of AMI offers a relatively high mortality. Revascularization by angioplasty or coronary artery bypass surgery (CABG) may be necessary to control the arrhythmia and prevent recurrent episodes.

D. **Accelerated idioventricular rhythm (AIVR).** Another ventricular arrhythmia that has been associated with AMI is nonparoxysmal VT or AIVR. Its incidence has been reported in between 10% and 30% of patients with AMI. Both anterior and inferior myocardial infarctions may be associated with this rhythm. It is probably best known as an arrhythmia secondary to reperfusion with thrombolytic therapy, although this relationship is also controversial. Hemodynamic changes with this rhythm are rare.

1. **Recognition.** AIVR has most of the characteristics of monomorphic VT except that the rate is slower, 60–100 bpm (Fig. 17-10).

2. **Treatment.** Of all ventricular arrhythmias accompanying AMI, AIVR appears to be the most benign and requires no specific treatment. Attempting to abolish the rhythm with lidocaine may cause asystole.

3. **Prognosis and chronic therapy.** AIVR, as stated earlier, represents a rhythm that has no prognostic significance. Its association with reperfusion from thrombolytics is transient.

E. **Ventricular fibrillation (VF).** The most devastating of all the ventricular arrhythmias associated with AMI is VF. It represents the most common mechanism of cardiac arrest resulting from AMI.

1. **Recognition.** Multiple foci of depolarization within the ventricles are responsible for the rapid, irregular waveforms varying in amplitude and configuration that are displayed electrocardiographically (Fig. 17-11). Various rhythms, which must be differentiated from VF, include polymorphic VT, ventricular flutter and asystole. Asystole may actually represent fine VF in some patients.

2. **Treatment.** The patient with pulseless VT or VF demands early electrical countershock. The treatment of such patients is outlined in Fig. 17-12 based on AHA recommendations. Variations of this treatment should be adapted to fit individual patient circumstances. For example, sodium bicarbonate may have some benefit in the patient with a prolonged arrest time. A brief

Fig. 17-10.   Accelerated idioventricular rhythm (AICR). (From Marriott H. *Practical Electrocardiography* (8th ed.). Baltimore: Williams & Wilkins, 1988.)

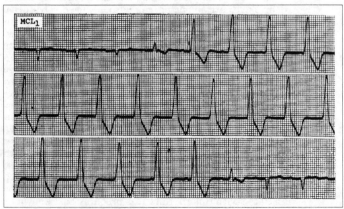

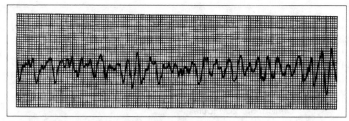

**Fig. 17-11.   Coarse ventricular fibrillation. (Repro-
duced with permission.** *Textbook of Advanced Cardiac
Life Support,* **1994. Copyright American Heart Association.)**

synopsis of the pharmacologic management of VF is
presented in Table 17-5.

3. **Prognosis and chronic therapy.** Although a high
   morbidity and mortality can be expected in those experiencing VF complicating AMI, long-term survival
   after hospitalization is not affected by its initial presence. Similar to sustained ventricular tachycardia,
   long-term therapy often consists of revascularization
   and in some cases the use of antiarrhythmics guided
   either by electrophysiologic studies or ambulatory
   monitoring. In some patients, implanted automatic
   defibrillators may be lifesaving.

VI. **Wide QRS tachycardia.** Wide QRS tachycardia is defined as
an arrhythmia occurring at a rate greater than 100 bpm and
having a QRS duration greater than 120 milliseconds. Three
causes for such arrhythmias include VT, SVT with aberrancy,
and preexcitation tachyarrhythmias. **Ventricular tachycardia,** as its name implies, is an arrhythmia originating in the
ventricles. **Supraventricular tachycardia (SVT) with
aberration** represents an arrhythmia whereby the impulse
is generated in structures at or above the AV node including
the sinus node and atria at a rate greater than 100 beats per
second. Abnormal conduction to the ventricles produces the
widened QRS. SVT may result from AV reentrant mechanisms, atrial flutter and fibrillation, atrial tachycardia, or
sinoatrial node reentrant mechanisms. Aberration of conduction may involve any point of the His-Purkinje system with
right and left bundle-branch block most common. **Preexcitation tachycardia** refers to arrhythmias in which the ventricles are depolarized earlier than would normally occur by
conduction through the AV node. The mechanism responsible
for such premature depolarization is the presence of an accessory pathway from the atria to the ventricles as seen in the
Wolff-Parkinson White (WPW) Syndrome and other preexcitation abnormalities.

In managing the patient with wide QRS tachycardia, the
clinician is confronted with this differential diagnosis for the
arrhythmia. Crucial differentiation must be made because incorrect diagnosis may lead to inappropriate therapy that can
result in death.

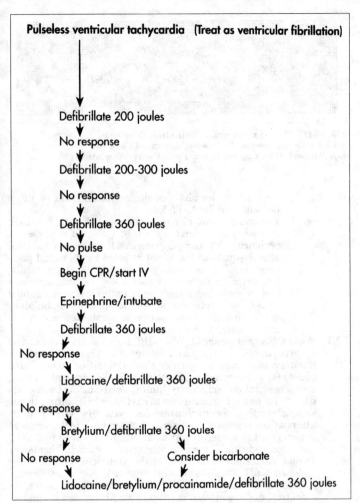

Pulseless ventricular tachycardia   (Treat as ventricular fibrillation)

Defibrillate 200 joules

No response

Defibrillate 200-300 joules

No response

Defibrillate 360 joules

No pulse

Begin CPR/start IV

Epinephrine/intubate

Defibrillate 360 joules

No response

Lidocaine/defibrillate 360 joules

No response

Bretylium/defibrillate 360 joules

No response   Consider bicarbonate

Lidocaine/bretylium/procainamide/defibrillate 360 joules

Fig. 17-12.   Treatment algorithm for pulseless ventricular tachycardia. (From Aufderheide TP, Gibler WB. *Emergency Cardiac Care*. St. Louis: Mosby–Year Book, 1994.)

A. **Patient presentation.** The history and physical examination in the patient with wide QRS tachycardia can differentiate the possible etiologies. Certain specific historic information and physical examination findings may lead to the correct diagnosis.

1. **History.** Historic clues to the presence of SVT with aberration or preexcitation are the age of the patient (usually <35 years old) and a history of long-standing recurrence of the tachyarrhythmia. Patients sometimes provide their diagnosis in the form of a

Table 17-5. Drug treatment: ventricular fibrillation

First-line drugs

Epinephrine

Initial dose	1.0 mg IVP (1:10,000)
Repeat dose	1.0 mg IV every 3 to 5 min.
	Consider high-dose epinephrine 0.1 mg/kg IV every 3 to 5 minutes.
End-points	Return of pulse with rhythm
	Severe arrhythmia generation

Lidocaine

Initial dose	1 mg/kg initial bolus (75–100 mg)
Repeat dose	Infusion may be given at 2–4 mg/min to prevent recurrence
Second bolus	15 to 20 minutes later, 0.5–0.75 mg/kg
End-points	Arrythmia terminated
	Toxic effects such as seizures, CNS changes, AV heart block

Second-line drugs

Bretylium

Initial dose	5 mg/kg IV bolus
Repeat dose	10 mg/kg IV bolus
	If arrhythmia is terminated, may infuse at 2 mg/min
End-points	Arrhythmia terminated
	Postural hypotension
	Nausea and vomiting

Sodium bicarbonate (NaHCO$_3$)

Initial dose	1 mEq/kg IVP
Repeat dose	0.5 mEq/kg IVP
End-points	Alkalotic pH
	Arrhythmia terminated

Procainamide

Initial dose	20 mg/min until arrhythmia is converted
Repeat dose	Infusion 1–4 mg/min to prevent arrhythmia recurrence
End-points	QRS duration is increased by 50% of original width
	Hypotension develops
	Total dose 1 g

Source: Gibler WB. Antiarrhythmics. In Barsan WG, Jastremski MS, Syverud SA (eds.), *Emergency Drug Therapy*. Philadelphia: Saunders, 1991.

"wallet-sized" ECG carried with them, or they may be aware they have WPW or some other named accessory pathway disease. Patients with VT are usually older (>50 years old) and have a history of previous MI, CHF, CABG, or valvular disease.

2. **Physical examination.** The physical examination also may aid in differentiating the source of the arrhythmia. One misconception is that the patient with VT will display hemodynamic instability; however, those with SVT with aberration and preexcitation will not. The blood pressure, pulse, and respiratory rate should not be used in this manner because all three vital signs may present in a stable or unstable condition. The physical examination should focus on the signs of AV dissociation, which in most cases will point to a diagnosis of VT. Such physical findings include **cannon A waves,** as well as variation in pulse and in the intensity of the first heart sound. Obviously, evidence of instability such as CHF must be elucidated since further therapy is guided by the presence of pump failure.

B. **Patient assessment.** Assessment of the patient with wide QRS tachycardia consists of a rhythm strip, 12-lead ECG, and other ancillary tests. These include serum electrolytes, chest x-ray, and cardiac enzymes as dictated by historic findings.

The **12-lead ECG** is helpful in differentiating VT from SVT with aberration in a number of ways. The presence of **AV dissociation, QRS width greater than or equal to 0.14 seconds,** and **left or right axis deviation** favors the diagnosis of VT. Likewise, the presence of **capture or fusion beats** as well as **concordance** (positive or negative) favors VT (Figs. 17-13 through 17-15). Concordance refers to deflection of the QRS complexes in the same direction. Although heart rate is of no value in differentiating the cause of wide-complex tachycardia, striking irregularity of the rhythm may suggest atrial fibrillation with aberrant conduction and not VT. Morphologic characteristics of the QRS wave have also been used to differentiate VT from SVT with aberrancy. In VT, the **morphology of the QRS in V1** is usually R, qR or RS instead of the characteristic triphasic rsR′ as seen in SVT with aberrancy. The **morphology of the QRS in V6** is usually S, or rS in VT versus RS as in SVT with aberrancy.

C. **Management.** Management, as with all patients exhibiting arrhythmias, includes securing the ABCs, connecting the patient to a monitor and a cardiac defibrillator, establishing at least one large-bore IV line, and providing the patient with oxygen. **Unstable patients** with wide QRS tachycardia require immediate cardioversion despite knowledge of the mechanism of the tachycardia. Synchronized electrical conversion starting with 50 joules and repeated at 100 and 200 joules is indicated in such situations. After 200 joules, the patient should be loaded with either procainamide or lidocaine and cardioverted with 360 joules (Fig. 17-16).

The **stable patient** may undergo carotid sinus message

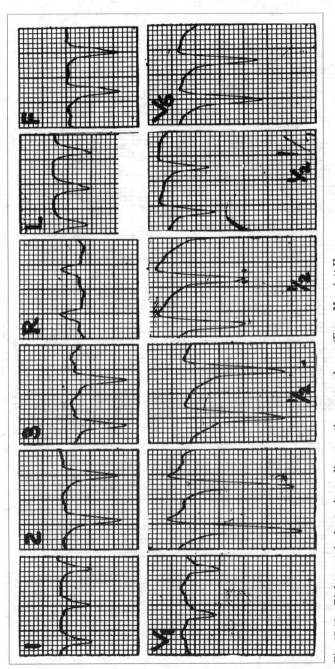

Fig. 17-13. Right ventricular tachycardia: negative concordance. (From Marriott H. *Practical Electrocardiography* (8th ed.). Baltimore: Williams & Wilkins, 1988.)

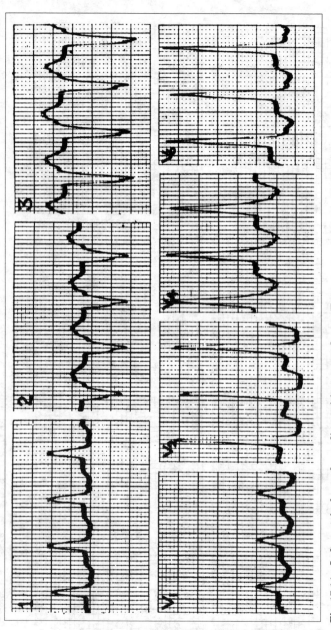

Fig. 17-14. Left ventricular tachycardia: positive concordance. (From Marriott H. *Practical Electrocardiography* (8th ed.). Baltimore: Williams & Wilkins, 1988.)

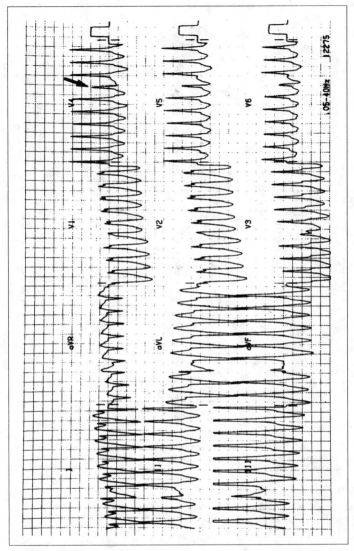

Fig. 17-15.   Ventricular tachycardia. (From Prystowsky E, Klein G. *Cardiac Arrhythmias.* **New York: McGraw-Hill, Inc., 1994. With permission.)**

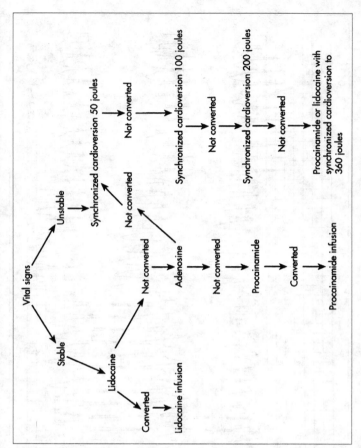

Fig. 17-16.   Treatment algorithm for wide complex tachycardia. (From Aufderheide TP, Gibler WB *Emergency Cardiac Care*. St. Louis: Mosby–Year Book, 1994.)

in order to block the AV node transiently and hence expose the underlying mechanism such as SVT with aberration. Likewise, **adenosine** may be administered at a 6-mg and then 12-mg dose intravenously to terminate the rhythm if SVT with aberrancy is present. The AHA suggests the stable patient should be loaded with **lidocaine** at less than or equal to 3 mg/min to a total of 1 g or until the arrhythmia is terminated. An infusion of 2–4 mg/min can then be used if conversion is successful. If unsuccessful, **procainamide** may be employed at 20 mg/min IV to a total of 1 g or until the arrhythmia is terminated. Again, if successful, a procainamide infusion may be administered at 1–4 mg/min. If still unsuccessful after procainamide, synchronized electrical **cardioversion** starting at 50 joules should be performed (see Fig. 17-16). Pharmacologic management of wide QRS tachycardia is summarized in Table 17-6.

In the pharmacologic management of wide QRS tachycardia, a few caveats exist. Assumption that the arrhythmia is SVT with aberrancy and subsequently treating it

Table 17-6. Drug treatment: wide QRS complex tachycardia

First-line drugs	
Lidocaine	
Initial dose	1 mg/kg initial bolus (75–100 mg)
Repeat dose	Infusion may be given at 2–4 mg/min to prevent recurrence
	Second bolus 15–20 min later, 0.5–0.75 mg/kg
End-points	Arrhythmia terminated
	Toxic effects such as seizures, CNS changes, AV heart block
Adenosine	
Initial dose	Adenosine 6 mg IV given by rapid (5 sec) push
Repeat dose	12 mg IV given by rapid (5 sec) push
End-points	Total dose 18 mg
	Prolonged asystolic interval after initial dose
	Arrhythmia terminated
Second-line drug	
Procainamide	
Initial dose	20 mg/min until arrhythmia is converted
Repeat dose	Infusion 1–4 mg/min to prevent arrhythmia recurrence
End-points	QRS duration is increased by 50% of original width
	Hypotension develops
	Total dose 1 g

Source: Gibler WB. Antiarrhythmics. In Barsan WG, Jastremski MS, Syverud SA (eds.), *Emergency Drug Therapy.* Philadelphia: Saunders, 1991.

as SVT with certain agents may be disastrous. Certain agents such as verapamil have been associated with acceleration of the tachyrhythmia; in particular atrial fibrillation to VF in the presence of an accessory tract. Thus, **verapamil should be avoided** even if clinical evidence points to the diagnosis of SVT with aberrancy. Procainamide, which slows conduction in the accessory pathway or suppresses ventricular ectopy, is the first-line drug in such situations, as is lidocaine.

After conversion, a repeat 12-lead ECG should be performed and compared to previous ones, specifically with reference to various etiologies including WPW, AMI, and atrial fibrillation/flutter.

D. **Patient disposition.** The patient who exhibits wide QRS tachycardia for the first time should be admitted for treatment and possibly electrophysiologic studies to determine the etiology. Consultation with a cardiologist should be obtained early in the course of treatment. Patients who have not been successfully converted or at some point during treatment exhibit signs of instability should be admitted to a critical care setting.

Patients with a long history of SVT with aberrancy or preexcitation may be released from the ED after successful conversion. Again, discharge is appropriate in such cases only after their cardiologist has been consulted, no signs of instability have been exhibited, and the event is typical for their presentation.

Bibliography

American Heart Association. *Textbook of Advanced Cardiac Life Support.* Dallas: American Heart Association, 1994.

Gibler WB. *Antiarrhythmias.* In Barsan WG, et al (eds.), *Emergency Drug Therapy.* Philadelphia: Saunders, 1991.

Gibler WB. Arrhythmias and Antiarrhythmic Therapy. In Gibler WR and Aufderheide TP (eds.), *Emergency Cardiac Care,* St. Louis: Mosby–Year Book, 1994.

Marriott HJ. *Practical Electrocardiography* (8th ed.) Baltimore: Williams & Wilkins, 1988.

Prystowsky EN, Klein GJ. *Cardiac Arrhythmias—An Integrated Approach for the Clinician.* New York: McGraw-Hill, 1994.

Right Ventricular Infarction

Andrew T. Guertler and William J. Brady Jr.

Right ventricular myocardial infarction (RVMI) most often occurs in the setting of an inferior wall myocardial infarction (IWMI) with a reported incidence ranging from 20% to 60% of IWMIs. Right ventricular involvement has been reported in up to 13% of patients with anterior wall myocardial infarctions (AWMI), but it rarely, if ever, accompanies lateral wall myocardial infarctions. Isolated RVMIs have been reported but are distinctly unusual.

The coronary arteries arise from the ascending aorta immediately above the aortic valve. The right coronary artery (RCA) and its branches supply the right atrium, the right ventricle (RV), portions of the inferior and posterior walls of the left ventricle, the posterior-inferior third of the intraventricular septum, and the sinoatrial node (75% of the time) and atrioventricular (AV) node. The right conus artery, which supplies the infundibulum and upper anterior wall of the RV, frequently originates from the aorta. Anterior ventricular branches, including the marginal branch, supply the anterior surface of the RV while posterior ventricular branches supply the RV diaphragmatic surface. The posterior descending artery (PDA) supplies a segment of the RV and the inferior wall of the left ventricle (LV), as well as provides branches to the posterior intraventricular septum. A septal branch of the PDA perfuses the AV node (Fig. 18-1). In 10% of people, the PDA is replaced by a branch of the left circumflex artery; such patients are termed "left dominant."

The extent of myocardial damage depends on the location of vessel occlusion. If the RCA is occluded, both the RV and LV inferior walls will likely infarct. Occlusion immediately proximal to the PDA will not affect the RV but will damage the LV inferior wall and posterior portion of the interventricular septum. Right ventricular infarct size is limited by a number of factors, including enhanced perfusion from extensive collateral flow, right coronary artery filling during systole, passive oxygen diffusion from blood in the RV, smaller RV muscle mass, and relatively low workload of the RV. When RV infarction occurs, it is usually transmural because the RV wall is thin.

Hemodynamic derangement in RV infarction depends on the extent of RV damage, the restraining effect of the pericardium, and the resulting interaction between the ventricles. Right ventricular myocardial infarction may cause acute RV dilatation and intrapericardial pressure elevation. There is reduced RV systolic pressure, LV end diastolic size, cardiac output, aortic pressure, and equalization of right and left ventricular diastolic pressures. Augmented atrial contractility is necessary to overcome the increased RV myocardial stiffness. Decreased preload (from either intravascular volume depletion or nitrate-induced venodilatation) and diminished atrial function by right atrial infarction or atrioventriculcar dyssynchrony may cause profound hypotension in patients with an RVMI. Associated LV infarction and loss of augmentation of RV systolic pressure by LV septal contractions may complicate these hemodynamic derangements.

Right ventricular infarction increases patient morbidity and mortality. Patients with IWMIs complicated by RV involvement have both a higher incidence of major in-hospital complications (64% vs.

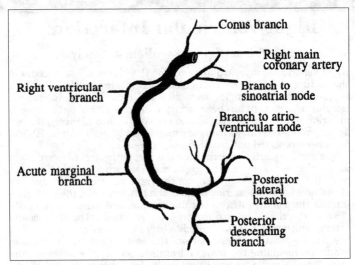

Fig. 18-1. Anatomy of the right coronary artery and its major branches. (From Cosby R. Clinicoarteriographic correlations in angina pectoris with and without myocardial infarction. *Am J Cardiol* 30:472–475, 1972. Adapted with permission from *American Journal of Cardiology.*)

28%) and higher in-hospital mortality rates (31% vs. 6%) than those without RV involvement. The subset of patients with RV infarction with decreased cardiac output and hypotension show increased early mortality. Although RV function typically returns to normal, patients sustaining severe RV damage have persistent RV dyskinesis and may develop chronic right heart failure.

I. Presentation

A. **History.** No particular historic facts indicate that RV infarction is occurring in patients with acute myocardial infarction (AMI). Historic findings mirror the typical MI (see Chap. 9). Right ventricular infarction typically complicates both inferior and anterior wall MIs. Therefore, patients with evidence of IWMI or AWMI should be evaluated for RV infarction. A history of hypotension following nitroglycerin use in a patient with an acute IWMI should increase suspicion for RV involvement. The occurrence of bradydysrhythmias or AV block also increases the likelihood of RV infarction. Such patients, in general, have larger infarcts and therefore are more likely to have RV involvement. Table 18-1 lists the clinical findings in patients with RV infarction.

B. **Physical examination.** Physical findings of RV infarction are present when there is marked RV involvement with RV failure. The triad of hypotension, clear lung fields, and jugular venous distension (JVD) in a patient with an IWMI is pathognomonic for RV infarction. This triad in patients with IMI is very specific but not sensitive

**Table 18-1. Clinical findings in patients
with right ventricular myocardial infarction**

Electrocardiogram

    Associated acute myocardial infarction (typically inferior wall leads II, III, and avf) with ST-segment elevations in V1 and right precordial leads (V2–6R).

    Advanced AV block, heart block, right bundle-branch block

Hypotension or shock, especially with an IMI

Hypotension following nitroglycerin therapy in a patient with an IMI

Hypotension, JVD, clear lung fields

JVD with inspiration (Kussmaul's sign)

Tricuspid regurgitation

Right-sided S_3 or S_4

Right atrial pressure >10 mm Hg and right atrial pressure to PCWP ratio >0.8

y descent $\geq x$ descent

for RVMI since significant hemodynamic compromise occurs infrequently. Other signs of RV infarction in patients include JVD upon inspiration (Kussmaul's sign), tricuspid regurgitation, and right-sided S_3 or S_4. Consider constrictive pericarditis, cardiac tamponade, pulmonary embolism with RV outflow obstruction, and restrictive cardiomyopathy in the differential diagnosis of elevated right-sided pressures. Although high-degree AV block commonly occurs with IWMI, complete heart block is more common when RVMI is present.

II. **Assessment**

  A. **Laboratory.** Since patients with RVMI can also have left ventricular failure and secondary hypoxemia, arterial blood gases or pulse oximetry are indicated to assess oxygenation. CBC, electrolytes, renal function, and glucose measurement are routinely done in the setting of RVMI, but their use is limited to assessment of cormorbid states. Creatine phosphokinase (CPK), CK-MB, myoglobin, and other serum markers for AMI should be assessed, as indicated for all patients with presumed MI (see Chap. 9). None of these tests is specific for RVMI.

  B. **Electrocardiogram.** Right ventricular myocardial infarction is diagnosed electrocardiographically when ST-segment elevation is noted in lead V1 or the right precordial leads, V3R and V4R. The ST-segment changes are frequently transient, lasting 12–72 hours, and may be absent in small RV infarctions. The degree of ST-segment elevation in the right-sided precordial leads may be small due to the relatively smaller RV muscle mass. An RVMI may cause ST-segment elevations in the standard precordial leads, mimicking an anteroseptal infarction. In RVMI, ST-segment elevation on a standard ECG decreases in magnitude from V1 to V5, whereas the opposite pattern is noted in anteroseptal infarction. Right-sided chest leads are needed to diagnose a RVMI, with the single best right-sided lead being V4R. Figure 18-2 is a standard 12-lead ECG in a patient with an IWMI complicated by RV involvement. This ECG demonstrates ST-segment elevations in the inferior leads (II and avf) and reciprocal changes (ST-segment depression and/or T-wave inversion) in the anterior (V2–4) and lateral leads (I, avl, V5, V6). Figure 18-3 depicts an ECG on the same patient with right-sided precordial leads (V2R–V6R). As can be seen in this example, ST segments are obviously elevated in leads V2R–V6R as well as in the inferior leads.

Right bundle-branch block and complete heart block are the most frequent conduction abnormalities associated with RV infarction.

C. **Echocardiography.** Two-dimensional echocardiography is useful in diagnosing RV involvement in patients with MI. Findings may include regional wall motion abnormality, decreased right ventricular systolic function, right ventricular dilatation, or paradoxical septal motion. These findings frequently are seen without hemodynamic abnormalities and are not specific for RV infarction (especially RV dilatation and decreased systolic function) since increased RV afterload due to extensive LV infarction also may result in these findings. Abnormalities in RV function may result from ischemia ("stunned" or "hibernating" myocardium) rather than infarction.

D. **Swan-Ganz catheter monitoring.** Hemodynamically unstable patients require right-sided cardiac pressure, or Swan-Ganz catheter monitoring, to direct and further adjust the effects of therapeutic interventions. Substantial RV infarctions produce right atrial pressures that equal or exceed pulmonary capillary wedge pressure (PCWP) resulting from a noncompliant RV and impaired left ventricular filling. This increased stiffness results in an altered venous pulse wave with the y descent being equal to or greater than the x descent. This finding can occur with a normal venous pressure and may be the most sensitive and specific hemodynamic criterion for RV infarction. A right atrial pressure of 10 mm Hg or more and a ratio of right atrial pressure to PCWP of 0.8 or greater has high specificity and sensitivity for RV infarction. These characteristic findings may become apparent only after volume loading, whereas patients with RV infarction and PCWPs greater than 20 mm Hg from extensive LV damage may demonstrate these characteristic hemodynamic findings only after LV filling pressures have been reduced. Patients with RV infarction without hemodynamic compromise meet clinical criteria for Forrester subset I, whereas those with hemodynamic abnormalities not resulting from extensive LV infarction meet subset III criteria (Table 18-2).

III. **Management** (Table 18-3)

A. **Initial resuscitation.** The evaluation of patients with an AMI begins with ensuring that an adequate airway and breathing exist and providing supplemental oxygen to maximize blood oxygen content. Hypoxemia due to

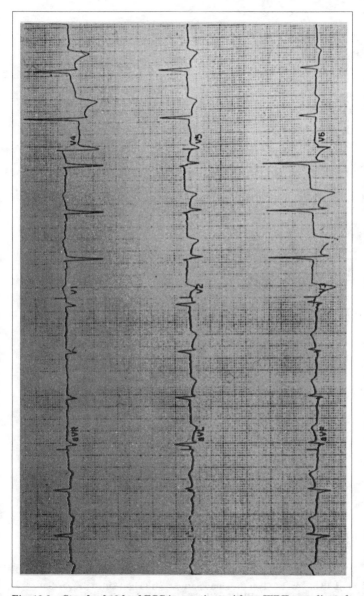

Fig. 18-2. Standard 12-lead ECG in a patient with an IWMI complicated by RVMI, demonstrating an acute infarction pattern with ST-segment elevation in the inferior leads (II and avf). Reciprocal changes (ST-segment depression and/or T wave inversion) in the anterior (V2–4) and lateral (I, avl, V5, V6) are also present.

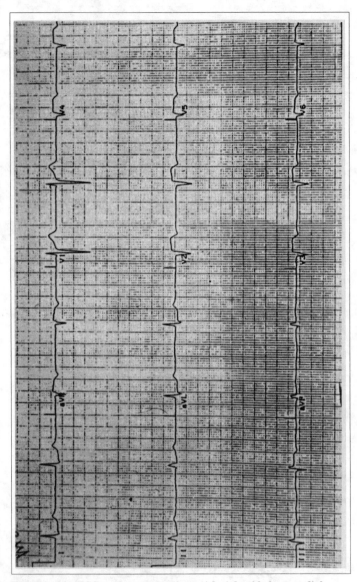

Fig. 18-3.   An ECG on the same patient with right-sided precordial leads showing acute RVMI with ST-segment elevation in leads V2R–V6R as well as the inferior leads.

Table 18-2. Relationship between clinical findings and hemodynamic parameters of cardiac index (CI) and pulmonary capillary wedge pressure (PCWP)

Subset	CI (liter/min per m²)	PCWP (mm Hg)
I. No pulmonary congestion or peripheral hypoperfusion	2.7 ± 0.5	12 ± 7
II. Isolated pulmonary congestion	2.3 ± 0.4	23 ± 5
III. Isolated peripheral hypoperfusion	1.9 ± 0.4	12 ± 5
IV. Pulmonary congestion and peripheral hypoperfusion	1.6 ± 0.6	27 ± 8

Source: Forrester JS. Correlative classification of clinical and hemodynamic function after acute myocardial infarction. *Am J Cardiol* 1977;39:137–145. Adapted with permission from *American Journal of Cardiology.*

pulmonary congestion ocurs in patients with RV infarction who also have significant LV involvement and may require diuresis and venodilatation. Arterial blood gases or pulse oximetry are indicated to guide oxygenation and ventilation decisions. Although typically unnecessary, endotracheal intubation may be required to maximize oxygenation. Pulse, blood pressure, and electrocardiographic monitoring should be instituted. Electrocardiographic monitoring is instituted to detect development of ventricular arrhythmias, bradycardia, AV block, and heart block. Intravenous lines should be established to allow fluid bolus therapy and to prepare for thrombolysis, if appropriate. Systemic hypotension and clear lung fields in the setting of IWMI are an indication for isotonic fluid boluses to maximize preload.

B. **Maintaining preload.** Patients with an RV infarction are at risk of developing hypotension, which may be avoided, minimized, or treated by maximizing preload. Hypotension is treated initially with isotonic fluid boluses (up to 3 liters) to achieve a blood pressure of 90 mm Hg or a PCWP of 15–18 mm Hg. Venodilators and diuretics should be avoided or used with extreme caution in asymptomatic patients with RV infarction to decrease the likelihood of hypotension.

When volume loading fails to increase cardiac output and correct hypotension, inotropic medication is required. Patients with an associated inferior or anterior myocardial infarction who may benefit from preload reduction and diuresis require central venous pressure monitoring to direct therapy.

C. **Inotropic support.** Inotropic medications are required if IV fluid therapy achieves a PCWP of 15 mm Hg with persistent hypotension. Swan-Ganz monitoring is very advantageous prior to initiating inotropic support to assure maximization of preload. Adrenergic inotropic agents such

Table 18-3.   Treatment of patients with an acute myocardial infarction complicated by right ventricular involvement

Supplemental oxygen
Maintaining preload
   IV isotonic fluid boluses (2–3 liters)
   Avoid nitrates and diuretics
Reperfusion
   Thrombolysis
   Angioplasty
Inotropic support*: hypotensive with PCWP >15 mm Hg
   Dobutamine (2–20 μg/kg/min)
   Dopamine (2–20 μg/kg/min)
Afterload reduction*
   Sodium nitroprusside† (0.5–10 μg/kg/min)
Heart rate control
   Atropine: 1 mg bolus repeated once
   Atrial pacing
   Maintain atrioventricular synchrony
      AV sequential pacing for complete heart block
      Prompt cardioversion for atrial fibrillation

---

* Central venous pressure monitored via Swan-Ganz catheter.
† Arterial line placed to monitor blood pressure.

as dopamine and dobutamine enhance RV function (see Chap. 14). The phosphodiesterase inhibitors (amrinone, milrinone, and enoximone) improve RV systolic function, decrease pulmonary vascular resistance, and improve cardiac output (see Chap. 14). Dobutamine, which does not increase LV filling pressure or cause tachycardia, is preferable if blood pressure is marginal with evidence of systemic hypoperfusion. However, if significant hypotension exists, dobutamine or phosphodiesterase inhibitors may further reduce arterial pressure due to systemic vasodilatation. In these cases dopamine, which maintains arterial pressure, should be initially considered.

   D. Afterload reduction. Severe right heart failure unresponsive to fluid boluses and inotropic support may respond to afterload reduction. Decreasing LV impedance by decreasing systemic vascular resistance with sodium nitroprusside may increase stroke volume and improve cardiac output. Patients requiring this therapy must have their central venous pressure monitored to direct titration of these medications. Right atrial pressure or PCWP should be maintained between 15–18 mm Hg initially using isotonic fluid boluses.

   E. Reperfusion. Any patient with a myocardial infarction that involves the right ventricle who has no contraindications to thrombolysis (see Chap. 10) should receive this therapy. Patients who have perfusion restored have a reduced incidence of RV infarction, better RV function, and lower incidence of complete heart block. If there are contraindications to thrombolysis or if thrombolysis fails to reestablish perfusion, angioplasty should be attempted to open the proximal RCA (see Chap. 12). Patients with hypotension or cardiogenic shock need reperfusion either by primary angioplasty or with thrombolytic agents followed by angioplasty.

F. Heart rate control. The presence of sinus bradycardia, junctional rhythm, high-degree AV block, or heart block and hypotension requires an increase of heart rate and an improvement in atrial-ventricular synchrony. Atropine, 1 mg IV, repeated once, is the initial treatment of choice followed by atrial pacing. Increasing heart rate does not establish synchrony between the atrial and ventricular contractions and therefore occasionally may fail to restore blood pressure. High-degree AV block may require atrioventricular sequential pacing to maximize ventricular filling. If atrial fibrillation occurs, early cardioversion should be accomplished to restore atrioventricular synchrony.

IV. Patient disposition. All patients sustaining an acute myocardial infarction should be admitted to a critical care unit with continuous cardiac monitoring and a dedicated staff that is able to interpret cardiac rhythms and has been trained in advanced cardiac life support. If these personnel and facilities are unavailable or if the patient requires angioplasty or bypass surgery, the patient should be transferred to a facility capable of providing this care. Transfer of a critically ill patient should occur only if the benefits of transfer outweigh the risks of not moving the patient. The transferring physician must discuss the risks and benefits of transfer with the patient and family, contact an accepting physician, stabilize the patient, and assure transfer is accomplished by appropriately trained individuals.

Bibliography

Berger PB, Ryan TJ. Inferior myocardial infarction: high-risk subgroups. *Circulation* 181:401–411, 1990.

Chatterjee K. Complications of myocardial infarction. *Curr Probl Cardiol* 7–79, 1993.

Forrester JS, Diamond GA, Swan HJC. Correlative classification of clinical and hemodynamic function after acute myocardial infarction. *Am J Cardiol* 39:137–145, 1977.

Kinch JW, Ryan TJ. Right ventricular infarction. *New Engl J Med* 330:1211–1217, 1994.

Roberts R, et al. Pathophysiology, recognition, and treatment of acute myocardial infarction and its complications. In Schlant RC and Alexander RW (eds.). *The Heart, Arteries, and Veins* (8th ed.) New York: McGraw-Hill, 1107–1184, 1994.

Williams JF. Right ventricular infarction. *Clin Cardiol* 13:309–315, 1990.

Mechanical Complications

Eric Drobny

When acute myocardial infarction (AMI) is accompanied by a mechanical cardiac complication, rapid diagnosis, stabilization, and aggressive therapy are necessary to ensure any chance of survival. Rupture of the left ventricular papillary muscles, the interventricular septum, or the free wall of the myocardium generally occurs within 1 week of AMI in patients older than 60 years. Frequently there is no prior history of cardiac disease. Sudden onset of rapid cardiovascular decompensation is the expected course with these complications. Rapid diagnosis and treatment may yield favorable outcomes in some cases, but in many cases cardiovascular death is the end result.

I. Papillary muscle rupture

A. **Pathophysiology.** Left ventricular papillary muscle rupture complicates myocardial infarction in approximately 1% of cases, accounting for up to 5% of related deaths. Rupture usually occurs 3 to 5 days after AMI, although it is not uncommon within the first 24 hours. Mortality approaches 90% with medical therapy alone; however, adequate stabilization and early surgical correction may reduce this to 30%–40%.

The posteromedial papillary muscle ruptures 6 to 12 times more frequently than the anterolateral muscle because its blood supply is from a single coronary artery. The anterolateral muscle is supplied by both the left anterior descending and circumflex arteries, whereas the posteromedial muscle is supplied by only the dominant coronary artery (right coronary in 90% of cases). Papillary muscles are predisposed to ischemia and infarction because of their significant metabolic requirements, their terminal location in the coronary circulation, and the high degree of tension sustained during the cardiac cycle. Frequently, rupture occurs distally and involves one of the small papillary heads; however, complete rupture of the papillary muscle may occur and is incompatible with life. Papillary muscle dysfunction may also cause acute mitral regurgitation. In this case papillary muscle ischemia or infarction contributes to valvular incompetence and regurgitation. This may occur with isolated papillary muscle ischemia or infarction, but usually requires concomitant contractile dysfunction of the underlying myocardium.

B. **Presentation.** Papillary muscle rupture generally occurs within 2 to 7 days of myocardial infarction in patients older than 60 years. It is more often associated with inferior or posterior AMI, and only one-third of patients have a history of cardiovascular disease. The severity of AMI and coronary artery disease varies. Close to 50% of patients suffer limited or subendocardial infarction, and nearly 50% have only single-vessel disease. Symptoms begin with **respiratory distress** secondary to acute mitral regurgitation (MR) and pulmonary congestion. Initially, a new loud apical holosystolic **murmur** is auscultated; however, it may be soft, nondescript, or absent. With equalization of left ventricular (LV) and left atrial (LA) pressure, the murmur may soften or disappear. Diffuse rales are usually present. In contrast to ventricular septal rupture, a precordial thrill is rarely palpated. Patients frequently experience rapidly progressive heart failure, hypotension, and cardiogenic shock.

C. **Assessment.** Papillary muscle dysfunction and rupture must be rapidly diagnosed and differentiated from other mechanical complications of AMI. In addition to a history and physical examination, electrocardiogram, chest x-ray, echocardiography, and the use of a Swan-Ganz catheter are necessary to diagnose and manage papillary muscle dysfunction and rupture (Table 19-1).

1. **Laboratory studies.** Cardiac enzymes are often elevated because of AMI.
2. **Electrocardiogram.** An inferior or posterior AMI is usually seen, although an anterior MI may be present in 25% of cases.
3. **Chest x-ray.** Pulmonary congestion is present. Because of the direction of the regurgent jet, the upper

Table 19-1. Clinical profile of mechanical complications of myocardial infarction

Variable	Ventricular septal defect	Free-wall rupture	Papillary muscle rupture
Mean age (yr)	63	69	65
Days after MI	3–5	3–6	3–5
Anterior MI	66%	50%	25%
New murmur	90%	25%	50%
Palpable thrill	Yes	No	Rare
Echo findings			
2D	Visualize defect	May have pericardial effusion	Flail or prolapsing leaflet
Doppler	Detect shunt	—	Regurgitant jet in LA
PA cath	Oxygen step-up in RV	Equalization of diastolic pressure	Prominent v wave in PCW tracing
Incidence	2–4%	Up to 10%	1%
Mortality			
Medical	90%	90%	90%
Surgical	50%	Case reports	40%–90%

MI = myocardial infarction, 2D = two-dimensional, LA = left atrium, PA = pulmonary artery, RV = right ventricle, PCW = pulmonary capillary wedge.

Source: Braunwald E. *Heart Disease: A Textbook of Cardiovascular Medicine* (4th ed.). Philadelphia: Saunders, 1992:1257.

lobes have greater involvement, particularly the right upper lobe. This localized congestion may be confused with a pulmonary infiltrate.

4. **Echocardiography.** Immediate bedside echocardiography (echo) should be employed in all patients presenting with acute MR or new holosystolic murmur after recent AMI. Echo will help distinguish between papillary muscle rupture and ventricular septal rupture, which may be difficult to distinguish clinically. In addition, echo will help to determine whether acute MR is secondary to papillary muscle dysfunction or rupture. Papillary muscle rupture is characterized by one or more of the following using two-dimensional (2D) echo: (1) abnormal cut-off of one papillary muscle, (2) a mobile mass attached to chordae and to the mitral valve, (3) a pattern of mitral prolapse or a flail mitral leaflet, and/or (4) moderate to severe MR. The specific mitral leaflet abnormality may be determined by the direction of the resultant regurgitant jet seen on color-flow Doppler. Transthoracic echo may not definitively diagnose papillary muscle rupture in the setting of chronic mitral valve disease, previous myocardial infarction, or when the patient requires mechanical ventilation. In such cases transesophageal echo has been employed successfully to make the diagnosis.

5. **Swan-Ganz catheter.** Hemodynamic monitoring is useful in the bedside diagnosis of acute MR and is essential in its management. Findings may include an elevated pulmonary capillary wedge pressure (PCWP) and a large v wave on tracings of the pulmonary arterial pressure. The PO_2 step-up from the right atrium (RA) to the right ventricle (RV) should be determined through blood gas sampling from the respective Swan-Ganz catheter ports. There should be little or no PO_2 step-up in the case of papillary muscle rupture. A step-up greater than 10% is diagnostic of septal rupture.

D. **Management**
   1. **Airway, breathing, and circulation (ABCs).** A stable airway should be secured. Oxygenation and ventilation should be maintained. Continuous cardiac monitoring, frequent monitoring of vital signs, and pulse oximetry should be initiated.
   2. **Pharmacologic management**
      a. **Vasodilators.** By decreasing afterload through arteriolar dilation, vasodilators increase aortic outflow and reduce MR. **Sodium nitroprusside** is an excellent vasodilator that is easy to titrate because of its rapid onset and short half-life. Continuous infusion should be started at 10–20 µg/min and increased by increments of 10 µg q15 min until the PCWP is lowered to 15–20 mm Hg. Sodium nitroprusside can cause significant hypotension; systolic blood pressure (SBP) should be maintained above 90 mm Hg. Hypotension may be associated with reduced coronary blood flow and reflex tachycardia, both contributing to myocardial ischemia.

Thiocyanate toxicity is another complication of sodium nitroprusside therapy. **Intravenous nitroglycerin** can also be used for afterload reduction; however, significant arteriolar dilatation is not obtained until the rate is over 2 μg/kg/min. Infusion is begun at 10 μg/min and increased by 10–20 μg q10 min, with the SBP kept over 90 mm Hg. Nitroglycerin may increase coronary blood flow and may have less risk of causing myocardial ischemia when compared with nitroprusside. Side effects include headache, reflex tachycardia, paradoxical bradycardia, arterial desaturation, methemoglobinemia, and hypotension.

b. **Inotropes. Dobutamine** supports blood pressure through increased stroke volume and cardiac output via beta-adrenergic agonism. Unlike dopamine, it has no appreciable vasoconstrictive effect even at high doses. This is an important consideration because vasoconstriction decreases aortic outflow, thereby worsening MR. Infusion is begun at 2–5 μg/kg/min and titrated by 50–75 μg to keep the SBP over 90–100 mm Hg. Complications include tachycardia, arrhythmias, worsening myocardial ischemia, nausea, headache, and increased atrioventricular (AV) conduction. Mitral regurgitation may worsen with increased cardiac output.
Dopamine augments blood pressure at low doses (2–5 μg/kg/min) by increasing cardiac output and stroke volume through $beta_1$ agonism. Although systemic pressure may improve, increased cardiac output may exacerbate MR. At higher doses (>5 μg/kg/min) alpha-adrenergic mediated vasopressor effects are present, resulting in vasoconstriction and worsened MR. A dopamine drip is administered via central venous access at 2–3 μg/kg/min. The drip should be titrated to keep the SBP over 90–100 mm Hg and the heart rate in the 110- to 115-bpm range. Complications include worsening MR, at which time the drip must be decreased. Additionally, one may see tachycardia, arrhythmias, myocardial ischemia, necrosis at the infusion site, nausea and vomiting, or decreased AV conduction time.

c. **Vasopressors.** There is no role for vasopressor use in the treatment of papillary muscle rupture.

3. **Mechanical support.** Mechanical circulatory support is used when cardiogenic shock is unresponsive to pharmacotherapy. The intraaortic balloon pump is ideally suited for stabilization of patients with surgically correctable lesions such as papillary muscle rupture. It is inserted through percutaneous puncture of the femoral artery and advanced so that it lies distal to the left subclavian artery and proximal to the renal arteries. It reduces ventricular afterload by deflating during systole, thus increasing blood flow into the aorta and reducing MR. The pump also augments diastolic

aortic pressure through inflation during diastole, thus increasing coronary perfusion pressure. Complications occur in nearly 30% of patients and include compromise of extremity or abdominal vasculature, aortic or femoral artery damage, infection, hemolysis, or embolism.

E. **Patient disposition.** All patients with papillary muscle rupture should be admitted to an intensive care unit for stabilization prior to emergent cardiac catheterization and subsequent surgical repair. When medical therapy is used alone, mortality is 50% in the first 24 hours and 94% after 8 weeks. Some patients may appear to do well with medical therapy, but eventually deteriorate after a brief period of improvement. Early surgical intervention may improve survival to nearly 70%.

II. **Ventricular septal rupture.** Ventricular septal rupture occurs in 2%–4% of AMIs, accounting for up to 5% of infarct-associated deaths. The septum may rupture during the first 24 hours or as late as 2 weeks after MI; however, most occur within 3–5 days. Mortality is greater than 90% with medical therapy alone and ranges from 25%–75% with surgical therapy. Two-thirds of septal ruptures occur with anterior MI. They are usually associated with significant coronary artery disease but may occur with single-vessel disease. Decompensation and cardiogenic shock occur secondary to the increased load placed on the right ventricle. Preexisting right ventricular dysfunction portends a worse outcome.

A. **Presentation.** Septal rupture tends to occur 3–5 days after MI. Twenty-five percent of patients have had previous MI, and the mean age at rupture is 63. Symptoms include significant chest pain and dyspnea. Signs of systemic venous congestion are out of proportion to those of **pulmonary congestion.** A new holosystolic **murmur** is auscultated in 90% of patients, and it does not soften or disappear with decompensation. A thrill is palpated over the precordium. The usual course is progressive **cardiogenic shock.**

B. **Assessment.** The clinical presentation of septal rupture cannot always be differentiated from that of papillary muscle rupture. Both occur soon after MI and are associated with a holosystolic murmur and heart failure. The palpable thrill and minimal pulmonary congestion seen with septal rupture are not always present.

1. **Electrocardiogram** will likely demonstrate an infarct pattern consistent with the location of septal rupture. Apical and anterior septal ruptures are associated with anterior infarcts, whereas posterior ruptures tend to occur with inferior infarcts. Two-thirds of septal ruptures occur with anterior infarctions.

2. **Chest x-ray** demonstrates congestive heart failure.

3. **Swan-Ganz catheter.** A step-up in oxygen saturation greater than 10% from the right atrium to the right ventricle is essentially diagnostic of ventricular septal rupture (compare PO_2 of blood gas samples sent from the RA and RV ports). Hemodynamic monitoring may

also be of some prognostic value because elevated right atrial pressure (>15 mm Hg) coupled with hypotension (SBP < 90 mm Hg) predicts poor surgical outcome.

4. **Echocardiography.** Immediate bedside echo should be obtained in all cases of suspect rupture. Careful examination provides an estimation of both the size and location of the septal defect and an assessment of RV function. Although 2D echo usually identifies the defect, color-flow Doppler is the most accurate mode of echo in the evaluation of septal rupture. Transesophageal echo is useful when the surface image is inadequate. Since the outcome of septal rupture repair appears to be unaffected by concomitant coronary artery bypass, some feel that a good echo study precludes the need for cardiac catheterization in unstable patients prior to surgery.

5. **Cardiac catheterization.** Ventriculography will readily identify the size and location of the septal defect. Since unstable patients and those with renal insufficiency may not tolerate this procedure, the surgeon may elect to repair a septal rupture without this study.

C. **Management**
   1. **Pharmacologic**
      a. **Vasodilators.** By decreasing afterload through arteriolar dilatation, vasodilators increase aortic outflow, thus decreasing the left-to-right shunt across the septal defect. However, if pulmonary vasodilation is greater than systemic vasodilation, the left-to-right shunt may worsen. Severe hypotension often does not allow for the use of vasodilators; however, some patients may receive significant benefit. **Sodium nitroprusside** and **intravenous nitroglycerin** produce reproducible and titratable afterload reduction when used as continuous infusions. Doses and side effects are discussed in sec. **I.D.2.a.**
      b. **Inotropes. Dobutamine** supports blood pressure through increased stroke volume and cardiac output via beta-adrenergic agonism. The shunt across the septal defect may worsen as cardiac output increases, so its use must be monitored closely. Doses are listed in sec. **I.D.2.b. Dopamine,** at low doses (2–5 μg/kg/min), augments blood pressure by increasing cardiac output. Although systemic pressure may improve, the increased cardiac output may worsen the shunt. The shunt also worsens at higher doses as vasoconstrictive effects increase. Drip via central venous access should be administered at 2–3 μg/kg/min. It should be titrated to keep the SBP over 90–100 mm Hg while avoiding significant tachycardia.
   2. **Mechanical support.** Mechanical circulatory support is used when cardiogenic shock is unresponsive to pharmacotherapy. The intraaortic balloon pump is

ideally suited for stabilizing patients with surgically correctable lesions like septal rupture.

D. Patient disposition
  1. **Medical.** Patients should be managed in an intensive care unit until they are taken to either the operating room or catheterization suite. Prognosis is poor, with over 90% mortality with medical therapy alone.
  2. **Surgical.** Because of the high rate of early mortality, some advocate immediate surgery without preoperative cardiac catheterization regardless of the patient's condition. The ability to maintain adequate systolic blood pressure, low right atrial pressure, and short cardiopulmonary bypass time is associated with greater survival. With aggressive early surgery, survival ranges from 48% to 75% initially, with a late mortality of 5%–14%.

III. Free-wall cardiac rupture. Myocardial free-wall rupture, or cardiorrhexis, is the third most common cause of death from AMI after arrhythmias and cardiogenic shock. It accounts for 8%–24% of infarct-related deaths. Free-wall rupture occurs much more frequently than papillary muscle or septal rupture, complicating approximately 10% of myocardial infarctions. Rupture may occur during the first 24 hours; however, most ruptures occur 2–7 days after infarction. Infarctions are transmural and generally involve the lateral wall of the left ventricle. Infarct expansion, a regional thinning and dilatation of the infarct zone, predisposes the ventricular free wall to rupture. It is believed that increased stress secondary to contraction of adjacent papillary muscles may also contribute to lateral wall rupture. Rupture tends to occur in the location of high shear force, such as the interface between infarcted and functioning myocardium. Mortality approaches 100%, and only with immediate recognition and aggressive surgical management is long-term survival possible.

A. Presentation. Cardiac rupture commonly occurs 2–7 days after transmural infarction of the left ventricular lateral wall. As with septal and papillary rupture, patients are usually older than 60 years and have no history of previous MI. Cardiac rupture occurs more frequently in women and is associated with preexisting hypertension. Early administration of thrombolytics may reduce the incidence of ventricular rupture; however, when given late in the course of MI, thrombolytics may increase the risk of rupture. Early ambulation after MI, anti-inflammatory medications, and anticoagulants may also be associated with cardiac rupture.

Cardiac rupture may present as either acute or subacute. Usually patients complain of the sudden onset of a sharp or tearing **chest pain.** It is often associated with several hours of recurrent angina as well as profound agitation and confusion. On examination, patients are often hypotensive and tachycardic with vagally mediated bradycardia suggesting impending complete cardiovascular collapse. They may be cyanotic with signs of tamponade, including distended neck veins and distant heart tones, and may have pulsus paradoxus. Cardiovascular collapse ensues rapidly with the development of pulseless electrical activity (PEA). A subacute form of cardiac rupture has been described in which patients develop worsening signs of **tamponade** (increased venous pressure, muffled heart tones, electrical alternans, and paradoxical pulse) over several hours or days. A high index of suspicion is required for timely diagnosis and treatment before rapid decompensation occurs. Rarely, patients may develop a pseudoaneurysm in which overlying pericardium and thrombus act to contain the rupture. In this case, flow through a ventricular wall defect may be heard as a systolic and/or diastolic murmur. Cardiac rupture must be considered in cases of sudden cardiovascular collapse because immediate therapeutic intervention is necessary for survival.

B. Assessment
1. **Electrocardiogram** frequently demonstrates anterolateral transmural infarction. In the case of rupture contained by pseudoaneurysm, the ECG may demonstrate persistent ST-segment elevation overlying the area of infarction. On rare occasions, electrical alternans or low voltage can be seen.
2. **Chest x-ray.** Cardiac rupture with tamponade is not associated with any specific CXR findings. However, an abnormal bulge may be present along the left heart border if rupture is contained by a pseudoaneurysm.
3. **Echocardiography** should be performed emergently if cardiorrhexis is suspected. Since patients often expire before an echo can be performed, there are few data on the evaluation of free-wall rupture with echo. The subacute form of rupture is associated with echocardiographic signs of tamponade. These include pericardial effusion, right ventricular compression, diastolic collapse of the right ventricle, and dynamic compression of the right atrium. On occasion an echodense mass representing thrombus will be seen in the pericardium. In the rare case of pseudoaneurysm, echo demonstrates a thin-walled aneurysm communicating with the ventricle through a narrow ventricular wall defect. Color-flow Doppler demonstrates flow through the defect.
4. A **Swan-Ganz catheter** will demonstrate features consistent with tamponade. These include equalization of right- and left-sided filling pressures, prominent systolic x-descent, and blunted y-descent on right atrial pressure tracing.

C. Management. The successful management of cardiac rupture requires prompt diagnosis and near heroic measures. Once the airway is secure and ventilatory support initiated, management is dictated by the patient's condition.
1. **Cardiovascular collapse.** When cardiac rupture presents as an acute terminal event with cardiovascular collapse and/or PEA, patients should be treated per advanced cardiac life support (ACLS) guidelines and should undergo emergent pericardiocentesis. Pericar-

diocentesis should include placement of a catheter in the pericardial space to allow for continuous drainage.

2. **Subacute rupture and evolving rupture.** In the event that the rupture is suspected, it may be possible to diagnose and initiate management prior to cardiovascular collapse. Pharmacologic management includes intravenous fluid loading, dobutamine, and finally dopamine to maintain blood pressure. The **intraaortic balloon pump** may be useful for preoperative stabilization; however, its use is controversial. Some authors argue that it is without clinical benefit and merely delays definitive repair, while others believe that this stabilizing therapy is necessary. Similarly, **cardiac catheterization** is deemed unnecessary and time-consuming by some, while others believe that it is helpful in determining LV function and the anatomy of the lesion and in planning surgical repair if the patient's hemodynamic condition allows.

D. **Disposition.** If cardiac rupture is detected and initial resuscitation efforts are effective, an aggressive surgical approach may result in survival. There are an increasing number of reports in which the rupture has been repaired successfully. Immediate thoracic surgical consultation should be made as soon as rupture is diagnosed. Generally, the patient should go directly to the operating suite.

Bibliography

Amin DK, Shah PK, Swan HJC. The Swan-Ganz catheter: indications for insertion. *J Crit Illness* 1:54–61, 1986.

Braundwald E. *Heart Disease.* (4th ed.). Philadelphia: Saunders, 1992:1249–1291.

Buda AJ. The role of echocardiography in the evaluation of mechanical complication of acute myocardial infarction. *Circulation* 84(Suppl I):109–121, 1991.

Cercek B, Shah PK. Complicated acute myocardial infarction: heart failure, shock, mechanical complications. *Cardiol Clin* 9:569–593, 1991.

Come PC, et al. Echocardiographic detection of complete and partial papillary muscle rupture during acute myocardial infarction. *Am J Cardiol* 56:787–789, 1985.

Held AC, et al. Rupture of the interventricular septum complicating acute myocardial infarction: a multicenter analysis of clinical findings and outcome. *Am J Heart* 116:1330–1336, 1988.

Meister SG, Helfant RH. Rapid bedside differentiation of ruptured interventricular septum from acute mitral insufficiency. *N Engl J Med* 287:1024–1025, 1972.

Pappas PJ, et al. Ventricular free-wall rupture after myocardial infarction. *Chest* 99:829–895, 1991.

Smyllie JH, Sutherland GR, Geuskens R. Doppler color flow mapping in the diagnosis of ventricular septal rupture and acute mitral regurgitation after myocardial infarction. *J Am Coll Cardiol* 15:1449–1455, 1990.

Cardiac Emergencies (Non-Myocardial Infarction)

Stable and Unstable Angina

Robert F. McCurdy and Brian J. Zink

I. **Significance.** Angina has been defined as a "spasmodic choking or suffocative pain" while angina pectoris is described as a "pain or oppression about the heart." Angina pectoris presents a diagnostic and management challenge routinely seen by the primary care and emergency physician. In 1991, according to the National Center for Health Statistics, the diagnosis of angina accounted for 570,000 hospital admissions. New onset angina involves significant mortality and morbidity. Recent trials evaluating the natural history of angina show a 10% to 15% incidence of myocardial infarction (MI) and 1% to 5% incidence of death within 3 to 6 months of initial onset. Prompt diagnosis of angina and initiation of treatment can reduce the risk of MI and death and improve the patient's quality of life.

II. **Pathophysiology.** Angina pectoris occurs when ischemic myocardial cells stimulate visceral afferent nerve fibers. The major underlying pathologic feature is atherosclerotic coronary artery disease. The pathologic changes that lead to stable angina develop insidiously over many years. Unstable angina, however, is the result of acute plaque fissuring or rupturing with development of a distal thrombus. Disruption of coronary artery endothelium releases subendothelial materials such as collagen, fibronectin, laminen, Von Willebrand's factor (VWF), and thrombospondin. These agents are potent activators of the coagulation cascade and inducers of platelet activation, adhesion, and aggregation. The end result is thrombin activation with thrombus formation. Thrombin stimulates additional recruitment of platelets potentiating thrombin growth. Additionally, thromboxane A_2, which is released from activated platelets, is a potent vasoconstrictor. The release of antiaggregatory and vasodilator agents such as prostacyclin and nitric oxide also is induced by thrombin formation; however, the effect of these substances is attenuated in diseased endothelium.

Coronary vasospasm in the absence of significant thrombus formation also has been shown to cause ischemia. This is known as variant angina or Prinzmetal's angina. Vasospasm may be associated with loss of endothelial integrity and resulting attenuation of endothelial releasing factor (EDRF) production.

Angina is primarily an intracoronary process, but it also may be exacerbated by any factors that increase myocardial oxygen demand or impair oxygen delivery. Determinants of oxygen demand include heart rate, inotropic state, and wall stress. Wall stress is primarily influenced by preload and afterload. Table 20-1 lists examples of conditions that may induce angina. In evaluating angina, exacerbating factors should be ruled out by history, physical examination, and appropriate laboratory testing.

III. **Differential diagnosis.** The differential diagnosis for patients presenting with angina-like symptoms is extensive and

**Table 20-1.   Clinical conditions
leading to secondary forms of angina**

Increase in myocardial oxygen demand

Tachycardia
    Fever
    Supraventricular tachycardia
    Ventricular tachycardia
    Thyrotoxicosis

High inotropic state
    Endogenous hyperadrenergic state
    Use of sympathomimetic amines

High afterload
    Aortic valvular stenosis
    Supravalvular aortic stenosis
    Hypertrophic cardiomyopathy
    Severe hypertension

High preload
    Left ventricular dilatation
    Severe congestive heart failure
    High output states

Impaired oxygen delivery

Anemia

Hypoxemia

Polycythemic states

Hyperviscosity

---

includes noncardiac causes of chest pain such as thoracic aortic dissection and pulmonary embolism, which are potentially life-threatening. Table 20-2 lists disease processes commonly included in the differential diagnosis of angina. A careful history, physical examination, ECG, and chest radiograph are important in establishing the presence of unstable angina, acute myocardial infarction (AMI), or other life-threatening diseases. Angina may appear concurrently with or as a result of other diseases. A pulmonary embolism with typical pleuritic-type chest pain also may induce angina, if there is significant hypoxia or reduction of venous return to the heart with reflex tachycardia.

IV. **The clinical syndrome of angina**
   A. **Presentation**
      1. **History.** Angina is primarily a clinical diagnosis. The patient's history is the most useful aspect of the clinical evaluation. The primary complaint is most often a description of some quality or type of **chest discomfort.** Classically, the discomfort is substernal and described as "squeezing," "pressure," or a sensation of "fullness." The patient may also describe the discomfort by fist clenching and placing it on the chest. This action is termed Levine's sign. If chest pain is the chief complaint, it is more likely to be described as dull or

Table 20-2. Differential diagnosis of angina

Cardiovascular
  Acute myocardial infarction
  Aortic dissection
  Myocarditis/pericarditis
  Aortic stenosis
  Hypertrophic cardiomyopathy

Pulmonary
  Pulmonary embolism
  Pneumothorax
  Pneumonia
  Pleuritis
  Neoplasm

Gastrointestinal
  Esophageal perforation, mediastinitis
  Pancreatitis
  Cholecystitis/biliary colic
  Acute peptic ulcer disease
  Esophagitis/reflux/spasm

Other
  Herpes zoster
  Musculoskeletal disorders/costochondritis

---

achy. A description of a sharp or stabbing pain is more likely to be pleuritic in origin. A burning sensation in the chest is often described with esophageal reflux. The classic location of anginal complaints is substernal or at the left breast; however, patients may complain of primarily shoulder, neck, jaw, arm, or back pain. Patients also may report numbness and tingling of the face, arm, or hand.

Associated symptoms of dyspnea, diaphoresis, dizziness, anxiety, and nausea may be described during anginal attacks. Infrequently, one or more of these symptoms may be present without accompanying chest discomfort during periods of ischemia. These may be considered anginal equivalents and can be present in patients with an autonomic neuropathy such as with long-standing diabetes.

In obtaining a history it is very important to elucidate the duration, timing, and precipitating and alleviating factors of anginal symptoms. Anginal attacks usually have a gradual onset with a duration of **less than 10 to 15 minutes.** Transient pain lasting a few seconds or constant pain lasting hours to days is more likely to be noncardiac in origin.

The primary precipitating factor in angina is exertion. However, other common provocative factors include ingestion of food, heat or cold stresses, and anxiety. Anginal symptoms most commonly are relieved by rest or the use of sublingual nitroglycerin. Nitroglycerin can also relieve esophageal spasm pain that can mimic anginal symptoms and is not, by itself, diagnostic of angina.

Additional history that is important to obtain and consider when making the diagnosis of angina includes **past medical history.** Patients should be questioned regarding any history of diabetes, hypertension, and previously diagnosed coronary artery disease (CAD). Those with known CAD should be asked about previous stress testing, angiography, angioplasty, and coronary artery bypass grafting (CABG). Family history, current and past medications, and cardiac risk factors such as tobacco use and hyperlipidemias are also important in the evaluation of angina.

The diagnosis of **unstable angina** should be suspected in any patient who describes an evolving character of chest discomfort that departs from a usual pattern. Patients may describe an increase in frequency, severity, or duration of pain. They also may describe increasing refractoriness to sublingual nitroglycerin, decreasing threshold of exercise tolerance, or pain occurring at rest. New onset angina is generally classified as unstable angina.

In contrast, patients with **stable angina** will describe transient, episodic chest discomfort that is quite predictable. The quality and frequency of attacks is relatively constant.

2. **Physical examination.** The physical examination generally does not play a major role in the diagnosis of angina. Patients with ongoing chest discomfort may appear anxious, uncomfortable, short of breath, or diaphoretic. Vital signs may reveal an elevated blood pressure and pulse rate. The cardiac examination may reveal a transient third or fourth heart sound or murmur, which indicates possible ventricular or valvular dysfunction. Arrhythmias such as atrial fibrillation, ventricular ectopy, or bradycardia may be noted. The pulmonary examination may reveal moist rales if pulmonary edema indicative of left ventricular failure is present. Jugulovenous distension and pedal edema may also be seen and may be indicative of some degree of left ventricular dysfunction. Other pertinent physical findings that are highly suggestive of vascular disease are cutaneous or mucocutaneous cholesterol plaques and the presence of bruits.

B. **Patient assessment.** Following a thorough history and physical examination, diagnostic studies and laboratory testing should be obtained on all patients suspected of having a cardiac etiology for their complaint. An assessment should be made regarding the likelihood of the patient having CAD and the risk for an adverse outcome. If the patient is determined to have a high probability of CAD, an attempt should be made to assign the patient to a diagnostic category: stable angina, unstable angina, or AMI. Unstable angina may be classified further by clinical presentation, background, and specific forms (Table 20-3).

1. **ECG.** The ECG is routinely obtained on all patients with suspected angina. In patients with stable angina, 75% of resting ECGs are abnormal. A variety of changes may be seen, including patterns of old MIs such as Q waves, conduction disturbances, left ventricular hypertrophy (LVH), and nonspecific ST-T abnormalities. These changes indicate the existence of previous coronary artery disease but are not diagnostic for stable or unstable angina.

   Patients with complaints of anginal-type symptoms should have an immediate 12-lead ECG reading obtained, ideally while they are still symptomatic. Continuous ST-segment monitoring, when available, is helpful in detecting the ST-segment changes over time with ischemia. The predictive value of an ECG is greatly enhanced if transient changes can be documented with ongoing chest pain. An ECG should be obtained for comparison when the patient is symptom free. An attempt should also be made to obtain ECGs from previous hospital, emergency department (ED), or clinic visits.

   The ST-T abnormalities associated with angina, in order of decreasing sensitivity and increasing specificity, are T wave inversion, ST depression, and ST elevation. Pseudonormalization of a previously inverted T wave can also be seen in angina. In general, ST elevation is seen with subepicardial injury and transmural ischemia. ST depression and T wave inversion indicate ischemia that is limited to subendocardial zones. See Figs. 20-1 and 20-2 for examples.

Table 20-3. Clinical classification of unstable angina

Clinical presentation

   Recent onset angina (within the previous 60 days)

   Crescendo angina pectoris

   Angina pectoris at rest

   Prolonged chest pain (with or without enzyme
   elevation)

Clinical background

   Postmyocardial infarction angina

   Postcoronary angioplasty angina

   Postbypass surgery angina

Specific forms

   Prinzmetal's variant angina

   Cocaine intoxication

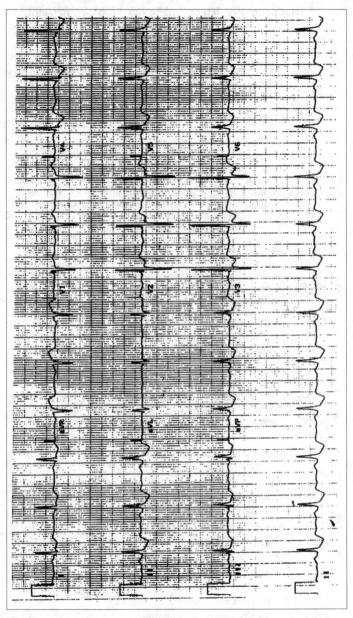

Fig. 20-1. ECG changes of unstable angina: ST depression of subendo-cardial ischemia.

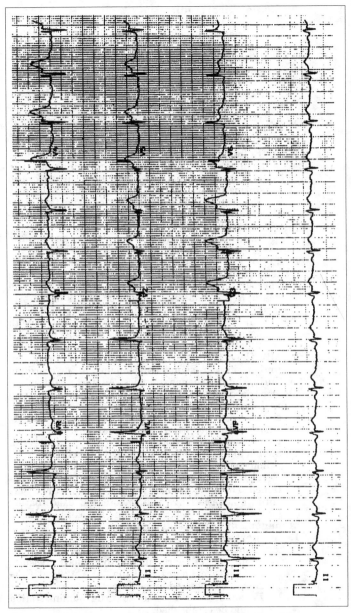

Fig. 20-2. ECG changes of unstable angina: ST elevation of transmural ischemia.

2. **Radiological studies**
   a. **Chest roentgenogram.** The chest radiograph is not particularly useful in the diagnosis of angina. An enlarged cardiac silhouette may indicate cardiomegaly or may be secondary to a chronic pericardial effusion. Vessel or valve calcification may be seen and is probably indicative of concomitant CAD, but it is not diagnostic. The chest radiograph is most useful in narrowing the differential diagnosis by detecting abnormalities such as an effusion, infiltrate, pneumothorax, pneumomediastinum, or a widened mediastinum.
   b. **Echocardiography.** Echocardiography provides a qualitative evaluation of left ventricular function, on both a regional and global basis. If performed during episodes of angina, echocardiography may detect wall motion abnormalities indicating areas of ischemic myocardium. Transesophageal echocardiography is also useful in diagnosing aortic dissection, pericardial effusion/tamponade, intracardiac neoplasm, and infectious vegetations.

3. **Laboratory studies.** Cardiac enzymes and other proteins found within myocardium are released into the bloodstream when prolonged ischemia leads to cell death. Serial, quantitative measurements of CK-MB, lactate dehydrogenase (LDH), and myoglobin are valuable in excluding the diagnosis of MI in patients with stable or unstable angina. Serial measurements over 9 to 12 hours are required to detect an increase in CK-MB. The patient with angina pectoris does not, by definition, lose a significant amount of myocardium during brief ischemic episodes. As such, cardiac enzymes are not typically elevated, even in serial testing in these patients. There have been reports, however, of small elevations of CK-MB and troponin T in patients who are subsequently diagnosed with unstable angina. Cardiac enzymes should be measured in patients with angina to rule out MI as an etiology of their pain.

Routine laboratory studies such as blood cell count, electrolytes, and arterial blood gases should also be obtained. These studies may aid in narrowing the differential diagnosis or revealing potential exacerbating factors of angina (e.g., anemia and hypoxia).

C. **Management of unstable angina**
   1. **Supportive care**
      a. **Monitoring.** All patients should have continuous monitoring of heart rate, rhythm, blood pressure, and pulse oximetry if available. A 12-lead ECG should be obtained immediately.
      b. **IV access.** An IV line for drug administration should be established.
      c. **Oxygen.** Oxygen should be applied to maintain an adequate hemoglobin saturation by pulse oximetry.
   2. **Pharmacologic therapy.** Pharmacologic therapy of angina is directed at (1) controlling the thrombotic

process, (2) decreasing myocardial oxygen demand, (3) affecting coronary artery tone, and (4) increasing oxygen delivery.

a. **Aspirin. Dose:** 160–325 mg, chewed immediately.

Salicylates reduce thrombosis through irreversible inhibition of the cyclooxygenase pathway in platelets and endothelial cells. The result is decreased thromboxane A_2 synthesis that effectively inhibits platelet function. Low-dose aspirin has been shown to have the same benefits as high-dose aspirin in decreasing the risk of fatal and nonfatal MI with fewer side effects. Relative contraindications to aspirin administration include hypersensitivity, active bleeding, or severe bleeding risk.

Ticlopidine inhibits platelet aggregation by interfering with fibrinogen receptors and the adenosine diphosphate (ADP) platelet activation mechanism. This drug may be useful in patients with aspirin hypersensitivity or intolerance. Ticlopidine has no proven advantage over aspirin in the inhibition of platelets and is considerably more expensive. Aspirin also has fewer side effects.

b. **Nitroglycerin. Sublingual dosing:** 0.4 mg q5min as needed up to 3 doses. **Intravenous dosing:** IV dosing should be considered in patients who are unresponsive to initial therapy. Use a starting dose of 10–20 µg/min and titrate by 5 µg/min, q3 to 5min with the end-point being relief of pain or development of undesirable side effects (e.g., hypotension). **Transdermal dosing:** Patients who respond well to initial oral therapy may be started in the ED on transdermal nitroglycerin that provides continuous dosing. A variety of patch and paste concentrations is available.

Nitroglycerin is extremely useful in the treatment of both stable and unstable angina. Sublingual nitroglycerin is rapidly absorbed and systemically converted to nitrous oxide that stimulates the production of cyclic guanosine monophosphate (cGMP). Cyclic GMP causes the relaxation of vascular smooth muscle. The resulting coronary vasodilation increases the oxygen supply to the ischemic myocardium. Systemically, arterial and venous vascular relaxation occur. The resulting decrease in preload and afterload reduces wall stress and myocardial oxygen requirements. Nitroglycerin and cGMP also have been shown to inhibit thrombin-induced platelet aggregation. For chronic management of angina with long-acting nitrates, a drug-free period must be provided each day to prevent tolerance. Adverse effects of nitrates include hypotension, headache, dizziness, and palpitations.

c. **Heparin. Dose:** An initial bolus of 80 U/kg (5,000–10,000 U) of heparin is given intravenously followed by an infusion of 18 U/kg/hr (1,000–1,500

U/hr). Therapeutic levels are reached when the patient's prothrombin time (PTT) is 1.5–2.5 times
higher than the control. A PTT should be obtained
6 hours following the initial bolus and then again
following any dosing changes.

Heparin therapy is generally accepted as beneficial in the management of unstable angina. Heparin acts by forming a complex with antithrombin
III, accelerating the antithrombotic effect. There is
an overall inhibitory effect of thrombin and factors
IX, X, XI, and XII. Therapy is by IV infusion following an initial fluid bolus. The use of heparin is
relatively contraindicated in patients with active
bleeding, severe bleeding risk, recent stroke, or a
history of heparin-induced thrombocytopenia.
Heparin has no role in the treatment of stable
angina.

d. **Beta-adrenergic blockers. Metoprolol:** Initial
IV bolus of 5 mg over 1 to 2 minutes. May repeat
dose q5min up to 15 mg. An oral dose of 25–50 mg
is given 1 to 2 hours following IV bolus and then
q6h. **Propranolol:** Initial IV bolus of 0.5–1.0 mg
over 1 to 2 minutes. An oral dose of 40–80 mg is
given 1 to 2 hours following IV bolus and then
q4–6h. **Esmolol:** Starting dose 0.1 mg/kg/min IV.
Titrate dose by 0.05 mg/kg/min for desired therapeutic effect up to 0.2 mg/kg/min maximum dose.

Beta-blockers have been shown to be useful in the
treatment of stable and unstable angina. Blockade
of myocardial beta$_1$ receptors inhibits catecholamine binding, resulting in decreased activation of adenyl cyclase and calcium influx. The
physiologic effects of beta$_1$ blockade are decreased
myocardial contractility, heart rate, and systolic
blood pressure. Blockade of beta$_2$ receptors in the
peripheral vasculature, allows alpha-adrenergic receptor activation to exert the predominant effect on
vascular tone, resulting in vasoconstriction. Beta$_2$
receptors are also present on bronchiolar smooth
muscle, and blockade may cause bronchospasm. Although beta-blockers are helpful in reducing anginal symptoms, they have not been shown to reduce
the risk of MI. Beta-blockers are contraindicated in
patients with AV block, bradycardia, hypotension,
congestive heart failure, left ventricular dysfunction, or severe reactive airway disease.

e. **Calcium channel-blockers. Nifedipine:** For
vasospastic angina, the patient may be given an
initial dose of 10 mg orally. Dosing may be repeated q4–6h as needed. A single dose should not
exceed 30 mg. **Verapamil:** Initial bolus of 5–10
mg over 2 to 5 minutes. May repeat bolus if needed
in 30 minutes. IV rate is 0.4 μg/kg/min. Also
useful in conversion of paroxysmal supraventricular tachycardia to normal sinus rhythm except
those associated with accessory bypass tracts.

Diltiazem: Initial bolus 0.25 mg/kg over 2 minutes. Second bolus of 0.35 mg/kg may be given 15 minutes later if needed. IV rate 10–15 mg/hr.

Calcium antagonists may be helpful in the treatment of stable and unstable angina, particularly if the suspected etiology is vasospasm. These drugs block the influx of extracellular calcium ions through membrane channels into the cells. This results in relaxation of vascular smooth muscle that includes the coronary vasculature. Peripherally, arterial vasodilation causes a reduction in afterload. In coronary vessels, vasodilation improves blood flow and oxygen delivery to the myocardium. Calcium antagonists also act directly on the myocardium, decreasing contractility and heart rate, and resulting in reduction of myocardial oxygen demand. Calcium channel blockers that act primarily on smooth muscle, such as nicardipine and nifedipine, may cause a reflex tachycardia by decreasing peripheral vascular resistance. Verapamil and intravenous diltiazem have a less potent effect on smooth muscle and act primarily on the myocardium, slowing AV nodal conduction and decreasing contractility. Calcium channel antagonists are contraindicated in patients with AV block, pulmonary edema, and left ventricular dysfunction.

f. Narcotic analgesics. Morphine: 2–10 mg IVP, titrated to pain relief. Morphine or other parenteral analgesics may be used during anginal attacks to reduce pain and anxiety. This reduces sympathetic discharge and stimulation of the myocardium. Morphine is contraindicated in patients with hypotension, confusion or obtundation, or respiratory depression.

g. Thrombolytic therapy. Thrombolytic therapy in acute angina is currently under investigation. Large clinical trials have shown that thrombolytic therapy has no benefit in the treatment of unstable angina and is possibly harmful.

2. Invasive interventions

a. Coronary artery bypass grafting (CABG). In patients with angina, most studies have shown similar 2-year mortality and incidence of MI in those treated surgically or medically. Some evidence exists, however, for improved 5-year survival with surgical therapy in a subset of patients with 3-vessel disease and abnormal left ventricular (LV) function. These patients may have an improved quality of life with fewer hospitalizations, fewer medications, and improved exercise tolerance. Vascular bypass grafting may also be useful in patients with recurrent angina on optimal medical therapy.

b. Coronary angioplasty. Angioplasty may be an option for management in patients with suitable anatomy. Preferably, it should be performed semi-

electively following medical stabilization, but may
be needed more acutely in cases of angina that are
refractory to pharmacologic therapy. Angioplasty is
associated with up to a 10% risk of complications
including MI, emergency bypass, in-hospital mortality, and the need for repeat angioplasty.

  c. Intra-aortic balloon counterpulsation (IABC).
  Intra-aortic balloon counterpulsation is a useful
  temporizing measure in patients with angina refractory to medical therapy. The balloon is inserted
  through the femoral artery and positioned in the
  descending thoracic aorta. Inflation of the balloon
  during diastole increases coronary perfusion by
  augmenting diastolic pressure. Deflation of the balloon during systole reduces cardiac work by lowering ventricular pressure and afterload. IABC has a
  10%–20% complication rate, which is usually related to local vascular injury at the site of insertion.

D. Patient disposition: unstable angina

  1. Admission and in-hospital care. In new onset or
  unstable angina, the risk of complications and progression to AMI is increased. Patients should continue
  to be monitored vigorously and ruled out for MI by serial cardiac enzyme determination. Consultation with
  a cardiologist who can monitor and coordinate care, as
  well as facilitate coronary angiography, is warranted.
  ICU, CCU, or telemetry unit admission is mandatory.
  Patients with unstable angina should proceed with
  their care depending on their clinical status. Patients
  with controlled angina on medical regimens are
  treated less aggressively than those with uncontrolled
  angina symptoms.

    a. Controlled angina. Elective coronary angiogra-
    phy to assess degree and distribution of coronary
    disease is usually indicated. Consideration of med-
    ical therapy, percutaneous transthoracic coronary
    angioplasty (PTCA), or CABG for treatment de-
    pends on angiographic findings.

    b. Continued angina or ECG changes. Urgent
    coronary angiography is indicated. Consideration
    of intra-aortic balloon counterpulsation is a tempo-
    rizing measure. If an acute thrombus is present on
    angiography, consideration is for thrombolytic
    therapy or PTCA.

  2. Chronic therapy

    a. Pharmacology

      (1) Aspirin

      (2) Sublingual nitrates as needed; chronic therapy
      with oral or transdermal nitrates can be con-
      sidered.

      (3) Chronic therapy with oral beta-blockers or cal-
      cium channel blockers can be considered.

    b. Lifestyle changes. Patients should receive coun-
    seling on reducing risk factors in an effort to stabi-
    lize angina, limit CAD progression, and alter plaque
    composition as follows.

> (1) Cessation of tobacco use
> (2) Dietary and pharmacologic control of hyperlipidemia
> (3) Control of hypertension through weight loss, diet, stress management, and pharmacologic therapy
> (4) Cardiovascular conditioning; new exercise programs should be rigorously monitored by qualified personnel.

E. **Patient disposition: stable angina.** The initial management of stable angina is identical to that of unstable angina. The goal is complete alleviation of chest pain. Assessment should include a complete history and physical examination. Patients who clearly have stable angina may be managed on an outpatient basis unless coexisting medical illnesses require in-hospital management. Consultation with the patient's primary care physician is desirable to schedule follow-up care. The primary physician can provide ongoing care, prescribe antianginal medications, and coordinate further cardiac evaluation. Chronic care is similar to the care of patients with unstable angina (see sec. **IV.D.2.**).

Bibliography

Braunwald E, et al. Effects of tissue plasminogen activator and a comparison of early invasive and conservative strategies in unstable angina and non-Q-wave myocardial infarction: results of the TIMI IIIB trial. *Circulation.* 89:1545–1555, 1994.

Braunwald E, et al. Diagnosing and managing unstable angina. *Circulation.* 90:613–622, 1994.

Catherwood E, O'Rourke D. Critical pathway management of unstable angina. *Prog Cardiovasc Dis.* 37:121–145, 1994.

Theroux P, Lidon R. Unstable angina: pathogenesis, diagnosis, and treatment. *Curr Probl Cardiol.* 18:162–231, 1993.

Waters D. A practical approach to diagnosis and treatment of unstable angina. *Heart Dis Stroke.* 3:159–163, 1994.

Pericarditis

Richard N. Nelson

Few medical conditions are mistaken for as many acute life-threatening disorders as is pericarditis. Although potentially serious in its own right, pericarditis should be diagnosed only after similarly presenting, more immediately deadly conditions—such as myocardial infarction, aortic aneurysm, aortic dissection, and pulmonary embolism—have been carefully ruled out.

Pericarditis includes any one of a number of inflammatory processes involving the pericardium, a dense and somewhat elastic structure that envelops the heart and the origins of the great arteries and veins. The most common causes of pericarditis are listed in Table 21-1. Most forms of pericarditis can eventually result in restriction of cardiac filling either via compression from blood or fluid trapped under pressure in the pericardial sac (see tamponade in Chap 22) or from thickening and hardening of the pericardium (constrictive pericarditis). Both conditions are life threatening but can be either prevented or managed early by appropriately diagnosing and treating the underlying pericarditis.

I. **Viral and idiopathic pericarditis.** Viral infections probably represent the most common cause of acute pericarditis, particularly among young and previously healthy individuals. Coxsackie group B and echoviruses often are implicated; however, other viruses are possible. Many cases of so-called idiopathic pericarditis probably are caused by viruses as well, but the difficulty and expense involved in confirming this usually precludes definitive diagnosis.

   A. **Presentation. Chest pain** is the hallmark of acute pericarditis. The pain is typically substernal, sometimes radiating to either or both trapezius muscle ridges. The pain often is exacerbated by breathing, coughing, movement, swallowing, and lying supine. Relief may be achieved by sitting up or bending forward. Often concomitant viral symptoms such as fever, malaise, and myalgias coincide with or precede the chest discomfort by one to two weeks.

   Pericardial friction rub is often though not always heard. It is best to auscultate the heart with the stethoscope's diaphragm firmly applied to the chest wall. Friction rubs are best heard at the lower-left sternal border, just medial to the cardiac apex. Having the patient lean forward or lie in the left lateral position during auscultation may accentuate the rub. Also, since friction rubs typically are variably present and absent, repeat examinations in a quiet room are indicated. Occasionally the friction rub is augmented during inspiration, particularly when the pleura is involved. This finding is referred to as a **pleuropericardial friction rub.**

   The classic friction rub has three components: atrial, ventricular, and diastolic. Thus the rub may be heard just prior to S_1 (atrial), following S_1 (ventricular), and following

Table 21-1. Causes of pericarditis

I. Idiopathic
II. Infections
  A. Viral
    1. Coxsackie B_5, B_6
    2. Echovirus
    3. Human immunodeficiency virus (HIV): opportunistic infections, malignancies, and associated myocarditis
  B. Bacterial
    1. Staphylococcus, *Streptococcus pneumoniae,* β-hemolytic streptococcus, *Hemophilus influenzae,* meningococcus, salmonella, psittacosis, tuberculosis, syphilis
  C. *Mycoplasma pneumoniae*
  D. Fungal
    1. Histoplasmosis, blastomycosis, aspergillosis, coccidioidomycosis
  E. Others
    1. Rickettsia, amebiasis, echinococcus
III. Neoplasms
  A. Primary
    1. Mesothelioma, angiosarcoma, teratoma, angioma, fibroma, lipoma, leiomyofibroma
  B. Metastatic
    1. Lung, breast, leukemia, lymphoma, melanoma, Kaposi's sarcoma, head and neck, colon
IV. Connective tissue disorders
  A. Lupus, rheumatic fever, vasculitis, scleroderma, rheumatoid arthritis, polyarteritis nodosa, dermatomyositis
V. Drug-induced
  A. Hydralazine, procainamide, cromolyn sodium, dantrolene, methysergide, daunorubicin
VI. Uremic
VII. Myxedema
VIII. Postmyocardial injury
  A. Trauma
    1. Postsurgical
    2. Postprocedure (e.g., pacemaker, cardiac catheterization)
  B. Postmyocardial infarction, Dressler's syndrome
X. Sarcoidosis
XI. Postradiation

S_2 (diastole), although only one or two of these components may be heard at any single examination. The sound itself is typically coarse, grating, or leathery and seems more superficial and less smooth than does a heart murmur.

Other signs associated with pericarditis include **fever, tachycardia,** and, if tamponade or constrictive pericarditis supervene, Kussmaul's sign (increased jugular venous distention with inspiration), jugular venous distension, pulsus paradoxus, and electrical alternans.

B. Assessment. Presence of a pericardial friction rub in the setting of typical symptoms of pericarditis is virtually diagnostic of the disorder. However, absence of friction rub does not exclude the diagnosis.

1. **ECG.** An ECG should be obtained on any patient suspected of having pericarditis. This is important not just to assist in the diagnosis, but also to help rule out more serious conditions such as myocardial infarction. The ECG in the setting of acute pericarditis typically shows diffuse ST-segment elevation (concave up), particularly in the limb and precordial leads. ST depression may occur in leads avr and V1. In addition, diffuse PR segment depression is seen often (Fig. 21-1). After several days, ST-segment elevation normalizes, and diffuse T-wave inversion may occur. ECG changes from acute pericarditis must be differentiated from these caused by myocardial infarction and early repolarization variant (Table 21-2).

2. **Chest x-ray.** A chest x-ray should be obtained if pericarditis is suspected. Most chest x-rays will be normal in patients with pericarditis; however, cardiac enlargement, particularly if it is a new finding, suggests the presence of pericardial effusion.

3. **Laboratory studies.** Most laboratory studies are not helpful. White blood cell count and erythrocyte sedimentation rate may be elevated, but these are nonspecific findings. Cardiac enzymes such as creatinine phosphokinase CK-MB isoenzyme fractions may be elevated if the pericardial inflammation extends to the surface of the myocardium.

4. **Echocardiogram.** Pericardial effusion often develops with idiopathic or viral pericarditis. An echocardiogram should be obtained to confirm and monitor pericardial effusion in any patient suspected of having effusion or tamponade.

C. Management

1. **Supportive care.** Much of the initial management of the patient presenting with signs and symptoms consistent with pericarditis should be aimed at ruling out more life-threatening causes of chest pain. Patients considered at risk for myocardial infarction should receive an IV line, oxygen, and continuous cardiac monitoring during the course of their work-up. Abnormal pulse oximetry or arterial blood gas results may suggest the possibility of pulmonary embolus. Aortic aneurysm or dissection is suggested by widened mediastinum on chest x-ray, unequal upper extremity pulses, and the presence of aortic insufficiency murmur. Finally, additional tests may be warranted in certain patients in whom the diagnosis of pericarditis is certain, but in whom the specific etiology (e.g., uremic, collagen vascular) is in question (see sec. **IV.**).

2. **Specific therapy.** Treatment consists of **nonsteroidal anti-inflammatory agents** (ibuprofen 400–600 mg qid, indomethacin 25–50 mg qid, or aspirin

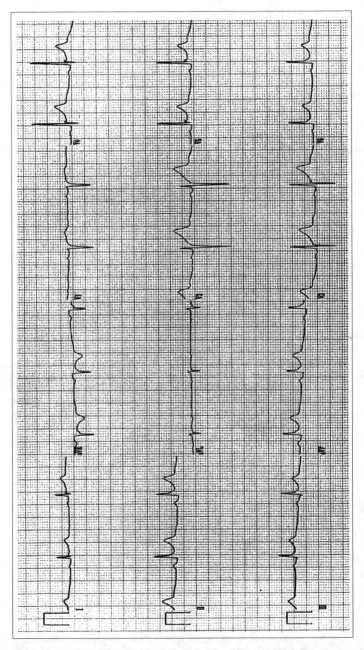

Fig. 21-1.   ECG ST elevation and PR depression from pericarditis.

Table 21-2. Differentiating pericarditis, myocardial infarction, and early repolarization variant

	Pericarditis	Myocardial infarction	Repolarization
ST/T ratio	>0.25	Variable	<0.25
ST elevation/ reciprocal depression	Diffuse/avr, V1	Regional/opposite	Anterior and inferior/avr
ST shape	Concave up	Flat or convex up	Concave up
Notched S wave	No	No	Yes
PR-segment depression	Yes	No	No

325–500 mg q4h). If discomfort is not adequately managed by nonsteroidal medications, consider adding a short course of prednisone, starting at 60 mg/d and tapering over one week.

   D. Patient disposition. Most patients with uncomplicated viral or idiopathic pericarditis may be discharged to home. Patients with large pericardial effusions as seen by echocardiogram, where tamponade is a possibility, should be admitted for observation until stabilized, probably to a monitored bed.

II. Uremic pericarditis. Up to one-third of patients with end-stage renal disease develop uremic pericarditis. Pericarditis is more likely in patients not undergoing dialysis therapy; however, those undergoing such therapy are still at risk. Factors identified as causes of uremic pericarditis include elevated concentrations of blood urea nitrogen, uric acid, calcium, and other unidentified blood toxins. The clinician also must recognize that the uremic patient is at risk of developing pericarditis from other causes, such as viral or bacterial infection, concomitant drug therapy, and postmyocardial infarction. In addition, pericarditis may occur secondary to the same disease process that caused the renal failure in the first place (e.g., lupus, Wegener's granulomatosis).

   A. Presentation. Most patients with uremic pericarditis present with chest pain characteristic of pericarditis (see above). Presence of a pericardial friction rub in a uremic patient without chest pain is not unusual, however, and still indicates the presence of pericarditis. Many patients present with dyspnea—with or without pain or friction rub—and a chest x-ray showing cardiac enlargement. In this scenario, pericarditis with pericardial effusion should be strongly suspected.

   Diminished cardiac sounds may be indicative of a large pericardial effusion. Kussmaul's sign, pulsus paradoxus, electrical alternans, and systemic hypotension and tachycardia all suggest cardiac tamponade.

B. **Assessment.** When evaluating a uremic patient for pericarditis, other causes of both chest pain and pericarditis must be ruled out. The same underlying process that causes renal failure (e.g., diabetes, hypertension) may predispose the patient to myocardial infarction. Also, not only may the underlying disease process (lupus) that causes renal failure also cause the pericarditis, but also the treatments for these processes (dialysis, immunosuppression) may result in a septic pericardial effusion.

Assessment should include chest x-ray, ECG, and appropriate renal blood chemistries. The **ECG** in patients with uremic pericarditis often is normal or shows only nonspecific changes. Low voltage suggests the possibility of a large pericardial effusion. **Chest x-ray** showing new cardiac enlargement also suggests, though doesn't confirm, pericardial effusion. **CK-MB** enzyme studies are obtained if myocardial infarction is suspected, but these levels may be chronically elevated in patients with renal failure. Blood and sputum cultures should be obtained on all febrile patients.

An **echocardiogram** is indicated when there is significant pericardial effusion or suspicion of septic pericardial effusion. Pericardiocentesis is indicated to rule out the latter.

C. **Management.** Besides the usual supportive measures, treatment of uremic pericarditis consists of intensive **dialysis** therapy. Dialysis may be needed daily during the acute phase of pericarditis and should be done with a minimum of heparin to avoid intrapericardial bleeding and tamponade. Anti-inflammatory medications probably do not substantially affect the course of the illness and may predispose to bleeding complications. Some patients may benefit from systemic steroids.

Patients with uremic pericardial effusion should undergo **serial echocardiograms** to monitor the size of the effusion and its hemodynamic effects. Those patients with expanding effusions despite dialysis therapy should undergo pericardiocentesis and possibly pericardiotomy and pericardiectomy.

D. **Patient disposition.** All patients with uremic pericarditis should be admitted to the hospital and monitored closely for expanding pericardial effusion and tamponade while they undergo dialysis.

III. **Postmyocardial injury.** Pericarditis may follow injury to the myocardium by a mechanical event (e.g., surgery, pacemaker wire perforation, blunt or penetrating trauma) or a pathophysiologic event (i.e., acute myocardial infarction). Postmyocardial injury pericarditis is postulated to be caused by either (1) an autoimmune phenomenon secondary to sensitization by myocardial or pericardial tissue antigens released in the circulation at the time of injury, or (2) a viral infection, either acute or reactivation.

Approximately 20% of patients suffering transmural myocardial infarction develop pericarditis. Most cases occur within one week of infarction, but some may develop weeks or even months later. The latter situation is referred to as **Dressler's syndrome.** Patients who have undergone mechanical trauma to the heart may develop pericarditis in a similar timeframe.

A. **Presentation.** Patients present with chest pain that they describe as of a different quality than that of the preceding myocardial infarction postoperative or post-traumatic discomfort. Pain is generally pleuritic and improves with sitting forward. Low-grade fever and pericardial friction rub often are present.

B. **Assessment.** An **ECG** should be obtained, but often it does not show ST-segment elevation typical of pericarditis. The **chest x-ray** may show evidence of increased heart size, suggestive of pericardial effusion, although absence of this finding does not rule out effusion. Elevations of **leukocyte count** and **sedimentation rate** may occur, but they are nonspecific findings. **Echocardiogram** should be obtained if pericardial effusion is suspected.

   The diagnosis is made based on both a constellation of history and physical findings and the history of recent myocardial injury.

C. **Management.** Uncomplicated postmyocardial injury pericarditis is treated with **nonsteroidal anti-inflammatory medications.** Corticosteroids may be considerd in refractory cases. Presence of hemodynamically significant pericardial effusion necessitates surgical intervention.

D. **Patient disposition.** Most patients with postmyocardial injury pericarditis who are not already hospitalized will require admission, mostly to rule out other causes of the chest discomfort as well as to monitor for the development of pericardial tamponade.

IV. **Other causes of pericarditis**

A. **Infectious pericarditis.** Numerous organisms can infect the pericardium, myocardium, and pericardial fluid, resulting in pericarditis. The most important of these are listed in Table 21-1.

   1. **Bacterial infection.** Purulent pericarditis is a rapidly fatal disorder if left untreated. The source is often pneumonia, although any septic process (endocarditis, peritonitis, urinary tract infection, septic abortion, mediastinitis from esophageal perforation, or necrotizing soft-tissue infections of the head and neck) have been implicated. Elderly or immunocompromised individuals are more at risk, although any age group with or without underlying disease could be affected. Diagnosis is made by pericardial fluid culture, and treatment consists of aggressive antibiotic therapy and surgical drainage. Special attention should be given to the possibility of tubercular pericarditis, in which the diagnosis is made by the presence of acid-fast bacilli in samples of pericardial fluid or biopsy.

   2. **Fungal infection.** Fungal infection of the pericardium is due usually to histoplasmosis, but other etiologies are possible (see Table 21-1). Diagnosis,

which may be difficult, is made by pericardial fluid culture and/or significant rise in histoplasmosis, serologic titers to greater than 1:32.

   3. **Human immunodeficiency virus (HIV) infection.** Pericarditis and pericardial effusion are not uncommon in the setting of acquired immunodeficiency syndrome (AIDS). Often evidence of pericarditis and effusion are absent during life and picked up only at autopsy. Etiologies include opportunistic infections, malignancies such as Kaposi's sarcoma involving the pericardium, and associated myocarditis.

B. **Connective tissue disorders.** Various connective tissue disorders and vasculitides can produce pericarditis. With the exception of that caused by lupus, many of the other disorders in this category produce pericarditis that is often clinically and electrocardiographically silent. Lupus, on the other hand, frequently causes symptomatic pericarditis with ECG changes, pericardial effusion, and occasionally tamponade. In fact, pericarditis secondary to lupus may precede the actual diagnosis of lupus. For this reason, lupus should be ruled out in patients with new onset idiopathic pericarditis, particularly if the patients are female.

   Treatment for pericarditis in this group of patients generally involves treating the underlying disorder. Nonsteroidal anti-inflammatory drugs and sometimes steroids are prescribed.

C. **Other causes of pericarditis.** Other etiologies of pericarditis include neoplastic, drug-induced, myxedematous, postradiation, and that caused by sarcoidosis. These and others are listed in Table 21-1.

V. **Complications of pericarditis.** The two main complications of pericarditis are cardiac tamponade and constrictive pericarditis.

A. **Cardiac tamponade.** Cardiac tamponade occurs when pericardial effusion, either from fluid or blood, accumulates to the extent that the resultant pressure impairs diastolic filling of the encased heart. Once this occurs, cardiac output and stroke volume are significantly reduced, and shock ensues. This is discussed more thoroughly in Chap. 22.

B. **Constrictive pericarditis.** Constrictive pericarditis occurs when the pericardial space is replaced by granulation tissue and scarring due to a previous or ongoing process. Hardening, shrinking, and decreased elasticity of the scarred pericardium results in restriction of myocardial motion, particularly during diastole. Causes of constrictive pericarditis include tuberculosis; viral, bacterial, fungal, or idiopathic pericarditis; uremia; neoplasm; collagen-vascular disease; previous mediastinal irradiation; previous surgery to the pericardium; and cardiac trauma.

   1. **Presentation.** Signs and symptoms of constrictive pericarditis generally appear over a longer time period than those of cardiac tamponade. Symptoms include dyspnea on exertion, orthopnea, fatigue, nausea,

abdominal discomfort, anorexia, and weight gain or loss (depending on the extent of peripheral and central edema). Physical findings include jugular venous distension without respiratory variation, absent pulsus paradoxus in the majority of cases, hepatomegaly, splenomegaly, and ascites. Lower-extremity edema often is present. Lungs are generally clear to auscultation, although decreased breath sounds at the bases usually indicate pleural effusions.

Patients with constrictive pericarditis may or may not have a friction rub on cardiac auscultation. However, approximately one-half will manifest a **pericardial knock.** Pericardial knock is a diastolic sound occurring shortly after the second heart sound that corresponds to the ventricle suddenly reaching its filling limit. Pericardial knock, if present, is a highly specific finding for constrictive pericarditis.

2. **Assessment.** Patients with constrictive pericarditis often resemble patients with chronic congestive heart failure, right ventricular infarct, restrictive cardiomyopathy, pericardial tamponade, and cirrhosis. Several simple tests help differentiate these conditions.

   Jugular venous distension in the presence of ascites and lower-extremity edema should alert the clinician to the possibility of constrictive pericarditis rather than cirrhosis. Relatively clear lung fields and pericardial knock further support this diagnosis. **ECG** often shows sinus tachycardia, nonspecific ST and T-wave changes, and generally low voltage. Atrial fibrillation is a common late finding. **Chest x-ray** shows a normal or slightly enlarged cardiac silhouette, and up to 50% of cases show pericardial calcifications. Lung fields are generally clear, although pleural effusions are common. **Echocardiogram** may or may not be helpful in diagnosing constrictive pericarditis. Findings include associated pericardial effusion if present, thickened pericardium, and paradoxical septal motion. Other potentially helpful studies include CT and MRI scans and chest fluoroscopy. **Cardiac catheterization** may be necessary to make the diagnosis; it typically shows equalization of left atrial, right atrial, and pulmonary artery wedge pressures. Other catheterization findings include decreased cardiac output and markedly reduced ventricular end-diastolic volumes.

3. **Management and disposition.** The definitive treatment for constrictive pericarditis is **pericardial resection.** In addition, any underlying cause of the condition, such as tuberculosis, should continue to be treated. Temporary stabilization of the condition may be achieved with diuretics, sodium restriction, and digitalis.

Bibliography

Braunwald E. Pericardial Disease. In Wilson JD, et al. (eds.). *Harrison's Principles of Internal Medicine* (12th ed.). New York: McGraw-Hill, 1991:981–987.

Cox GR. Pericardial and Myocardial Disease. In Rosen P, et al. (eds.). *Emergency Medicine, Concepts and Clinical Practice* (3rd ed.). St. Louis: Mosby, 1992:1391–1400.

Rostard SG, Rutsky EA. Pericarditis in end-stage renal disease. *Cardiol Clin* 8:701–706, 1990.

Shabetai R. Pericarditis. *Cardiol Clin* 8:639–644, 1990.

Pericardial Tamponade

Ralph Battels

I. **Etiology.** Pericardial effusion leading to pericardial tamponade can occur from a variety of sources. Because tamponade often follows a rapidly degenerating course, swiftly progressing to decompensation and death, it is incumbent upon the physician to rapidly assess, diagnose, and treat this condition. As reported by Shoemaker et al., the incidence of acute hemorrhagic pericardial tamponade in a patient presenting with penetrating thoracic or abdominal trauma is 2%. In addition, a large number of underlying diseases may cause pericardial irritation and effusion with or without progressing to tamponade (Table 22-1). The most common causes of pericardial effusion are viral and idiopathic. Other common causes include malignancy, uremia, trauma, and radiation exposure. Less common but equally important etiologies are autoimmune disorders and adverse drug reactions. Hemopericardium may result from a number of conditions other than trauma, including aortic aneurysm, ventricular rupture, anticoagulant therapy, pseudoaneurysm, and iatrogenic cardiac perforation.

II. **Pathophysiology.** Although knowledge of the underlying causes of pericardial tamponade is important, it is also essential that the physician possesses an understanding of the basic pathophysiology of acute and chronic tamponade. The cardinal feature of tamponade is the accumulation of fluid within the pericardium, which leads to an increase in the pressure within the intrapericardial space. The ability of the body to tolerate pericardial effusion without producing tamponade is a function of the amount of time over which the fluid accumulates rather than the total amount of fluid present. Given adequate time over which to compensate, the body may be able to tolerate pericardial effusions of more than one liter without producing tamponade. In a more acute setting, however, an effusion as small as a few hundred milliliters may result in hemodynamic collapse and death.

The pericardium is a relatively nonelastic structure. As pericardial fluid accumulates, increased intrapericardial pressure compromises the ability of the atria and ventricles to adequately expand during diastole. Atrial and ventricular filling become mechanically limited by the expanding collection of extracardiac fluid. Decreased diastolic volume results in decreased stroke volume (SV), resulting in decreased cardiac output (CO) and a subsequent fall in atrial blood pressure. As cardiac output continues to drop, an additional problem arises in that the cardiac pump is no longer able to adequately handle the amount of blood returned to it by the venous system. This causes a rise in central venous pressure (CVP), resulting in many of the classic physical signs of pericardial tamponade.

The body attempts to compensate for the developing tamponade in a number of ways. First, the body responds to the decreased stroke volume by increasing the heart rate (HR) in an attempt to preserve cardiac output ($CO = SV = \times HR$). In

Table 22-1. Causes of acute pericarditis and tamponade

Trauma
  Direct or indirect penetrating thoracic trauma
  Blunt thoracic trauma
  Cardiac perforation secondary to central venous catheters or
    other intercardiac instrumentation
  Pacemaker wire perforation (either at insertion or later)
  Pericardotomy/pericardial window
Systemic disease
  Uremia (from any underlying disorder)
  Connective tissue disorders
  Sarcoidosis
  Amyloidosis
Drugs
  Procainamide
  Quinidine
  Hydralazine
  Cromolyn sodium
  Anticoagulants
Infections
  Bacterial
  Viral
  Fungal
  Parasitic
Neoplasms
Radiation
Myocardial infarction
  Dressler syndrome
  Ventricular rupture
Dissecting aortic aneurysm

addition, the body attempts to increase preload by increasing
peripheral vascular resistance in an effort to achieve a more
advantageous position on the Starling curve and increase the
force of contraction. It is worth noting that both of these
strategies significantly increase myocardial oxygen demand.
In the face of underlying cardiac pathology such as coronary
artery disease or diastolic dysfunction, these compensatory
mechanisms may cause significant additional morbidity, including the development of congestive heart failure (CHF),
angina, and infarction. As the cardiac output continues to
drop, the body attempts to maintain blood pressure by vasomotor contraction. Although this does serve to preserve blood
pressure, it also increases central venous pressure and further compromises cardiac function.

In the normotensive patient, the earliest sign of pericardial
tamponade is a rise in central venous pressure to a level

greater than 15 ml of water. This represents a compensated state in which the patient may also be tachycardic. Blood pressure then decreases, although the body is still able to preserve an elevated central venous pressure. As the compensatory mechanisms continue to fail, central venous pressure and blood pressure may rapidly fall, indicating that a poor outcome is likely. The patient may become bradycardic or, in some cases, exhibit EMD, signaling imminent cardiorespiratory arrest. Because of this association, bradycardia in the setting of pericardial tamponade is an indication for rapid and aggressive intervention to prevent the patient's otherwise certain death.

III. **Clinical pericardial tamponade**
   A. **Presentation**
      1. **History.** In pericardial tamponade, as with many other clinical conditions in medicine, a good history will often point toward the correct diagnosis. Unfortunately, pericardial tamponade may present so rapidly that adequate historical investigation may be impossible. In the acute setting, a history of penetrating chest or abdominal trauma, central venous instrumentation, or recent myocardial infarction are all risk factors associated with a possible diagnosis of tamponade. In the chronic setting, however, the historical clues may be much more subtle despite acute decompensation. The presence of malignancy, recent viral illness, autoimmune disorder, renal disease, or history of exposure to high levels of radiation should alert the physician to consider pericardial effusion or tamponade in the differential diagnosis.

      The **differential diagnosis** of pericardial tamponade includes conditions that may also produce the signs of increased central venous pressure, tachycardia, and hypotension. Tension pneumothorax, because of its impingement on the great vessels of the mediastinum and because of the increased intrathoracic pressure, can produce a triad of signs similar to those of pericardial tamponade. Pulmonary edema, whether from fluid overload or from biventricular failure, can produce tachycardia, hypotension, and increased CVP. This especially needs to be considered in the face of aggressive fluid management, as in a trauma resuscitation. It is easy to see why the clinical diagnosis of pericardial tamponade is often difficult. Its progression is often rapid, the classic physical findings are often absent, and its diagnosis is easily confounded by the presence of underlying diseases.

      2. **Physical examination.** The classic findings of pericardial tamponade were first described by Beck in 1937. **Beck's triad** consists of (1) muffled or distant heart sounds due to decreased sound transmission through the fluid-filled pericardium, (2) distended neck veins due to the rising central venous pressure, and (3) hypotension due to decreased stroke volume with decreased force of myocardial contraction. This triad, however, is often unreliable. Beck's original pa-

per was based on clinical research in patients with chronic effusions and tamponade involving large amounts of pericardial fluid. In the setting of acute tamponade, fluid accumulations are likely to be much smaller than those in Beck's original studies, resulting in a change or even complete absence of the classic signs and symptoms he originally described. This is especially true in the acute care setting, where a noisy work environment and the presence of confounding factors such as hypovolemic hypotension or coexisting cardiovascular or pulmonary disease may mask the expected physical findings.

Another often-cited sign of pericardial tamponade is the presence of a **pulsus paradoxus.** Pulsus paradoxus is defined as a drop in the systolic blood pressure by more than 10 mm Hg during inspiration. The presence of pulsus paradoxus is assessed by careful auscultation of the systolic blood pressure while the patient is slowly breathing. The first value noted is that point where the heartbeat is intermittently audible during expiration only. The next value is that point where the heartbeat is audible throughout the respiratory cycle. If the difference between these two points is greater than 10 mm Hg, then a pulsus paradoxus is present. While helpful in making the diagnosis of pericardial tamponade, the presence of a pulsus paradoxus is by no means specific. Many other clinical conditions may also result in a pulsus paradoxus, including chronic obstructive pulmonary disease (COPD), pneumothorax, acute asthma, pulmonary edema, and respiratory decompensation from other sources. In addition to being nonspecific, pulsus paradoxus may be masked by hypovolemia and may only become apparent after fluid resuscitation has been administered.

B. **Assessment.** In the evaluation of the patient with suspected pericardial tamponade, many different diagnostic modalities can be employed. ECGs, chest x-rays, echocardiograms, central venous pressure monitoring, and chemical and microbiological evaluation of the pericardial fluid all have a role in the diagnosis and treatment of pericardial tamponade.

1. **Central venous pressure monitoring.** As previously mentioned, an increase in central venous pressure is often a sentinel sign of pericardial tamponade. A rise of central venous pressure to a value greater than 15 ml of water is diagnostic of central venous hypertension and indicative of possible tamponade. Therefore, monitoring of the central venous pressure with a Swan-Ganz catheter can provide uniquely valuable data, and its use should be seriously considered. This is especially true in the case of penetrating trauma, where the central venous pressure monitor can also act as a guide to measure the adequacy of fluid resuscitation.

2. **ECG.** The ECG change most classically associated with pericardial tamponade is electrical alternans.

Electrical alternans is described as a change in both amplitude and morphology of the P wave, QRS complex, ST segment, or T wave with every other cardiac beat. The cause of this interesting phenomenon has been theorized to be the actual to-and-fro motion of the heart within the fluid-filled pericardial sac with each beat. Consequently, variation in the amplitude and morphology of the ECG tracing occurs as the myocardium rocks toward and then away from the anterior chest wall, with every other beat interpreted differently by the electrodes. When the quantity of pericardial fluid within the pericardial space reaches some critical point, the heart begins to oscillate at one-half the frequency of the heartbeat, producing the characteristic alternating pattern. Although highly specific to pericardial tamponade, electrical alternans is not very sensitive; therefore, its absence does not rule out pericardial effusion or developing tamponade. In addition, electrical alternans is more commonly seen with chronic effusions due to larger pericardial fluid volumes. Hence, electrical alternans is even less sensitive in the acute setting.

3. **Chest x-ray.** The chest x-ray, although not specifically diagnostic, is useful in diagnosing the presence of a pericardial effusion and ruling out other similarly present entities such as tension pneumothorax. The classic radiographic description of pericardial tamponade is that of a "water bottle heart" where the cardiac silhouette is somewhat globular and hangs down within the mediastinum. As with the other classic signs of tamponade, the "water bottle heart" is more commonly seen with chronic effusions than in the acute setting. To produce this radiological sign, at least 200–300 ml of pericardial fluid must be present. The longer time course of chronic effusion often allows the body to adapt and accept the necessary quantity of pericardial fluid without decompensation. Other radiographic signs of pericardial effusion and possible tamponade are splaying of the subcardinal angle beyond its normal range of 45–75 degrees, a change in heart size or contour on serial examinations, and an anterior displacement of the subpericardial fat pad line from the anterior chest wall on the lateral view. Signs such as radiographically evident pneumocardium or the appearance of air fluid levels after pericardiocentesis are certainly diagnostic of a significant pericardial fluid collection. However, these findings are rare and not sensitive enough to be relied upon to reach a proper diagnosis of significant pericardial effusion or tamponade.

4. **Laboratory studies.** Chemical and microbiologic assessment are restricted to evaluation of pericardial fluid after it has been obtained. Therefore, the main utility of laboratory testing is to elucidate the underlying etiology of the effusion. In the acute setting the most common pericardial fluid obtained is blood. The

cause of the pericardial tamponade in these settings is often readily apparent (i.e., trauma). Blood obtained from the pericardium should be nonclotting, since prolonged exposure to the turbulence within the pericardium depletes the clotting factors. If the blood obtained clots, an extrapericardial source is implied.

In the case of chronic effusion leading to pericardial tamponade, laboratory examination is the key to guiding treatment of the underlying disease after the acute crisis has been managed. Pericardial fluid should be sent for bacterial and mycobacterial cultures and Gram stain in order to evaluate for possible infectious etiologies. Cytological examinations should be performed to assess the presence of malignant processes. Proper chemical analysis of the pericardial fluid for etiologies such as uremia, autoimmune diseases, exudative processes, or other clinical entities (see Table 22-1) will provide valuable information and guide treatment.

5. **Echocardiogram.** Echocardiography is the gold standard for the diagnosis of pericardial effusion causing tamponade. Correctly performed, transthoracic echocardiography can visualize pericardial fluid collections as small as 20 ml. In addition, fairly accurate estimates as to both the amount and distribution of the pericardial fluid may be obtained. Echocardiography can also be used to characterize the presence of masses or foreign bodies within the pericardial space. Ventricular wall rupture, ventricular aneurysm, and pseudoaneurysm can be diagnosed using echocardiography. In addition to being a diagnostic tool, echocardiography can also aid in treatment with such procedures as echocardiogram-guided pericardiocentesis. It is important to note that in many centers the logistics of obtaining an echocardiogram may add significant delay to the treatment of a critically ill patient. In an unstable or decompensating patient, it is not justifiable to withhold potentially lifesaving treatments in order to obtain better diagnostics.

C. **Management**
   1. **Supportive measures.** The management of a patient with pericardial tamponade is very similar to the standard trauma resuscitation as proposed by the American College of Surgeons. After the patient's **airway and breathing** have been assesssed and patency ensured, the patient's circulatory status must be evaluated and appropriate stabilization and treatment measures promptly instituted. Medical management of pericardial tamponade is primarily supportive. A minimum of two large-bore **intravenous access** catheters should be introduced on opposite sides of the body to provide rapid access for drug administration and **fluid resuscitation** as needed. Increasing the preload by maximizing venous pressure with isotonic fluid administration is imperative prior to consideration of pressor agents or inotropic support. **Inotropic**

agents may be required to support the patient's blood pressure as a temporizing measure while more definitive treatments are being instituted. Dobutamine is usually the first drug of choice because it does not cause significant afterload increase. If the patient is stable enough and time permits, a central venous catheter may be helpful to monitor central venous pressure and to provide additional intravenous access.

2. **Pericardial drainage procedures.** When pericardial tamponade is suspected or diagnosed, the cardiothoracic surgical team should be alerted because more invasive and definitive procedures may be required. Pericardiocentesis and pericardial windows are both potentially lifesaving procedures. However, these procedures are not benign and carry significant iatrogenic risks. For this reason, they should be performed by individuals who have received proper training. With either of these two procedures, or indeed if the patient is stable enough to warrant immediate pericardial decompression, disposition of the patient should be made in consultation with the cardiothoracic team or similar specialists who can provide the skills and equipment necessary to ensure that prompt definitive treatment can be delivered as it becomes necessary.

   a. **Pericardiocentesis.** Pericardiocentesis is most often attempted from a subxiphoid approach. A 14- to 18-gauge spinal needle is attached to a 20-ml or larger syringe by way of a three-way stopcock. The needle is inserted in the area between the left costoxiphoid angle and the xiphoid process at an angle of approximately 30 degrees at the chest wall. The needle is then pointed toward the tip of the left shoulder or directly cephalad (Fig. 22-1). Aspiration is performed while the needle is introduced and advanced in the manner described. When the tip of the needle enters the pericardial sac, pericardial fluid may be removed. Aspiration of even a small amount of fluid may provide dramatic clinical improvement, especially in acute tamponade. It may be helpful to pass a catheter through the needle for repeated aspiration should symptoms recur. Similarly, the needle or catheter can be placed to gravity-drain. The **complications** of this procedure include penetration of the heart itself, laceration of a coronary artery, pneumothorax, hemothorax, arrhythmias, pneumopericardium, and death.

   If **ultrasound** is readily available, it may be used to guide the pericardiocentesis. A small amount of normal saline is added to the aspiration syringe and shaken vigorously to introduce echogenic air bubbles. When the operator believes that the pericardium has been entered, a small amount of the saline is injected. If placement is correct, the echogenic saline will enter the pericardium and outline the heart, ensuring correct placement prior to aspiration.

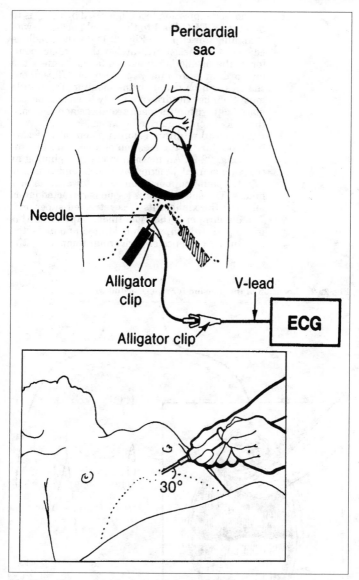

Fig. 22-1. Proper positioning of the pericardiocentesis needle.

Another aspiration technique used by many is to connect an **ECG lead** to the spinal needle by way of an alligator clip (see Fig. 22-1). As the needle is advanced, an assistant watches the cardiac monitor. If the needle is passed too far and enters the myocardium, an injury pattern of ST-segment changes will be noted on the monitor. The needle must then be withdrawn slightly to ensure proper placement within the pericardial sac and decrease the risk of ventricular penetration.

b. **Pericardial window.** Another potentially lifesaving procedure is the creation of a pericardial window (Fig. 22-2). An incision is made beginning at the xiphisternal junction and is extended in the sagittal plane no more than 6 cm toward the umbilicus. The subcutaneous tissue is retracted laterally and the xiphoid itself is retracted superiorly. The diaphragm is then identified. Superior to this is the pericardium, which is located and dissected out. In the presence of pericardial tamponade the

Fig. 22-2. Location of the incision for a pericardial window.

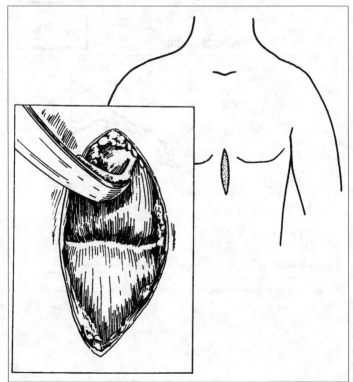

pericardium will be tense and bulging. A small incision is made in the pericardium and the contents evacuated. The patient should then be taken to the operating suite where a more definitive procedure may be performed.

Bibliography

Beck CS. Acute and chronic compression of the heart. *Am Heart J* 14:515, 1937.

Friedman HS, et al. The electrocardiographic features of acute cardiac tamponade. *Circulation* 50:260, 1974.

Reddy PS, Curtiss EI, O'Toole JD, Shaver JA. Cardiac tamponade: hemodynamic observation in man. *Circulation* 58:265, 1978.

Shabetai R. The pathophysiology of cardiac tamponade and constriction. *Cardiovasc Clin* 7:67, 1976.

Shoemaker WC, et al. Hemodynamic monitoring for physiologic evaluation diagnosis and therapy of acute hemopericardial tamponade from penetrating wounds. *J Trauma* 13:36, 1973.

Stein L, Shubin H, Well MH. Recognition and management of pericardial tamponade. *J Am Med Assoc* 225:503, 1973.

Acute Myocarditis

John M. Strayer

Myocarditis is an inflammatory process of the cardiac myocytes that may be focal or diffuse. It may manifest as a subclinical infection, cardiac failure, or cardiac dysrhythmias with ensuing sudden death (Fig. 23-1). Myocarditis may mimic many different disease processes; therefore, the clinician must have a high clinical suspicion to make the diagnosis.

I. **Incidence.** It is estimated that myocarditis is likely to occur in up to 15% of a given virus-infected population. It often occurs in epidemics, especially in pediatric populations. There is a male predominance of about 2:1. Most patients have subclinical disease and have a benign course, but as many as one-third of those who recover from myocarditis will have residual functional abnormalities ranging from nonspecific ECG changes to congestive heart failure. About 50% of those who present with heart failure will show improvement in cardiac function after the acute phase. In a 20-year review of sudden death of Air Force recruits, 20% had myocarditis upon autopsy, but no direct cause and effect relationship was proven. Neonatal Coxsackie myocarditis is frequently fatal with a mortality rate as high as 50%.

II. **Etiology** (Table 23-1). Causes of myocarditis include infection, toxic agents, and systemic disease. Infectious causes include viral, bacterial, rickettsial, and fungal infections. Echoviruses and enteroviruses are the most common causes of myocarditis in the United States and Europe, but in South America, Chaga's disease caused by *Trypanosoma cruzi* is most common.

In the United States, Coxsackie B virus has been implicated in approximately 50% of human cases based on serologic studies. Coxsackie A, echovirus, and adenovirus make up a smaller percentage. Coxsackie virus is also responsible for most cases of myocarditis in neonates and children who are less than 1 year of age. It becomes less common in older children, but then more common in adolescents and young adults. Many cases are labeled idiopathic since direct viral causation is difficult to prove.

III. **Clinical myocarditis**

A. **Presentation** (Table 23-2)

1. **History.** The diagnosis of myocarditis relies heavily on a thorough history and physical examination and a high clinical suspicion. About 60% of patients with active myocarditis will have typical systemic viral symptoms including malaise, myalgias, arthralgias, fatigue, or rash. The viral illness is usually gastroenteritis or upper respiratory tract infection. Other common symptoms include dyspnea, decreased exercise tolerance, and palpitations.

Cardiac manifestations usually occur 10 to 14 days following a viral infection, and may present as pericarditis, myocardial ischemia, or congestive heart fail-

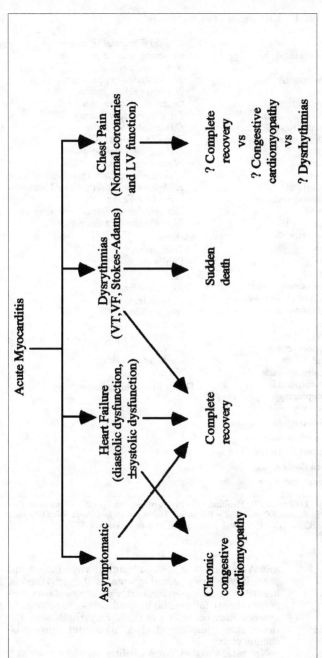

Fig. 23-1. Clinical presentation and outcome of acute myocarditis. (From Kereiakes DJ, Parmley WW. Myocarditis and cardiomyopathy. *Am Heart J* 108:1318. Reproduced with permission. *American Heart Journal.* Copyright American Heart Association.)

Table 23-1.   Etiologies of myocarditis

Viral
  Coxsackie (A, B)
  echovirus
  Influenza (A, B)
  Polio
  Herpes simplex
  Varicella-zoster
  Epstein-Barr
  Cytomegalovirus
  Mumps
  Rubella
  Rubeola
  Vaccinis
  Coronavirus
  Rabies
  Hepatitis B
  Arbovirus
  Junin
  HIV
Protozoal
  Trypanosoma cruzi
    (Chagas' disease)
  Toxplasma gondii
Fungal
  Aspergillosis
  Blastomycosis
  Candidiasis
  Cocidiomycosis
  Cryptococcosis
  Histoplasmosis
  Mucormycosis
Hypersensitivity
Systemic diseases
  Connective tissue disease
  Sarcoidosis
  Rheumatic fever

Bacterial, Rickettsial, Spirochetal
  Corynebactium diphtheriae
  Salmonella typhi
  β-hemolytic streptococci
  Neisseria meninguidis
  Legionella pneumophila
  Listeria monocytogenes
  Campylobacter jejuni
  Coxiella brunetti (Q fever)
  Chlamydia trachomatis
  Mycoplasma pneumoniae
  Chlamydia psittaci (psittacosis)
  Rickettsia rickettsii (Rocky Mountain
    Spotted Fever)
  Borrelia burgdoferi (Lyme disease)
  Mycobacterium tuberculosis
Metazoal
  Trichinosis
  Echinococcosis
Toxic
  Anthracyclines
  Catecholamines
  Interleukin-2
  α_2-interferon
  Lead
  Arsenic
  Carbon monoxide
  Venom
Drugs including cocaine

Source: O'Connell JB, Renlund DG. Myocarditis and Specific Myocardial Diseases. In Schant RC, Alexander RW (eds.), *The Heart, Arteries and Veins* (8th ed.). New York: McGraw-Hill, 1994. Reproduced with permission.

ure. A patient may have subclinical viral illness but present with unexplained symptoms of dysrhythmias, heart block, Stokes-Adams attacks, or new onset congestive heart failure. Light-headedness, dizziness, or syncope may occur due to cardiac dysrhythmias. Patients may complain of chest pain that mimics ischemic pain.

Neonatal Coxsackie myocarditis usually occurs at 5 to 10 days of age and presents with upper respiratory tract symptoms, fever, lethargy, poor feeding, and

Table 23-2. Clinical manifestations of acute myocarditis

Symptoms	Signs
Fatigue	Sinus tachycardia
Fever	Pericardial or pleuropericardial rubs
Orthopnea	Cardiac dysrhythmias
Paroxysmal nocturnal dyspnea	Conduction disturbances
Cough	Heart failure
Dyspnea	Apical murmur
Palpitations	Tachypnea
Precordial pain	Jugular venous distention
Dizziness	Peripheral edema
Syncope	Inspiratory rales
History or evidence of viral infection	

Source: Adapted from Reyes MP, Lerner AM. Coxsackie myocarditis. *Prog Cardiovasc Dis* 27:388, 1985 and Houghton JL. Pericarditis and myocarditis. Which is benign and which isn't? *Postgrad Med* 91, 1992.

tachycardia. This is followed by the acute onset of tachypnea, cyanosis, and circulatory collapse. Neonatal Coxsackie myocarditis should be considered in any baby with viral-like illness who suddenly develops signs of poor perfusion or heart failure. In older children the illness is less dramatic. About 50% of children with myocarditis complain of chest pain that is usually pleuritic and precordial in location. Fever and shortness of breath are common accompanying symptoms.

2. **Physical examination.** Sinus tachycardia out of proportion to temperature elevation should make the clinician suspect myocarditis. Physical examination may reveal tachycardia, faint heart sounds, cardiomegaly, hypotension, narrow pulse pressures, gallop rhythm, and tricuspid or mitral regurgitation murmurs. Jugular venous distention, pulmonary rales, hepatosplenomegaly and peripheral edema may be observed in severe cases that present as acute congestive heart failure. Pericardial or pleuropericardial rubs may be appreciated when there is concomitant pericarditis.

Symptoms of congestive heart failure of myocarditis are usually due to left ventricular dysfunction but may be due to right or biventricular dysfunction as well. Pulmonic and systemic embolization due to ventricular or atrial dysfunction is a potential complication that should be anticipated.

B. **Assessment** (Table 23-3)

1. **Laboratory.** There is no specific laboratory test for identifying myocarditis, but there are many lab and ancillary tests that may support the diagnosis. Mild to moderate leukocytosis, elevated erythrocyte sedimentation rate, and C-reactive protein can be found in the laboratory evaluation. Other lab evaluations should

Table 23-3.   Diagnostic testing for acute myocarditis

Myocardial enzymes	Elevated CK-MB, SGOT, LDH
Chest radiograph	Enlarged cardiac silhouette
ECG	Low-voltage QRS
Echocardiography	ST segment elevation or depression
Technetium pyrophosphate myocardial scintigraphy	T wave flattening or inversion
	Conduction disturbances
	Dysrhythmias
	Contractility dysfunction of the myocardium
	Generalized myocardial uptake (nonspecific)

Source: Reyes MP, Lerner AM. Coxsackie myocarditis. *Prog Cardiovasc Dis* 27;389, 1985.

include blood cultures, Mycoplasma cultures, arteriosclerosis obliterans (ASO) titers, hepatitis panel, monospot, and CMV serology to identify possible etiologic agents. Cardiac enzymes may be elevated depending on the amount of myocardial necrosis and transaminases and lactate dehydrogenase (LDH) may also be elevated.

2. **Chest x-ray (CXR).** Enlarged cardiac silhouette due to ventricular dilatation or accompanying pericardial effusion, as well as engorged pulmonary veins, interstitial pulmonary edema, and pleural effusion consistent with congestive heart failure, may be seen on chest x-ray. In younger patients, myocarditis is often misdiagnosed as acute pneumonia with bilateral infiltrates.

3. **ECG.** The ECG may reveal a wide variety of abnormalities, but most ECG changes are nonspecific. Cardiac dysrhythmias include premature atrial contractions (PACs), premature ventricular contractions (PVCs), supraventricular tachycardia (SVT), atrial fibrillation, and atrial flutter. Myocarditis involving the conduction system can lead to conduction disturbances such as first- or second-degree atrioventricular (AV) block, right or left bundle-branch block, and rarely, complete heart block. Rare cases of complete block may present with syncope or sudden death. ST-T segment changes may be global or localized depending on the extent of myocardial involvement. In rare cases, the ECG changes may mimic acute myocardial infarction (AMI).

   Scarring after recovery from acute myocarditis may result in Q waves similar to those seen with myocardial infarction (MI).

4. **Echocardiogram.** Echocardiograms may be used to rule out pericardial effusion only to reveal myocardial dysfunction, enlarged ventricular dimensions, and lo-

cal or global dyskinetic wall motion. Pericardial effusion and mural thrombi may be identified.

5. **Nuclear medicine studies.** Gallium-67 scans are sensitive but not specific for myocardial inflammation and leukocyte infiltration. False positives can result from MI and unstable angina.

The indium-111 antimyosin antibody scan has proven to be more specific for myocyte necrosis than the gallium-67 scan. It can identify myocarditis, but it cannot identify the etiology.

6. **Myocardial biopsy.** Myocardial biopsy has been advocated as a means for making antemortem diagnosis and guiding immunosuppressive therapy. Recently published Dallas Criteria define active myocarditis as inflammatory infiltrate of the myocardium with necrosis and degeneration of adjacent myocytes not typical of the ischemic damage associated with coronary artery disease. This has helped standardize the pathologic diagnosis of myocarditis. However, biopsy is still limited by sampling error, inadequate samples, and timing of samples during the course of illness. In some studies, myocardial biopsy confirmed the suspected diagnosis in less than 10% of the patients.

C. **Management**

1. **Supportive care.** Acute myocarditis can present in many different ways, therefore management is directed at the presenting signs and symptoms. The mainstay of therapy is supportive. Strict bed rest is recommended because exercise may exacerbate disease. Oxygen, nutrition, fever control, and correction of anemia will improve oxygen carrying capacity. Congestive heart failure should be treated with standard therapeutic measures that include salt and fluid restriction, diuretics, and angiotensin converting enzyme (ACE) inhibitors (see Chap. 14). Digoxin may be used if there is no evidence of impending heart block. Complicating dysrhythmias should be treated with appropriate antidysrhythmic agents. Central hemodynamic monitoring, inotropic support and pacemaker insertion may be needed in more severe cases. Heparinization should be considered to reduce the risk of thromboembolization in patients with dilated cardiac chambers.

2. **Immunosuppressive therapy.** Nonsteroidal anti-inflammatory drugs should be avoided during the first two weeks of illness because of a reported increase in myocardial cell necrosis and increased viral replication during the acute phase. Immunosuppressive therapy is controversial since improvement is seen with steroid therapy in patients with idiopathic or autoimmune myocarditis, but steroids may cause worsening of the disease in patients with viral myocarditis.

3. **Admission.** Admission to the intensive care setting should be guided by the patient's symptoms. Patients with severe heart failure, syncope, heart block, or

other dysrhythmias should be admitted to an ICU environment. If the diagnosis of MI has not been ruled out, ICU admission is indicated. In relatively asymptomatic or mildly symptomatic patients, step-down unit admission is warranted to observe for dysrhythmia development.

Bibliography

Cox GR. Pericardial and Myocardial Disease. In Rosen et al. (eds.), *Emergency Medicine: Concepts and Clinical Practice*. St. Louis: Mosby–Year Book, 1992:1403–1409.

Houghton JL. Pericarditis and myocarditis: which is benign and which isn't? *Postgrad Med*. 91:273–278, 1992.

O'Connell JB, Renland DG. Myocarditis and Specific Myocardial Diseases. In Schlant RC, Alexander RW (eds.), *The Heart, Arteries and Veins*. New York: McGraw-Hill, 1994:1591–1603.

Olinde KD, O'Connell JB. Inflammatory heart disease: pathogenesis, clinical manifestations, and treatment of myocarditis. *Annu Rev Med*. 45:481–490, 1994.

Wayne J, Braunwald E. The Cardiomyopathies and Myocarditides: Toxic, Chemical, and Physical Damage to the Heart. In Braunwald E (ed.), *Heart Disease: A Textbook of Cardiovascular Medicine*. Philadelphia: Saunders, 1992:1440–1469.

The Cardiomyopathies

Misty E. Arnold

There are two basic types of cardiomyopathies: dilated and hypertrophic. Dilated cardiomyopathy (DCM) is characterized by thinning of the myocardial wall and dilatation of all four cardiac chambers with gradual progression to cardiac failure. Hypertrophic cardiomyopathy (HCM) is characterized by cardiac enlargement secondary to hypertrophy of the ventricular walls and septum without dilatation of the chambers.

I. **Dilated cardiomyopathy.** Etiologies of DCM are numerous, but more common etiologies include alcohol toxicity, peripartum, ischemic, idiopathic, and myocarditis (Table 24-1).

Alcoholism has been associated with DCM for some time. It is believed that the alcohol or one of its metabolites is directly toxic to the myocardium. Thiamine deficiency may be a contributing factor. Remission or stabilization of this disease process may occur with total abstinence.

Peripartum cardiomyopathy occurs between one week and six months after delivery, but a few women develop symptoms during the last month of pregnancy. The exact cause is unknown, and symptoms usually are heralded by acute onset of pulmonary edema and left ventricular (LV) dysfunction. Black women with multiple parity, inadequate nutrition, and hypertension are at increased risk of developing peripartum DCM.

Idiopathic cardiomyopathy has no known cause but is inherited in some cases. Characteristics include dilatation of all four chambers with an association of increased thrombus formation. A decreased ejection fraction (EF) is secondary to hypokinesis of the LV. The mean age for onset of symptoms is between 20 and 50 years. Left ventricular failure gradually progresses to right heart failure. Blacks have a higher mortality rate than whites from idiopathic DCM. Other risk factors include smoking, uncontrolled hypertension, and diabetes.

Postmyocarditis cardiomyopathy is caused by a number of infectious agents of which coxsackieviruses are the most common. The major histologic features include myofibrillar necrosis and myocardial inflammation. Initially postmyocardial necroses (PMNs) infiltrate the myocardium, and then leukocytes predominate. Signs and symptoms of acute myocarditis include pleuritic chest pain and a pericardial friction rub. Diagnosis is made with an endomyocardial biopsy. Treatment usually includes immunosuppressive drug therapy.

Ischemic cardiomyopathy is caused by underlying coronary artery disease and previous myocardial infarctions (MIs). The resulting scar tissues become hypokinetic and remodeled, causing ventricular dilatation. This dilatation can lead to mitral regurgitation, which further lowers the ejection fraction. These patients have a higher risk of future myocardial infarction and congestive heart failure (CHF).

Table 24-1.   Etiologies of dilated cardiomyopathy

Ischemic
Peripartum
Toxic
  Alcohol
  Cobalt
  Catecholamines
  Carbon monoxide
  Lithium
  Hydrocarbon poisoning
  Arsenic
  Cyclophosphamide
  Doxorubicin
  Daunorubicin
Metabolic
  Hyper- or hypothyroidism
  Hyper- or hypokalemia
  Thiamine deficiency
  Hemochromatosis
  Hunter-Hurler syndrome
  Glycogen storage diseases
Neuromuscular diseases
  Friedreich's ataxia
  Muscular dystrophy
Infiltrative
  Leukemia
  Chagas' disease
  Carcinomatosis
  Sarcoidosis
Immunologic
  Post-transplant
  Viral myocarditis
Idiopathic
  Hereditary

A. **Presentation.** Patients with DCM usually present to the
   emergency department in varying degrees of CHF with
   complaints of dyspnea and/or chest pain. These patients
   may have a history of coronary artery disease, myocardial
   infarction, or no cardiac problems.
   1. **Symptoms.** In cases of ischemic DCM, patients may
      present with the classic historic findings of acute myo-
      cardial ischemia (see Chap. 9). Chest pain or tightness
      radiating to the jaw or arm, shortness of breath,
      and/or diaphoresis are common in this setting.
      Other causes of DCM rarely present with chest pain

as much as they present with symptoms of LV failure. In these patients, shortness of breath, dyspnea on exertion, orthopnea, or paroxysmal nocturnal dyspnea are common. In patients with further progression to right-sided heart failure, swelling in the feet or extremities and weight gain are common.

2. **Physical findings.** Depending on the severity of the cardiac failure, the patient may be experiencing anything from mild shortness of breath to florid respiratory failure. The respiratory rate often is elevated, while temperature is normal. Most patients are somewhat tachycardic, although this effect is variable depending on the severity of the failure and the medications that the patient may be taking. Blood pressure is often normal or slightly high in patients with early DCM, whereas in patients with end-stage disease, the blood pressure is often low, with systolics in the 80–90 mm Hg range despite left ventricular failure and pulmonary edema. Physical findings for patients with left heart failure include pulmonary basilar rales with an S4 or S3 gallop. A mitral regurgitant murmur often is present, as well as tricuspid regurgitation if there is right heart dilatation and failure. If right heart failure is present, there is often jugular venous distention, pedal edema, a right ventricular heave, or a widely slit S2.

B. **Assessment**
1. **Laboratory assessment.** Arterial blood gases should be obtained early to evaluate the patient's respiratory status, to determine the need for oxygen or mechanical ventilation, and to define the patient's acid-base status. Electrolytes should be evaluated since many of these patients are hypokalemic from diuretic use. Hypokalemia and hypomagnesemia can be associated with an increased risk of ventricular dysrhythmias. Renal function studies often show a high BUN consistent with prerenal failure from poor kidney perfusion. In patients with severe right-sided heart failure, the results of liver function tests may be elevated due to passive congestion of the liver. Elevated CPKs with elevated MB fractions indicate myocardial infarction in patients with ischemic DCM.

2. **Chest x-ray (CXR).** The chest x-rays show cardiomegaly with LV enlargement with or without RV enlargement. Left atrial enlargement may be detectable. Lung fields show redistribution of the vasculature and interstitial or alveolar edema, Kerley B lines, blunting of the costophrenic angles, and fluid in the fissures.

3. **ECG.** ECG findings are variable and often nonspecific. Acute ST elevation in contiguous leads is associated with myocardial infarction in patients with ischemic DCM. Abnormal Q waves also may be present secondary to a previous myocardial infarction. Bundle-branch blocks, especially left bundle-branch block (LBBB), are common in all types of DCM. Some ECGs may show left ventricular hypertrophy. Various

arrhythmias are possible, with atrial fibrillation being the most common.

4. **Swan-Ganz catheter.** The CVP often is elevated in patients with right-sided heart failure, but this is not a good measurement of left-sided failure. Swan-Ganz catheters are more sensitive for left-sided heart failure, demonstrating an increase in the pulmonary artery wedge pressure that is associated with CHF. Cardiac output usually is depressed.

5. **Echocardiography.** Echocardiography is useful for the diagnosis of DCM. All chambers are grossly dilated in DCM, with hypokinetic systolic wall function and a decrease in the ejection fraction. Ventricular wall thickness is usually normal. Patients with DCM are at risk for developing thrombi in the atria or ventricles, which may be seen on surface echocardiogram but are more easily identified on transesophageal echocardiography. The echocardiogram may show mitral regurgitation, which is secondary to the dilation of the mitral annulus. Tricuspid regurgitation also may be seen.

6. **Cardiac catheterization.** Cardiac catheterization with ventriculography demonstrates a depressed ejection fraction and diffuse hypokinesis with DCM. The underlying coronary artery disease of ischemic DCM, as well as mitral regurgitation, is detected by catheterization. Most of the nonischemic causes of DCM have normal coronary arteries by cardiac catheter.

C. **Management**

1. **Congestive heart failure (CHF).** Therapy for DCM consists of positive inotropic agents, diuretics, vasodilators, and ACE inhibitors. Therapy is not significantly different than that for CHF due to other causes (see Chap. 14), with a few notable exceptions.

   Digoxin 0.125–0.25 mg daily is the most commonly used chronic positive inotropic agent in DCM, but its use in the treatment of acute pulmonary edema is limited. Treatment of patients with acute pulmonary edema from CHF secondary to DCM includes decreasing preload with diuretics and nitrates and decreasing afterload by controlling systemic hypertension with nitrates, ACE inhibitors, hydralazine, or nipride (see Chap. 14). Care must be taken not to depress the arterial blood pressure too much with these agents, because many end-stage DCM patients already have tenuous systolic blood pressures.

   In patients with CHF and low systolic blood pressure, IV dobutamine 0.5–5.0 mg/kg/min often is added for inotropic support, but only with caution, because dobutamine can exacerbate ventricular arrhythmias and increase ischemia. The effects of dobutamine can last for weeks, even after discontinuing treatment, allowing for the intermittent use of "dobutamine tune-ups" for patients with end-stage DCM.

2. **Arrhythmias.** Atrial fibrillation is common in patients with DCM and may precipitate CHF. Ventricular rate is best controlled with digoxin (see Chap. 16).

Calcium channel blockers should be avoided if possible, because they can exacerbate the heart failure; beta-blockers also are used with caution. Ventricular arrhythmias are treated with quinidine or procainamide (see Chap. 17). Disopyramide should be avoided because it also may precipitate failure by its negative inotropic effects. The need for systemic anticoagulation with warfarin may be necessary if chronic atrial fibrillation is present, or if the ejection fraction is extremely low.

D. Disposition

1. **Admission.** Admission is advocated in patients with worsening CHF. The need for IV dobutamine infusions, intubation for mechanical ventilation, IV nitrate infusions, or continuous treatment for dysrhythmias warrant admission to the CCU or ICU. Patients with known coronary artery disease and those presenting with chest pain require admission to "rule out" myocardial infarction with serial CPKs and ECGs. If these patients are hemodynamically stable and if the likelihood of myocardial infarction is low, they may be admitted to telemetry. If unstable, or if the patient is at high risk for infarction, then admission to the CCU is advocated.

   It is possible to aggressively treat patients with mild CHF in the emergency department and subsequently discharge them to home. Discharge should be done only after they have responded to emergency department treatment. They must be hemodynamically and cardiac-rhythm stable, be capable of oxygenating adequately on room air, and be compliant with outpatient treatment regimens. In addition, the etiology of their DCM must have been previously documented such that they are not at risk for myocardial infarction.

2. **Transplantation.** Transplantation is the therapy of choice in patients with end-stage heart failure from DCM. It should be considered for patients in New York Heart Association (NYHA) class IV or severe class III who are refractory to other surgical or medical interventions. Patients considered for transplantation are those with a life expectancy of less than one year who have normal or reversible renal or hepatic dysfunction. Patients also must be free of infection or systemic diseases like sarcoidosis or systemic lupus erythematosus (SLE). Recent malignancy and HIV infections are absolute contraindications to transplantation, as are pulmonary hypertension, current alcoholism, or drug addiction. Relative contraindications include recent history of pulmonary embolism, pulmonary infarction, and insulin-requiring diabetes. Patients eligible for transplant also must demonstrate psychosocial stability.

II. Hypertrophic cardiomyopathy (HCM). The second type of cardiomyopathy is called hypertrophic cardiomyopathy. Other designations include asymmetrical septal hypertrophy, idiopathic hypertrophic subaortic stenosis, and hypertrophic obstructive cardiomyopathy. HCM is a familial disease characterized by cardiac enlargement secondary to hypertrophy of the ventricular walls and septum without dilatation of the chambers. Outflow tract obstruction may or may not be present. Characteristic histology includes a disarray of the myofibrils in the myocardium. Obstruction is caused by the anterior leaflet of the mitral valve obstructing the outflow tract of the left ventricle during systole, causing a high pressure gradient across the outflow tract and increased end-diastolic pressure in the left ventricle. Increasing cardiac contractility increases the degree of obstruction and decreases cardiac output. Inotropes and exercise increase both the myocardial contractility and the obstruction, thereby increasing the pressure gradient and the intensity of the murmur associated with HCM. Drugs and maneuvers that decrease the murmur include beta-blockers and squatting. Squatting increases LV filling, whereas beta-blockers decrease myocardial contractility.

The pathophysiology of HCM is diastolic dysfunction, as opposed to the systolic dysfunction of DCM. In HCM, the left ventricle is stiff and noncompliant, hindering LV filling. Increased LV filling pressures lead to lower cardiac output and poor coronary perfusion pressure with subsequent myocardial ischemia.

The etiology of HCM is unknown, but there is a definite autosomal dominance inheritance pattern in some families. Patients with HCM are at high risk for sudden death, with an annual mortality rate of 2%–3%. The usual causes of sudden death are lethal ventricular arrhythmia and a decrease in cardiac output.

A. Presentation

1. Symptoms. Symptoms of HCM include dyspnea, fatigue, angina, palpitations, syncope, and sudden death. Sudden death may or may not be related to exertion, and it is not always related to the degree of outflow obstruction. Angina can occur at rest or with exertion and may not be relieved with nitrates; nitrates often will increase the obstruction. Syncope in HCM has three causes: (1) secondary to ventricular tachycardia or fibrillation; (2) secondary to an increase in the outflow tract obstruction, causing a decrease in the cardiac output and blood pressure; or (3) secondary to decreased diastolic filling, resulting in a decrease in the cardiac output and systemic blood pressure.

Patients with severe outflow tract obstruction or poor ventricular filling also may present with shortness of breath, orthopnea, and paroxysmal nocturnal dyspnea due to left heart failure.

2. Physical examination. Vital signs are variable, with blood pressure ranging from hypertensive to hypotensive, depending on the degree of outflow tract obstruction and LV failure. Hypotension is a sign of severe LV dysfunction, especially in patients with signs of elevated LV filling pressures. Lungs are often clear, unless LV failure is present. Cardiac findings include a hyperdynamic apical pulse and carotid upstroke. An S3 may be heard with LV failure, and an S4 is very common due to the stiff, noncompliant ventricles. Paradoxical splitting of S2 is associated with a fixed and severe obstruction. There are two types of murmurs associated with HCM: (1) an LV outflow obstruction murmur with ejection that is a crescendo/decrescendo in quality heard at the left sternal border between the third and fourth intercostal spaces, and (2) a mitral regurgitation murmur, which is a soft, blowing holosystolic murmur best heart at the apex. Valsalva maneuvers increase the intensity of the systolic murmurs, whereas squatting decreases the intensity.

B. **Assessment**
1. **Laboratory.** The initial assessment of the patient with HCM should include arterial blood gases or pulse oximetry to document the degree of hypoxemia, especially with symptoms or signs of LV failure. Electrolytes, renal function, and CBC are rarely helpful in HCM except in ruling out comorbid states. Electrolyte disorders can precipitate cardiac dysrhythmias. Patients presenting with chest pain or dysrhythmias may have elevated CPKs, with elevated MB fractions due to myocardial infarction.
2. **ECG.** The most common ECG finding in HCM is LV hypertrophy with or without strain (Fig. 24-1). Large negative T waves also may be seen across the precordium. Abnormal Q waves in the inferior or lateral leads may be associated with "pseudoinfarction." The etiology is unknown, but usually it is not secondary to previous infarction but instead is related to the hypertrophied septum. If the left atrium is enlarged, wide P waves in lead II are seen. Approximately 5% of the patients will have an LBBB or RBBB. Atrial fibrillation is also common in patients with HCM.
3. **Chest x-ray.** The heart size on chest x-ray may be mildly enlarged or normal. Usually left ventricular enlargement is seen. Signs of pulmonary edema or pulmonary congestion are seen on CXR in patients in CHF.
4. **Echocardiography.** Echocardiography is the gold standard for diagnosis of HCM because it best demonstrates the presence of left ventricular hypertrophy. The interventricular septum is often massive. The ejection fraction is usually normal or may be increased, while the stroke volume is relatively small. An echocardiogram also can demonstrate the outflow obstruction caused by the mitral valve leaflets contacting the septum during systole. Doppler studies also provide estimates of the outflow tract pressure gradients. Exact pressure gradients must be measured during a cardiac catheterization. Mitral regurgitation also can be diagnosed by echo studies.
5. **Cardiac catheterization.** As stated previously, echocardiography is the gold standard, and cardiac catheterization is reserved for three groups of patients with HCM:

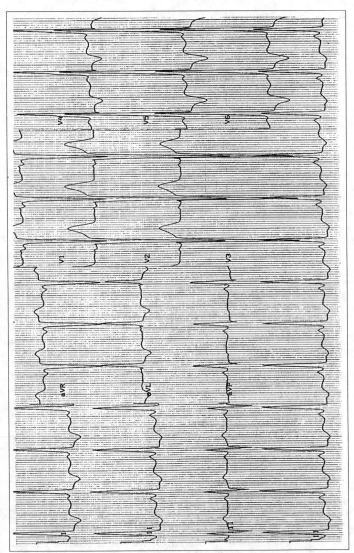

Fig. 24-1. ECG tracing illustrating the changes seen with LVH due to HCM.

  a. patients with suspected coexisting cardiac disorder such as coronary artery disease,
  b. failure of medical management with subsequent evaluation of possible surgical candidacy, and
  c. patients for whom diagnosis is not certain.

  Catheterization usually shows elevated left ventricular end-diastolic pressures and increased left atrial pressures. Ventriculography may be useful in screening for the outflow causes by the mitral valve leaflets. Ventriculography also can assess the magnitude of mitral regurgitation and determine the pressure gradient of the outflow tract.

C. Management. The acute management of patients with HCM includes treatment of angina, hypotension, syncope, and pulmonary edema. Patients with any of these conditions should be monitored continuously for cardiac dysrhythmias. Oxygenation and IV access should be established early.

  Patients with HCM and pulmonary edema cannot be treated with diuretics, afterload reducers, and preload reducers with the same aggressiveness as with typical CHF patients (see Chap. 14). Care must be taken to very slowly reduce pulmonary capillary wedge pressure (PCWP) with diuretics or nitrates. Rapid reduction in preload can exacerbate the outflow obstruction and precipitate ischemia, hypotension, or cardiovascular collapse. If nitrates are to be used, they should be carefully titrated intravenously to avoid hypotension.

  In hypotensive patients, small fluid boluses can be used to maximize LV filling pressures. Care should be taken to avoid precipitating pulmonary edema. If pressors are needed to control hypotension, a pure alpha-agonist such as phenylephrine or methoxamine should be used. Dopamine and dobutamine cause increased contractility and obstruction and can worsen the outflow obstruction and hypotension.

  Patients with angina can be treated with aspirin, nitrates, and beta-blockers. Again, care must be taken not to reduce preload too much with nitrates, since lowering preload may increase ischemia, or precipitate syncope or cardiovascular collapse.

  Atrial fibrillation is poorly tolerated in patients with HCM because of the lack of atrial contraction. However, digoxin is contraindicated due to its positive inotropic properties, which increase obstruction and may increase symptoms. Patients in atrial fibrillation may need cardioversion or quinidine for conversion to normal sinus rhythm. Beta-blockers can be used to control the heart rate.

D. Disposition
  1. Admission. Any patient with HCM who presents to the emergency department with syncope or presyncope should be admitted to a monitored bed for evaluation of potentially lethal arrhythmias. Patients who present with angina should be admitted to a monitored bed to "rule out" MI and carefully manage their

ischemia. Patients who present in pulmonary edema should be admitted to the CCU for careful titration of diuretics and nitrates, watching for the development of hypotension. If a patient presents in new-onset atrial fibrillation, immediate cardioversion is often necessary to prevent CHF, followed by admission to a monitored bed to watch for recurrence and initiate antiarrhythmic therapy.

2. **Medical and surgical management.** Chronic treatment of HCM involves decreasing the outflow obstruction and diastolic dysfunction with negative inotropic agents, which increase the ventricular compliance. Beta-blockers inhibit the sympathetic stimulation and decrease contractility, heart rate, and wall stress. Calcium channel blockers like verapamil and diltiazen also are used. Verapamil is used most commonly and has the greatest effect on the outflow pressure gradients and obstruction secondary to its negative inotropic effects. Heart block and hypotension are contraindications to verapamil. Disopyramide (an Ic antiarrhythmic) may be used as well, since it has negative inotropic properties. It is also useful in the treatment of ventricular arrhythmias.

Sudden death is unrelated to the degree of obstruction. Twenty-four-hour Holter monitors are useful in detecting asymptomatic dysrhythmias that are potentially fatal. Amiodarone and other antiarrhythmics like sotolol, disopyramide, and procainamide also may be used. An automatic implantable cardioverter-defibrillator (AICD) may be necessary in patients with a history of ventricular arrhythmias refractory to medical therapy.

Surgical intervention includes myomotomy and myomectomy of the hypertrophied septum. Surgery is reserved for symptomatic patients with significant outflow obstruction. Mitral valve replacement may be done at the same time, depending on the degree of mitral regurgitation.

Bibliography

Acquantella H, Rodriguez-Salas LA. Doppler echocardiography in restrictive cardiomyopathies. *Cardiol Clin* 8:349, 1990.

DeRosa JJ, Banas JS Jr, Winters SL. Current perspectives on sudden cardiac death in hypertrophic cardiomyopathy. *Prog Cardiovasc Dis* 6:475, 1994.

Johnson RA, Fifer MA, Palacios IF. Dilatated and restrictive cardiomyopathies. *The Practice of Cardiology*. Boston: Little, Brown, 1989.

O'Gara PT, DeSanctis RW, Powell WJ Jr. Hypertrophic Cardiomyopathy. *The Practice of Cardiol.* Boston: Little, Brown, 1989.

Sasson Z, et al. Echocardiographic and Doppler studies in hypertrophic cardiomyopathy. *Cardiol Clin* 8:217, 1989.

Infectious Endocarditis

Christina E. Hantsch and Daniel J. DeBehnke

I. **Definitions.** Infectious endocarditis is the result of infection of the heart valves and/or endocardium. It is usually characterized by positive blood cultures and any new or changing heart murmur. Previously, endocarditis was subdivided into acute and subacute classifications. This chapter uses terminology that is based primarily on the cardiac valve involved and not on the timing and duration of the infectious process.

When the infectious process involves a previously normal valve, it is termed **native valve endocarditis (NVE).** **Right-sided endocarditis (RSE)** is a subgroup of NVE and commonly affects IV drug abusers. When artificial valves are involved, the process is termed **prosthetic valve endocarditis (PVE).** Clinical signs and symptoms of infectious endocarditis with persistently negative blood cultures are termed **culture-negative endocarditis (CNE).**

II. **Epidemiology.** Infectious endocarditis has become a very different disease than it was in the preantibiotic era. Changes in the susceptible population and the introduction of effective chemotherapeutic agents now can treat the infection early in its course. Rheumatic heart disease previously was the most common predisposing cause for infectious endocarditis, but its prevalence has been steadily decreasing. Children with congenital heart disease are now surviving heart surgery and are becoming a population at risk. The elderly are also increasingly at risk because of acquired valvular disease and surgical valve replacement. In the preantibiotic era, streptococci were by far the most common infecting organisms. Now, the proportion of cases caused by gram-negative organisms, fungi, and other unusual organisms has increased. The classification of infectious endocarditis by valve type and common infecting organisms is detailed in Table 25-1.

III. **Pathophysiology.** Several events are prerequisites for the development of infectious endocarditis. The first is some degree of turbulent blood flow from a high to a low pressure zone in the heart. This usually occurs because of abnormal flow from a valvular orifice or a septal defect. This flow then damages the endocardial surface and initiates a series of events that results in the development of a sterile platelet-fibrin thrombus. Bacteremia is then needed to seed the platelet-fibrin thrombus, and subsequent bacterial growth on the thrombus occurs. Bacteremia can be caused by many different events, including sepsis, IV drug abuse, or instrumentation of the oral cavity, gastrointestinal, or genitourinary systems. There may also be some degree of immunologic compromise in susceptible individuals that allows the infectious process to continue.

IV. **Specific endocarditis subgroups**

    A. **Native valve endocarditis (NVE).** Since rheumatic heart disease has decreased in prevalence, NVE has become a disorder of individuals with congenital or acquired cardiac abnormalities (Table 25-2). The most common infecting organism in NVE is *Streptococcus,* with *S. viridans*

Table 25-1.   Infectious endocarditis classification by valve involved and common infecting organisms

Native valve endocarditis (NVE)
   Streptococcus viridans
   S. bovis
   S. fecalis
   Staphylococci
   Gram-negative organisms
   Fungi
Right-sided endocarditis (RSE)
   Staphylococci
   Streptococci
   Pseudomonas
   Gram-negative organisms
   Fungi
   Diphtheroids
Prosthetic valve endocarditis (PVE) (early and late)
   Staphylococci
   Streptococci
   Gram-negative organisms
   Fungi
   Diphtheroids
Culture-negative endocarditis
   "HACEK" group
      Hemophilus
      Actinobacillus
      Cardiobacterium
      Eikenella
      Kingella
   Fungi
   Rickettsiae
   Acid-fast bacilli

and *S. bovis* most frequently isolated. Staphylococci are the next most commonly found organisms. Other organisms that can cause NVE are summarized in Table 25-1. NVE most commonly involves the left side of the heart, and the mitral valve is more commonly involved than the aortic valve.

B. **Right-sided endocarditis (RSE).** RSE is most commonly seen in IV drug abusers. Other patients at risk include patients with central venous catheters or transvenous pacing wires. In IV drug abusers the infecting organisms usually arise from the skin or from an infection at an injection site (abscess, cellulitis, or phlebitis). Injection of contaminated material is less often a cause for RSE. The most common organism in RSE is *Staphylococ-*

**Table 25-2. Cardiac lesions at
risk for infectious endocarditis**

Aortic valve disease
Mitral insufficiency
Mitral stenosis
Mitral valve prolapse
Patent ductus arteriosus
Ventriculoseptal defect
Coarctation of the aorta
Marfan's syndrome
Pulmonary valve disease
Tricuspid valve disease
Idiopathic hypertrophic subaortic stenosis
Calcific aortic stenosis

cus aureus; Pseudomonas and fungi are also seen (more
commonly in IV drug abusers). The most frequently involved valve in RSE is the tricuspid valve. Pulmonary
valve endocarditis is quite rare.

C. **Prosthetic valve endocarditis (PVE).** Infection of
prosthetic valves that occurs within 2 months of cardiac
surgery is called early PVE, and infection occurring later
than 2 months postoperatively is classified as late PVE.
Early PVE usually results from intraoperative contami-
nation and postoperative wound infection. Late PVE results from similar etiologies as NVE. The infecting
organism in early PVE usually is *Staphylococcus,* with *S.
epidermidis* the most common. Gram-negative organisms
and fungi are also seen. Organisms of late PVE are similar to those of NVE, with streptococci most commonly
found. Staphylococci and gram-negative organisms can
also be seen. In PVE, the aortic valve is more often infected than the mitral valve. This is in direct contrast to
NVE, where the mitral valve is more often infected.

D. **Culture-negative endocarditis (CNE).** Inflammation
of the endocardium with negative blood cultures is termed
CNE. This can occur in patients who have been partially
treated with prior antimicrobial therapy or infected with
fastidious organisms (see Table 25-1). Since true infection
is occurring in these patients, a more appropriate term for
this disorder is "apparent" culture-negative endocarditis.

V. **Clinical endocarditis**

A. **Presentation**

1. **History.** Recognition of the susceptible population
and supportive historical evidence in their presentation are important for the prompt diagnosis of infectious endocarditis. Dental extraction, periodontal
surgery, genitourinary or gastrointestinal instrumentation, or a surgical procedure within 3 months prior
to patient presentation is significant, especially if the
patient did not receive antimicrobial prophylaxis.

Additional factors include current intravascular device infection, recent valvular surgery, or a prior episode of endocarditis. IV drug abusers have a high risk for endocarditis involving previously normal valves. Further risk, however, has not been detected in the subset of IV drug abusers who are HIV-positive.

Patients with infectious endocarditis may develop constitutional signs and symptoms of infection or a specific complication of the disease. The acuteness of presentation is generally indicative of the virulence of the responsible pathogen. Organisms such as *S. viridans* and *S. bovis* have an insidious onset of more than 4 to 8 weeks. Malaise, arthralgias, and myalgias are among the earliest symptoms to develop. These symptoms are associated with a low-grade fever (<39.0°C) and night sweats. Gastrointestinal manifestations include anorexia and weight loss; neurologic manifestations include headache and mental status changes. Endocarditis due to *Staphylococcus aureus* or *Neisseria gonorrhoeae* progresses more rapidly and typically presents within 2 weeks of infection. Patients develop high fever (>39.5°C) and associated rigors as well as signs of peripheral vascular occlusion or embolic phemomena. Furthermore, patients with infections secondary to these organisms are more likely to complain of shortness of breath, dyspnea on exertion, orthopnea, or palpitations suggestive of congestive heart failure and valvular incompetence.

2. **Physical examination.** On initial evaluation, patients may appear acutely or chronically ill. In either situation, fever, pallor, and a new or changing murmur are common findings. Approximately 90% of patients will be febrile on initial evaluation. Lack of a fever, however, should not preclude the consideration of endocarditis, especially with the overall upward shift of the age of patients with the disease and the decreased ability of the geriatric population to demonstrate a febrile response to infection. About 80% to 90% of patients will have an appreciable murmur at presentation, and virtually all will develop a **murmur** at some point during their clinical course. Usually the murmur is consistent with mitral or aortic insufficiency, reflecting the increased incidence of left-sided valvular involvement. Maneuvers to increase the intensity of right-sided murmurs are beneficial in IV drug abusers or other patients at increased risk for tricuspid or pulmonic valve involvement. The emergency physician should pay close attention to other features of the cardiac examination. Irregularities of cardiac rhythm may indicate invasion of the conducting system by a myocardial abscess. A new, third heart sound or basilar rales may be indicative of early congestive heart failure.

On abdominal palpation, **splenomegaly** is frequently appreciable. This finding is detected in one-third to one-half of patients with endocarditis and becomes more predominant in those with long-standing infections. There is typically no associated abdominal tenderness unless a recent embolic event to the spleen has occurred.

The physical examination should also include a thorough search for complications of infectious endocarditis. Major **embolic events** are well known and have been increasingly reported as a presenting symptom. Coronary artery obstruction secondary to vegetative fragmentation may lead to chest pain characteristic of a myocardial infarction. Peripheral vascular occlusions may result from showered emboli, and patients may present with a painful and cold extremity. Similarly, alterations of cerebral blood flow may result in transient or progressive focal neurologic deficits. These most commonly occur in the middle cerebral artery; however, they are not exclusively embolic events. Mycotic aneurysms or vasculitic changes may lead to intracerebral or subarachnoid hemorrhage. Emboli may damage numerous organ systems, including the pulmonary, renal, and gastrointestinal systems. This may confuse the diagnosis of infectious endocarditis by mimicking primary noncardiac disease processes. Five peripheral lesions have classically been associated with endocarditis and are attributed to either microembolic or immunologic changes. **Janeway lesions** are flat, nontender, blanching, red lesions with an irregular border that occur on the palms and soles. **Osler's nodes** are erythematous, nodular lesions that appear on the extremities and are characteristically painful. Most often they occur on the pulp of the fingers. **Splinter hemorrhages** are subungual lesions that have a linear form and end prior to reaching the distal edge of the nail bed. Ophthalmologic signs include **conjunctival petechiae** and **Roth spots.** The latter represent a form of retinal hemorrhage with a pale center surrounded by an irregular red border.

B. Assessment

    1. Laboratory evaluation. Routine studies performed in the emergency department are suggestive but not diagnostic of infectious endocarditis. Patients with longer courses prior to presentation will have a greater degree of **anemia.** This is typically a normochromic normocytic anemia secondary to a hypoproliferative state, but may be hemolytic secondary to mechanical destruction. Hemolysis induced by normal prosthetic valves may be difficult to distinguish from this. Elevation of the **leukocyte count** with prevalence of immature forms is also supportive information. Abnormalities on urine analysis are indicative of insult to the renal system. Hematuria, red cell casts, and proteinuria may all be seen. An elevated **erythrocyte sedimentation rate** (ESR) to the level of 50 mm/hour or more is also typically seen.

        Blood cultures are paramount, not only in the diagnosis but also in the treatment of infectious endocarditis. Consequently, attention must be paid to the manner in which blood cultures are obtained. An aerobic and anaerobic set, each containing at least 10 ml of blood, should be obtained in the emergency department. There does not appear to be an increased yield with arterial sampling as opposed to venous sampling. Significant detection rates are noted, however, with increased quantities of blood culture. It is currently recommended that three sets should be obtained in the first 24 hours of a patient's hospital course. These should be obtained at intervals of at least 1 hour and be drawn from separate sites. Positive identification of the causative organism will be made in up to 90% of blood cultures obtained in the above fashion. This rate is decreased to approximately 75% if antibiotics have been taken by the patient within 2 weeks prior to presentation. Antibiotics should not be administered until the three sets of blood cultures have been obtained. In critically ill patients who require the administration of antibiotics in the emergency department, the interval between blood cultures should be reduced to no less than 15 minutes.

2. **ECG assessment.** There are no diagnostic changes seen on the electrocardiograms of patients with endocarditis. Rather, abnormalities may represent secondary complications such as ischemia or infarction, conduction disturbances, or pericarditis. Progression of any abnormality or development of abnormalities in previously normal ECGs is useful in following the course of the disease.

3. **Diagnostic radiology**
   a. **Chest radiography.** The chest radiograph may identify valvular calcifications of an abnormal valve that is at high risk for infection. Alternatively, chest radiography may identify complications in patients with known or suspected endocarditis. Specific clues include vascular redistribution, Kerley B lines, and pleural effusions suggestive of congestive heart failure or multiple pulmonary infiltrates suggestive of septic emboli.
   b. **Echocardiography.** Echocardiography provides a reliable, noninvasive means of confirming the diagnosis of infectious endocarditis. All patients with clinical evidence suggestive of infectious endocarditis should be screened with transthoracic echocardiography (TTE). This technique is limited in patients with preexisting valve abnormalities or prosthetic valves. Adequate two-dimensional TTE scans can be obtained in up to 80% of patients, and the overall detection rate for vegetations is approximately 50%. In addition to diagnostic capability, echocardiography has prognostic value. Patients with endocarditis detected by TTE, especially if the vegetation is greater than 1 cm, have a predictably higher risk for complications (e.g., congestive heart failure, emboli).

A greater diagnostic and predictive yield is obtained by transesophageal echocardiography (TEE). Inadequate TTE, negative TTE despite high clinical suspicion, and abnormal TTE are indications for further evaluation by TEE. The improved image quality with this semi-invasive procedure increases the sensitivity to more than 90%. Evaluation for related perivalvular abnormalities and valvular dysfunction assists in surgical planning and identifies patients who are likely to fail medical management. The technology has advanced significantly since this procedure was first used to evaluate for endocarditis. Although a negative scan currently does not exclude the diagnosis of endocarditis, a positive scan with clinical support can be diagnostic.

C. **Management.** Management of the patient with endocarditis should be centered on treating the underlying infection while continuously anticipating and aggressively treating any complications of the disease that may occur. Congestive heart failure, cardiac arrhythmias, and septic shock are common complications of endocarditis. The treatments for these complications are covered in other chapters of this text.

  1. **Medical therapy.** The mainstay of treatment for endocarditis is antimicrobial therapy. Because of the unique nature of the disease, successful treatment differs from that for most bacterial infections. First, valvular vegetations consist of a mesh of fibrin strands in which bacteria replicate freely and reach high concentrations. Phagocyte cell penetration into the mesh is limited, and this normal host defense is rendered ineffective. Antibiotics must be bactericidal in order to eradicate the infection. Second, once the bacteria have reached their high concentrations, their metabolic rate decreases. Reduced susceptibility to antimicrobial action results, mandating a prolonged duration of treatment. Consistent serum levels of appropriate agents are necessary for sterilization. Therefore parenteral administration is the most reliable route.

  Bacteriologic confirmation of the diagnosis of endocarditis should be achieved prior to initiation of antibiotics in patients who are medically stable. However, in those with an acute presentation, empiric therapy is necessary and may be initiated in the emergency department. Despite the urgency of the situation, sufficient blood cultures usually should be obtained as described previously: prior to administration of an antibiotic. Antimicrobial selection is based on the suspected organism involved. A **penicillinase-resistant penicillin** in combination with an **aminoglycoside** is the combination of choice in patients with NVE. In patients with prosthetic valves or added risk due to IV drug abuse, methicillin resistance should be considered and the penicillin replaced by **vancomycin.** Hypersensitivity to penicillin also necessitates the use of vancomycin. Adjunctive therapy with rifampin is controversial but may be added in patients whose course is complicated by meningitis or prolonged bacteremia. Table 25-3 summarizes the recommended initial antimicrobial therapy.

A second issue to be considered is anticoagulation. Previous belief supported the use of heparin in an effort to decrease the thrombotic valvular vegetation size. However, the risk of significant hemorrhage from a mycotic aneurysm or intracranial embolus has been recognized more recently and the practice of routine anticoagulation discontinued. Patients with prosthetic valves who present on oral anticoagulants should be continued on the medication with close monitoring and maintenance of their prothrombin time in the low therapeutic range.

2. **Surgical therapy.** Surgical intervention is an important adjunct to medical management in endocarditis. Several indications for valve replacement may be discovered during the emergency department course. The emergency physician should evaluate the patient for these indications and promptly obtain consultations as appropriate. In NVE, the leading indication for operative intervention is refractory **congestive heart failure.** When the aortic valve is involved, hemodynamic instability is common. Other indications include conduction abnormalities associated with **intracardiac abscesses,** recurrent or **major systemic emboli,** and **large, mobile vegetations** detected by echocardiography. In PVE, moderate to severe heart failure secondary to valve dysfunction and acute obstruction must be treated with emergent valve replacement. Surgery will be necessary in about 50% of patients with PVE. Other indications for surgical intervention in endocarditis, such as fungal or gram-negative endocarditis, may become evident during the patient's hos-

Table 25-3. Recommended initial antimicrobial treatment for bacterial endocarditis

Native valve endocarditis

Patients not allergic to penicillin

Nafcillin or oxacillin 2g IV q4h + gentamicin 1 mg/kg (80 mg maximum) IV q8h

Patients with hypersensitivity to penicillin

Vancomycin 30 mg/kg IV q6h to q12h (2 gm/24 hr maximum) + gentamicin 1 mg/kg (80 mg maximum) IV q8h

Prosthetic valve endocarditis or IV drug abusers

Vancomycin 30 mg/kg IV q6h to q12h (2 g/24 hr maximum) + gentamicin 1 mg/kg (80 mg maximum) IV q8h ± rifampin 300 mg PO q8h

Nafcillin or oxacillin 2 g IV q4h + gentamicin 1 mg/kg (80 mg maximum) q8h ± rifampin 300 mg PO q8h

pital course. These organisms are less responsive to antimicrobial therapy, and patients at risk for such infections may also benefit from prompt surgical consultation.

   D. Disposition. All patients with suspected or known endocarditis should be managed as inpatients with continuous cardiac monitoring. Furthermore, if there is evidence of a secondary complication such as congestive heart failure or a major embolic event, admission to the intensive care unit is appropriate. The patient should be primarily cared for by an internist, cardiologist, or infectious disease specialist. Consultation by a cardiothoracic surgeon is required for the indications previously discussed.

VI. Endocarditis prophylaxis. Since endocarditis results from bacteremia and bacteremia is associated with certain health care procedures, prophylaxis of at-risk individuals has become routine. However, no prospective study has shown prophylaxis to be effective. The American Heart Association has developed criteria for prophylaxis in certain at-risk populations, and these are summarized in Tables 25-4 and 25-5. The usual antibiotic regimen for prophylaxis is **amoxicillin** 3.0

Table 25-4. Cardiac conditions*

Endocarditis prophylaxis recommended

Prosthetic cardiac valves, including bioprosthetic and homograft valves

Previous bacterial endocarditis, even in the absence of heart disease

Surgically constructed systemic-pulmonary shunts or conduits

Most congenital cardiac malformations

Rheumatic and other acquired valvular dysfunction, even after valvular surgery

Hypertrophic cardiomyopathy

Mitral valve prolapse with valvular regurgitation

Endocarditis prophylaxis not recommended

Isolated secundum atrial septal defect

Surgical repair without residua beyond 6 months of secundum atrial septal defect, ventricular septal defect, or patent ductus arteriosus

Previous coronary artery bypass graft surgery

Mitral valve prolapse without valvular regurgitation†

Physiologic, functional, or innocent heart murmurs

Previous Kawasaki disease without valvular dysfunction

Previous rheumatic fever without valvular dysfunction

Cardiac pacemakers and implanted defibrillators

* This table lists selected conditions but is not meant to be all-inclusive.
† Individuals who have a mitral valve prolapse associated with thickening and/or redundancy of the valve leaflets may be at increased risk for bacterial endocarditis, particularly men who are 45 years of age or older.
Source: Dajani AS, et al. Prevention of bacterial endocarditis: recommendations by the American Heart Association. *JAMA* 264:2919–2922, 1990. Copyright 1990, American Medical Association.

Table 25-5.   Dental or surgical procedures*

Endocarditis prophylaxis recommended

Dental procedures known to induce gingival or mucosal bleeding, including professional cleaning

Tonsillectomy and/or adenoidectomy

Surgical operations that involve intestinal or respiratory mucosa

Bronchoscopy with a rigid bronchoscope

Sclerotherapy for esophageal varices

Esophageal dilatation

Gallbladder surgery

Cystoscopy

Urethral dilatation

Urethral catheterization if urinary tract infection is present†

Urinary tract surgery if urinary tract infection is present†

Prostatic surgery

Incision and drainage of infected tissue†

Vaginal hysterectomy

Vaginal delivery in the presence of infection†

Endocarditis prophylaxis not recommended‡

Dental procedures not likely to induce gingival bleeding, such as simple adjustment of orthodontic appliances or fillings above the gum line

Injection of local intraoral anesthetic (except intraligamentary injections)

Shedding of primary teeth

Tympanostomy tube insertion

Bronchoscopy with a flexible bronchoscope, with or without biopsy

Cardiac catheterization

Endoscopy with or without gastrointestinal biopsy

Cesarean section

In the absence of infection for urethral catheterization, dilatation and curettage, uncomplicated vaginal delivery, therapeutic abortion, sterilization procedures, or insertion or removal of intrauterine devices

---

* This table lists selected procedures but is not meant to be all-inclusive.

† In addition to a prophylactic regimen for genitourinary procedures, antibiotic therapy should be directed against the most likely bacterial pathogen.

‡ In patients who have prosthetic heart valves, a previous history of endocarditis, or surgically constructed systemic-pulmonary shunts or conduits, physicians may choose to administer prophylactic antibiotics even for low-risk procedures that involve the lower respiratory, genitourinary, or gastrointestinal tracts.

Source: Dajani AS, et al. Prevention of bacterial endocarditis: recommendations by the American Heart Association. *JAMA* 264:2919–2922, 1990. Copyright 1990, American Medical Association.

PO 1 hour prior to the procedure followed by 1.5 g 6 hours after the initial dose. In penicillin-allergic patients, **erythromycin** ethylsuccinate 800 mg or erythromycin stearate 1.0 g PO 2 hours before the procedure and then one-half that dose 6 hours after the procedure can be used. **Clindamycin,** 300 mg PO 1 hour before the procedure and 150 mg 6 hours after the initial dose, can also be used in penicillin-allergic patients.

Bibliography

Bayer AS. Infective endocarditis. *Clin Infect Dis* 17:313–320, 1993.

Durack DT. Prevention of infective endocarditis. *N Engl J Med* 332:38–43, 1995.

Fowler VG, Durack DT. Infective endocarditis. *Curr Opin Cardiol* 9:389–400, 1994.

Maisch B, Drude L. Value and limitations of transesophageal echocardiography in infective endocarditis. *Heiz* 18:341–360, 1993.

Molavi A. Endocarditis: Recognition, management, and prophylaxis. *Cardiovasc Clin* 23:139–174, 1993.

Valvular Heart Disease

Carlos A. A. Torres

There are a variety of degenerative and congenital abnormalities that may affect the heart valves (Table 26-1). Valvular disease can also result from several systemic disorders, some of which will be mentioned, although not discussed in detail, in the sections on each individual valvular disease.

The most common complication of valvular heart disease is congestive heart failure (CHF). The following discussion will point out differences in treatments and the advantages of certain approaches to the treatment of CHF for each valvular disorder. Guidelines for the general treatment of CHF may be found in Chap. 14.

I. **Rheumatic heart disease.** Rheumatic fever (RF) deserves special mention because of its historic significance and worldwide importance. Although rheumatic fever continues to be the leading cause of heart disease in many developing countries (25 to 30 million cases per year), the incidence in the United States for the past decade has been only 0.23–1.14 cases/100,000 school-age children per year. Despite these relatively low numbers, there was a resurgence in rheumatic fever in the mid-1980s, causing concern among many health professionals.

Although the pathogenesis of RF is not totally clear, the weight of evidence points to its being a connective tissue disorder brought on as a consequence of the interaction between a group A beta-hemolytic streptococcal pharyngeal infection and the immune response of the host. Contributing environmental factors that enhance dissemination of streptococcal infection include low socioeconomic status, poor nutrition, poor hygiene, and overcrowding.

RF is characterized by an inflammatory process that involves the heart (carditis) and to a lesser degree, joints and other structures. Carditis can present itself in varying degrees from fulminant myocarditis to undetectable inflammation with resultant valve scarring as a late consequence.

A. **Presentation.** Clinically, cardiac manifestations may vary from new onset of murmurs or pericardial rub to overt CHF. Extracardiac manifestations include subcutaneous nodules, erythema marginatum, Sydenham's chorea, fever, and abdominal pain.

The diagnosis of RF is mostly clinical, with the laboratory being used for verification of clinical suspicion. Physical and historic findings are divided into major and minor manifestations as established by the revised Jones criteria (Table 26-2).

B. **Assessment.** Laboratory studies should be centered on making the diagnosis as well as ruling out the complications of RF. The CBC is nonspecific, although during the acute infection the WBC count may be elevated. Later in the disease, the WBC count is usually normal. Renal function tests should be obtained to rule out renal involvement

Table 26-1. Causes of valvular heart disease

Acute	Chronic
Infective endocarditis	Rheumatic valve disease
Rheumatic carditis	Calcifications
Blunt and penetrating trauma	Myxomatous degeneration
Prosthetic paravalvular leak	Dilatation of the left ventricle
Prosthetic component escape or failure	Carcinoid syndrome
	Syphilis
Thromboembolism	Rheumatoid arthritis
Papillary muscle or chordal rupture	Connective tissue disorders
	Blunt trauma
	Turbulent flow with prosthetic valves
	Prosthetic component dysfunction
	Papillary muscle dysfunction
	Congenital

with poststrep immune complex disease. The urinalysis can also be used to screen for renal involvement. X-rays can demonstrate cardiomegaly, and the ECG may display an increased P-R interval in cases of carditis. Antistreptolysin O titers are usually used to verify the previous streptococcal infection. Additional testing with antihyaluronidase, antistreptokinase, and antiDNase B antibodies may increase the laboratory sensitivity for the disease. The echocardiogram is the most common tool used to visualize the valvular or wall motion abnormalities of rheumatic carditis.

C. **Management.** In mild cases, if the diagnosis rheumatic carditis is unclear and evidence of carditis is not present, treatment should consist of analgesics and symptomatic therapy only. Once the diagnosis is established, **salicylate therapy** with aspirin at 100 mg/kg/d usually will

Table 26-2. Jones criteria (modified in 1984)

Major manifestations	Minor manifestations
Carditis	Fever
Polyarthritis	Arthralgia
Chorea	History of rheumatic fever or rheumatic heart disease
Subcutaneous nodules	Elevated ESR, CRP, or white blood cells
Erythema marginatum	Prolonged PR interval

Note: Two major or one major and one minor manifestations, with supporting evidence of a recent streptococcal infection, indicate the probable presence of rheumatic fever.

improve symptoms dramatically. It will not, however, impact the course of the disease. Most doctors also recommend the use of **corticosteroids** with prednisone at 40–60 mg/d if signs of carditis are present.

All patients should be treated with **antibiotics** to eliminate any residual streptococcal infection. The usual recommendation is a single dose of 1.2 million units of benzathine penicillin administered intramuscularly (I.M.).

Prognosis is usually good if there is minimal clinical evidence of carditis. The prognosis worsens with the severity of the acute attack and the recurrence of episodes. For this reason, prophylaxis for future infections is crucial. Rheumatic carditis patients usually receive monthly injections of benzathine penicillin G at 1.2 million units I.M. after the acute episode has resolved. The length of prophylaxis is controversial and should be tailored to each patient.

II. **Aortic stenosis.** The hallmark of aortic stenosis (AS) is an obstruction to left ventricular outflow. Valvular stenosis is the most common cause of this outflow obstruction; however, obstruction may result from subvalvular or supravalvular etiologies. The primary etiologies of valvular AS are degenerative (now the most common cause in the United States), rheumatic, and congenital.

The timing of the clinical manifestations of AS are related to the underlying etiology. Clinically significant AS before the third decade more often is due to congenital malformations, whereas disease manifesting itself around the seventh decade usually is due to degenerative changes. AS presenting between these two extremes of age is often due to degenerative changes occurring on a congenitally bicuspid valve (most common etiology in young adults) or a rheumatic etiology.

Despite the etiology, the consequences of AS on cardiovascular physiology are the same. Stenosis of the valve creates an outflow obstruction to the left ventricle. This obstruction usually progresses slowly and allows the left ventricle to adapt to the increase in pressure gradient across the valve by means of concentric hypertrophy. If there is no relief of the outflow obstruction, compensating mechanisms are eventually overcome, and myocardial fibrosis, decreased diastolic compliance, and decreased contractility lead to symptoms of congestive heart failure.

Once patients with AS become symptomatic, their average survival, if left untreated, is approximately 2 to 3 years.

A. **Presentation**

1. **History.** In the majority of cases, initial symptoms begin around the sixth decade of life, and consist mainly of angina pectoris, exertional syncope, dyspnea on exertion, and congestive heart failure.

Angina occurs in approximately 60% of patients. Although its clinical symptoms are similar to those caused by coronary artery disease (CAD) and are intensified by exertion and relieved by rest, it does not always imply any underlying CAD. Subendocardial ischemia results from a combination of increased oxygen demand by the hypertrophied muscle and decreased coronary artery flow reserve. Approximately

50% of patients presenting with AS will have significant CAD in addition to left ventricular hypertrophy, which adds to the imbalance of myocardial oxygen supply and demand.

Exertional syncope is thought to result from the inability of the heart to increase its output proportionately to the systemic vasodilatation that occurs normally during exertion. As a result of the outflow obstruction, the heart is unable to maintain adequate arterial blood pressure and cerebral perfusion, resulting in hypotension and syncope.

CHF due to AS outflow obstruction results in **dyspnea on exertion,** shortness of breath at rest, orthopnea, paroxysmal nocturnal dyspnea, and chest tightness (see Chap.14).

2. **Physical exam.** The **pulse** pressure in AS is typically narrow, displaying a slow rise with sustained duration (pulsus parvus et tardus). It may be normal in elderly individuals. The jugular venous pulse can show prominent a waves secondary to decreased compliance from a hypertrophied right ventricle. The lung examination may demonstrate rales in the bases in patients with CHF.

On the **cardiac examination,** a sustained cardiac impulse is characteristic, and occasionally a precordial a wave may be visualized. With the onset of CHF, the apex becomes displaced inferiorly and to the left. With the patient in full expiration and leaning forward, a systolic thrill may be palpable. The characteristic **murmur** of AS (Fig. 26-1) is a crescendo-decrescendo diamond-shaped systolic ejection murmur, heard best

Fig. 26-1. Heart murmurs in valvular disease.

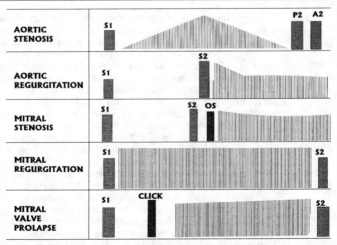

at the right upper sternal border and radiating up into the carotid arteries. In young adults it may be preceded by a sharp aortic ejection sound. A_2 closure is delayed and in some cases may result in a paradoxically split S_2 sound. In the elderly, the murmur may present itself as a cooing musical sound.

B. **Assessment**
1. **ECG.** In about 90% of cases, the ECG will be abnormal, showing signs of left ventricular hypertrophy (LVH). These include increased QRS voltage and ST-segment depression with asymmetric T-wave inversion in the lateral leads.
2. **Chest x-ray (CXR).** The CXR may display prominence of the aorta due to poststenotic turbulence. Enlargement of the heart is not usually seen on the CXR until CHF ensues.
3. **Echocardiogram.** Typical echocardiographic findings include calcification and thickening of the aortic valve with decreased mobility of the leaflets. Doppler echocardiography provides an accurate determination of the pressure gradient and aortic valve cross sectional area translating the degree of progression of the disease.
4. **Cardiac catheterization.** Cardiac catheterization can be useful to demonstrate the aortic valve gradient and cross-sectional area when the echocardiogram is equivocal. It can also delineate concomitant CAD.

C. **Management.** Patients who present with dyspnea, CHF, or cardiac arrhythmias should be placed immediately on continuous cardiac monitoring. An IV access should be established and baseline laboratory tests should be obtained. If endocarditis or acute rheumatic fever is suspected, blood cultures and ASO titers should also be drawn.

CHF and anginal episodes should be treated accordingly (see Chaps. 14 and 20, respectively), with the following alterations:
1. A reversible cause of the sudden onset of dyspnea or overt CHF such as atrial fibrillation or cardiac ischemia must be aggressively pursued and treated (see Chap. 16). When premature atrial contractions are frequent, the physician should be more aggressive in attempting medical prophylaxis with an atrial antidysrhythmic. The loss of an atrial contraction, such as can be seen in atrial fibrillation, can cause significant lowering of ventricular filling pressure in patients with AS, causing secondary hypotension and CHF.
2. Diuretics should be used with caution in patients who have evidence of fluid overload because they may induce hypotension by lowering the left ventricular preload and reducing cardiac output. It is recommended to start with lower dosages (20 to 40 mg IV of furosemide) and to closely observe the patient's hemodynamics. Digitalis is usually helpful only for controlling ventricular rate in atrial fibrillation/flutter or if there is evidence of increased ventricular volume or decreased ejection fraction as with dilated cardiomyopathy. Beta-blockers are

indicated for the treatment of angina associated with
AS, but can aggravate left ventricular failure.

3. Left atrial enlargement is not common until late in the
course of AS. The presence of atrial arrhythmias or left
atrial enlargement by CXR should prompt further investigation for concomitant mitral valve disease.

D. Patient disposition. Asymptomatic patients require adequate arrangements for follow up. They should be instructed to report to their physicians the onset of any
symptoms of AS and to present to the emergency department (ED) if they have any concerns. All AS patients require endocarditis prophylaxis education.

Cardiology consultation and admission should be obtained for symptomatic patients with angina, CHF, or syncope. Medical therapy can be very tenuous because of
difficulties between balancing preload and correcting fluid
overload. Average survival in symptomatic patients who
do not undergo surgery is very poor. Most symptomatic
adults with angina also require admission to rule out
myocardial infarction (MI), with subsequent cardiac catheterization to rule out CAD.

Surgical consultation should be obtained because surgical therapy is the most definitive treatment for AS. Indications for surgery are based on the patient's age and the
severity of the stenosis. In adults, an aortic orifice less
than 0.4 cm^2/m^2 or less than 0.75 cm^2 is considered severe
and warrants surgical correction.

Balloon aortic valvuloplasty is advised only in young
patients who have noncalcific stenosis or in those who
refuse surgery. Patients who are expected to have a high
surgical mortality rate due to their general condition may
also be considered for this procedure.

III. Aortic insufficiency. Aortic insufficiency (AI) is caused by
the inadequate coaption of the aortic valve leaflets. It has
many etiologies, some of which are mentioned in Table 26-3.
With such a wide range of causes, the natural history of the
disease is varied, and it may parallel that of the underlying
disorder for years before it becomes clinically manifest. Regardless of its nature, in chronic AI, the backflow of blood to
the ventricle causes significant left ventricular volume over-

Table 26-3. Causes of aortic regurgitation

Cusp abnormalities	Aortic vessel abnormalities	
	Inflammatory	**Noninflammatory**
Rheumatic fever	Rheumatoid arthritis	Marfan's syndrome
Rheumatoid arthritis	Ankylosing spondylitis	Myxomatous degen-
Endocarditis	Syphilis	eration
Congenital	Reiter's syndrome	Aortic dissection
		Chronic hypertension

load. This eventually leads to compensatory dilatation and hypertrophy. Chronic severe AI will lead to exhaustion of compensatory mechanisms and consequent CHF.

A. Presentation

1. **History.** AI may present in the acute or chronic form. **Acute AI** is the result of either infective endocarditis, trauma, or aortic dissection. It is characterized by severe dyspnea, hypotension, and signs of cardiovascular collapse. A wealth of physical findings like those seen in chronic AI is not found. Instead, patients appear acutely ill, with peripheral vasoconstriction, cyanosis, tachycardia, shock, and pulmonary congestion.

    Patients with **chronic AI** may remain asymptomatic for many years before CHF develops. The most common complaints are palpitations with a sensation of pounding in the chest due to a very enlarged heart (cor bovinum), exertional dyspnea, paroxysmal nocturnal dyspnea, and orthopnea.

    Decreased coronary filling resulting from AI can also lead to angina. Its most classic presentation is that of nocturnal angina, prompted by the decreased diastolic pressure and decreased heart rates that occur during sleep.

2. **Physical examination.** The **pulse** is characteristically described as being intense with an abrupt collapse. It is also known as Corrigan's pulse or water-hammer pulse. The absence of a widened pulse pressure in a patient without CHF makes the diagnosis of AI unlikely. This widened pulse pressure is responsible for a variety of peripheral findings. For example, auscultation of the femoral artery may reveal loud systolic and diastolic sounds (pistol shots), or proximal compression of the artery may elicit a humming sound distally (Durozier's sign). In addition, shining a light through or applying gentle pressure at the patient's fingertips may reveal capillary pulsation (Quincke's sign), and on occasion a characteristic "head bobbing" with each pulse may be seen (de Musset's sign).

    In advanced AI, a diffuse inferior and laterally displaced apical impulse is felt. At times, a systolic thrill may also be noticed because of the increased stroke volume. The classic aortic regurgitant **murmur** (see Fig. 26-1) is best heard on the sternal borders around the third or fourth intercostal space. It is a high-pitched murmur that begins shortly after A_2, and is best heard during expiration while the patient leans forward. In general, the longer the duration of the murmur, the more severe the regurgitation. Early closure of the mitral valve during forward blood flow may lead to a diastolic rumbling murmur, known as the Austin Flint murmur, which is best heard at the apex.

B. Assessment

1. **ECG.** Early findings include increased QRS voltage and amplitude with tall T waves in the precordial leads. As aortic regurgitation progresses, T waves be-

come inverted and ST-segment depression may develop.

2. **X-ray.** The most prominent finding in AI is cardiomegaly. The heart typically is enlarged downward and to the left. Dilatation of the aorta commonly is found and is more pronounced than in AS. Because aortic root diseases may present as AI, marked dilatation should raise the suspicion of such disorders.

3. **Echocardiogram.** Echocardiography is the best, noninvasive diagnostic tool in the evaluation of AI. On M-mode, diastolic fluttering or premature closure of the mitral valve is characteristic. Two-dimensional echo is most helpful in determining if the etiology of the AI is the valve itself or the aortic root. Assessment of left ventricular dimensions and function also may be obtained with echo.

Doppler echocardiography has superior sensitivity and accuracy compared to the previously mentioned echo methods. It is capable of detecting aortic regurgitation, and it will also approximate the size of the valve orifice and quantify the regurgitant flow.

In cases where valve replacement is deemed necessary, heart catheterization should be performed.

C. **Management.** Patients should be managed according to the severity of the regurgitation and the compromise of hemodynamic conditions. Acute aortic regurgitation requires immediate hemodynamic stabilization. Treatment is similar to other forms of CHF or cardiogenic shock (see Chap. 14). Medical management is aimed at afterload reduction and is a temporizing measure only until surgical treatment can be performed.

Patients with severe chronic AI and decreased cardiac reserve should be treated with cardiac glycosides as well as diuretics and dietary salt restriction. Treatment of hypertension is fundamental because the increased afterload will worsen the regurgitant flow. Judicious use of vasodilator therapy has proven to be the most useful approach of all toward managing these patients, both for treatment of hypertension and CHF. It also has been shown to slow the progression of the disease.

The use of beta-blockers is discouraged in most chronic cases because they may precipitate or aggravate CHF.

D. **Patient disposition.** Asymptomatic patients should be referred for cardiology follow up. They also should be instructed regarding endocarditis prophylaxis.

Patients who are symptomatic usually require admission and cardiology consultation. Consultation with the cardiovascular surgery service may be indicated in acute and severe cases.

Unlike in AS, no individual measurement can be used to precisely time surgery for AI. Instead, careful individual follow up is the key. In general, patients with normal left ventricular function require only subsequent testing. Patients with abnormal left ventricular function should be assessed in terms of their exercise tolerance and clinical progression over time. If deterioration is present, surgery is usually indicated, taking into account the operative risks as well as the presence of concomitant CAD.

Patients who refuse surgery or cannot undergo surgery may benefit from long-term vasodilator therapy and other medical interventions aimed at treating CHF.

IV. Mitral stenosis. Mitral stenosis (MS) is characterized by the obstruction of blood flow from the left atrium into the left ventricle. The most common cause of mitral stenosis is RF. Other less frequent causes include congenital heart disease, connective tissue disorders, and methysergide therapy. Obstruction to flow may also be caused by nonvalvular mechanisms such as atrial myxomas, thrombus and cor tritriatrium.

An average of 2 years is required for the development of MS after the onset of RF. Progression seems to be slower in temperate areas than in tropical zones near the equator. In the United States, approximately 10 years is required before signs of MS become clinically evident.

Stenosis of the mitral apparatus results in elevated diastolic pressures in the left atrium that are greater than left ventricular diastolic pressure. This pressure elevation is transmitted back into the pulmonary vasculature. The sequence of events that follows if left untreated involves enlargement of the left atrium, hyperplasia and hypertrophy of the pulmonary vessels, and pulmonary hypertension with eventual overload and failure of the right ventricle. Complicating events include atrial fibrillation, systemic embolus, hemoptysis, and infective endocarditis.

By the time patients develop orthopnea, they usually have critical obstruction of the mitral apparatus. These patients are at increased risk for pulmonary edema precipitated by atrial fibrillation, exertion, fever, sexual intercourse, or any other event that places demands on the cardiovascular system. Elevations in heart rate decrease the time for blood flow to occur across the mitral valve and cause an elevation of the pressure gradient across the mitral valve with subsequent left atrial hypertension. The resulting pulmonary edema can be treated to an extent by decreasing the ventricular rate.

Once patients develop severe, disabling symptoms, progression is fairly rapid. Patients with New York Heart Association (NYHA) class IV failure have approximately a 15% 5-year survival rate.

A. Presentation

1. **History.** The most common presenting symptom of a patient with mitral stenosis is dyspnea. This is the result of pulmonary venous hypertension and reduction in the compliance of the lungs secondary to interstitial edema and dilated vessels. The intensity of dyspnea varies with the degree of CHF.

   In more advanced cases of MS, occasional hemoptysis can be seen due to erosion of the bronchial veins. This can at times be life threatening. Thromboembolism is also a frequent complication of MS due to a dilated left atrium. The initial presentation of a patient with MS may be a stroke or a coronary embolus, especially in the elderly population. Infective endocarditis, hoarseness, and signs of right-sided heart failure may also be present in MS patients.

2. **Physical examination.** The **pulse** in MS is usually normal with no characteristic findings. Neck veins may be distended if right-sided heart failure is present. In those patients in sinus rhythm, a prominent a-wave is detectable. In atrial fibrillation, a prominent cv-wave can be seen.

   Palpation of the heart in advanced cases of MS may disclose a prominent right ventricular heave against the left sternal border. A diastolic thrill may be felt at the apex of the heart. This is best identified by asking the patient to assume the left decubitus position. **Auscultation** of the heart (see Fig. 26-1) reveals a prominent S_1, an opening snap, a diastolic rumble, and, in those cases where pulmonary hypertension is present, a prominent P_2. The opening snap, considered to be the most typical finding in MS, appears to be caused by abrupt stop of the stenotic mitral valve. Valves that are very rigid or immobile will not produce the snap. The diastolic rumble that follows is best heard at the apex with the bell of the stethoscope and can be increased by exertion and the left decubitus position.

   In patients with pulmonary hypertension, a diastolic blow that is caused by pulmonic regurgitation may be heard at the right sternal border. This is called a Graham Steell murmur. As right-sided heart failure develops, edema, ascites, hepatomegaly, and signs of pleural effusions can be seen.

   Associated murmurs, including those of concomitant aortic valve disease and mitral regurgitation, are not uncommon.

B. **Assessment**
   1. **ECG.** Early mitral stenosis is associated with a normal ECG. With progression of the disease and subsequent left atrium enlargement, the P wave duration increases and may appear biphasic in V1. Atrial fibrillation is very common in the later stages of the disease. Signs of right ventricular hypertrophy develop if there is right ventricular pressure elevation to 70 mm Hg.
   2. **X-ray.** The CXR typically displays an enlarged left atrium without any increase in the size of the left ventricle. Displacement upward of the left main stem bronchus may result as a consequence of the enlarged left atrium. Enlarged pulmonary arteries and right atrium may also be present. Special attention should be paid to examination of the lung fields for signs of interstitial edema such as Kerley B lines.
   3. **Echocardiogram.** The echocardiogram is the most sensitive noninvasive tool for detection of mitral valve stenosis. In M-mode, a decreased EF slope is characteristic. Thickening of the leaflets and calcifications may also be visualized. Two-dimensional studies will often disclose the presence of thrombi, calcifications, and the decreased orifice in the mitral valve. Doppler

echocardiography is very accurate in estimating the transvalvular gradient and the orifice cross-sectional area.

C. **Management.** Once MS has been identified in a patient, treatment will depend on the degree of congestive heart failure. In asymptomatic patients, strenuous exertion should be avoided. Patients who are relatively symptomatic may improve with mild **diuretics** and **sodium restriction.** Digitalis is not recommended except to slow the ventricular rate in patients with atrial fibrillation and in advanced cases of right-sided ventricular failure.

Mitral stenosis is one of the rare valvular diseases in which **beta-blockers** may prove beneficial by reducing heart rate during exertion and increasing patients' tolerance for heavy activity (even in those patients in sinus rhythm).

Anticoagulation is indicated in patients with atrial fibrillation. An international normalized ratio (INR) 2.0 to 3.0 is recommended in patients without history of embolism. In patients who have experienced an episode of embolism, an INR of 3.0 to 4.5 is recommended.

Atrial fibrillation of recent onset may be treated by electrical or chemical **cardioversion** if significant atrial enlargement is not present. A preparatory course of anticoagulants is given in preparation for elective cardioversion (see Chap. 16). Subsequently, patients may be maintained on quinidine. If attempts at cardioversion are unsuccessful, anticoagulation and control of ventricular rate is necessary. Digitalis and either diltiazem or verapamil may be used for the latter purpose. A ventricular rate of 60 to 65 bpm is optimal. A low-dose beta-blocker (atenolol 25 mg once a day) sometimes can be added to patients on digitalis to achieve this rate.

D. **Patient disposition.** Cardiology follow-up is required for all patients, including those who are asymptomatic. In symptomatic cases, the severity of their symptoms should determine whether admission is indicated. Mitral valve surgery is indicated in symptomatic patients with a valve area less than 1.2 cm.^{2} Patients who have a significant decrease in exercise tolerance should also be considered for surgery. Emboli or hemoptysis are also viewed as indications for surgery.

Percutaneous balloon mitral valvuloplasty is more successful than aortic valvuloplasty and is seen as an alternative to surgery in many cases, with better results in younger patients. In the elderly, because of debilitating conditions that may coexist with mitral stenosis, valvuloplasty may be attempted when surgery is not indicated or the risk is very high.

V. **Mitral regurgitation (MR).** MR is defined as the return of part of the left ventricle's output to the left atrium. There are several etiologies for this entity, all of which result in the inadequate functioning of the mitral valve apparatus. This intricate structure consists mainly of the annulus, the leaflets, the chordae tendinae, and the papillary muscle. In a competent mitral valve, all components act harmoniously to produce timely opening and complete closure of the valve. If any of the components is damaged or does not function adequately, regurgitation may result. The mitral valve annulus has a sphincter-like function. It can undergo calcification and suffer compromise of this action, or the ventricle may dilate and cause the annulus to expand, keeping the leaflets from adequate closure.

The papillary muscles may suffer from ischemia and lead to dysfunction or, more dramatically, they may rupture and cause severe cardiovascular impairment and cardiogenic shock. The posterior papillary muscle is particularly prone to suffer ischemia during an inferior MI because of its terminal and single blood supply by the right coronary artery. The anterior muscle, by contrast, usually is supplied by both the left anterior descending and the circumflex arteries.

Chordae tendinae, which attach to the papillary muscles, may elongate or rupture as a consequence of mechanical strain, connective tissue disease, or as a result of a series of disorders below, causing MR.

RF, trauma, or endocarditis may affect many of the structures causing significant alterations in their shape and function. Whatever the etiology, the natural history of MR is twofold: (1) If the events occur over a long period of time, the left atrium will slowly become dilated and thin. It becomes capable of accommodating almost all of the regurgitant flow. The left ventricle then dilates and increases its wall thickness to compensate for the decreased forward blood flow. These two factors enable early diastolic filling of the left ventricle with little or no backflow into the pulmonary system. (2) If the events occur over a short period of time, adequate adaptation does not happen, the increased pressures are reflected towards the pulmonary system, and massive pulmonary edema and cardiogenic shock follow.

A. Presentation

1. **History.** Acute MR in a patient with a history of CAD or recent MI suggests papillary muscle involvement. Abrupt onset of pulmonary edema or cardiogenic shock in these patients should raise suspicion of acute MR.

   Chronic MR usually takes 2 to 3 decades before it becomes manifest. Initial symptoms are easy fatigue and dyspnea. In more advanced cases orthopnea will be present as well. If undiagnosed, a full-blown case of CHF (involving both right and left ventricles) will develop. The onset of atrial fibrillation will speed up the development of symptoms, but its impact is not as significant as in MS.

2. **Physical examination.** The **pulse** in MR may be normal, but in some cases an increased intensity on the initial phase of the carotid pulse can be felt. The jugular venous pulse is frequently not affected. In advanced stages, as right heart failure ensues, neck veins become distended.

   In the early phases of MR or in acute MR, inspection and palpation are unremarkable. As the disease progresses, the apex is displaced to the left and a "lift" may be felt or even seen. A systolic thrill may be felt in advanced cases. The typical **murmur** (see Fig. 26-1) is usually a loud, holosystolic murmur with a "blowing" characteristic to it, heard best at the apex with radiation to the axilla. It is accentuated by isometric exercise, which may be used to differentiate it from the murmur of AS. It may obscure the first and second heart sounds. Keep in mind that intensity of the murmur does not correlate with severity of the disease, and in some patients who are obese or who have an enlarged anterior-posterior chest diameter it can barely be heard.

B. Assessment

   1. ECG. Common findings are those of atrial enlargement and left ventricular strain. Atrial fibrillation is a common finding in advanced cases, and right ventricular hypertrophy may be present. In acute MR, which is of ischemic origin, the ECG may display findings consistent with AMI or severe ischemia.

   2. X-ray. Left atrial enlargement and left ventricular enlargement may be seen on CXR. In acute MR, signs of pulmonary edema may be the only findings.

   3. Echocardiogram. Echocardiography may be used to determine the etiology and extent of mitral regurgitation, but bidimensional echo is more useful for this purpose. Doppler echocardiography can be used to perform an estimate of the degree of MR.

C. Management. The acute management of CHF due to MR does not differ from the treatment of CHF due to MS. The mainstay of therapy is diuretics, salt restriction, and afterload reduction. If atrial fibrillation is present, rate control with either digoxin, diltiazem, or verapamil is indicated. Digoxin is helpful in alleviating symptoms of CHF as well. The use of vasodilators is the most beneficial nonsurgical intervention in most cases. Because the mitral and aortic valves are almost parallel to each other, reducing impedance to aortic flow by afterload reduction will decrease regurgitation and significantly improve patient condition. In acute MR, IV nitroprusside and intraaortic balloon counterpulsation can be used as a temporizing lifesaving intervention until definite treatment is possible (see Chap. 14).

D. Patient disposition. All patients with confirmed MR should be referred for cardiologic follow-up and should be educated regarding endocarditis prophylaxis. CHF and atrial fibrillation are the most common indications for admission to the hospital. The degree of symptomatic involvement usually determines the need for admission. If MI is suspected or confirmed, admission to the CCU is indicated.

   Indications and timing for surgery for MR are controversial. In general, when symptoms are disabling, surgery is made available as an option to consider. Replacement or, in many cases, reconstruction of the valve can be possible, with the return of the patient's functional capabilities. Results are dependent on the degree of ventricular dysfunction and adequate timing of the surgery itself.

VI. Mitral valve prolapse. Mitral valve prolapse (MVP) is the billowing or prolapse of the mitral valve leaflets into the left atrium during ventricular systole. Various degrees of this process may occur from simple protrusion of the mitral valve to prolapse and redundancy of the mitral leaflets resulting in inadequate coaption and MR.

The prevalence of this valve abnormality is approximately 6% in the general population. It has been argued that the denomination of MVP or Barlow syndrome be utilized only when these valvular abnormalities are associated with other symptoms such as palpitations, abnormal T waves, and cardiac arrhythmias. Symptoms are seen in only a small proportion of these patients. It is predominant in women, but men tend to have more severe forms of MVP.

MVP may be caused by several mechanisms. CAD with secondary papillary muscle dysfunction and rheumatic disease have been associated with this disorder, but the most common etiology is myxomatous degeneration of the mitral valve. There appears to be a hereditary component to the syndrome. Some researchers believe that MVP is at one end of a spectrum of connective tissue disorders that has its full expression in Marfan's syndrome.

The majority of patients with MVP are asymptomatic, but 10% to 15% of patients will develop progressive MVP. Complications of MVP include MR, infective endocarditis, arrhythmias, cerebral embolisms, and sudden death.

A. Presentation
1. **History.** MVP may be an unexpected finding during a routine physical examination, or it may be associated with complaints such as easy fatigability, palpitations, postural orthostasis, syncopal episodes, and chest discomfort. The chest pain of MVP may resemble that of CAD, but it is usually atypical, stabbing in nature, prolonged, and not related to exertion. It is seen most often in young thin women.
2. **Physical examination.** Patients with MVP may have a marfanoid habitus with long slender limbs and a "flat" or concave chest, but the general inspection may be unremarkable as well. The **pulse** is usually normal unless significant MR is present, in which case the carotid pulse may have a sharp upstroke. The jugular venous pulse is also normal unless MR is present.

   Auscultation provides the key to diagnosis in most cases. A characteristic **systolic click** can be heard. It may or may not be associated with a crescendo mid-to-late systolic murmur. It is best heard at the left sternal border, but various positions should be attempted. Expiration and lying down tend to promote a delay in the click as well as decrease the intensity of the murmur. Standing and straining (valsalva) will bring the click earlier in systole and increase the murmur. These findings may be intermittent and change on different occasions.

B. Assessment
1. **ECG.** In most cases the ECG is normal. Inverted T waves may be present in leads III and avf. A prolonged

Q-T interval and arrhythmias can also be found. Although SVT is the most common sustained tachydysrhythmia found, premature atrial contractions (PACs) and premature ventricular contractions (PVCs) are frequently found. Occasionally, more malignant ventricular arrhythmias are present. Most arrhythmias associated with MVP are benign, but some are of significance and require therapeutic intervention.

2. **X-ray.** The CXR is usually normal unless severe MR is present.

3. **Echocardiogram.** This is the most reliable noninvasive method for diagnosing MVP. The most typical finding is a late or pansystolic prolapse of the mitral valve leaflets into the left atrium. Both M-mode and bidimensional echocardiography may be utilized, but the latter is usually more sensitive.

C. **Management and disposition.** Patients should be reassured that MVP is a benign disease in the majority of cases. Those who are asymptomatic with no ECG abnormalities or signs of arrhythmias may be scheduled for elective follow-up. Patients with syncope, palpitations, chest pain, arrhythmias, inverted T waves, or prolonged Q-T intervals on the ECG may require Holter monitoring and stress testing.

The use of beta-blockers has been advocated to treat patients in whom palpitations or pain are a source of anxiety, with variable results. Prolonged Q-T intervals and ventricular arrhythmias also respond favorably to beta-blockers in most cases.

Antiplatelet therapy such as aspirin is indicated for those patients with cerebral emboli in whom MVP is suspected to be the source of embolization. Anticoagulation is indicated for refractory cases.

Prophylaxis for infective endocarditis is indicated by most research in all patients with click and murmur, but is controversial for those with only a click.

VII. **Tricuspid insufficiency (TI).** TI or tricuspid regurgitation is defined as an inadequate coaption of tricuspid leaflets, resulting in backflow of blood into the right atrium during systole. The most common cause of TI is not a primary valvular abnormality (organic tricuspid insufficiency) but rather the dilatation of the tricuspid annulus secondary to a dilated right ventricle (functional TI). Organic TI is rare and seen mostly as a result of infective endocarditis in IV drug abusers. Other causes include RF, carcinoid syndrome, papillary muscle dysfunction, trauma, and congenital abnormalities. Right ventricular hypertension of any cause (congenital, cor pulmonale, right ventricular infarction or MS) may lead to functional TI, which is usually more amenable to medical treatment.

TI is well tolerated as long as pulmonary hypertension is absent. The onset of pulmonary hypertension leads to right ventricular failure and decreased cardiac output.

A. **Presentation**

1. **History.** The presentation of TI is dependent on its etiology. Finding TI in an IV drug abuser should

prompt suspicion of infective endocarditis. In the context of pulmonary hypertension and left ventricular failure, patients initially may experience an improvement in pulmonary symptoms but soon develop edema, congestive hepatomegaly, and other signs of right-sided failure. As cardiac output decreases, complaints of increased weakness and fatigability also are found.

2. **Physical examination.** Edema, ascites, cachexia, and cyanosis may be present. Hepatomegaly and occasionally a pulsatile liver can be felt. The arterial **pulse** may be normal or have decreased intensity and amplitude if CHF is present. The jugular veins are distended in right-sided failure; prominent c-v waves with a sharp y-descent may be seen. A venous thrill can, on occasion, be palpated. Hepatojugular reflux can be elicited.

A right ventricular impulse may be palpated at the right sternal border. On auscultation, a holosystolic **murmur** that characteristically increases with inspiration and decreases with expiration is heard best at the lower right sternal border. S_3 and an increased P_2 are present when there is pulmonary hypertension and failure. Atrial fibrillation is common.

B. **Assessment**
   1. **ECG.** Findings include right ventricular hypertrophy, right bundle-branch block, and R waves in V1. Atrial fibrillation is not unusual.
   2. **X-ray.** Cardiomegaly with an increased right atrium occurs frequently. Enlarged pulmonary arteries and azygos veins can also be noticed. In more advanced cases, pleural effusion may also be present.
   3. **Echocardiogram.** Echocardiograms may reveal dilation of the annulus, paradoxical movement of the ventricular septum, and deformities or prolapse of the valve. Contrast echocardiograms performed by injecting a bolus of saline or dye peripherally, will reveal a characteristic back and forth movement of contrast through the tricuspid valve that is diagnostic. Color Doppler also is extremely sensitive in detecting and assessing the degree of tricuspid regurgitation.

C. **Management and disposition.** If pulmonary hypertension and right ventricular hypertension are not present, there is no indication for treatment. Functional TI is best managed by treating the underlying cause. It usually will improve without surgical intervention. If surgery is indicated, annuloplasty techniques that have been developed for dilated tricuspid annulus are currently the most common surgical approach. Organic TI disease, when advanced, usually requires surgical replacement of the valve. The treatment of tricuspid endocarditis is discussed in Chap. 25.

VIII. **Prosthetic valve disease.** Prosthetic valve disease arises as a result of disorders in structure or function (or both) of artificial valves in the human heart (Fig. 26-2).

The etiology depends on the type of valve and the structure

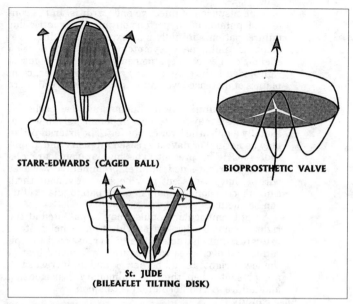

STARR-EDWARDS (CAGED BALL)

BIOPROSTHETIC VALVE

St. JUDE
(BILEAFLET TILTING DISK)

Fig. 26-2.   Common artificial valve types.

involved. In bioprosthetic valves, the most common cause of
valvular insufficiency is structural degeneration. This occurs
to a certain degree in all implanted biologic valves and over
time may become clinically significant (e.g., calcification of
valve structures and leaflet tears). In mechanical prostheses,
common problems are prosthetic component failures and or
component escape.

Regardless of valve type, the risk of paravalvular lead, infective endocarditis, and thromboembolism is always present.
Prosthetic endocarditis is discussed in Chap. 25.

A. Presentation. Degeneration of porcine valves usually becomes clinically significant approximately one decade after implantation. Its presence may result in valvular
stenosis, valvular regurgitation, or hemolytic anemia. In
mechanical valves, regurgitation may be a result of disk
or ball fracture or variance—events less likely to occur
with the use of modern pyrolitic carbon materials. More
dramatically, a disk or ball may escape from its restraining structures because of failure of the valve. This leads to
embolization of the disk or ball with resulting cardiogenic
shock.

Paravalvular leak may occur with either type of valve.
Its timing is an important factor in establishing the diagnosis. Early after implantation, deficiencies relating to
surgical technique and fixation should be suspected,
whereas later episodes should always raise the suspicion
of infective endocarditis.

Thrombosis and embolism occur with both types of valves, but are more common with mechanical valves. Thrombosis of the valve is usually heralded by dyspnea at rest, CHF, angina or auscultatory changes. Physical findings vary for each patient. Previous knowledge and documentation of the auscultatory findings for each patient will greatly enhance the diagnostic yield in early cases.

Hemolytic anemia is a complication common to any prosthetic valve that is related to the generation of excessive blood turbulence by the valvular structures.

B. Assessment

1. **Laboratory.** The CBC is helpful in diagnosing hemolytic anemia and screening for infection. Blood cultures should be obtained in all cases in which infective endocarditis is a possibility; PT and partial thromboplastin time (PTT) test are crucial in assessing anticoagulation status, especially in patients taking oral anticoagulants.

2. **ECG.** The ECG is usually not helpful except when ischemia is suspected.

3. **X-ray.** The CXR may show signs of CHF, and may delineate the type of valve by location. It also can be useful in diagnosing broken mechanical valves. Cineradiography is a valuable diagnostic tool in diagnosing valve abnormalities and in assessing efficacy of treatment in some cases.

4. **Echocardiogram.** Transesophageal echocardiography as well as Doppler echocardiography are the most valuable noninvasive tools in assessing and diagnosing prosthetic valve disease. In many instances, by employing these methods the underlying etiology and the decision to undergo surgical versus medical treatment may be made.

C. Management and disposition. Thromboembolic events are best avoided by maintaining adequate **anticoagulation.** In patients with mechanical valves, an INR of 2.5–3.0 is recommended. In those in whom embolism occurs despite adequate anticoagulation, dipyridamole at 400 mg/d can be added. For bioprosthetic valves, anticoagulation is recommended for the first 3 months for all adult patients. An INR of 2.0–3.0 is desirable. Continuous anticoagulation should be maintained in those patients with a history of embolism, presence of thrombi in the atrium during surgery, or atrial fibrillation.

Once the valvular thrombus forms and is diagnosed, thrombectomy must be performed surgically, especially if hemodynamic instability cannot be controlled. In hemodynamically stable patients, some research has advocated the use of thrombolytics with monitoring of valvular function in an attempt to avoid surgery.

Surgical treatment is indicated for symptomatic cases of valvular stenosis or regurgitation or if there is severe regurgitation on Doppler. Surgery is also indicated in those cases in which hemolysis is severe and the hematocrit cannot be maintained despite iron and folate therapy.

Consultation with a cardiologist or cardiovascular surgeon is necessary and should be obtained as soon as prosthetic valvular dysfunction is suspected.

Bibliography

Braunwald E. *Heart Disease: A Textbook of Cardiovascular Medicine* (4th ed.). Philadelphia: Saunders, 1992.

Burge DJ, DeHoratius RJ. Acute Rheumatic Fever. In Brest AN, Frankl WS (eds.), *Valvular Heart Disease: Comprehensive Evaluation and Treatment.* Philadelphia: F. A. Davis, 1993.

Hancock EW. Valvular Heart Disease. In Federman DD, Rubenstein E (eds.), *Scientific American Medicine.* New York: Scientific American, Inc., 1992.

Hurst WJ, Schlant J. *The Heart, Companion Handbook* (7th ed.). New York: McGraw-Hill, 1990.

Khan SS, Gray RJ. Valvular emergencies. *Cardiol Clin* 9:689–709, 1991.

Pacemakers and Implantable Defibrillators

Charles J. Love

I. **Pacemaker emergencies.** Since the first pacemaker was implanted in 1958, the features and complexity of pacing systems have evolved rapidly. The primary purpose of the pacemaker continues to be the delivery of an electrical stimulus via an electrode (also known as the "lead") to the myocardium. Though true malfunction of the pacemaker is relatively uncommon, the pacing lead continues to be the source of many problems. However, the most common source of pacemaker-related consults is now "pseudomalfunction" of the pacing system. This is due to a general lack of understanding regarding the function of the newer, sophisticated pacing systems, as well as from artifacts generated by the newer ECG monitoring systems.

Pacemaker technology continues to advance rapidly. Many of the newer devices now pace both the atrium and ventricle (dual-chamber pacemakers). In addition, newer devices are capable of changing the pacing rate by using an independent sensor. Sensors may increase the paced rate in response to body vibration, body movement, increased minute ventilation, increased blood temperature, or other physiologic changes depending on the sensor type. Many of the currently implanted pacing systems use a bipolar lead that results in a small and sometimes invisible pace artifact. If the pace artifact is not noted on the ECG, misinterpretation of the ECG is common. It is even possible to misdiagnose an increased pacing rate as ventricular tachycardia.

A. **Indications for permanent pacing.** The most recent guidelines for implantation of permanent pacemakers were published jointly in the *Journal of the American College of Cardiology* and in *Circulation* in 1991. The recommendations are summarized in Table 27-1. These guidelines cover most situations for which pacemakers will be implanted. One newer and evolving indication is the use of pacing in patients with idiopathic hypertrophic subaortic stenosis (IHSS). The use of pacing to "preexcite" the apical portion of the heart has been shown to reduce the aortic outflow gradient in these patients.

B. **Classification of pacemakers.** Pacemaker function is classified through the NBG code (**N**orth American Society of Pacing and Electrophysiology/**B**ritish Pacing and Electrophysiology **G**roup). This is a 5-position code that denotes the pacing, sensing, sensor, and antitachycardia functions of a pacemaker (Table 27-2). Most pacemakers can be described using the first three letters of the code, with addition of the fourth letter "R" only when a sensor is active. Other letters in the fourth position are not routinely used. Letters in the fifth position are added only if antitachycardia functions are present. Thus, a dual-chamber pacemaker with pacing and sensing functions in both atrium and ventricle would be de-

Table 27-1.   Pacemaker implant guidelines

Symptomatic sinus node dysfunction
Symptomatic AV block
Persistent AV block post MI
AV block to catheter ablation
Bradycardia-tachycardia syndrome
Carotid sinus hypersensitivity
Neuro-cardiogenic syncope (severe cardioinhibition)
Bi- or trifascicular block with syncope

Table 27-2.   NASPE/BPEG codes

First position indicates the chamber paced.
  V = ventricle
  A = atrium
  S = single*
  D = dual
  O = no pacing
Second position indicates the chamber sensed.
  V = ventricle
  A = atrium
  S = single*
  D = dual
  O = no sensing
Third position indicates the response to a sensed event.
  I = inhibited
  T = triggered/tracking
  D = dual
  O = no response
Fourth position indicates programmability and rate response.
  O = not programmable
  P = simple programming (3 functions or fewer)
  M = multiprogrammable (more than 3 functions)
  C = communicating (M + telemetry capabilities)
  R = rate responsive
Fifth position indicates antitachyarrhythmia functions.
  O = none
  P = pacing
  S = shock
  D = dual

* Manufacturer's designation for single-chamber device that may be
implanted in either the atrium or ventricle.

scribed as "DDD." The same device with an activated sensor would be a "DDDR."

DDD and VDD pacing modes are capable of "tracking" or following the sensed atrial rhythm by following each atrial sensed event with a pace into the ventricle. The behavior of a pacemaker programmed to a tracking mode is quite similar to a normal AV node. One can see Wenckebach (Mobitz-I) and 2:1 (Mobitz-II) type blocks. Other dual-chamber modes such as DDI and DVI may pace both chambers but are not able to track the atrial rhythm. These modes are useful in patients with intermittent atrial arrhythmias. To allow the use of DDD in patients with intermittent atrial dysrhythmias, automatic mode switching is now used. This allows the pacemaker to follow the atrial rate in most conditions. However, if a pathologic atrial rate is detected (e.g., atrial fibrillation or flutter), the pacemaker will temporarily change to a nontracking mode such as VVI or DDI. The device resumes tracking function if and when the atrial rate falls back into an acceptable rate range.

There are two types of **lead configurations:** unipolar and bipolar. In a unipolar configuration, the cathode (negative electrode) is in the heart and the anode (positive electrode) is provided by the metal pacemaker case. This results in a large "spike" on the ECG when a pace output occurs. In a bipolar configuration the anode is also in the heart. Due to the very small inter-electrode space, the pace artifact on the ECG is usually quite small. One must recognize that even though a bipolar lead is present, pacing and sensing may not be bipolar. Most newer pacemakers allow independent programming of pacing and sensing in each chamber to unipolar or bipolar.

C. **Etiology and types of pacing system problems.** Pacemaker problems may be due to a number of different causes. The time of malfunction discovery relative to the implant may provide a clue as to the most likely etiology. It is extremely helpful, if not essential, to obtain information about the model of the pacemaker and the current programming of the device. The model may be obtained from an identification card that most patients carry. If they do not have this card with them, the implanting physician or hospital may be able to provide the implant data. Programmed information is carried by some patients with their card, or it may be obtained from the pacemaker using the programming device. If the manufacturer and model are not known, a radiograph of the device will allow its identification by radio-opaque logo or by the characteristic appearance of the circuitry.

Pacing problems tend to fall into several broad categories: **failure to output, output with failure to capture, failure to sense, oversensing,** and **pacing rate problems.** A logical method of dealing with a suspected malfunction is to identify which of these conditions exists, confirm that the behavior is abnormal, and then seek to provide the appropriate corrective action.

II. Approach to the patient with pacemaker complications

A. Pacemaker failure to output.
This is a potentially life-threatening situation if the patient is completely or almost completely dependent on the pacemaker to maintain an adequate heart rate. The patient may present with syncope, presyncope, palpitations, or seizure or else be asymptomatic. The causes of failure to output are listed in Table 27-3.

A patient presenting with a slow heart rate and syncope, seizure, or presyncope may require emergent heart rate support. This may be accomplished with an external cutaneous pacemaker or by transvenous temporary pacing. In some situations where the cause of the bradycardia is due to failure to pace from oversensing, **a strong magnet may be placed over the device to force asynchronous pacing.** It is important to note that a multiple-lead ECG recording may be necessary to differentiate between no output conditions and output with failure to capture (see below). The pacemaker "spike" may be quite difficult or impossible to see in some leads, especially in those programmed to a bipolar output. Definitive therapy usually requires surgical intervention to replace the device or lead in most no-output conditions. Rarely, the device has been reset or reprogrammed to an "OOO" mode and can be programmed back to a functional state.

Crosstalk is an uncommon cause of failure to output a ventricular pulse after an atrial pulse is delivered. This may occur when the ventricular lead senses and is inhibited by its own atrial output. As the ventricle is "looking" for a QRS in the range of 2 mV, and the atrial output is typically 2.5 V (2500 mV) or higher, it can be seen that sensing of the latter could easily occur. The pacemaker has features to prevent this (ventricular blanking period) or to detect this problem and deliver a rescue pulse (safety pacing). Though now this is rarely seen, it should be considered when atrial pacing is seen without ventricular output.

Table 27-3.   Causes of failure to output

Battery failure

Circuit failure

Lead conductor coil failure

Lead insulation failure

Oversensing

Crosstalk

Improper positioning of lead in the pacemaker

Pseudomalfunction

   Bipolar spike not seen

   Hysteresis

   Unrecognized intrinsic activity

Table 27-4. Causes of failure to capture

Lead movement
Elevated capture threshold
Myocardial infarction
Metabolic/electrolyte disturbance
Antiarrhythmia drugs
Defibrillation
Electrocautery
Myocardial perforation
Inappropriate lead placement
Poor electrical connection of lead
Lead conductor coil failure
Lead insulation failure
Battery failure
Circuit failure
Pseudomalfunction
    Recording artifacts
    Pace during physiologic refractory period

B. Pacemaker stimulus present but fails to capture.
This condition may occur as a result of many causes (Table 27-4). The emergency physician should be especially alert to metabolic and electrolyte abnormalities such as those occurring after a cardiac arrest, renal insufficiency, and diabetic ketoacidosis that may increase the amount of energy required to pace the heart. This may cause an apparent malfunction because loss of capture resolves as the metabolic problem is corrected.

The ECG will show pacemaker artifact but a failure of the stimulus to capture the heart (Fig. 27-1). One must be aware that a stimulus may fall into the physiologic refractory period of the myocardium and therefore would not be expected to capture. The latter is usually the result of undersensing the intrinsic beat and is not related to a capture problem. One also must be aware of the propensity of modern ECG recording systems to place false artifacts on

Fig. 27-1. Failure to capture. Note the presence of pace artifact occurring at the appropriate time (programmed VVI at 75 bpm) without evidence of ventricular capture.

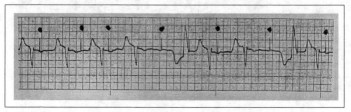

a recording due to their pacemaker enhancement circuitry. This feature artifically enhances the pacemaker artifact to make it more visible. However, any electrical transient (such as a loose recording electrode) or strong electromagnetic interference may cause the system to place additional artifacts on the recording.

If the patient is unstable because of bradycardia, action to establish an adequate heart rate utilizing temporary pacing as described above should be initiated. If the output pulse of the pacemaker was set too low to consistently capture the heart or if the lead has dislodged, increasing the energy output of the pacemaker may establish consistent capture. Correction of metabolic derangement or hypoxemia may restore capture rapidly as noted above. Because each manufacturer has a proprietary programmer for their pacemakers, the necessary equipment to change the pacemaker programming may not be readily available in many settings. A manufacturer's representative or the hospital's pacemaker service may be called to adjust the device if necessary. It would be a good policy to have the phone numbers of the appropriate personnel readily available should adjustment be required.

C. **Failure to sense.** Some patients present with undersensing of the QRS or P wave, causing the pacemaker to deliver a stimulus even though the patient has a beat of his or her own. This may cause constant or intermittent asynchronous pacing, which should not be confused with fusion or pseudofusion. **Fusion** occurs when a pacemaker output and intrinsic beat occur at the same time (Fig. 27-2). Patients may note palpitations or "skips" due to the extra systoles caused by the pacemaker's failure to sense intrinsic beats. Failure to sense is rarely a medical emergency. However, there is a possibility that a critically timed pacemaker stimulus could initiate an arrhythmia in a susceptible patient. Treatment for this malfunction usually requires reprogramming the pacemaker to a more sensitive setting, repositioning the lead to a more optimal position, or replacing a defective lead. Some undersensing

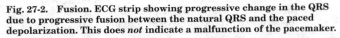

Fig. 27-2. Fusion. ECG strip showing progressive change in the QRS due to progressive fusion between the natural QRS and the paced depolarization. This does *not* indicate a malfunction of the pacemaker.

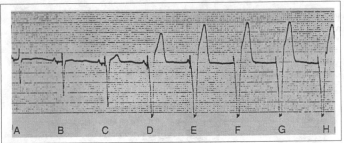

may be transient, such as that seen with electrolyte abnormalities or after the patient is defibrillated.

D. Oversensing. Oversensing of external or internal electrical signals has become increasingly uncommon with the use of bipolar pacing systems. Since unipolar systems use the pacemaker can as the anode, it is possible to sense the electrical activity of the pectoralis (or abdominal muscles if the device is located in the abdominal region). This is termed **myopotential oversensing.** In general, the device cannot distinguish between a sensed electrical event that is not a P wave or QRS (e.g., myopotentials) and an actual cardiac event. Therefore, it will respond to any sensed event as if it were a true cardiac event. If the sensed event is in the ventricle, inhibition of the ventricular output will occur. If the sensed event is in the atrium, no atrial output will occur and the device will attempt to "track" the event and deliver a pace impulse to the ventricle. Patients seizing or shivering would be likely to experience this situation. **One may acutely overcome the inhibition by placing a strong magnet over the pacemaker.** This will disable the device's ability to sense and produce asynchronous pacing. Elimination of the source of the false signals also will allow the device to resume normal function. If this is a recurrent problem, the pacemaker may be reprogrammed to a less sensitive setting.

Strong sources of **electromagnetic interference (EMI)** may cause inhibition of a pacemaker. Older devices frequently were affected by the "leaky" nature of older microwave ovens and the design of the pacemakers. Newer pacemakers are encased in metal that reflects most EMI. In addition, the pacemaker circuitry is designed to identify and reject or compensate for nonphysiologic signals. Other strong sources of EMI, such as large electric motors, transformers, and arc welders, may affect pacemaker function. The most common source of pacemaker EMI inhibition in the hospital is the use of surgical electrocautery. This may cause inhibition, tracking behavior, or reprogramming of the device. When present, the inhibition occurs only during power application and ceases when the power is turned off. Cellular telephones currently pose only a minor EMI threat to persons with pacemakers. Generally it is agreed that the pacemaker will be affected only when the antenna of the cellular phone is placed over the device. However, the newer "digital" technology (such as that already used in Europe and soon to be introduced in the United States) may be a significant threat. Devices may be inhibited by phones operating several feet away from the patient. Fortunately, the effect of EMI is usually transient, with normal pacemaker function resuming after the source of EMI is turned off or when the patient gets farther from the source.

E. Rate-related problems. Rate-related problems fall into two categories: pacing too slowly and pacing too rapidly. The reasons that a pacemaker may pace too slowly are listed in Table 27-5. Though battery depletion may cause

Table 27-5. Causes of slow pacing

Circuitry failure
Battery failure
Battery depletion
Magnet mode
Unrecognized or undocumented programming change
Oversensing
Device reset due to interference or electrocautery
Hysteresis

a **slow pacing rate,** most pacemakers will continue to operate normally until the battery is nearly exhausted. One of the more confusing causes of a patient's rhythm falling below the pacing rate is the use of hysteresis. This allows the patient's intrinsic rate to fall below the normal pacing rate. When a secondary lower rate (hysteresis rate) is reached, the pacemaker resumes pacing at the higher rate until the patient's intrinsic rate inhibits the device. When this occurs the device will not pace again until the hysteresis rate is reached again.

Pacing at high rates may have multiple causes (Table 27-6). In the DDD mode the ventricular pacing rate may increase in response to tracking of the P waves. This is normal behavior. However, if the patient develops atrial fibrillation or flutter, most pacemakers will try to track the abnormal atrial rate to the upper pacing rate that has been programmed into the device. In addition, dual-chamber pacemakers are subject to the development of "endless-loop tachycardia." This may occur in susceptible patients, those who are capable of retrogradely conducting a ventricular event to the atrium. When a premature ventricular event occurs and conducts retrogradely to the atrium, the pacemaker senses the retrograde P wave. When the retrograde P wave is sensed, the pacemaker delivers a stimulus to the ventricle, thus perpetuating the

Table 27-6. Causes of fast pacing

Circuitry failure
Battery depletion
Sensor-driven response
Magnet mode
Unrecognized or undocumented programming change
Tracking of atrial rhythms (tracing)
Triggered mode
Oversensing on the atrial channel
Runaway pacemaker
Endless-loop tachycardia

cycle. Another common cause of higher pacing rates is the activation of the rate response sensor. These sensors may respond to vibration, temperature, or increased minute ventilation. As an example, a patient with a vibration-based sensor who is shivering or seizing may experience an increased rate.

F. **Postoperative issues.** There are two common approaches to the insertion of a transvenous pacing system: subclavian venipuncture and cephalic vein cutdown. If the subclavian approach is used, there is a possibility of pneumothorax, hemothorax, and (rarely) chylothorax. With either approach, venous thrombosis, myocardial perforation, pericarditis, pericardial tamponade, and infections may occur. Hematoma formation around the site of the pacemaker insertion is also not uncommon and may be misdiagnosed as infection. Though aspiration of the pocket to differentiate between hematoma and infection may be performed, it should not be performed routinely without other suggestive physical signs or evidence supporting infection due to the possibility of introducing an organism. As more pacemaker insertions are performed in outpatient and ambulatory settings, emergency departments may be seeing more of these complications.

III. **Assessment and treatment of pacemaker complications**
   A. **Assessment**
      1. **Electrocardiogram.** A 12-lead ECG and rhythm strip are mandatory for evaluation. Many of the pacemakers implanted are bipolar (cathode and anode in the heart) and produce only a very small pace artifact. This may be easily missed, even with a 12-lead ECG. Some devices produce extra electrical artifacts due to specialized features. If the ECG recorder used has pace artifact enhancing circuitry, many additional "pacing spikes" may be seen. This can be mistaken as **runaway pacemaker,** a rare catastrophic malfunction during which the device paces at high rates. The artifact may be eliminated by disabling the enhancement circuitry, repositioning the ECG electrodes, or monitoring a different lead configuration. Because true runaway pacemakers result in rapid heart rates, differentiation between artifact and true pacemaker outputs is usually not difficult.
      2. **Chest x-ray.** A posteroanterior and lateral chest x-ray may be useful if malfunction is suspected. During the first month following implant, **lead dislodgment** may occur, resulting in any one of a number of abnormalities. Pacing of the "wrong" heart chamber, frequent ectopic beats, and diaphragm stimulation may occur in addition to sensing and capture problems. After the first month, lead dislodgment is uncommon, and attention should be paid to the integrity of the conductor coils. **Insulation faults** may be difficult to see by x-ray. Any break or discontinuity of the coils requires further evaluation. Some **leads may appear to be fractured** due to the type of construction used.

This is referred to as a "pseudofracture." Without knowledge of the specific lead type and normal x-ray appearance for that lead model, this may be difficult to determine. Particular attention should be paid to the area where the leads pass under the clavicle. This is the most common site of fracture due to compression of the lead between the clavicle and first rib.

B. **Management.** The first priority is to determine if the patient appears to be pacemaker dependent. If pauses are noted without escape rhythm, either transvenous or external **temporary pacing** should be instituted. If oversensing is suspected, placing a **strong magnet over the pacemaker** should cause resumption of pacing. The resultant pacing rate and mode with the magnet over the device will vary with the model of the pacemaker. For most devices, pacing will be asynchronous in the programmed mode. If magnet placement does not cause pacing to resume, oversensing is probably not the sole cause for the failure. If available, the approriate pacemaker programmer should be used to **interrogate the pacemaker.** This may not only allow diagnosis of the problem, but also allow one to "program around" the problem. If the capture threshold has exceeded the programmed output of the pacemaker, then the output may be increased. On newer devices the polarity can be changed from bipolar to unipolar, allowing pacing even if there has been a partial wire fracture in a bipolar lead.

Beyond these remedies, one may have to perform a **surgical intervention** to replace one or more components of the pacing system. Only in the rare occurrence of "runaway pacemaker" must this be done urgently. If this malfunction is present and the ventricle is being paced very rapidly, one must open the pacemaker insertion site and cut the ventricular lead. If the patient is pacemaker-dependent, ventricular asystole will occur and temporary pacing must be established immediately.

Infections are almost always due to *Staphylococcus aureus* or *epidermitis.* Treatment of a pacemaker wound infection (if it is other than superficial) involves removal of the pacing system. As long as the foreign body remains in place, the infection is virtually impossible to clear. Superficial infections of the incision may be treated with antibiotics but often are a sign of more extensive infection. Pocket infections, sepsis, and endocarditis must be treated with device removal and IV antibiotics.

Finally, one must be sure that what is seen is truly a malfunction. The presence of hysteresis, "sleep mode," sensors, and other features that affect the pacing rates and beat-to-beat intervals makes interpretation of the paced ECG very challenging. Before a pacemaker is removed or a determination of malfunction is made, consultation with a qualified pacemaker service or the company representative should be made. Many pacemakers have been condemned as defective and removed, only to find that a special feature was enabled that clearly explained the behavior of the device.

C. **Patient disposition.** If the pacemaker malfunction is corrected by a minor programming change, there is no need to admit the patient to the hospital. However, most other situations will require admitting the patient for a surgical repair. Some patients who are not dependent on the pacemaker or who pace very infrequently may be admitted electively for revision. Data are usually available for patients who are followed closely by a qualified pacemaker center and/or physician. If little is known about the patient, then admission is advisable to prevent abrupt onset of patient symptoms.

D. **Special considerations**
1. **External defibrillation.** When using an external defibrillator for either atrial or ventricular arrhythmias, the paddles should be placed as far from the pacemaker as possible. Most manufacturers recommend a distance of at least 6 cm from the pacemaker. Whenever possible, anterior-posterior paddle or patch placement is preferred. Capacitive coupling from the shock can cause a current to be induced into the lead and can affect the pacemaker or the lead/myocardial interface. Therefore, any time that external defibrillation is performed, it is recommended that the pacing system be evaluated completely by qualified personnel to assure that no damage to the pacemaker or lead system has occurred.

2. **Magnetic resonance imaging (MRI).** The current recommendation by all manufacturers is that MRI should not be performed on patients who have implanted pacemakers. Placement of some pacemakers in the strong magnetic field with pulsing RF energy may result in inappropriate pacing, absence of pacing, or damage to the pacemaker. However, there is new evidence that MRI may be acceptable on newer generation of pacemakers. However, until the manufacturers change their recommendations, it would be wise to avoid this diagnostic modality unless it is absolutely critical to the diagnosis and management of a patient. Should MRI be needed, consultation with qualified pacemaker clinic personnel or a manufacturer's representative is mandatory so that appropriate precautions may be taken and special programming of the pacing system may be performed.

IV. **Implantable cardioverter/defibrillator (ICD) emergencies.** Use of the ICD as a therapeutic modality for patients at risk for life-threatening ventricular arrhythmias has increased at an exponential rate since its introduction in the mid-1980s. This is due in part to the phenomenal efficacy of the ICD in treating sudden cardiac death in high-risk populations, as well as the reduced size and simpler implant techniques that are now available. Early devices were triggered when the ventricular rate increased above a nonprogrammable cutoff rate. Once this occurred, the device charged to its peak output and delivered a shock to the heart. The shock was delivered through patches that were placed directly on the heart through a median sternotomy or lateral thoracotomy. Patients were typically in the hospital for 7 to 10 days after the insertion of the device.

The new devices are now half the size of the original devices and are getting smaller. The therapy they are capable of delivering is far better than that of the original ICDs. Current devices are able to provide "tiers" of therapy that can be tailored to the individual patient's needs, including **backup bradycardia pacing, antitachycardia pacing, low energy cardioversion,** and **high-output defibrillation.** Advances in the energy waveforms now allow reliable defibrillation below 10 joules in many patients. The ICD now can reconfirm the presence of the arrhythmia to avoid shocking a patient who may have had a nonsustained event. Extensive telemetry and diagnostics allow the device to record and play back the intracardiac electrograms that preceded the delivery of therapy. New lead systems are implanted using transvenous techniques, which allows patients to be discharged within 24 hours of device implantation.

A. **Indications for ICDs.** ICDs are indicated for a small number of patients who have survived sudden cardiac death that was not due to an acute myocardial infarction or reversible cause. The approved indications are listed in Table 27-7.

B. **ICD function.** Normal function of an ICD consists of several stages. First, the device constantly monitors the ventricular rate. If the rate drops below the programmed lower rate, ventricular pacing will occur if this function is available on the device. Once the rate exceeds the tachycardia detection rate, the device may allow a delay or a confirmation algorithm and then begin to apply therapy. Tachycardias may even be stratified into "slow," "fast," and "fibrillation" zones. This allows for specific and different types of therapy to be delivered to arrhythmias based on their rate, hemodynamic stability, and patient need. If a monomorphic tachycardia is present, the device may be programmed to use pacing stimuli to "overdrive" the arrhythmia without the need for a shock. If pacing therapy fails or accelerates the rhythm, then shock therapy is delivered. For more rapid tachycardias or fibrillation, shock therapy is delivered immediately. Older devices were "committed" and not able to abort therapy once detection had occurred and charging had begun. This resulted in

Table 27-7.   ICD implant guidelines

Episode(s) of hemodynamically significant VT/VF

Recurrent syncope with VT/VF induced at EPS; no other etiology found

For ICD to be indicated:

No effective/tolerated drug available

Failed drug, ablation, or surgical therapy

Inability to predict efficacy by electrophysiologic testing

Arrhythmia not due to acute MI (within 24 hours of VT/VF)

No reversible cause present (e.g., digitalis toxicity, hypokalemia)

unnecessary shocks to patients who had nonsustained arrhythmias. Newer ICDs allow noncommitted shocks that reconfirm the presence of the arrhythmia during the charging period or just before the shock is delivered.

C. **Postoperative issues.** Consideration of postoperative complications for transvenously inserted ICDs are essentially identical to those listed for permanent pacemakers (see sec. **II.F.**).

D. **Etiology of ICD malfunction.** As with pacemakers, ICDs are very reliable. The lead systems present the major source of malfunction. Problems with ICDs fall generally into two categories: **unnecessary shocks** and **failure to shock.** In our clinic the delivery of inappropriate shocks is the most common type of malfunction.

The overwhelming cause of spurious shocks is the presence of atrial arrhythmias, notably atrial fibrillation. When an atrial rhythm such as sinus tachycardia, atrial flutter, atrial fibrillation, or other rapid atrial rate leads to a rapid ventricular rate, the ICD usually is not able to differentiate this from a true malignant ventricular arrhythmia. This frequently leads to patient shock and presentation to the physician. Some ICDs have additional detection algorithms that require either a sudden onset of the rapid rhythm or stability of the rate to filter out sinus tachycardia and atrial fibrillation, respectively. Though these add specificity, they may decrease sensitivity to arrhythmias that require therapy.

E. **Approach to the patient with ICD discharge.** First, it is imperative to document whether or not a shock truly occurred. Many patients experience what they think is a shock, only to be proven wrong by the shock count telemetered by the device. One common cause is a nocturnal myoclonus that disturbs the spouse who then thinks that a shock has been delivered. Once it is determined that the device has shocked the patient, a determination must be made as to whether it was an appropriate shock. Symptoms such as lightheadedness, palpitations, and chest pain, may provide valuable clues to the presence or absence of a preceding tachyarrhythmic event. The lack of symptoms does not exclude the possibility of tachycardia triggering the device. Most new ICDs have the capability of recording the intracardiac ECG to document the event that led to the shock. Using these tools, ventricular fibrillation and tachycardia may be differentiated from atrial fibrillation with rapid ventricular response, electrical noise, and lead fractures causing false signals.

If the shock was appropriate, evaluation of secondary causes is indicated. **Electrolytes** (including potassium and magnesium) and **antiarrhythmic drug levels** may be obtained as appropriate. An **ECG** to evaluate the patient for acute ischemia is also useful. It is critical to maintain the patient on a monitor and save any rhythm strips that document arrhythmia. **Rhythm strips** that are recorded in the emergency department (ED) or by the emergency squad should be placed on the chart for future reference. The decision to admit the patient to the hospital is made easier in that the patient is "protected" by the ICD. One must remember that the device was placed because the patient was considered to be at high risk for an arrhythmic event. A single event that was terminated by a single shock does not require admission unless a secondary factor requiring correction is present. However, multiple events over a short period of time, or one event that required multiple shocks to terminate, may be indicative of a change in patient substrate or a problem with the system. Patients who receive shocks for no apparent reason should have the system thoroughly tested by qualified personnel. Any evidence of lead failure or device malfunction would require admission for correction if programming the device will not resolve the problem.

When a patient presents with spurious shocks that do not remit, the device should be deactivated using the programmer. If a programmer is not available, a pacemaker magnet may be placed over the middle of the device. The magnet will turn off the antitachycardia functions on some devices after 30 seconds of magnet placement. Other devices are inhibited only as long as the magnet remains in place. Regardless which device used, placing the magnet on the device terminates any antitachycardia therapies but will have no effect on the backup pacemaker function of the device. This is important for patients who utilize the ICD's pacemaker function to prevent severe bradycardia.

An ICD that does not shock the patient or deliver antitachycardia therapy when appropriate may lead to sustained tachycardia and possibly death. The most common cause of failure to shock is a tachycardia that does not exceed the minimum rate at which the device will detect. Changes in drug therapy that cause the tachycardia rate to slow or inappropriate programming of the device are not uncommon. This situation may be corrected by proper reprogramming of the ICD to the appropriate rate detection range.

Bibliography

Barold SS (ed.). *Modern Cardiac Pacing.* Mt. Kisco: Futura, 1985.
Benditt DG (ed.). *Rate Adaptive Pacing.* Boston: Blackwell Scientific, 1993.
Ellenbogen KA (ed.). *Cardiac Pacing.* Boston: Blackwell Scientific, 1992.
Ellenbogen KA, Kay GN, Wilkoff BL (eds.). *Clinical Cardiac Pacing.* Philadelphia: Saunders, 1995.
Furman S, Hayes DL, Holmes DR (eds.). *A Practice of Cardiac Pacing* (3rd ed.). Mt. Kisco: Futura, 1993.

Cardiac Emergencies in the Pediatric Patient

Daniel G. Rowland and David P. Chan

Congenital heart disease accounts for the majority of pediatric cardiac emergencies in infancy, whereas acquired heart disease is more prevalent in late childhood and adolescence. Cardiac arrhythmia, another significant cause of heart disease, can occur at any age. Congenital heart defects have a reported incidence in the range of 5–8 cases per 1000 live births, excluding bicuspid aortic valve and mitral valve prolapse. Many infants with significant cardiac anomalies may be asymptomatic in the first 24 to 48 hours after birth and may not present prior to discharge from the hospital. Since the number of structural, functional, and acquired cardiac conditions is far too great to discuss in detail in this chapter, the discussion will focus on the general presenting pathophysiology: congestive heart failure (CHF) secondary to large shunt lesions or left-sided obstructive lesions, cyanotic congenital heart disease, arrhythmias, and, briefly, acquired heart disease. Many of the acquired disease processes are not unique to children and are discussed separately in other chapters.

I. **Approach to the pediatric patient with congestive heart failure (CHF).** Heart failure is a pathophysiologic condition that results when the pump function of the myocardium is unable to meet the metabolic demands of the body. In infancy and childhood, this condition usually occurs from abnormal work imposed on a normal myocardium from excessive volume or pressure loads, or from intrinsic alterations in myocardial contractile performance. Both physiologic states can exist as a result of congenital or acquired diseases. Table 28-1 lists the various causes of heart failure in infants and children based on the underlying physiologic mechanisms.

A. **Presentation.** The age at presentation can provide important information regarding the specific etiology of the CHF. The timing of key events in the transition from fetal to postpartum circulation has a significant influence on the onset of heart failure when certain underlying structural defects exist. **Closure of the ductus arteriosus** typically occurs in the first few days of life; however, it may remain patent for a few weeks. In coarctation of the aorta or hypoplastic left heart syndrome, as in the fetus, the ductus arteriosus permits perfusion of the systemic circulation by output from the right ventricle. Constriction of the ductus results in decreased systemic perfusion to all or portions of the body, with resultant CHF. In isolated coarctation, the left ventricle may experience a severe, acute rise in afterload as the result of an increase in the degree of obstruction caused by closure of ductal tissue in the juxtaductal aorta. Development of signs and symptoms of heart failure follow closely.

Another major alteration in transitional circulation is the progressive decrease in **pulmonary vascular resis-**

Table 28-1. Etiology of heart failure in infants and children

Excessive volume load

Ventricular septal defect (VSD)

Atrioventricular septal defect (AV canal defect, endocardial cushion defect)

Patent ductus arteriosus (PDA)

Aorticopulmonary septal defect (AP window)

Single ventricle

Valvular insufficiency

Total anomalous venous connection

Arteriovenous malformation

Excessive pressure load

Aortic stenosis

Coarctation of the aorta or interrupted aortic arch

Hypoplastic left heart syndrome

Critical pulmonary stenosis

Alterations of myocardial function

Myocarditis

Cardiomyopathy

   Hypoxia

   Toxins

   Drugs

   Severe anemia

   Carnitine deficiency

Endocarditis

Anomalous left coronary artery from the pulmonary artery

Coronary insufficiency secondary to Kawasaki's disease

Arrhythmias

Supraventricular tachycardia

Atrial flutter or fibrillation

Congenital heart block

tance that occurs over the first few weeks to months of life. In cardiac anomalies characterized by left-to-right shunts, the degree of shunting is directly related to the relaxation of the pulmonary vascular bed. It is unusual for heart failure to develop in patients even with large defects before the third week of life. The presence of associated lesions, atrioventricular valve regurgitation, and anemia may hasten the development of symptoms. Another congenital anomaly that may present with the fall in pulmonary vascular resistance is anomalous left coronary artery from the pulmonary artery.

Table 28-2 outlines the causes of heart failure as a function of age in early infancy. Older infants and children

**Table 28-2. Causes of heart
failure presenting in early infancy**

First 7–10 days of life
Structural anomalies
  Hypoplastic left heart syndrome
  Critical aortic stenosis
  Coarctation
  Interrupted aortic arch
  Obstructed total anomalous pulmonary venous return
  Critical pulmonary stenosis
  Ebstein's anomaly
Arrhythmias
  Supraventricular tachycardia
  Congenital complete heart block

First 4–8 weeks of life
Structural anomalies
  Ventricular septal defect
  Atrioventricular septal defect
  Single ventricle
  Patent ductus arteriosus
  Aorticopulmonary window
  Truncus arteriosus
  Tricuspid atresia without pulmonary stenosis
  Anomalous left coronary artery from pulmonary artery
Arrhythmias
  Supraventricular tachycardia
  Congenital complete heart block

rarely present with CHF secondary to undiagnosed congenital heart disease. Diagnoses such as new-onset cardiomyopathy, myocarditis, or pericarditis are more likely (see Chap. 23).

The clinical manifestations of heart failure in infants and children may be quite different from those of adolescents and adults. A detailed discussion of the compensatory mechanisms, such as myocardial hypertrophy, ventricular dilatation, and increased adrenergic activity, are beyond the scope of this chapter and are discussed elsewhere. The specific signs and symptoms that result from failure of these adaptive mechanisms vary with the underlying pathologic process.

1. **History.** A careful, detailed history can often be the most useful information in helping the clinician determine the presence of congestive heart failure. Many of the physical findings, particularly in infants, can mimic those of more common pediatric ailments such as bronchiolitis. Specific areas of investigation should

Table 28-3.   Signs and symptoms of heart failure in infants and children

History

Infants
  Take longer to feed with frequent breaks
  Fall asleep shortly after beginning to feed
  Sweat excessively with feeds, cry
  Breathe harder and faster than normal
  Not gaining weight well
Older children
  Anorexia
  Decreased exercise tolerance
  Orthopnea
  Chronic nonproductive cough

Physical findings

Infants
  Tachypnea
  Retractions, grunting, nasal flaring
  Wheezing
  Tachycardia
  Gallop rhythm
  Hepatomegaly
  Cool extremities
  Decreased capillary refill
  Diminished peripheral pulses
  Mottled skin
  Peripheral cyanosis
  Central cyanosis (if CHF severe)
Older children and adolescents
  Rales
  Peripheral edema
  Ascites
  Systemic venous distention

be the patient's feeding habits and intake, the presence of significant sweating, the breathing pattern, and growth (Table 28-3).

Feeding represents the most significant form of exercise and energy expenditure for an infant. In the presence of heart failure, the infant's cardiovascular system is already functioning at a higher basal level using the previously mentioned compensatory mechanisms. As a result, the activity of feeding may pose an additional stress that cannot be compensated for by the limited or nonexistent cardiac reserve. The earliest sign is increased respiratory effort during feeding that may or may not exist during rest. The increased respiratory demands often result in the need for frequent breaks between sucking and thus prolong the time required for feeding. A normal feeding time of 15 to 20 minutes may take as long as 45 to 60 minutes. In some cases, the duration of the feeds may not be significantly altered; however, the amount consumed may be diminished because of the infant becoming easily fatigued and falling asleep. The act of feeding may also be accompanied by significant diaphoresis caused by the increased energy expenditure and increased adrenergic state. Older children and adolescents in CHF often complain of anorexia.

Somatic growth, particularly weight, is often affected. Infants with chronic CHF typically are underweight and undernourished. There are several underlying causes of this phenomenon. The alterations in feeding usually result in decreased caloric intake, while the increased work of the heart and respiratory muscles creates a state of increased metabolic demand. Congestion of the gastrointestinal tract results in malabsorption of nutrients. Finally, the redistribution of regional blood flow seen in severe heart failure results in decreased flow and perfusion to organs such as the skin and skeletal muscle. In older children and adolescents, there may be weight loss due to anorexia or weight gain secondary to fluid retention.

2. **Physical findings. Tachypnea** is one of the most consistent physical findings in infants with CHF regardless of the underlying etiology. It is caused by the presence of interstitial pulmonary edema, which can be the result of increased pulmonary blood flow, obstructed pulmonary venous return or left ventricular inflow, left ventricular dysfunction or outflow obstruction, or any combination of the above. As the degree of CHF increases, alveolar and bronchiolar edema result in more labored respiratory effort, accompanied by the development of retractions, nasal flaring, and grunting. It is extremely important to note that wheezing can be a sign of heart failure in infants and should not be simply excused as bronchiolitis or viral syndrome in this age group. The presence of rales is rare in infants and becomes more common with advancing age. Chronic cough may also be present at any age.

Central **cyanosis** can be seen as the result of impaired gas exchange due to the presence of edema at the alveolar level. This is typically an indicator of moderately severe CHF. Peripheral cyanosis can also be seen secondary to poor peripheral perfusion.

Sinus **tachycardia** represents a compensatory mechanism resulting from increased adrenergic tone. In pathologic conditions where there is diminished stroke volume (i.e., dilated cardiomyopathy) or congenital defects with large left-to-right shunts, systemic cardiac output is maintained by increased heart rate. Caution should be taken not to confuse a compensatory sinus tachycardia with a supraventricular tachyarrhythmia presenting with heart failure. In general, infants with sustained heart rates of more than 230 bpm should be strongly suspected of having an arrhythmia. A gallop rhythm may be due to the presence of a third and/or fourth heart sound.

Cardiac **murmurs** can be highly variable depending on the underlying lesion and are typically nondiagnostic. The absence of these findings in no way excludes heart disease, because infants and children with significant dilated cardiomyopathy may have few to no auscultatory abnormalities. Palpation of the chest may demonstrate a hyperactive precordium with displacement of the left ventricular (LV) impulse or the presence of a right ventricular (RV) heave or tap. These findings are also nonspecific and can be found in numerous cardiac etiologies.

Peripheral **pulses** may be diminished to some degree in all infants and children with congestive heart failure. In infants less than 1 month of age, the finding of markedly diminished, absent, or differential pulses between upper and lower extremities should strongly suggest obstructive lesions of left ventricular outflow. In lesions such as patent ductus arteriosus (PDA) and arteriovenous malformations, peripheral pulses may be bounding. There is a wide pulse pressure because of the large diastolic runoff into the low-resistance pulmonary or venous circulations. Other findings of low systemic perfusion include cool extremities, mottled skin, and delayed capillary refill.

Peripheral **edema,** venous distention, and ascites in older children, as in adults, are signs of systemic venous congestion associated with significant right heart failure. These findings are extremely unusual in infants. Enlargement of the liver due to passive congestion is the most common finding in infancy and can be seen in both right and left heart failure. Hepatomegaly should be distinguished from liver displacement secondary to lung hyperinflation and flattening of the diaphragm seen with bronchiolitis. In addition to an increased span, the liver may be pulsatile in the presence of significant right atrioventricular valve regurgitation. In newborns with severe CHF, jaundice may be secondary to liver congestion and impaired bilirubin metabolism.

B. **Assessment**
   1. **Radiologic studies.** Any patient suspected of having CHF should have a routine chest x-ray (CXR) performed, including any infant presenting with wheezing for the first time. With the exception of obstructed total anomalous pulmonary venous return, cardiomegaly should be present. If the patient is known to have existing heart disease, careful comparison with previous films is necessary to evaluate any incremental changes. There should be a variable degree of pulmonary vascular congestion depending on the severity of

the heart failure and the underlying pathology. Significant cardiomegaly in the absence of pulmonary vascular congestion should raise the possibility of a large pericardial effusion. Other findings may include hyperinflated lung fields and pleural effusions.

2. **Electrocardiogram.** There are no specific ECG findings that are diagnostic of CHF. Ventricular hypertrophy, atrial enlargement, axis deviation, and T wave changes are relatively nonspecific indicators of the underlying etiology. An exception would be the presence of significant left axis deviation with a mean frontal-plane QRS axis between -60 and -150 degrees, which strongly suggests the presence of an atrioventricular septal defect, either as an isolated defect or as part of a more complex condition. The ECG can be extremely helpful in determining the presence of an underlying arrhythmia or myocardial ischemia, which can be seen in anomalous left coronary artery from the pulmonary artery or Kawasaki disease.

3. **Laboratory studies.** In patients with evidence of significant respiratory or cardiovascular compromise, an arterial blood gas (ABG) analysis can detect the presence and degree of metabolic or respiratory acidosis, hypoxemia, and the presence of impending respiratory failure. Serum electrolytes may reveal underlying life-threatening derangements, especially hypokalemia in patients already receiving chronic therapies such as furosemide and digoxin. Hyponatremia may be present secondary to excessive water retention. A complete blood count with differential analysis can demonstrate evidence of severe anemia or infection as an underlying cause. It should be noted that patients in CHF can have a leukocytosis with a slight left shift.

C. **Management.** Because of the large number of potential underlying etiologies, CHF cannot be treated uniformly in all pediatric patients. After the diagnosis of heart failure has been established, therapeutic interventions should be aimed at removing any precipitating or aggravating causes, decreasing metabolic demands, relieving pulmonary congestion, and improving systemic perfusion and oxygen delivery (Table 28-4). Treatment of the underlying cause requires identification of the specific diagnosis and often surgical intervention, both of which may not be available in the emergency setting.

1. **Remove precipitating or aggravating causes.** Treat any underlying **arrhythmias** when present. Tachyarrhythmias should be converted to normal sinus rhythm by medical therapy, electrical cardioversion or defibrillation. The specific treatment for various arrhythmias is discussed later in the chapter. Life-threatening bradyarrhythmias should be treated with an external pacemaker or with temporary transvenous pacing when available. Correct significant **anemia.** Restrict **fluid** and salt intake.

2. **Decrease metabolic demands.** Endotracheal **intubation** with mechanical ventilation is crucial. In

Table 28-4.   Medical management strategies of CHF in pediatric patients

1. Remove any precipitating or aggravating factors.
   Transfuse for severe anemia.
   Treat arrhythmias.
   Restrict fluid and salt.
2. Reduce metabolic demands.
   Reduce fever.
   Bed rest
   Sedate agitated patients.
   Endotracheal intubation and ventilation
3. Relieve pulmonary congestion.
   Diuresis (furosemide 1 mg/kg IV/PO)
   Mechanical ventilation with PEEP
   Morphine sulfate (0.05–0.10 mg/kg IV/IM)
4. Improve myocardial performance and oxygen delivery.
   Inotropes (dobutamine, dopamine)
   Afterload reduction (nitroprusside)
   Preload reduction (nitroprusside, nitroglycerin)
   Oxygen (use cautiously in suspected left-to-right shunt lesions)
   Prostaglandin E_1 (0.1 µg/kg/min) for left heart obstructive lesions
   Correct metabolic acidosis with $NaHCO_3$ (1–2 mEq/kg).

patients with significant respiratory effort, this can significantly diminish the demands on the myocardium. Patients who are not in need of intubation should be oxygenated by whatever means possible, guided by blood gases or pulse-oximetry. In cases of severe pulmonary edema, endotracheal intubation with the use of positive end-expiratory pressure (PEEP) may help control the pulmonary edema and improve gas exchange.

Reduce **fever** if present using antipyretics. **Agitated** patients should be sedated. Morphine sulfate administered in doses of 0.05–0.10 mg/kg IV or IM can be used for patients who are particularly restless.

3. **Relieve pulmonary congestion.** Diuresis should be initiated by pharmacologic therapy. Loop **diuretics,** such as furosemide and ethacrynic acid, act by inhibiting active reabsorption of chloride in the distal loop of Henle, ultimately causing excretion of excess sodium and water. They have the advantage of existing in both oral and parenteral forms with relatively rapid onset of action. Furosemide 1 mg/kg given IV or IM should be used in cases of severe CHF with pulmonary edema. In less severe failure, oral dosing at 1–2 mg/kg 2 to 4 times daily should be adequate. Other diuretics, such as thiazide diuretics and aldosterone antagonists, should be reserved for chronic therapy. Aggres-

sive treatment with loop diuretics will increase potassium loss and may result in significant hypokalemia. Electrolytes should be monitored closely.

Morphine therapy can be used to improve pulmonary hemodynamics. In addition to the previously mentioned sedative effects, morphine both reduces systemic arterial resistance and increases systemic venous capacitance. This will decrease both the afterload and preload imposed on the myocardium and may improve pulmonary edema.

4. **Improve systemic perfusion and oxygen delivery.** Systemic perfusion or cardiac output is determined by the physiologic principles of preload, afterload, contractility, and heart rate. Therapy aimed at improving cardiac output should address these determinants.

   a. **Inotropic agents.** In the acute setting, parenteral agents are most efficacious in augmenting myocardial performance. Beta$_1$-adrenergic receptor agonists are the inotropic agents of choice. **Dobutamine** infused at rates of 10–20 μg/kg/min produces a positive inotropic effect with minimal chronotropic changes. Stimulation of beta$_2$-adrenergic receptors produces peripheral vascular dilatation, reducing left ventricular afterload and further augmenting cardiac output. Other agents, such as isoproterenol, have similar effects, but their potent chronotropic effects often limit their use.

   Low-dose **dopamine** (3–6 μg/kg/min) also produces vasodilation through stimulation of dopaminergic receptors with selectivity for the renal, mesenteric, cerebral, and coronary vascular beds. Higher-dose dopamine should be avoided because of the potential negative effects on intracardiac shunting and increased afterload placed on the ventricular myocardium. Digoxin should be reserved for more stable patients and long-term therapy.

   b. **Vasodilator therapy.** Vasodilators can influence afterload and/or preload, depending on their site of action. Arterial vasodilators can effectively reduce systemic vascular resistance and thus afterload while improving peripheral perfusion. Venous vasodilators can dramatically reduce preload by increasing venous capacitance and venous pooling. As with inotropic agents, IV vasodilators that are titratable and short-acting are preferable. **Sodium nitroprusside** affects both the arterial and venous vascular beds. **Nitroglycerin** has primarily venodilatory properties. The major adverse reaction to initiation of any vasodilator is hypotension. Sudden changes in preload may result in inadequate filling pressures and decrease cardiac output. In the setting of decreased contractility, the myocardium may be unable to increase cardiac output adequately in response to significant arterial vasodilation. Therefore, careful monitoring of blood pressure is essential during therapy. Hypotension can be avoided by

initiating low-dose therapy and titrating as tolerated. An initial infusion of nitroprusside at 0.5
µg/kg/min can be used safely in most patients. If hypotension occurs, treating with volume expansion
and concurrently decreasing or discontinuing therapy is usually adequate. In rare situations, vasoconstrictors may be necessary.

c. **Oxygen therapy.** As CHF worsens, gas exchange
at the alveoli becomes progressively impaired. Administration of humidified oxygen may improve
oxygen delivery to the peripheral tissues. It should
be emphasized strongly that oxygen therapy in patients with large left-to-right shunt lesions such as
ventricular septal defect, PDA or atrioventricular
septal defect may actually result in acute worsening of their condition. This occurs as a result of
oxygen's ability to lower pulmonary vascular resistance and raise systemic vascular resistance, both
serving to increase the amount of left-to-right
shunting.

d. **Prostaglandin therapy.** When there is evidence
from the history and clinical findings to suggest a
ductal-dependent circulation such as in coarctation, interrupted aortic arch, critical aortic stenosis, or hypoplastic left heart syndrome in a
newborn infant, **prostaglandin E$_1$** (PGE$_1$) is often
lifesaving. Ductal dilation permits improved systemic perfusion via the right ventricle while decreasing pulmonary congestion. PGE$_1$ should be
administered by continuous IV infusion at a rate of
0.1 µg/kg/min. The major side effects of PGE$_1$ administration are hypotension secondary to vasodilation, respiratory depression with apnea, and
irritability, with the latter two symptoms related to
central nervous system effects. If the patient is not
already intubated prior to initiation of therapy, the
patient should be placed on cardiorespiratory monitors and the equipment and personnel should be
readily available in anticipation of potential apnea.
Any patient who will require transfer to another
hospital should be electively intubated and ventilated before transport.

5. **Correct metabolic derangements.** Many infants
with left-sided obstructive lesions present with metabolic acidosis due to poor tissue perfusion and lactic
acid production. Often, reestablishing distal perfusion
with prostaglandin will have a major influence on correcting this problem. In the setting of severe acidosis,
however, myocardial performance is greatly diminished and correction of the acidosis with sodium bicarbonate in 1–2 mEq/kg aliquots is necessary.

D. **Disposition.** The prognosis for an infant or child presenting with congestive heart failure is highly variable and depends a great deal on the underlying pathology. The
long-term outlook, therefore, relies upon a specific and accurate diagnosis. This may not always be available in the

emergency setting because of the need for specialized diagnostic testing such as two-dimensional echocardiography and cardiac catheterization, and the need for trained physicians, including pediatric cardiologists and cardiothoracic surgeons, to interpret and implement more diagnosis-specific interventions. Unfortunately, these personnel and technologies are typically available only at regional tertiary care pediatric centers. Regardless of the etiology, however, the morbidity and mortality of CHF can be significantly altered by appropriate recognition and initial management in the emergency department.

II. **Approach to the pediatric patient with cyanosis.** The presentation of a child who is cyanotic can be dramatic. Appropriate management requires a logical approach to reach a general division of the various diagnoses that can be associated with cyanosis. Differentiation must be made to determine if the etiology of the hypoxemia is secondary to respiratory or cardiac disease. Pneumothorax, airway obstruction, and severe bronchospasm are examples of the most common respiratory causes for cyanosis. A complete discussion of the other causes is beyond the scope of this chapter. This section will address the general approach to the cyanotic child with suspected cardiac disease. Understanding some general concepts of cardiac physiology in each of the cyanotic heart lesions will guide the emergency physician to the appropriate management plan.

Children with a cyanotic heart defect are hypoxic because systemic venous blood bypasses the alveolar capillary bed and enters the systemic circulation. The degree of cyanosis is partly determined by the amount of pulmonary venous blood that mixes with the desaturated systemic return. This mixing can occur at various levels, in the atrium, in the ventricles, or across the ductus arteriosus. For most of the lesions with decreased pulmonary blood flow, the major determinant to the degree of desaturation is the severity of obstruction of flow to the pulmonary circulation. For the other lesions, the amount of mixing of saturated and desaturated blood will dictate the degree of cyanosis.

A. **Presentation.** As with acyanotic and obstructive lesions, the age of the child at the time of presentation with previously unrecognized cyanosis is helpful in narrowing the list of differential diagnoses. Children with cyanotic congenital heart disease usually present within the first few months after birth. Infants with simple transposition of the great arteries, tricuspid atresia, or pulmonary atresia with intact ventricular septum will usually present in the first week after birth, if not shortly after delivery. Associated lesions such as large ventricular septal defects may lessen the degree of cyanosis and thus delay presentation. The timing of presentation for some lesions is determined by the development of obstruction to pulmonary blood flow. In tetralogy of Fallot, the initial degree of pulmonary stenosis may be quite mild and the patient may experience signs and symptoms related to the left-to-right shunt from the large ventricular septal defect. The infundibular stenosis, however, can be a progressive phenomenon that will eventually result in right-to-left shunting. In an older, previously healthy child who acutely develops cyanosis, it is extremely unlikely to be the result of an undiagnosed cyanotic heart lesion.

1. **Patient history.** Obtaining a careful history from the parents is important in the evaluation of the patient. In the newborn, there may not be much history apart from the cyanosis. Obviously, any suggestion of respiratory symptoms should clue the physician toward a pulmonary process; however, this does not exclude cardiac disease. The history can be of great importance in the child who has known congenital heart disease. Information regarding the underlying **cardiac defect,** current **medications,** and most importantly previous **surgeries** altering the physiology can be crucial in guiding the emergency physician to the appropriate treatment. Table 28-5 lists some of the more common surgical procedures with a brief description of each. If the child is chronically cyanotic, most families will know the "baseline" **oxygen saturation** for their child. Comparing this information with the measured saturation in the emergency department will help determine if there is any acute disease process or interval change. Specific problems seen in children who have undergone corrective or palliative surgery will be discussed separately.

2. **Physical examination.** The examination should always include an accurate documentation of the pa-

Table 28-5. Common operations for congenital heart disease

Procedure	Description
Blalock-Taussig shunt	Subclavian artery to pulmonary artery shunt
Central shunt	Ascending aorta to main pulmonary artery shunt with artificial graft
Waterston shunt	Direct ascending aorta to right pulmonary artery anastomosis
Potts shunt	Direct descending aorta to left pulmonary artery anastomosis
Glenn shunt	Superior vena cava to right pulmonary artery anastomosis
Mustard procedure	Artificial baffle of systemic venous return to the mitral valve (surgery for TGA)
Senning procedure	Similar to the Mustard procedure but uses primarily atrial tissue to construct baffle
Fontan operation	Direct anastomosis of systemic venous return to the pulmonary artery. Modified Fontan includes intra-atrial tunnel of inferior vena cava flow to pulmonary artery.
Rastelli operation	Closure of VSD and an extracardiac conduit for the RVOT

tient's **vital signs.** Shock can present with cyanosis because of poor perfusion and venous stasis of the distal extremities. Examination of the oral mucosa will usually determine the presence or absence of central **cyanosis.** It should be noted that central cyanosis can be masked by the presence of significant anemia. Auscultation of the **lung fields** will determine if there is evidence of pulmonary disease. Children with cyanotic heart defects most often have clear lung fields, with the possible exception of total anomalous pulmonary venous connection, when rales may be present. Many infants with significant cyanosis will also have an increased **respiratory rate** without signs of distress—so-called happy tachypnea—caused by the central nervous system response to hypoxemia.

Surprisingly, auscultation of the heart may not be helpful in arriving at the correct cardiac diagnosis during the general evaluation. The absence of a **heart murmur** does not exclude the presence of congenital heart disease. The presence of a specific type or location of a murmur simply may indicate an associated defect such as a ventricular septal defect or pulmonary stenosis and not the primary anomaly. In the majority of cyanotic defects, the second heart sound is single; total anomalous pulmonary venous connection and Ebstein's malformation of the tricuspid valve are the exceptions, where the second heart sound is usually widely split. In transposition of the great arteries, the second heart sound also may be quite loud because of the position of the aortic valve just below the sternum.

B. Assessment
   1. Pulse-oximetry and arterial blood gas measurement. First and foremost, the presence or absence of central cyanosis needs to be confirmed, and if present, to what degree. Transcutaneous pulse-oximetry is usually readily available and accurate. In some situations a transcutaneous saturation cannot be obtained or the accuracy of the measurement is doubtful, such as in a poorly perfused child. In these situations, an arterial blood gas analysis is essential to determine the oxygenation, ventilation, and acid-base status of the patient.

   2. Radiographic findings. A CXR is important to differentiate the varied cyanotic congenital heart defects as well as to exclude the presence of pulmonary disease. It should be obtained on all patients with the initial presentation of cyanosis. The importance of comparing the present study to any previous CXRs, if available, cannot be more strongly emphasized. Chronic pulmonary changes may mimic an infiltrate, and progressive changes in cardiac size and pulmonary vascularity in the patient with known heart disease may be diagnostic of the underlying pathology.

   On the initial examination, careful attention should be paid to the arrangement of the vital organs. The presence of the stomach on the opposite side of the cardiac silhouette, as in left-sided stomach bubble with dextrocardia, suggests a high probability of a complex heart defect.

Sometimes the shape of the cardiac silhouette may guide the physician to the correct cardiac diagnosis. Patients with tetralogy of Fallot classically have a "boot-shaped" heart because of absence of the pulmonary artery knob and upturned apex. In transposition of the great arteries, the silhouette has been described as an "egg on a string," a shape caused by the narrow mediastinum resulting from the abnormal orientation of the aorta and pulmonary artery. The cardiac shape on the CXR should be used only to collaborate the physical findings and history of the patient.

Unlike the anomalies presenting with CHF, the pulmonary vascularity in cyanotic lesions can be normal, increased, or decreased. The appearance of the pulmonary vascular markings will reflect the physiology of the patient and is critical in the division of the differential diagnoses. Table 28-6 lists the various diagnoses of cyanotic heart disease based on the pulmonary vascular appearance.

3. **Electrocardiogram.** As in the patient with acyanotic heart disease with CHF, the ECG is rarely diagnostic. It may help supprt a diagnosis suspected from the history and physical findings. The presence or absence of sinus rhythm should be determined. Any ventricular hypertrophy, atrial enlargement, and axis deviation should be noted. It should be emphasized that the age of the patient will determine the normal criteria in interpreting any ECG from a child. Tachyarrhythmias do not typically present with cyanosis. However, when present it should be diagnosed and treated appropriately.

4. **Oxygen challenge test.** The patient who presents to the emergency department with cyanosis should be

Table 28-6.   Pulmonary blood flow in cyanotic congenital heart defects

Decreased pulmonary blood flow
Tetralogy of Fallot
Tetralogy of Fallot with pulmonary atresia
Pulmonary atresia with intact ventricular septum
Critical pulmonary stenosis
Ebstein's malformation of the tricuspid valve
Tricuspid atresia with pulmonary stenosis

Normal to slightly increased pulmonary blood flow
Transposition of the great arteries

Increased pulmonary blood flow
Total anomalous pulmonary venous connection
Truncus arteriosus
Tricuspid atresia without pulmonary stenosis

treated with oxygen supplementation. However, a few caveats should be noted. First, children with pulmonary pathology usually have a greater response to oxygen supplementation than children with cyanotic heart disease. Second, in older patients with pulmonary hypertension (Eisenmenger's physiology) as the etiology of their cyanosis, oxygen may blunt their respiratory drive. Such patients should be closely monitored. Finally, as noted in the previous section, oxygen supplementation in the patient with cyanosis and evidence of CHF should be used cautiously. However, if cyanotic heart disease is suspected, especially in a young infant, an oxygen challenge test should be performed. The oxygen challenge test requires documentation of the patient's arterial oxygen level in room air. Oxygen at a concentration at or near 100% is then delivered. After approximately 10–20 minutes, a repeat PO_2 is measured. If the PO_2 increases to greater than 100 mm Hg, the most likely cause of the cyanosis is pulmonary disease. The lack of a significant rise in oxygen tension strongly suggests an underlying cyanotic heart lesion.

5. **Laboratory studies.** Measurement of the hemoglobin and hematocrit is important for several reasons. As mentioned earlier, the presence of anemia can mask partially or completely the presence of significant cyanosis. The finding of polycythemia strongly supports the presence of long-standing hypoxemia, whether secondary to cardiac or to pulmonary disease.

C. **Management.** The specific management of the cyanotic infant or child depends considerably on the underlying pathology. This section briefly reviews several of the more common cyanotic lesions listed in Table 28-6. The difficulty of this type of discussion is the variability in the anatomy within each type of congenital heart defect. For example, in tetralogy of Fallot, the degree of obstruction is extremely variable and is the key determinant of the degree of cyanosis. Furthermore, any surgical intervention may markedly change the expected physiology of the individual lesion. The general approach to these defects will be based on the underlying pathophysiology.

1. **Cyanotic lesions with decreased pulmonary blood flow.** The general pathophysiologic aberration in this group is a decrease in blood flow to the lungs for oxygenation. This results in a relatively smaller amount of oxygenated pulmonary venous return mixing with the desaturated systemic venous blood. The ratio of the two will determine the oxygen level in the systemic circulation. The most common lesions in this category include **tetralogy of Fallot, tricuspid atresia with pulmonary stenosis, pulmonary atresia with intact ventricular septum,** and **critical pulmonary stenosis.** Any therapy for this group of patients should enhance the pulmonary blood flow either by decreasing the degree of obstruction or by augmenting the pulmonary blood flow. The former effect is usually difficult to

produce on an acute medical basis and requires an interventional catheter or surgical procedure. Augmentation of pulmonary blood flow may also be quite difficult medically in the older infant and child, with the possible exception of tetralogy of Fallot, which will be discussed separately.

Newborn infants presenting with severe cyanosis and decreased pulmonary blood flow often can benefit greatly from opening or dilation of the ductus arteriosus with **prostaglandin E₁** (PGE₁). The patent ductus can supply an alternative source of flow to the pulmonary circulation, bypassing any existing central obstruction. As in the critical left-sided obstructive lesions discussed earlier, PGE₁ is administered by continuous intravenous infusion at a rate of 0.1 μg/kg/ min. The major side effects of PGE₁ administration are hypotension secondary to vasodilation, apnea, and irritability. All patients receiving PGE₁ should be carefully monitored for these adverse effects. The medical staff should be prepared to intervene in anticipation of potential apnea or hypotension. Again, any patient who will require transfer to another hospital should be electively intubated and ventilated prior to transport.

a. **Tetralogy of Fallot.** Patients with unrepaired tetralogy of Fallot can be at risk for a hypercyanotic or **"tet" spell.** Hypercyanotic episodes usually occur in the early waking hours. With agitation, the infant may become tachycardic and cyanotic. As a result of the hypoxemia, the infant may become more agitated and thus more cyanotic. Accompanying respiratory distress is usually present. Some clinicians hypothesize that there is constriction of the right ventricular outflow tract (RVOT), which causes further compromise in pulmonary blood flow. Regardless of the mechanism, the relative amount of blood that exits the heart consists of a progressively smaller proportion of oxygenated blood. With continued agitation, this cycle can perpetuate and may lead to death. The presence of a hypercyanotic episode is truly a medical emergency.

The approach to the management of the patient with a hypercyanotic spell is given in Table 28-7. After an initial episode, the child is at marked risk for having recurrent episodes. Therefore, the occurrence of a hypercyanotic spell is an indication for surgical intervention, and appropriate arrangement for admission to a tertiary center should be made.

b. **Ebstein's malformation of the tricuspid valve.** Most patients are diagnosed with this condition in the newborn period because of cyanosis and the presence of a murmur. The cyanosis tends to improve in the first few days of life as pulmonary vascular resistance decreases. The CXR will typically demonstrate marked cardiomegaly even in a newborn infant because of severe insufficiency of the

Table 28-7.   Treatment of hyper-cyanotic spells in tetralogy of Fallot

Knee-to-chest position
Supplemental oxygen
Morphine sulfate (0.1 mg/kg IM or SQ)

If not responding to above:

Obtain IV access.
Repeat morphine sulfate if agitated.
IV fluid bolus (10 ml/kg)
Phenylephrine infusion (0.5–5.0 μg/kg/min—titrate to effect)
NaHCO$_3$ (1 mEq/kg IV)
Propranolol (0.05–0.10 mg/kg IV—maximum dose 1 mg)

If remains critical:

Consider general anesthesia and paralytic agent.
Urgent consultation with cardiothoracic surgery is needed for emergent intervention.

abnormal tricuspid valve and right atrial dilation. Cyanosis, particularly associated with exercise, can return when the child is older. Treatment is limited and most often involves anticongestive therapy with diuretics and digoxin if CHF exists.

There is a 5% to 20% incidence of an accessory bypass tract resulting in Wolff-Parkinson-White (WPW) syndrome in patients with Ebstein's anomaly. These patients can present with peripheral cyanosis if tachyarrhythmias are present. As in all patients with WPW, the presence of atrial flutter/fibrillation secondary to the stretched atrium is especially concerning. Rapid antegrade conduction via the bypass tract can result in ventricular fibrillation. A patient with Ebstein's anomaly and hemodynamic instability should have an ECG to evaluate for any evidence of WPW and tachyarrhythmias.

2. **Cyanotic lesions with normal to slightly increased pulmonary vascularity.** Complete **transposition of the great arteries (TGA)** is the primary congenital heart defect in this category. The primary reason for the cyanosis in the newborn is the presence of parallel circulatory pathways instead of the pulmonary and systemic circulations functioning in series. The systemic venous blood flows through the right atrium and through the right ventricle, and then is ejected back into the systemic circulation. Parallel to this, the pulmonary venous blood circulates through the left atrium, the left ventricle, and then the pulmonary artery. The degree of mixing between the circulations across the foramen ovale, ductus arteriosus, and/or ventricular septal defect, if present, will deter-

mine the level of cyanosis. Almost all patients with simple TGA will present as newborns with intense cyanosis. Children with complicated forms of TGA can present at a later age from a lesser degree of cyanosis.

The lack of mixing of blood between the parallel circulation can lead to death. The immediate therapy should be oriented at improving the mixing of blood. Again, **prostaglandin E₁** (PGE₁) infusion represents the major therapeutic advance that can be lifesaving. In this situation the patent ductus is not necessary to augment diminshed pulmonary or systemic blood flow, but serves as a site to allow oxygenated blood to reach the systemic circulation and vice versa. The dosage and side effects are similar to those previously outlined. Rarely, the administration of PGE₁ does not result in a rise in oxygen levels. In these patients, immediate transfer to a center with expertise in pediatric cardiology for balloon atrial septostomy is needed. Administration of fluid boluses and aggressive correction of metabolic acidosis are intermediate palliative resuscitative maneuvers.

3. **Cyanotic lesions with increased pulmonary vascularity.** In this group of defects, the cyanosis is often variable and can be quite mild, depending on the amount of pulmonary blood flow. CHF often develops in those patients with unrestricted pulmonary blood flow. This category includes **persistent truncus arteriosus, tricuspid atresia without pulmonary stenosis,** and **total anomalous pulmonary venous return.** In patients presenting with mild cyanosis, CHF, and increased pulmonary vascularity on CXR, treating with high-concentration oxygen may result in a rapid decompensation caused by worsening of the CHF. This is similar to the infant or child with a large left-to-right shunt lesion without cyanosis. The hypoxemia is usually mild in this situation and not life-threatening. Immediate management should be directed toward improving the CHF, primarily with **diuretics** (see sec. **I.C.**).

III. **Special problems in the postoperative cardiac patient.** Since congenital heart disease represents a vast collection of anomalies with a variety of surgical approaches used to treat it, it is not surprising that there are unique long-term sequelae. Table 28-5 lists some of the more common operations (past and present) with descriptions of the resulting hemodynamics. Some of the long-term problems can be attributed to the altered hemodynamics and anatomy, and others are the result of the surgical process itself.

A. **Arrhythmias.** Significant atrial and ventricular arrhythmias can be seen in patients regardless of their surgical results. Any patient with previous surgery involving the atrium is at risk for developing rhythm disturbances such as atrial flutter or fibrillation, junctional ectopic tachycardia, and sinus node dysfunction (sick sinus syndrome). These arrhythmias are more prevalent in patients undergoing extensive atrial surgery such as a Senning or Mustard procedure for transposition of the great arteries and are rare after simple secundum atrial septal defect repair. Other conditions, such as atrioventricular valve stenosis or regurgitation, may result in marked atrial enlargement and predispose the patient to these arrhythmias. Ventricular tachycardia is rare in children; however, it can be a significant cause of morbidity and mortality in patients with a previous ventriculotomy. This is certainly true in the patient with previous repair of tetralogy of Fallot, particularly if there is moderate residual RVOT obstruction and pulmonary insufficiency.

B. **Single-ventricle physiology.** In infants born with only one functioning ventricle or atrioventricular valve [e.g., tricuspid atresia, hypoplastic left heart syndrome (HLHS), complex single ventricle, unbalanced atrioventricular septal defect (AVSD)], the surgical approach is oriented toward an ultimate single-ventricle palliative repair, the Fontan procedure. The **Fontan procedure** results in a unique physiologic state not encountered in any other illness. The systemic venous blood is separated from the pulmonary venous return and directed into the pulmonary circulation without the assistance of a ventricle. Staging operations to this final physiology can include a systemic-to-pulmonary arterial shunt or a Glenn anastomosis. Systemic oxygen saturations with a systemic-to-pulmonary shunt, such as a Blalock-Taussig shunt, can vary from as low as the 60s to the high 80s, depending on the size of the graft and the growth of the child. Patients with a Glenn anastomosis usually have saturations in the 80s to low 90s. After the Fontan procedure, if there are no further shunts or fenestrations, saturations should be near normal.

In patients with Glenn shunts, cyanosis with edema of the head and upper thorax warrants evaluation for the presence of an **obstructed superior vena cava.** If this is an acute change, there is a high probability that a clot is present and the patient may be at significant risk for a pulmonary embolism. Fontan patients are also at risk for pulmonary embolism, particularly older patients who have not had a lateral tunnel modification. The right atrium can become markedly dilated over time, creating an ideal situation for clot formation. Most, if not all, patients with a Glenn or Fontan physiology should be on some form of antiplatelet or anticoagulant therapy to prevent this complication.

Protein-losing enteropathy (PLE) is another known complication of Fontan physiology. Patients with PLE can present with CHF marked by significant fluid retention with ascites, peripheral edema, and pleural effusions. These are usually chronic changes and do not present acutely unless ignored by the patient.

C. **Shunt-dependent lesions.** Patients with defects such as pulmonary atresia where pulmonary circulation is totally or predominately dependent on flow across a systemic-to-pulmonary shunt can present with sudden and severe cyanosis and acidosis. Careful auscultation for a continuous shunt murmur should be done. In the absence of a

murmur, the cyanosis should be considered the result of
shunt occlusion until proven otherwise and represents a
life-threatening emergency. The patient should be treated
with fluid boluses and sodium bicarbonate for any existing
acidosis and transported immediately to the closest tertiary care institution where pediatric cardiothoracic surgeons are available.

D. Cerebral vascular accidents. Patients with existing
right-to-left shunts, both pre- and postoperatively, are at
risk for stroke. This risk is significantly increased in patients with chronic cyanosis and secondary polycythemia.
It should be remembered that air emboli from IV lines
may also cause strokes and that filters should be used on
all lines to prevent this occurrence.

E. Bacterial endocarditis. Any patient with an existing jet
lesion, valvular lesion, or prosthetic material (valve, graft,
or patch) is at increased risk for infective endocarditis. Patients in this category who present with persistent low-
grade fever without an obvious source or a history of a
recent dental procedure or poor dental hygiene should be
evaluated for endocarditis (see Chap. 25).

F. Postpericardiotomy syndrome. This syndrome occurs
approximately 1–4 weeks after cardiac surgery in which
the pericardium has been entered (most often open heart
surgery). There is evidence to suggest an autoimmune etiology. The syndrome is characterized by persistent fever,
irritability, and pleural and pericardial effusions. A pericardial friction rub may be noted on examination but may
be absent in large effusions. A CXR may demonstrate
pleural fluid and/or enlargement of the cardiac silhouette
due to an effusion. A leukocytosis with a left shift and elevated sedimentation rate are often present. Treatment for
small to moderate pericardial effusions involves bed rest
and anti-inflammatory agents. Both nonsteroidal agents
and steroids have been advocated. Although rare, the pericardial effusions can become large enough to cause tamponade that requires pericardiocentesis.

**IV. Approach to the pediatric patient with tachyarrhyth-
mias.** The majority of pediatric arrhythmias originate from
the atrioventricular (AV) node or above. These tachyarrhythmias are characterized by normal QRS complexes, with the
exception of WPW syndrome, which may have a widened QRS
complex due to antegrade conduction down the bypass tract.
Ventricular arrhythmias are characterized by wide QRS complexes.

The mechanisms of tachyarrhythmias in children are similar to those described in previous chapters devoted specifically to the various types of electrophysiologic disturbances
(see Chap. 16). This section presents some unique caveats on
tachyarrhythmias for children.

A. Presentation. Supraventricular tachycardia (SVT)
is the most common form of tachyarrhythmia among
pediatric patients. The majority of these children have
structurally normal hearts. The mean age of initial presentation is approximately 3 years of age. Typically, the
heart rate at presentation is greater than 230 bpm. Higher

rates tend to occur in younger children and also in children with accompanying congestive heart failure. Sinus tachycardia needs to be differentiated from SVT. An infant with sepsis or severe respiratory distress can have sinus tachycardia with rates that approach 220 bpm. Characteristically, the heart rates in SVT tend to be quite stable with very little variation. In contrast, sinus tachycardia due to anemia, sepsis, or dehydration will tend to fluctuate.

Rarely, newborns can also present with atrial flutter. They usually have structurally normal hearts. In contrast, 75% of older children who present with atrial tachycardia have underlying heart disease. The rate of the tachyarrhythmias can vary between 100 and 400 bpm depending on the atrial rate and the degree of AV block.

Wolff-Parkinson-White (WPW) syndrome is diagnosed by identifying an initial slur or delta wave in the QRS complex on the surface ECG. This represents antegrade conduction down the bypass tract with preexcitation of the ventricular myocardium. The majority of cases present in infancy. Interestingly, during a tachycardic episode, most patients with WPW usually have normal-duration QRS complexes. Frequent recurrences usually warrant chronic medical therapy or, more recently, radiofrequency ablation of the bypass tract.

Ventricular arrhythmias are rare in the pediatric population without a history of underlying heart disease and/or intracardiac surgery. The exceptions are cardiac trauma, illicit drug exposure, and prolonged QT-interval syndrome. Calculation of the corrected QT interval (QTc) is important and can be done by measuring the QT interval in milliseconds divided by the square root of the immediately preceding R-R interval. A normal QTc is less than 440 milliseconds. If prolonged, these patients have a risk for developing Torsades de Pointe and sudden death.

Isolated uniform **premature ventricular contractions (PVCs)** and premature atrial contractions (PACs) are common among infants and children and are usually benign. Treatment is rarely required.

1.   **Patient history.** Typically, an infant or young child with a tachyarrhythmia will present with a history of irritability, paleness, decreased appetite, and/or lethargy for several hours to days. An older child may be able to verbalize complaints of chest pain, palpitations, lightheadedness, and/or nausea. If significant cardiac compromise is present, syncope and/or cardiac arrest may be the initial presentation.

2.   **Physical findings.** The assessment of a child with suspected SVT must include an evaluation of the child's perfusion. Assessment of vital signs and the child's capillary refill can usually be done quickly and efficiently to determine the absence or presence of shock or CHF.

B. **Assessment.** A 12-lead **ECG** is the most accurate way to diagnose arrhythmias. Most patients with SVT have normal-appearing QRS complexes. P waves may or may not be identified. Attention should be directed to identifying any evidence of preexcitation (i.e., WPW) or flutter waves (i.e., atrial flutter). An irregular narrow-complex tachycardia should alert one to the possibility of atrial flutter or fibrillation with variable conduction. Ventricular tachycardia is usually recognized with the presence of wide QRS complexes. In ventricular tachycardia, P waves can occasionally be identified and have no temporal relationship to the QRS. One caveat to remember is that if the patient has a partial bundle-branch block, which is common in postoperative patients, the QRS duration will also be prolonged. However, a direct relationship between the P wave and the QRS complexes usually can be identified.

C. **Management**
  1. **Supportive measures.** In all children with tachyarrhythmias, some basic principles should be followed. The child's airway should be secured if emergency resuscitation is required. Real-time monitoring of the rhythm is needed to determine the effect of any therapeutic intervention. Electrolyte disturbances, if present, should be corrected.
  2. **Specific therapy**
     a. **Supraventricular tachycardia (SVT).** Treatment will depend on the duration of the tachycardia, the heart rate, and the hemodynamic status of each patient. A child who is in shock or CHF represents a true emergency. If an ECG or rhythm strip confirms the diagnosis of SVT, then **synchronized cardioversion** (0.5 joule/kg) should be performed. The amount of energy can be doubled if this is unsuccessful.

     If the patient is not hemodynamically compromised, IV access should be established. **Adenosine** can be given. An initial dose of 50–100 µg/kg (adult dose is 6 mg) should be used. It must be administered as a rapid bolus and followed immediately by a flush with normal saline. If no effect is noted within 1–2 minutes, the dose should be doubled. This can be repeated again within minutes with increasing doses to a maximum dose of 300 µg/kg or 12 mg total in adolescents and young adults. If the drug is effective, a very short episode of bradycardia or asystole will be observed, usually with return to normal sinus rhythm. If the patient converts briefly but reverts back to tachycardia, it is not necessary to increase the dose. Occasionally, flushing of the skin tones and minor coughing may be associated with administration of adenosine. By blocking AV node conduction, adenosine may also unmask atrial flutter waves that may not have been evident when the child was tachycardic. Rare reports have described adenosine administration with deterioration to a ventricular tachycardia or fibrillation in patients with WPW.

     Vagal maneuvers have been used extensively in the past to end an episode of SVT and can be attempted only if the patient is stable and IV access is unavailable. The most common method is to apply an ice bag to the patient's face near the nose bridge for approximately 30 seconds. The success of this procedure is quite variable. The application of direct ocular pressure, another previously described maneuver, is strongly discouraged because of reports of resulting retinal detachment.

Chronic therapy for these patients will need to be individualized to each patient. Cardiology consultation should be sought prior to discharge from the emergency department to ensure appropriate follow-up. Infants with new-onset SVT probably should be admitted for observation and possible initiation of chronic therapy.

b. **Atrial flutter or fibrillation.** Atrial flutter or fibrillation usually requires inpatient management. If the tachycardia is long-standing, the presence of an atrial thrombus needs to be excluded prior to conversion to normal sinus rhythm because of the risk of embolic events. The diagnostic test of choice is echocardiography, from either the transthoracic or transesophageal approach. If hemodynamic compromise is present, especially in the young infant, **synchronized cardioversion** as previously described should be performed. In more stable patients, conversion with medical therapy may be achieved with digoxin and/or **class Ia antiarrhythmic agents.**

c. **Ventricular arrhythmias.** Pulseless ventricular tachycardia and ventricular fibrillation require direct **cardioversion** starting at 2 joule/kg. If unsuccessful, the energy should be doubled to 4 joule/kg and may be repeated a second time at this energy. **Lidocaine** therapy should be initiated. A loading dose of 1 mg/kg should be given followed by a continuous infusion at 20–40 µg/kg/min. In patients with ventricular tachycardia with a palpable pulse but with signs of shock, synchronized cardioversion should be attempted. The initial energy dose should be 0.5 joule/kg. Again, this can be doubled if tachycardia persists.

Patients who are not hemodynamically compromised can be treated with lidocaine at the doses described above. Once stabilization is achieved, the patient will require a thorough hemodynamic and electrophysiologic evaluation so that an appropriate management plan can be developed.

V. **Approach to the pediatric patient with acquired heart disease**

A. **Kawasaki syndrome**

1. **Etiology and presentation.** Kawasaki syndrome is a generalized immune-mediated vasculitis process of unknown etiology. There is a seasonal tendency, with most cases presenting in the winter and early spring

months. About 85% of cases involve children less than 5 years of age, and there is preferential incidence among males.

2. **History and physical findings.** The diagnostic criteria are listed in Table 28-8. The most common presentation is a child with fever and a generalized exanthem. Typically, these children are extremely irritable.

3. **Assessment**
   a. **Radiographic studies.** The CXR is usually normal. Mild cardiomegaly may be seen in the presence of myocarditis.
   b. **Electrocardiogram.** The ECG may show evidence of carditis with prolongation of the PR interval, nonspecific ST-T wave changes, and sinus tachycardia. Evidence of acute coronary insufficiency is usually not present during the acute presentation.
   c. **Laboratory studies.** A CBC may demonstrate a leukocytosis and thrombocytosis. The thrombocytosis may not be present until the subacute phase of the illness, usually in the second week. The erythrocyte sedimentation rate should be elevated. Other signs of generalized inflammation may also be present, including elevated liver enzymes, sterile pyuria, and CSF leukocytosis.

4. **Management.** The major thrust of therapy is directed toward preventing cardiovascular involvement. During the early stages, myocarditis may develop. Approximately 1–2 weeks after the initiation of symptoms, there may be involvement of the coronary arteries that may lead to coronary artery aneurysm formation and later coronary insufficiency. There is strong evidence that administration of IV **gamma globulin** within the first 10 days of the illness decreases the incidence of coronary aneurysm development. This therapy should be administered on an inpatient basis. This will allow for monitoring of any potential arrhythmias and signs of heart failure that can be associated with inflammation of the myocardium. Appropriate anti-inflammatory doses of **aspirin** (80–100 mg/kg/d) should be initiated and continued until all evidence of acute inflammation has subsided. Low-dose aspirin

Table 28-8. Kawasaki syndrome diagnostic criteria

1.	Fever >5 days
2.	Four of the following findings:
	Palmar or plantar erythema and/or digital desquamation
	Polymorphous exanthem
	Bilateral conjunctival erythema
	Erythematous oral cavity (strawberry tongue)
	Cervical lymphadenopathy

(3–5 mg/kg/d) should be continued for antiplatelet effect until resolution of the thrombocytosis.

Close monitoring by a pediatric cardiologist is required for all patients diagnosed with Kawasaki syndrome. A baseline echocardiogram delineating the ventricular function and coronary anatomy should be performed during the acute phase of the disease.

B. Acute rheumatic fever (ARF)

1. **Etiology and presentation.** There is clearly a resurgence of rheumatic heart disease. The incidence of new-onset ARF is currently estimated at 0.5–3.1 cases per 100,000 population. The majority of the cases are seen in school-age children. No sex differentiation has been noted. With a previous history of ARF, the incidence of a recurrence approaches 50%, with subsequent streptococcal pharyngitis.

2. **History and physical findings.** The diagnostic criteria are listed in Table 28-9. It should be emphasized that the diagnosis of rheumatic fever requires documentation of a recent or ongoing group A streptococcal infection. Careful auscultation for the presence of a previously undiagnosed murmur consistent with mitral regurgitation or aortic insufficiency should be performed. The absence of a murmur does not exclude the presence of carditis because there may be subclinical changes detectable only by echocardiography. Tachycardia in the absence of fever may also be a sign of carditis. In severe carditis, there may be signs and symptoms of CHF.

3. **Assessment**

   a. **Radiographic studies.** The CXR is usually normal. Cardiomegaly may be seen in the presence of significant valvular involvement due to aortic or mitral regurgitation.

   b. **Electrocardiogram.** The ECG may show evidence of carditis with prolongation of the PR interval and sinus tachycardia.

   c. **Laboratory studies.** A CBC may demonstrate a leukocytosis; however, it may be normal in a significant number of patients with ARF. The

Table 28-9. Jones criteria for rheumatic fever

Major criteria	Minor criteria
Erythema marginatum	Prolonged PR interval
Carditis*	Elevated ESR
Sydenham's chorea*	Elevated C-reactive protein
Subcutaneous nodules	Arthralgias
Migratory polyarthritis	Fever

To make a diagnosis, one needs two major criteria or one major and two minor criteria plus documented recent streptococcal infection.

* Can assume a diagnosis if present alone with proven streptococcal infection.

erythrocyte sedimentation rate should be elevated. Laboratory evidence of a recent streptococcal infection by rapid strep screen, throat culture, and/or elevated serum antibody titers for streptococcal antigens (ASO, anti-DNAse B, antihyaluronidase, and streptozyme) should be obtained.

4. **Management.** Patients diagnosed with ARF probably should be hospitalized and observed for any signs of carditis. Consultation with cardiology, infectious disease, and rheumatology should be sought. Treatment of patients with ARF is divided into two areas: (1) symptomatic therapy on presentation and (2) long-term prophylaxis. All therapeutic regimens should start with eradication of any ongoing strep infection. This can be accomplished with a 10-day course of oral **penicillin** at 250 mg tid. It may be more effective in some patients to administer a single dose of penicillin G benzathine (1.2 million units if >25 kg and 600,000 units if <25 kg). Erythromycin (50 mg/kg/d; maximum 1 g/d; divided into 3–4 doses) can be used if there is a history of penicillin allergy.

Symptomatic therapy is directed toward decreasing the inflammation associated with this disease and any cardiovascular morbidity. The mainstay of anti-inflammatory therapy involves the use of either **aspirin** or **corticosteroids.** In patients with signs of CHF, inotropic agents, diuretics, afterload reduction, and digoxin may be necessary. Bed rest is required in all patients with ARF, especially in children with evidence of cardiac involvement.

Long-term prevention of recurrent episodes of ARF requires chronic penicillin maintenance therapy. This can be accomplished with IM penicillin G benzathine (1.2 million units every 4 weeks) or with oral penicillin (250 mg bid). Alternative therapy with sulfadiazine or erythromycin can be used.

Bibliography

Chameides L, Hazinski MF (eds.). *Textbook of Pediatric Advanced Life Support.* Dallas: American Heart Association, 1994.

Emmanoulides GC, Riemenschneider TA, Allen HD, et al. (eds.). *Moss and Adams Heart Disease in Infants, Children, and Adolescents, Including the Fetus and Young Adult.* Baltimore: Williams & Wilkins, 1995.

Garson A Jr, Bricker JT, McNamara DG (eds.). *The Science and Practice of Pediatric Cardiology.* Philadelphia: Lea & Febiger, 1990.

Noncardiac Chest Pain

Eric Anderson

Patients presenting to the emergency department (ED) with chest pain represent a significant diagnostic challenge to the emergency physician. The potential catastrophic consequences of a missed diagnosis, in addition to patient and physician anxiety, make the accurate evaluation of this complaint paramount. Properly diagnosing conditions such as unstable angina, myocardial infarction, pulmonary embolus, and acute aortic dissection are lifesaving. These entities will be covered in detail in other chapters. This chapter will center on non-life-threatening causes of chest pain. These clinical entities can cause significant morbidity, expense, and anxiety for the patient if not accurately diagnosed. In all cases, the life-threatening conditions as listed above should be thoroughly ruled out prior to entertaining non-life-threatening diagnoses.

The exact incidence of non-life-threatening chest pain is difficult to ascertain. However, chest pain is the chief complaint in approximately 5% to 10% of ED visits nationwide. It is estimated that approximately 600,000 to 1 million cardiac catheterizations are performed yearly to evaluate chest pain. Approximately one-third of these patients are found to have normal or nonstenotic coronary arteries. These 200,000 or so patients represent only the tip of the iceberg of noncardiac chest pain. The number of patients with noncardiac chest pain who do not undergo cardiac catheterization is staggering. Despite reassurance that the cause of the patient's pain is noncardiac or non-life-threatening, noncardiac chest pain still contributes significantly to patient disability and loss of productivity.

Clinical entities discussed in this chapter include gastroesophageal reflux disease, lower esophageal spasm, musculoskeletal chest pain, psychiatric chest pain, pneumothorax, pneumonia, bronchitis, pleural disorders, sickle cell disease, acute chest syndrome, and herpes zoster. However, there are many other causes of noncardiac chest pain that are beyond the scope of this text (Table 29-1).

I. Gastrointestinal causes of chest pain

A. Gastroesophageal reflux disease. Originally, it was felt that esophageal motility disorders caused esophageal-related chest pain. However, studies with ambulatory esophageal manometry have failed to show a consistent association between pain and esophageal motor anomalies. Ambulatory esophageal pH monitoring, however, has shown a relationship between pH drops that are less than or equal to 4 and chest pain. This implies that gastroesophageal reflux and not esophageal spasm is the primary cause of esophageal chest pain.

1. Presentation. Pain of gastroesophageal reflux disease has been described as burning, squeezing, or tightness in the chest region. Some patients describe it as heartburn. When severe, it can radiate to the neck, jaw, and sides of the chest. Because these symptoms mimic cardiac ischemia, it is imperative to rule out a

Table 29-1.   Common causes of chest pain

Life-threatening causes of chest pain
Coronary ischemia or myocardial infarction
Pulmonary embolism
Tension pneumothorax
Dissecting aortic aneurysm
Borehaave's syndrome

Non-life-threatening causes of chest pain
Mediastinal causes
  Pericarditis
  Mediastinal emphysema
  Valvular disease—mitral valve prolapse
Gastrointestinal causes
  Gastroesophageal reflux disease
  Esophageal motility disorders—Nut-cracker esophagus, diffuse esophageal spasm, hypertension of the lower esophageal sphincter, achalasia
Pulmonary causes
  Pneumonia or bronchitis
  Pleural disorders—cancer, empyema, pleurisy
  Acute chest syndrome of sickle cell anemia
Chest wall causes
  Trauma—contusion, rib fracture
  Costochondritis
  Cervical or thoracic spinal diseases
  Herpes zoster
Psychogenic causes of chest pain
  Anxiety or hyperventilation

---

cardiac etiology of the chest discomfort before pursuing a gastrointestinal evaluation course. Often the pain of esophageal reflux is exacerbated by eating or by drinking hot liquids. Patients often describe a sensation of food caught in their chest.

2. **Assessment.** The typical laboratory and plain x-ray studies available in the ED do not aid in the diagnosis of esophageal chest pain. It is an ED diagnosis of exclusion. Testing patients with a "GI cocktail" of antacids, with or without lidocaine, may ease the pain, but its use as a definitive test should be discouraged because patients with myocardial disease have also reported pain relief with this testing. Further non-ED testing includes:

   a. **Barium swallow.** Esophagitis involves the superficial mucosa; therefore, it cannot be diagnosed by simple barium swallow.

  b. **Endoscopy.** Endoscopic diagnosis of esophagitis is
     confirmed by the presence of friable mucosa, linear
     erosions, or ulcerations.
  c. **Acid challenge.** The Bernstein test is performed
     by installation of 0.1 N HCl into the distal esopha-
     gus in an effort to produce the characteristic pain.
     This test is useful, but not diagnostic, if results are
     positive. Negative results are nondiagnostic.
3. **Management**
  a. **Medications**
     (1) H$_2$ blockers are administered on bid dosage
         schedules. Cimetidine, Ranitidine, Famotidine,
         and Nizatidine are all possible (Table 29-2).
     (2) An alternative is the proton pump inhibitor
         omiprizole, 10–20 mg/d.
     (3) Antacids administered 1 hour after meals and
         especially before bedtime are optional.
  b. **Body position.** The head of the bed should be ele-
     vated and the body should remain in upright posi-
     tion after meals.
  c. **Dietary.** Smaller meals, low-fat meals, and no
     meals before bedtime limit reflux. Weight loss and
     alcohol and smoking cessation are also helpful.
  d. **Surgery—fundoplication.** Surgical therapy
     should be limited to patients with intractable pain
     and anatomic strictures, who are unresponsive to
     medications.
B. **Esophageal motility disorders.** A variety of esophageal
   motility disorders from achalasia to spasmodic conditions
   of the body in the esophagus and lower esophageal sphincter can cause chest pain. These conditions usually are

**Table 29-2. Treatment of
gastroesophageal reflux disease**

Medications
   Cimetidine 800 mg bid
   Ranitidine 150 mg bid
   Famotidine 20 mg bid
   Nizatidine 150 mg bid
Body position
   Elevate head of bed
   Remain upright for at least 1 hr after meals
Dietary
   Small meals
   Low-fat meals
   No eating before bedtime
   Cessation of smoking
   Cessation of alcohol use
Surgery—fundoplication

associated with food intake and dysphagia or odynopha-gia. Dysphagia is the sensation of obstruction when a food or water bolus is swallowed. Odynophagia is painful swal-lowing. Odynophagia is common in nonreflux esophagitis as well as in inflammatory conditions such as monilial or herpes esophagitis, or in esophageal peptic ulcer diseases (i.e., Barrett's esophagitis). Carcinoma of the peri-esophageal tissues can cause a steady, deep, boring type of chest pain.

1. **Achalasia.** Achalasia is a condition caused by defec-tive innervation of the smooth muscle of the distal body of the esophagus. This results in vigorous, unor-ganized esophageal muscular contractions and a hy-pertensive lower esophageal sphincter that does not open normally in response to an esophageal food bolus. The esophageal muscular contractions are prolonged and of greater than normal amplitude. The underlying pathophysiology of achalasia is defective innervation of the smooth muscle portion of the esophageal body and lower esophageal sphincter. Vigorous achalasia has less denervation than classic achalasia. Secondary achalasia may be caused by carcinoma, lymphoma, Shogert's disease, and radiation therapy.

   a. **Presentation.** Symptoms of this condition include chest pain, dysphagia, and regurgitation. Symp-toms are typically brought on by eating or drink-ing. Symptoms are made worse by eating quickly, emotional distress, and the amyl nitrite test. Acha-lasia can affect both genders and all ages.

   b. **Assessment.** In the ED, the chest x-ray may show a dilated fluid level adjacent to the trachea. An emergency barium swallow classically may show a dilated distal esophagus with a very narrow, non-relaxing lower esophageal sphincter.

      At endoscopy, installation of cholecystokinin (CCK) causes contraction of the lower esophageal sphincter. In a normally innervated lower esopha-geal sphincter this would cause a marked decrease in lower esophageal sphincter pressure; however, in the abnormally innervated esophagus of achala-sia this causes a paradoxic contraction.

   c. **Management.** Emergency treatment involves re-assuring the patient that the chest pain is not of coronary or other life-threatening origin. Sympto-matic treatment includes recommendations that the patient take small swallowing boluses of solids and liquids. Gastrointestinal referral is indicated. Definitive treatment involves lower esophageal and lower esophageal sphincter balloon dilatation. Surgical treatment involves a Heller's extramu-cosal myotomy.

2. **Diffuse esophageal spasm, nut-cracker esopha-gus, lower esophageal sphincter spasm, and nonspecific motility disorders.** The pathophysio-logic etiologies of these conditions is poorly un-derstood. Pathophysiologic observations in diffuse

esophageal spasm include diffuse esophageal contractions, only some of which are propulsive. Spontaneous, repetitive, high-pressure, contractile waves of prolonged duration often occur. In nut-cracker esophagus, there are very high amplitude 400 mm Hg propulsive contractions (normal is 0 to 80 mm Hg). In spasm of the lower esophageal sphincter, also known as hypertensive lower esophageal sphincter, pressures exceed 45 mm Hg (normal is 0 mm Hg) during relaxation of the lower esophageal sphincter with swallowing. Hypertensive lower esophageal sphincter may be associated with other esophageal motility disorders. It tends to be associated with nut-cracker esophagus more than with diffuse esophageal spasm. See Table 29-3 for the incidence of each condition.

a. **Presentation.** Symptoms of the above esophageal motility disorders include substernal chest pain that is brought on by eating or emotional stress. The pain may have a cardiac type of radiation pattern (i.e., across the chest, radiating to both arms, or radiating to both sides of the jaw). Dysphagia for solids or liquids may occur with or without chest pain.

b. **Assessment.** Barium swallow demonstrates a normal proximal esophagus; however, the distal esophagus demonstrates multiple peristaltic waves and uncoordinated simultaneous contractions. There may be a "corkscrew" appearance of the esophagus that is typical of the diffuse esophageal spasm. Esophageal manometry may show the typical prolonged high amplitude contractions of the lower esophagus. Lower esophageal sphincter tone is normal or below normal. These abnormalities tend to be episodic and thus, the initial manometry may be normal. Several techniques have been developed to precipitate spasm. The most reliable is ergonovine. However, ergonovine can also cause coronary artery spasm with resultant coronary ischemia. This would not only confuse a diagnostic picture but also cause significant risk to a patient with known prior history of coronary artery disease (CAD). Other precipitating maneuvers or medications tend to produce the esophageal spasms less reliably.

Table 29-3. Frequency of esophageal motor abnormalities

Nut-cracker esophagus	48%
Nonspecific motility disorders	35%
Diffuse esophageal spasm	10%
Hypertensive lower esophageal sphincter	4%
Achalasia	2%

      c. **Management.** In the ED, medications can be initiated including isosorbide dinitrate, 2.5–10.0 mg sublingually before meals, or nifidipine, 10–20 mg before meals. Reassurance and arrangement of follow-up with a gastroenterologist are also indicated. Balloon dilation and longitudinal myotomy of the esophageal circular muscle are also treatment modalities often employed by gastroenterologists and surgeons.

II. **Chest wall pain.** Chest pain secondary to chest wall abnormalities tends to be sharper and more focal in character than chest pain secondary to CAD. This pain typically is elicited by certain body movements or manipulations during the physical exam. Pain of neurologic origin (shingles and cervical disk disease, and paraspinal pathologies) will tend to be radicular and dermatomal. Pain patterns vary with the causative condition (Table 29-4). The following are common causes of chest wall pain.

    A. **Costochondritis.** Inflammation of costochondral and costosternal articulations are the most common cause of musculoskeletal anterior chest wall pain. This condition is often caused by unusual physical activity and occasionally is accompanied by, or preceded by, a viral illness. This chest pain is sharp, focal, and exacerbated by sternal or parasternal compression. Upper extremity movements that cause the pectoralis muscle to contract and place traction on the costosternal area can often reproduce this pain. Tietze's syndrome is the rare objective finding of localized redness, swelling, and heat in the area of the involved costochondral/costosternal articulation. Treatment includes nonsteroidal anti-inflammatory agents and rest. If patients are unable to tolerate nonsteroidals, acetaminophen with codeine is an alternative.

    B. **Shoulder girdle anomalies.** Arthritis, subacromial bursitis, and biceps tendinitis may cause chest discomfort that is typically exacerbated by movement of the involved shoulder. Symptoms are decreased by resting the involved shoulder. Initial treatment involves the use of nonsteroidal anti-inflammatory agents and rest of the involved shoulder. Acetaminophen with codeine is an option for patients with intolerance to nonsteroidals.

    C. **Spinal/paraspinal disease.** Spinal and paraspinal causes of chest pain include osteoarthritis of the thoracic spine, herniated cervical or thoracic disk, costovertebral joint dysfunction, and interspinous ligament disruption. Typically this pain is posterior and paraspinal, sharp and stabbing. The patient may have a recent history of minor trauma or muscular strain. The area is tender to palpation with radicular pain that will follow a dermatomal distribution. Pain is also increased when assuming certain body positions or during deep breathing. There is total relief of symptoms with lidocaine 1% costal nerve block. This is a diagnostic and therapeutic procedure for the condition, but nonsteroidal anti-inflammatory agents are the initial treatment of choice.

Table 29-4. Causes of chest wall pain

	Symptoms	Physical exam	Treatment
Costochondritis	Painful parasternal region	Tender parasternal region to compression (rarely Tietze's syndrome)	Rest Analgesics
Shoulder girdle anomalies	Painful shoulder	Shoulder tender on exam	Rest Analgesics
Spinal/paraspinal conditions	Posterior paraspinal pain with anterior radiation	Involved area is tender to palpation Local skin hyperalgesia/dysesthesia	Lidocaine Intercostal nerve block
Trauma	History of trauma Local pain	Local bruises, swelling, tenderness	Rest, ice, analgesics
Shingles	Painful unilateral (determatomal) chest pain	Normal for 2 to 3 days, then development of vesicular rash in involved dermatome	Analgesics (often narcotic strength) Dameboro soaks Acyclovir

D. Trauma. The aftereffects of trauma may leave the patient with residual chest pain. Rib fractures or chest wall contusions may leave the patient with a painful, tender chest for several weeks. The diagnosis is often apparent from recent history or physical examination. Some patients may require an in-depth inquiry into the patient's recent activities in order to elicit the information to confirm a diagnosis. Treatment is with symptomatic analgesics and rest. Chest wall binders are controversial, and may contribute to atelectasis and subsequent pneumonia.

E. Herpes zoster. Shingles is caused by reactivation of the *Varicella zoster* virus that manifests as painful vesicles in a unilateral dermatomal distribution. There is a prodromal period of pain in the dermatomal distribution before the rash appears. This prodromal pain syndrome might deceive the physician into thinking that the patient may have one of the painful radicular entities identified in sec. **D.** above. The appearance of the rash and culture of the virus from the vesicles is diagnostic. The incidence of shingles is approximately 5 to 10 cases per 1000 persons in the sixth through eighth decades of life. It is most common in the elderly or immunocompromised individuals (i.e., AIDS, chemotherapy, steroids, bone marrow transplant). The pain of shingles, which can be intense and involve the whole dermatome, is not particularly affected by movement or deep inspiration.

Treatment involves the liberal use of analgesics like acetaminophen with codeine. Dameboro soaks provide local soothing and limit secondary infection. Acyclovir therapy, 800 mg PO 5 times daily for 7 to 10 days, accelerates cutaneous healing. It also accelerates the resolution of zoster ophthalmicus for patients with fifth cranial nerve involvement. There is also a decrease of posttherapeutic neuralgia with acyclovir use.

III. Psychiatric chest pain. It has been estimated that 30% of patients presenting to EDs with chest pain have a concurrent psychiatric disorder. It has also been established that approximately 20% of patients with acute cardiac ischemia have a concurrent psychiatric disorder. Emergency physicians must be cognizant of these estimates and be prepared to evaluate these patients.

Panic disorder and depression are commonly seen in patients who present to EDs with noncardiac chest pain. Patients with these disorders will tend to return to the ED for recurrent episodes of chest pain more often than patients without psychiatric disease. In fact, patients with panic disorder are more likely to return to the ED than patients with cardiac ischemia. Patients with depression have also been found to utilize the ED more often than patients with cardiac ischemia. The reasons for this apparent paradox is that patients with these psychiatric disorders are more sensitive to their physical status. This heightened awareness and anxiety about their symptoms tends to lower the decision threshold regarding an ED visit.

Patients with chronic medical illness tend to have a higher rate of psychiatric illness. There are also higher rates of psychiatric illness in patients in which chest pain is part of their chronic medical illness. One study reported that over one-half of the cardiology clinic patients with known CAD and atypical chest pain had panic disorder.

Emergency physicians recognize only a small fraction of psychiatric illness in chest pain patients. At present there is no reliable screening tool to distinguish between patients with psychogenic chest pain and patients with cardiac chest pain. This is an active area of research. Until reliable objective measures for myocardial ischemia have been developed, the physician will have to rely on a good history and physical examination, clinical acumen, and present diagnostic adjuncts (e.g., ECG, chest x-ray) when evaluating patients with chest pain.

One of the more common presentations for psychiatric chest pain is **hyperventilation syndrome.** These patients tend to be young, female, and without underlying disease. They may or may not be under significant stress. They present with chest tightness, shortness of breath, dizziness, light-headedness, and sometimes syncope. Classically they hyperventilate, causing systemic alkalosis, with resultant fingertip and circumoral numbness, light-headedness, and carpal-pedal spasms. Treatment includes reassurance, instructions and coaching to slow breathing, and sometimes anxiolytics.

IV. **Acute chest syndrome of sickle cell anemia.** The acute chest syndrome is common in patients who suffer from sickle cell anemia. The overall incidence for all ranges and genotypes is approximately 29%. The syndrome is most common in the 2- to 5-year-old age range with the SS genotype. The overall incidence of the syndrome decreases as age increases. Repeated episodes of the acute chest syndrome can lead to pulmonary fibrosis and pulmonary hypertension.

A. **Presentation.** The acute chest wall syndrome consists of the constellation of chest pain, fever, leukocytosis, and pulmonary infiltrates in patients with sickle cell disease. Predisposing factors include infection, dehydration, hypoxia, and acidosis. Analgesics have been implicated in adults and adolescents with sickle cell anemia. It has been suggested that cigarette smoking is also a predisposing factor in this patient population in the development of acute chest syndrome.

B. **Assessment.** Diagnosis is based on the clinical picture as described above (i.e., the sickle cell patient with chest pain and fever). Chest x-ray and CBC will confirm the infiltrates and leukocytosis. At this initial diagnostic stage in the evaluation, it is difficult to distinguish acute chest syndrome from pneumonia or pulmonary infarction.

C. **Management.** The respiratory management of these entities is similar. Oxygenation and ventilatory status must be assessed (arterial blood gas). Respiratory status is maintained by supplemental oxygen, and if necessary, intubation. Generally, antibiotics will be initiated pending sputum culture results, which in the case of acute chest syndrome will be negative. Acute chest syndrome will resolve with supportive care; however, antibiotics should be

used because it is virtually impossible to distinguish between acute chest syndrome and pneumonia in the early
stages. Acute chest syndrome should be considered in all
sickle cell patients presenting with fever and chest pain.

V. Pulmonary causes of chest pain

   A. Pneumonia and bronchitis. These conditions typically
   cause a pleuritic or bronchial type of chest pain due to the
   inflammatory response to infection. **Pleuritic pain** is
   sharp, localized, and markedly worse with deep inspiration. **Bronchial pain** is burning, raw, aching pain that is
   localized substernally and made worse with cough or deep
   inspiration. Diagnosis of either of these conditions is by
   history, physical examination, and chest x-ray. Treatment
   is with appropriate antibiotics, antitussives, and analgesics, taking into account the patient's age, underlying
   medical problems, and present clinical status. Admission
   or discharge of the patient is based on a combination of
   the above factors. An in-depth discussion of the management of pneumonia, bronchitis, and pleural effusion is beyond the scope of this text. These entities are mentioned
   only to remind the reader of their possible presence in the
   patient with chest pain.

   B. Carcinoma. Lung or mediastinal carcinoma causes typically a deep, boring, steady pain. It is caused by traction
   or pressure on pain-sensitive structures in the chest. Involvement of the pleura can cause pleuritic, sharp chest
   pain as well. The pain of carcinoma can be intense and often requires narcotic analgesics.

   C. Pleural effusion. A pleural effusion is an abnormal collection of fluid in the pleural cavity. This can be secondary
   to infection, malignancy, congestive heart failure, renal
   failure, collagen vascular diseases, and many other conditions. This fluid collection can cause compression on the
   lungs and compromise respiratory efforts. If respiratory
   compromise occurs, drainage of the fluid becomes necessary. Empyema is another condition that may require
   drainage. An empyema is a collection of pus in the pleural
   space. See Table 29-5 for indications and contraindications for thoracentesis.

   D. Pneumothorax. A pneumothorax occurs when air is
   trapped in the pleural space, causing collapse of the involved lung. Pneumothorax may be spontaneous or secondary to trauma. Spontaneous pneumothorax occurs
   commonly in patients with emphysema with ruptured
   blebs, in HIV positive patients with pneumocystis carinii
   pneumonia, in patients on mechanical ventilators, and in
   patients with focal abnormalities of lung tissue. Rarely,
   spontaneous pneumothoraces may progress to a tension
   pneumothorax, which is a cardiovascular emergency. In a
   tension pneumothorax, the leaking lung forms a one-way
   valve effect whereby air escapes into the pleural cavity
   and is trapped. Eventually, a high-pressure pneumothorax is formed that causes lateral shift of the mediastinum,
   crimping the vena cava, and limiting venous return to the
   heart. The result is a mechanical distributive form of circulatory shock.

**Table 29-5. Thoracentesis/thoracostomy:
indications and contraindications**

	Needle thoracentesis	Tube thoracostomy
Indications	Pleural fluid evacuation and examination Tension pneumothorax (temporary) prior to chest tube placement	Traumatic hemo/ pneumothorax Tension pneumothorax Iatrogenic pneumothorax Empyema
Contraindications	Insertion of needle through an area of infection Positive-pressure ventilation Knowledge that a chest tube is going to be placed Bleeding diathesis	Bleeding Diathesis Pleural adhesions
Complications	Pneumothorax Hemothorax Puncture of lung parenchyma Infection Bleeding	Intraparenchymal placement of chest tube Infection Bleeding

1. **Presentation.** Patients present classically with one-sided pleuritic chest pain and shortness of breath. Cyanosis may be present as well. Breath sounds are decreased on the involved side. If a tension pneumothorax is present, jugular venous distension, deviation of the trachea, hypotension, and tachycardia are also seen.

2. **Assessment.** Diagnosis is made by characteristic physical findings and confirmed by chest x-ray.

3. **Management.** Very small spontaneous pneumothoraces can be managed expectantly with serial daily chest x-rays and observation. Larger pneumothoraces require serial needle aspirations or chest tube thoracostomy.

4. **Disposition.** All patients who undergo chest tube thoracostomy require admission to the hospital. Recurrent spontaneous pneumothoraces are an indication for thoracotomy to resect the defective lung tissue or pleurodesis to scar down the pleura and avoid further episodes.

VI. **Tube thoracostomy: the procedure**

A. The patient is positioned with an arm behind the head or at least abducted to allow access to the lateral aspect of the chest. The patient should be sitting in a semi-Fowler's position, up approximately 30 to 45 degrees. When the patient is supine, it is more difficult for the physician doing the procedure because in the supine position the diaphragm will tend to move higher, increasing the risk of iatrogenic diaphragm, liver, or spleen injury.

B. The length of chest tube is estimated from insertion to lung apex. A clamp is placed at the estimated length required for proper placement and set aside.

C. The skin is prepped with povidone-iodine (Betadine) from the midchest down to the sheet and from the twelfth rib up to the axilla.

D. The area of tube insertion is the fourth or fifth intercostal space between the anterior and midaxillary lines (Fig. 29-1A).

Fig. 29-1. Tube thoracostomy. *A.* Proper incision placement for chest tube thoracostomy. *B.* Blunt dissection using a clamp to create an opening through the chest wall subcutaneous fat and muscle *C.* Advancing the closed clamp through the chest wall and parietal pleura. *D.* Sweeping of the pleura with a finger. *E.* Placement of the thoracostomy tube into the chest cavity. (Parts A–D reprinted with permission from Symbas PN. *Cardiothoracic Trauma.* Philadelphia: W. B. Saunders, 1989. Part E from Millikan JS. Complications of tube thoracostomy for acute trauma. *Am J Surg* 140:738–741, 1980. Reprinted with permission from American Journal of Surgery.)

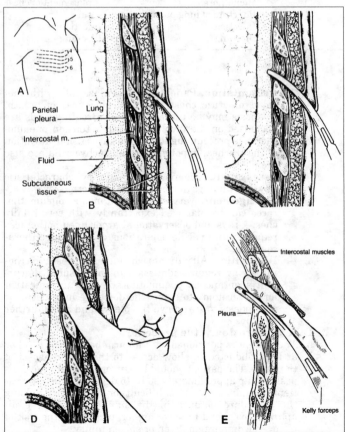

E. Sterile drapes or fenestrated sterile sheets are placed around the chosen site for the incision.

F. The area of tube insertion is anesthetized with 1% or 2% lidocaine on a long, small gauze needle (25-gauge or 27-gauge). Skin, muscle, periosteum, and parietal pleura are anesthetized at the site of insertion.

G. Using a No. 10 scalpel, a 2- to 2½-cm incision is made in the skin 1 rib below the planned penetration into the thoracic cavity (see Fig. 29-1A). Feel free to increase the length of this incision, if necessary. Using blunt clamps, bluntly dissect up over the rib superior to the point of the incision. Keep clamps on this rib and bluntly dissect (by spreading the clamps) to the parietal pleura (Fig. 29-1B). Make sure to keep the clamps on the top of the rib and not let them drift up to the bottom of the next superior rib because a neurovascular bundle runs under and behind the ribs at this level. Lacerating an intercostal artery at this level will cause brisk bleeding because these vessels come directly off the aorta.

H. A finger is placed on the clamp approximately 1½ to 2 cm from the skin edge, and the closed clamp is pushed through the parietal pleura (Fig. 29-1C). The finger prevents overinsertion of the clamp and potential resultant lung injury. When the clamp is opened, a rush of air or fluid indicates proper placement in the pleural cavity. If air or fluid are not obtained, check placement with the finger and try again.

I. Clamps are removed and a finger is placed in the incision to sweep the pleura and assure placement in the pleural cavity and that there are no local pleural adhesions (Fig. 29-1D).

J. Using a clamp attached to the tip of the chest tube and using a finger as a guide, the tube is placed into the thoracic cavity (Fig. 29-1E). The tube is angled to the patient's back and superiorly. The tube is inserted until the initial clamp in step 2 is at the skin insertion site. The tube is then attached to the drainage system.

K. The tube is secured with large suture material. It is covered with petrolatum-impregnated gauze and then layered with 4 × 4 gauze. Tape is placed over the gauze. The mesenteric tape technique is used to secure the tube that protrudes from the gauze.

L. A postprocedure chest x-ray is obtained to confirm tube position and fluid or air drainage. Breath sounds and vital signs are reassessed.

Bibliography

Arroyo JF, et al. Costavertebral joint dysfunction: another misdiagnosed cause of atypical chest pain. *Postgrad Med J* 68:655–659, 1992.

Castro O, et al. The acute chest syndrome in sickle cell disease: incidence and risk factors. *Blood* 84:643–649, 1994.

Murata GH. Evaluating chest pain in the emergency department. *West J Med* 159:61–68, 1993.

Richten JE. Investigation and management of noncardiac chest pain. *Bailliere's Clinical Gastroent* 5:281–306, 1991.

Richter JE. Overview of diagnostic testing for chest pain of unknown origin. *Amer J of Med* 92(suppl SA), 1992.

Shima MA. Evaluation of chest pain. *Post Grad Med* 91:155–164, 1992.

Swarnjit S, et al. The contribution of gastroesophageal reflux to chest pain in patients with coronary artery disease. *Ann of Int Med* 117:824–830, 1992.

Wilson LR, Yinling K. Psychiatric aspects of chest pain in the emergency department. *Med Clin North Am* 75:1175–1188, 1981.

V

Toxicologic Cardiovascular Emergencies

Digitalis Toxicity

Marcel J. Casavant

Digitalis compounds (the cardiac glycosides) are among the ten most commonly prescribed drugs in the United States. Not surprisingly, overdose of these agents is also common. In 1992, the American Association of Poison Control Centers received reports of 2310 toxic exposures to digitalis medications resulting in 19 deaths and 211 moderate or major adverse outcomes, and 2937 exposures to plants that contain cardiac glycosides (Table 30-1), resulting in no deaths but 18 moderate or major adverse outcomes.

I. **Digitalis pharmacology**
   A. **Mechanism of action.** The primary action of the digitalis compounds is to block the sodium-potassium ATPase pump, which normally maintains the transcellular sodium and potassium gradient. When the pump is blocked, sodium is no longer actively extruded from the cell and thus accumulates in the intracellular fluid. As the sodium accumulates intracellularly, it begins to exit passively through the membrane sodium-calcium exchange channel, resulting in higher intracellular concentrations of calcium. This extra calcium results in increased force of contraction (inotropic effect).

   Accompanying the increased intracellular sodium concentration is an increased extracellular concentration of potassium. Although the total body load of potassium is unchanged, the shift to the extracellular space leads to hyperkalemia, which in acute overdose serves as a marker for the extent of digitalis effect. Chronically, however, the increased proportion of extracellular potassium leads to an increase in renal potassium losses and a decrease in the total body potassium load. Hyperkalemia may not be seen in chronic overdose. In the heart, the increased extracellular potassium contributes to slowing of Purkinje conduction and enhanced automaticity of junctional and atrioventricular (AV) nodal tissue. In overdose, these effects contribute to ventricular ectopy and re-entrant tachycardias.

   Besides increasing contractility, digitalis compounds also slow the rate of conduction and contraction. This slowing appears to result from an increased potentiation of the vagus nerve, a slowing of sinoatrial (SA) node firing, and a slowing of AV node conduction, mediated by an increase in the refractory period. Automaticity of the Purkinje fibers is increased. The increased vagal tone from digitalis results from stimulation of brainstem centers, which also leads to generalized sympathetic hyperactivity.
   B. **Therapeutic benefits.** Increased intracellular calcium results in increased inotropy, which is useful in heart failure. Prolonged AV nodal refractoriness and delayed conduction to the ventricles are useful in atrial

Dr. Casavant is supported by grant number ED 05651 from the National Institute of Environmental Health Sciences, NIH.

Table 30-1.   Digitalis-like intoxications

Plant	Animal	Drug
Dogbane	Toad skin (may protect toad from predators)	Declanoside
Foxglove	Toad venom (used in some Chinese medicaments)	Digitalis
Lily of the valley		Digitoxin
Oleander		Digoxin
Red squill		Gitalin
Rhododendron		Lanatoside C
		Oubain

tachydysrhythmias to limit the ventricular rate. Increased vagal tone and decreased automaticity of the SA and AV nodes may result in true antidysrhythmic effect, leading to conversion of some atrial dysrhythmias (including fibrillation and flutter) to a sinus rhythm.

C. **Kinetics.** The behavior of the digitalis compounds in the body is best described by a two-compartment model with first-order elimination. After the drug is absorbed from the GI tract into the bloodstream (the central compartment), it distributes into muscle and other tissue (the peripheral compartment), where it has its effect. The apparent volume of distribution (V_d) for digoxin is 5–10 liter/kg; digitoxin is distributed in a smaller volume to (0.5 liter/kg). The distribution phase lasts 6–12 hours. The elimination half-life of digoxin is 30–50 hours; for digitoxin it is 5–8 days. Whereas digoxin is excreted primarily in the urine, digitoxin undergoes enterohepatic recirculation and hepatic elimination, with a small fraction eliminated by the kidneys.

Therapeutic serum levels for digoxin are 0.5–2.0 ng/ml; for digitoxin, 10–25 ng/ml. Approximately 20% of the digoxin in serum is protein-bound; more than 90% of digitoxin in serum is protein-bound.

D. **Indications for digitalis.** Digitalis and related compounds (cardiac glycosides) are indicated for the treatment of atrial tachyarrhythmias, including atrial fibrillation, atrial flutter, and paroxysmal atrial tachycardia. The glycosides are indicated also in the management of low-output congestive heart failure, especially if associated with left ventricular insufficiency.

II. **Etiologies of digitalis overdose**

A. **Overdose.** In 1992, accidental overdose accounted for 4686 digitalis exposures, and intentional overdose comprised 445 exposures. Most acute overdoses result from accidental or suicidal ingestion.

B. **Hypokalemia.** A patient taking steady-state doses of digitalis may develop digitalis toxicity as a result of hypokalemia. The hypokalemia may result either from increased renal losses due to higher concentrations of extracellular potassium resulting from the use of digitalis or from concurrent diuretic use. Digitalis appears to compete with potassium for membrane binding sites, and hypokalemia therefore results in increased digitalis binding and toxicity. Further, hypokalemia and digitalis toxicity have synergistic effects on myocardial automaticity.

C. **Renal failure.** Chronic digoxin overdose often is associated with continuing a previous digoxin dose while renal failure worsens. This results in decreased digoxin clearance and increased serum levels. This can happen chronically over a period of months or subacutely over a period of days to one week. One mechanism of acute deterioration involves slowly worsening renal function and slowly climbing digitalis levels until the area postrema of the brainstem is stimulated by the digitalis. The resultant nausea, vomiting, and prerenal failure contribute to acute-on-chronic digitalis intoxication.

D. **Drug interactions.** Chronic and acute-on-chronic digitalis intoxications also result from therapeutic errors, such as addition of drugs that can decrease clearance (quinidine blocks renal clearance of digoxin; erythromycin and cimetidine decrease hepatic metabolism of digitoxin; verapamil, spironolactone, and amiodarone increase the half-life and serum levels of digitalis compounds) or can increase bioavailability (erythromycin and tetracycline kill gut bacteria that degrade glycosides), and such as removal of medications that increase clearance (such as cholestipol and other steroid-binding resins).

III. Digitalis toxicity
A. Presentation
1. **Acute intoxication.** Acute digitalis overdoses most often occur because of accidental ingestion (such as by a toddler) or intentional overdose (in a suicide attempt). Usually the victim has no underlying cardiac pathology and is taking no other medicines. Anorexia, nausea, vomiting, and diarrhea are common early symptoms. Lethargy and seizures are reported, the latter only rarely.

2. **Chronic intoxication.** Chronic digitalis overdoses are often iatrogenic (failure to monitor levels and adjust dosage after adjusting other medications that can affect digoxin levels) or result from worsening coexisting disease (chronic renal insufficiency). Often the patient has been taking the glycosides because of underlying cardiac disease (congestive heart failure) and is also on other medicines (e.g., diuretics). GI effects are less prominent, but patients complain of malaise, weakness, and dizziness. Other CNS changes include confusion and headache. Visual disturbances occur, including blurring and a pathognomonic yellow-blue halo around objects (xanthopsia).

3. **Acute-on-chronic intoxication.** This category of overdose results from a dosing error or suicide attempt by a patient maintained on digitalis. Any combination of the above two presentations may occur.

B. Assessment

1. **Laboratory.** Measurement of serum electrolytes, especially potassium, calcium, and magnesium, is critical. These should be monitored during the course of treatment because clinically significant changes may develop at any stage of digitalis poisoning. Serum potassium is almost always elevated in acute overdose, whereas in chronic overdose, hypokalemia or hypomagnesemia often are seen as precipitating factors. An initial serum creatinine and BUN help to assess renal function as another precipitating factor in digitalis toxicity.

   Because patients with chronic overdose often have pre-existing medical problems and have been taking numerous medications, more laboratory studies may be indicated (CBC, liver enzymes, glucose, other drug levels).

2. **ECG or cardiac rhythm.** Electrocardiographic findings in acute intoxication include bradydysrhythmias, including sinus bradycardia, sinus arrest, and AV block. These are more common than the tachydysrhythmias, but both ventricular tachycardia and fibrillation may occur. Any type of ventricular dysrhythmia is possible, including premature ventricular contractions (PVCs), bigeminy, and trigeminy.

   In chronic overdoses, although bradydysrhythmias are possible, the tachydysrhythmias (including accelerated junctional tachycardia or junctional escape, ventricular bigeminy, trigeminy, tachycardia, or fibrillation, bidirectional tachycardia, and atrial tachycardias with block) are more common (Fig. 30-1).

3. **Digoxin levels.** In acute overdose, postdistribution levels (drawn at least 6 hours after the overdose) correlate best with toxicity. Still, the acute level is helpful to confirm the overdose, and may indicate a worse-possible-case level. In chronic overdose an early level is predictive of toxicity. The level may appear falsely high after administration of digoxin-specific antibody fragments (see later).

Fig. 30-1.   Atrial flutter is one of the dysrhythmias associated with chronic digitalis intoxication.

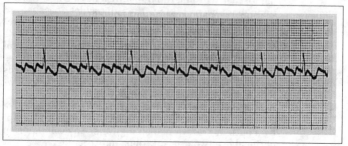

Digoxin-like immunoreactive substance (DLIS) is an endogenous compound that gives false elevations on immunoassays for digitalis compounds. It is present in significant levels, however, only in neonates and in patients with severe renal insufficiency. In the setting of possible overdose, therefore, the role of DLIS often can be ignored.

C. Management

1. **General management.** All patients with a possible overdose of a digitalis compound require prompt attention, careful cardiac monitoring, and aggressive intervention. Although effects after acute overdose may not appear early (due to the distribution time from the central compartment), they can develop suddenly without warning. Toxicity can occur after ingestion of only a few pills (or leaves) by children.

   Although respirations and spontaneous airway usually are maintained even in the face of significant digitalis toxicity, careful monitoring remains indicated. Vomiting frequently occurs in this setting, and airway protective reflexes are lost when poorly perfusing rhythms occur. Securing an airway is indicated whenever consciousness is impaired or cardiovascular stability is apparent. Because of potassium release, which may accompany use of succinylcholine, this agent is relatively contraindicated in the setting of digitalis overdose.

   Frequent vital-sign measurement and continuous cardiac rhythm monitoring are important. Securing adequate IV access early saves time should antiarrhythmics or the specific antidote, digoxin antibody fragments, become needed. Monitoring should continue for at least 24 hours after significant overdose.

2. **Decontamination.** Following acute oral overdose, early decontamination is indicated. Although some authorities still recommend ipecac for gastric emptying (15 ml PO for children aged 12 months to 12 years; 30 ml PO for patients older than 12 years), this should be used only if available in the minutes following overdose, before digitalis-induced vomiting and significant vagal effects can occur. The need for gastric lavage is also controversial; prompt administration of gram doses of activated charcoal (the larger of 1 g charcoal for each kg of patient weight or 10 g charcoal for each gram of drug ingested) with cathartic should suffice, unless there is a possibility of coingestion of substances not adsorbed to charcoal (e.g., lithium, iron, ethanol). Following chronic oral overdose or acute parenteral overdose, activated charcoal is indicated only if:

   1. An oral dose may have been taken in the last 6–8 hours.
   2. The overdose involves digitoxin, which has significant enterohepatic recirculation.
   3. The patient has chronic renal failure, because the small additional clearance to be gained from char-

coal will be large in comparison to the limited renal clearance.

4. Other substances that can be adsorbed to charcoal have been ingested.

Repeat dose charcoal (0.5 g charcoal for each kg of body weight q4h) is indicated for digitoxin overdose.

Because vagal tone is already increased by digitalis overdose, pretreatment with atropine (0.01–0.04 mg/kg) should occur before orogastric lavage, nasogastric tube placement, or endotracheal intubation occur. This may help to prevent episodes of bradycardia and sinus node arrest reported in the setting of digitalis overdose.

Steroid-binding resins (cholestyramine or cholestipol) given orally are also effective in interrupting enterohepatic recycling of digitoxin and, in patients with renal insufficiency, of digoxin.

There is no role for dialysis or charcoal hemoperfusion in the clearance of the cardiac glycosides, due to their large volumes of distribution and their serum protein binding.

3. **Electrolyte management.** In digitalis overdose, hyperkalemia usually indicates only a shift of potassium from intracellular to extracellular space. Correction depends on reversing the shift, with glucose (0.5 g/kg IV bolus), insulin (0.1 U/kg IV bolus), and bicarbonate (1 mEq/kg IV0. Avoid potassium-binding sodium polystyrene sulfonate unless hyperkalemia is unresponsive to these measures and cardiac irritability accompanies hyperkalemia; the resultant loss of potassium could later lead to hypokalemia and increased susceptibility to digitalis effect. Calcium is contraindicated as a potassium antagonist because the intracellular calcium level is already increased by digitalis effect and worsened ventricular dysrhythmia, or else loss of myocardial contractility ("stone heart") may result.

Hypokalemia increases the risk of digitalis toxicity and should be treated early and aggressively with IV and oral potassium supplementation and frequent monitoring of serum levels and the QRS and T waves on the cardiac monitor.

Hypomagnesemia is a common electrolyte disturbance accompanying chronic digitalis overdose, probably because of long-term diuretic use. Some authorities feel correction of hypokalemia is impossible in the face of uncorrected hypomagnesemia. Correction (with $MgSO_4$ 1–2 g IV over 30 min) is indicated, unless heart block is present. In digitalized patients, conduction delays and blocks may occur with administration of parenteral magnesium.

4. **Antiarrhythmics.** Prophylactic administration of atropine (0.01–0.04 mg/kg IV bolus) is indicated before lavage, nasogastric (NG) tube placement, or intubation. Atropine also is indicated to treat bradydysrhythmias, heart block, and sinus arrest. Prompt correction

of hypokalemia and hypomagnesemia is critical in management of dysrhythmias. Ventricular tachyarrhythmias are treated with Class Ib agents: lidocaine 1.0–1.5 mg/kg IV bolus, repeated to maximum of 3 mg/kg IV bolus and followed by a drip of 1–4 mg/min; or phenytoin 15–20 mg/kg slow IV (less than 1 mg/kg/min in children or 50 mg/min in adults), with subsequent doses (if needed) of 2.5 mg/kg/d, adjusted based on results of therapeutic drug monitoring. Propranolol or other beta-blocking drugs may lessen myocardial irritability and automaticity and can be used in the treatment of tachydysrhythmias.

Class Ia antiarrhythmics (procainamide, disopyramide, quinidine) are contraindicated since they may worsen digitalis-induced arrhythmias and AV blockade. Quinidine also elevates serum digoxin and digitoxin levels. Sympathomimetic agents (especially isoproterenol) should be avoided if possible, because they contribute to increased automaticity.

5. **Electrical therapy.** Temporary transcutaneous pacing may be needed in cases of sinus arrest, bradycardia, or AV block. If possible, avoid use of cardioversion for tachydysrhythmias, because this may provoke ventricular fibrillation in the setting of digitalis overdose. If cardioversion is used as a last resort, start with low energy levels. Early use of digoxin-specific antibody fragments (see below) may make these electrical therapies unnecessary.

6. **Fab fragments.** The treatment of digitalis overdose with antibody therapy represents one of the great recent advances in cardiovascular toxicology. Sheep are immunized with digoxin, and their antibodies are collected and cleaved. The Fab fragments are specific for digoxin but have some affinity for digitoxin and the other digitalis compounds. Administered intravenously, the antibody fragments bind and inactivate serum digoxin molecules. The decrease in free serum levels results in a gradient that draws tissue digoxin back into the central compartment, where it can be bound. This results in a reversal of digitalis effect, which begins in minutes and is complete within 4 hours.

   a. **Indications.** Digoxin-specific Fab fragments should be used when the following occur in the setting of possible digitalis overdose.

      (1) Life-threatening dysrhythmia (ventricular tachycardia, ventricular fibrillation, severe bradydysrhythmia or high-grade AV block)

      (2) Milder dysrhythmia refractory to electro-lyte replacement or Class Ib antiarrythmic drugs

      (3) Hyperkalemia (K+ >5.5 mEq/liter)

      (4) Digoxin-induced pump failure

      (5) Massive dose (>10 mg in an adult; >4 mg in a child)

      (6) Very high level (>4 ng/ml postdistribution, or >10 ng/ml during the distribution phase)

b. Dosage and administration. Each vial of Digibind (digoxin-specific antibody fragments) contains 40 mg and binds 0.6 mg of digoxin. There are five ways to calculate the dose.

(1) In an acute overdose where the ingested amount is known, multiply the dose ingested (in milligrams) by the bioavailability (average F=0.8 for digoxin, or use F for specific preparation, if known) to estimate the maximum number of milligrams absorbed; then divide by 0.6 (the number of milligrams of digoxin bound per vial of Fab fragments). A higher dose may be needed for the other digitalis compounds, against which digoxin-specific antibodies may be less potent.

(2) In an overdose where the amount ingested is unknown and postdistribution levels are unknown, an empirical dose of 10–20 vials may be given.

(3) In a chronic overdose, or in an acute overdose when a postdistribution level is known, the body's digoxin burden is estimated by this formula: digoxin level (ng/ml) × 5 liter/kg (Vd) × patient weight (kg) × 0.001 ml mg/liter ng. Dividing the estimated body burden by 0.6 (mg digoxin bound per vial) gives the dose.

(4) In a chronic overdose where a therapeutic level is still desired, one can theoretically lower the level back into the therapeutic range by subtracting the desired level from the measured level, multiplying by the Vd and patient weight, and dividing by the conversion factor (0.001 ml mg/liter ng) to estimate that part of the body burden we want to bind and inactivate. Dividing by 0.6 mg digoxin bound per vial gives the number of vials to use.

(5) When the patient's hemodynamic stability allows less rapid dosing, one-half the number of vials predicted by any of the above methods can be given initially, followed by 1 vial every 20 to 30 minutes, titrated to effect. This minimizes the risk of overdosage of antibody fragments, which is a concern only in the setting of chronic dependence on digoxin for management of congestive heart failure or dysrhythmia.

Because two of the above dose calculations use a population estimate for V_d, they are imprecise. Careful clinical monitoring is essential. Fab fragments are administered through a micropore filter (0.22 μm) and given over 30 minutes (if patient is sufficiently stable), or by IV push.

c. Precautions. Although derived from sheep serum, the Fab fragments have not proved a major cause of allergic and anaphylactic reactions. The major adverse effects of Fab fragment administration have been in patients previously dependent on digitalis: loss of myocardial contractility (when the patient had been maintained on digitalis for its inotropic effect) and rapid increase in heart rate (when the patient had been using digitalis to block AV conduction of an atrial tachydysrhythmia). Other adverse effects result from the success of Fab fragments in treating an intoxication for which other therapies have been initiated: sudden hypokalemia when glucose, insulin, bicarbonate, and possibly sodium polystyrone sulfonate have been used to lower the serum potassium. None of these possible adverse effects constitutes a contraindication to Fab fragment administration; they testify to the need for careful monitoring and observation, and for titrating the antidote to clinical effect when time (and the patient's cardiovascular status) permits.

D. Disposition
1. **Discharge criteria.** Following possible digitalis overdose, patients may safely be discharged home (if accidental) or to psychiatric or protective care (if intentional) if they remain asymptomatic, undergo successful GI decontamination (including passage of charcoal stool), and have a low serum drug level drawn at least 6 hours after the exposure. While in the ED, they should have continuous cardiac monitoring and close observation. At least 6 hours of ED observation are warranted unless presentation is delayed and the history is reliable.
2. **Admission criteria.** Any patient who develops symptoms, including vomiting, abdominal pain, CNS changes, hyperkalemia, or cardiac rhythm abnormality in the setting of possible digitalis overdose, deserves careful monitoring in the CCU. Observation should continue for at least 12 hours after all signs of toxicity have resolved.

Bibliography

Benowitz NI. Cardiac Glycosides. In Olson KR (ed.), *Poisoning and Drug Overdose* (2nd ed.). Norwalk, CT: Appleton & Lange, 1994.

Cummins RO (ed.). *Textbook of Advanced Cardiac Life Support.* Dallas: American Heart Association, 1994.

Lewin NA. Digitalis. In Goldfrank LR (ed.), *Toxicologic Emergencies.* Norwalk, CT: Appleton & Lange, 1994.

Litovitz TL, et al. 1992 Annual Report of the American Association of Poison Control Centers Toxic Exposure Surveillance System. *Am J Emerg Med* 11:494–555, 1993.

Menard RH. *Introduction to Arrhythmia Recognition.* California Heart Association, 1968.

Cocaine-Associated Chest Pain

Judd E. Hollander

The use of cocaine has reached epidemic proportions. Over 30% of men and 20% of women between the ages of 26 and 34 have used cocaine at least once. Twenty-three million Americans have used cocaine at some time, and 5 million use it regularly. Cocaine is the most common illicit drug of abuse in emergency department (ED) patients. In the United States, there are over 160,000 ED visits annually that are secondary to cocaine, and chest pain is the most common cocaine-related complaint. Additionally, many other symptoms may be secondary to myocardial ischemia (i.e., shortness of breath, palpitations, syncope). Most of these patients are admitted to the hospital, with the ensuing cost of hospitalization exceeding 83 million dollars annually.

I. **Pathophysiology.** Cocaine is a natural alkaloid found in *Erythroxylon coca,* a shrub indigenous to South America. The medicinal use of cocaine is based on the fact that it is the only local anesthetic that causes vasoconstriction.
   A. **Pharmacology.** The initial effect of cocaine on the cardiovascular system is vagotonic, producing a transient bradycardia. This effect is rapidly followed by increased sympathetic stimulation that results in tachycardia and hypertension. Peripherally, cocaine produces a sympathomimetic response by inhibiting the reuptake of epinephrine and norepinephrine while enhancing the presynaptic release of norepinephrine. The increased concentration of norepinephrine at the postsynaptic alpha receptors leads to the stimulatory effects of cocaine. Centrally, the mechanism is less well-defined. Cocaine may enhance the release of norepinephrine and/or block the neuronal reuptake of dopamine and excitatory amino acids.

   The Goldfrank-Hoffman model explains the relationship between the central and peripheral manifestations of cocaine toxicity (Fig. 31-1). CNS agitation stimulates increased neuronal firing, which, coupled with reuptake blockade, exaggerates the sympathetic response and leads to the peripheral manifestations of cocaine toxicity (including cardiovascular complications). Feedback may further enhance CNS excitation, leading to seizures and hyperthermia. According to this model, blockade of the peripheral effects will not reduce CNS toxicity.
   B. **Cardiotoxic effects.** Acutely, cocaine increases myocardial oxygen demand, causes coronary artery vasoconstriction, and enhances thrombus formation. Chronic use leads to accelerated atherosclerosis and left ventricular hypertrophy, which may further exacerbate the discrepancy between oxygen supply and demand (Table 31-1).

   The ability to increase myocardial oxygen demand and decrease coronary blood flow through vasoconstriction; enhance platelet aggregation and in situ thrombus formation; and cause premature atherosclerosis, left ventricular

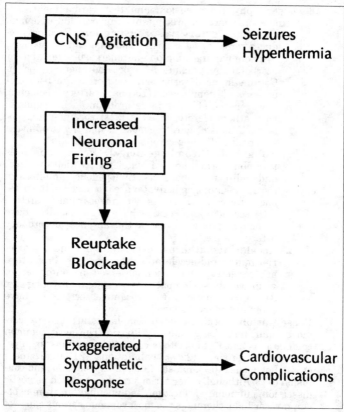

Fig. 31-1.   The Goldfrank-Hoffman model of cocaine toxicity. (From Goldfrank LJ, Hoffman RS. The cardiovascular effects of cocaine. *Ann Emerg Med* 20:165–175, 1991.)

Table 31-1.   Pathophysiologic mechanisms for cocaine-associated myocardial ischemia

Increased myocardial oxygen demand
    Hypertension
    Tachycardia
    Left ventricular hypertrophy
Coronary artery vasoconstriction
In situ thrombus formation
Accelerated atherosclerosis

hypertrophy, hypertension, and tachycardia makes cocaine a multifaceted precipitant of myocardial ischemia.

1. **Coronary artery vasoconstriction.** Cocaine produces coronary vasoconstriction that can be reversed
   by phentolamine, an alpha-adrenergic blocker, and exacerbated by propanolol, a beta-adrenergic blocker.
   Cocaine-induced vasoconstriction occurs in both diseased and nondiseased coronary artery segments;
   however, the effect is more pronounced in segments
   with atherosclerotic disease. Most cocaine-using patients are also cigarette smokers, and the two have a
   synergistic effect on coronary vasoconstriction.

2. **Enhanced thrombogenicity.** Cocaine enhances
   thrombus formation and platelet activation by direct
   and indirect mechanisms. Endogenous inhibitors of
   tissue plasminogen activator are increased in the presence of cocaine. Patients with myocardial infarction
   (MI) secondary to cocaine have been noted to have
   thrombus present even in the absence of coronary
   artery disease.

3. **Accelerated atherosclerosis.** Cocaine induces arterial injury and accelerates atherogenesis. Premature
   atherosclerosis has been observed in autopsies of
   young cocaine-using patients. Despite their young age,
   31%–67% of patients with cocaine-associated MI have
   coronary artery disease.

II. **Presentation.** Cocaine-related complaints are usually cardiovascular, neurologic, and psychiatric. The most common
complaint is chest pain. Other common symptoms are dyspnea (22%), anxiety (22%), palpitations (21%), dizziness
(13%), headache (10%), nausea (9%), psychosis (9%), and confusion (9%). Although other serious conditions, such as aortic
dissection, pulmonary infarction, and pneumothorax, may occur, myocardial ischemia is the most common serious cause of
chest pain. In addition, since many of the above symptoms are
suggestive of ischemic heart disease, the initial evaluation is
directed toward excluding MI.

A. **History.** The typical patient with cocaine-associated myocardial ischemia is a young male smoker with a history of
recurrent cocaine use and few other traditional cardiac
risk factors. The history should include the specific drugs
and estimated amount used; the frequency of use; the
presence of coingestants; an assessment of past medical
history; the present symptoms; and an assessment of the
patient's social support system. Cardiac risk factors, the
duration and frequency of cocaine use, a description of
chest pain, and associated cardiac symptoms may be useful historic information, although cocaine-associated MIs
have occurred with very aytpical presentations.

Signs and symptoms suggestive of ischemia other than
chest pain are frequently present; however, cocaine-
associated MI in the absence of chest pain appears very
rarely. Although cocaine-associated myocardial ischemia
may occur for several weeks after cessation of cocaine use,
most patients with myocardial infarction have the onset of
symptoms within 24 hours of cocaine use.

B. **Physical examination.** The physical examination may reveal signs of sympathetic stimulation, such as an altered mental status, hyperthermia, seizures, hypertension, tachycardia, mydriasis, diaphoresis, hypoactive bowel sounds, and possibly tachypnea.

A complete physical examination should be performed on all patients suspected of cocaine use. The initial examination should assess the airway, breathing, and circulation (ABCs), the vital signs, the cardiovascular system, bowel sounds, the pupils, the mental status, and the neurologic status. Agitation may be secondary to cocaine, underlying psychiatric disorders, or a postictal state. The cardiac examination may help identify patients with valvular disease, endocarditis, hypertrophic cardiomyopathy, congestive heart failure, or myocarditis secondary to acute or chronic stimulant use. Chest findings may suggest pneumonia, pulmonary infarction, pneumomediastinum, or pneumothorax. Abdominal examination should assess the possibility of visceral infarction. Because of the propensity of stimulants, in particular cocaine, to affect every organ system, it is imperative that all patients undergo a thorough physical examination.

III. **Assessment.** Patients with presumed cocaine-induced myocardial ischemia should undergo a rapid and efficient workup to rule out myocardial infarction.

A. **Laboratory testing.** Routine laboratory testing, including CBC, tests for electrolytes and glucose, and renal studies are usually of low yield in patients with cocaine use. The CBC may show an elevated white blood cell count due to demargination, but this is nonspecific. The glucose level may be elevated and potassium may be mildly depressed because of adrenergic stimulation. Arterial blood gases should be used to assess oxygenation and acid-base status in cases where the patient is short of breath or hypoxic by pulse-oximetry. Cocaine use has been shown to cause profound lactic acidosis because of peripheral vasocontriction and muscle ischemia.

B. **Chest radiography.** Chest radiography may help diagnose pneumonia, pulmonary infarction, pneumomediastinum, pneumothorax, or aortic dissection. It may provide useful information regarding cardiac size, silhouette, and congestive heart failure.

C. **Electrocardiography.** The ECG, though not very sensitive, has historically been the best early predictor of a myocardial infarction in patients with chest pain unrelated to cocaine. However, it is less sensitive and less specific for predicting MI in patients with cocaine-associated chest pain. ECGs are abnormal in 56%–84% of patients with cocaine-associated chest pain, and up to 43% of patients who are "ruled out" for MI have ECGs that meet standard TIMI criteria for thrombolytics use. Conversely, normal or nonspecific ECGs do not significantly reduce the likelihood of MI.

D. **Cardiac serum markers.** Following cocaine use, approximately 50% of patients with cocaine-associated chest pain have elevations in serum total creatine kinase (CK). Patients with acute myocardial infarction (AMI) are likely to have rising serum CKs. Patients with initial total serum CK elevations that subsequently decline are less likely to have an MI. Cocaine results in skeletal muscle injury, and as a result, false-positive elevations in CK-MB have been observed in the absence of MI. CK-MB remains the mainstay for the initial diagnosis of AMI due to cocaine use, although a high relative index of CK-MB to total CK or a rising level of CK-MB in serial testing is often needed to confirm the diagnosis. The immunoassay for cardiac troponin I has no detectable cross reactivity with human skeletal muscle troponin I, making it more specific than CK-MB for myocardial injury when concomitant skeletal muscle injury exists. Use of cardiac tropin I may, therefore, enhance the diagnostic accuracy of MI in patients with cocaine-associated ischemia. Unfortunately, assays for troponin I are not yet available in most hospitals or are not rapidly available for real-time emergency department use.

IV. **Management.** Patients should have IV access established, be placed on a cardiac monitor, receive supplemental oxygen, and undergo a thorough history and physical examination. Electrocardiography and chest radiography to identify myocardial ischemia, pneumonia, pulmonary infarction, pneumomediastinum, pneumothorax, congestive heart failure, or aortic dissection should follow. The treatment of pulmonary maladies secondary to cocaine does not differ from that secondary to other etiologies, and will not be discussed further in this chapter. Patients with chest pain that is clearly not cardiac in origin should be treated as dictated by their conditions.

The pharmacologic treatment of patients with potentially ischemic chest pain, hypertension, or tachycardia secondary to cocaine has several important differences from that of patients with myocardial ischemia or infarction unrelated to cocaine. When treatment strategies would be altered by recent cocaine use, rapid bedside toxicologic assays for cocaine or cocaine metabolites may be useful, since patient self-reporting is not entirely reliable.

A. **Ischemic chest pain.** Patients with potentially ischemic chest pain should be treated with oxygen, benzodiazepines, aspirin, and nitroglycerin, and IV access should be established. Calcium channel blockade or phentolamine can be considered as second-line therapy. If evidence of myocardial infarction continues and ECG criteria for thrombolytic therapy are met, reperfusion may be considered with either primary angioplasty or thrombolytic therapy. If the ST-segment elevations are new compared to old ECGs and chest pain is unabating, it is reasonable to give thrombolytic agents, in the absence of traditional contraindications. If the ECG ST-segment elevation is unchanged from old ECGs and if the chest pain persists despite pharmacologic therapy, it may be best to pursue diagnostic cardiac catheterization and mechanical reperfusion, as necessary.

   1. **Benzodiazepines.** Benzodiazepines attenuate the cardiac and central nervous system toxicity of cocaine, and therefore should be considered as first-line ther-

apy. They reduce anxiety, blood pressure, and heart rate, thereby decreasing the myocardial oxygen demand. Benzodiazepines are recommended for patients with cocaine-associated myocardial ischemia, anxiety, tachycardia, or hypertension. The typical dose is 2.5–5.0 mg of diazepam or 2–4 mg of lorazepam titrated intravenously.

2. **Aspirin.** Aspirin will prevent thrombus formation by its effects on the prostaglandin pathway. It has a good safety profile and demonstrated utility in patients with ischemic heart disease unrelated to cocaine, and should also be given to patients with cocaine-associated myocardial ischemia. The dose is 160 mg chewed.

3. **Nitroglycerin.** Nitroglycerin, administered sublingually or in a intravenously titrated dose sufficient to reduce mean arterial pressure by 10%–15%, reverses cocaine-induced coronary artery vasoconstriction and relieves symptomatic chest pain. Accordingly, nitroglycerin should be used as primary therapy for cocaine-associated myocardial ischemia, and may be helpful for the treatment of cocaine-associated hypertension and congestive heart failure.

4. **Phentolamine.** Phentolamine, an alpha-adrenergic blocking agent, reverses cocaine-induced coronary artery vasoconstriction. Cautions regarding the use of phentolamine stem from concerns regarding its marked vasodilatory effects; however, low doses (1 mg IV) may avoid the potential vasodilatory and hypotensive effects while still maintaining anti-ischemic effects. For patients with ischemic chest pain unrelieved by benzodiazepines and nitroglycerin, phentolamine may be useful.

5. **Calcium channel blockers.** In animal models of cocaine toxicity, calcium channel blockers prevent malignant arrhythmias, decrease the negative inotropic effects of cocaine, blunt the increases in systemic vascular resistance, and protect against myocardial infarction, although central nervous system toxicity and mortality may be increased. In general, calcium channel blocking agents are not considered useful in the treatment of acute myocardial infarction unrelated to cocaine. Verapamil, however, does reverse cocaine-induced coronary artery vasoconstriction, and therefore may have a role in the treatment of refractory myocardial ischemia secondary to cocaine. The dose is 2.5–10.0 mg titrated intravenously to reduce heart rate or chest pain.

6. **Beta-adrenergic blockers.** Beta-adrenergic blocking agents, one of the mainstays of treatment of acute myocardial ischemia unrelated to cocaine, are contraindicated in patients with recent cocaine use. They enhance cocaine-induced coronary vasoconstriction, increase the blood pressure, do not control heart rate, enhance the likelihood of seizures, and worsen survival. Beta-blockers should be avoided in patients with recent cocaine use.

7. **Combined alpha-beta blockers.** Some patients have been treated with labetalol without adverse consequences; however, current data do not support this use. The beta-adrenergic blocking effects of labetalol are much more potent than the alpha-adrenergic blocking effects, and complications from the unopposed alpha effects have occurred in patients with sympathetic storm (from pheochromocytoma) when labetalol has been used. Cocaine-induced coronary vasoconstriction is not improved by labetalol. As a result, labetalol is not recommended.

8. **Thrombolytic agents.** The enhanced thrombus formation secondary to cocaine makes treatment with thrombolytic therapy a theoretically attractive option. Concerns about the risk of intracranial bleeding appear to be less worrisome than originally believed. The reported complication rate in patients with cocaine-associated myocardial infarction is less than 3% (compared to 1.5%–2.0% in traditional patients with MI).

However, several concerns, besides safety, continue to limit the use of thrombolytic agents. The clinical benefit is unclear, the mortality from cocaine-associated myocardial infarction is extremely low in patients who reach the hospital alive, and young patients with cocaine-associated chest pain have a high incidence of early repolarization (J point and false-positive ST elevations) that may result in a high rate of administration of thrombolytic agents to patients without MI. Care must be taken to avoid giving thrombolytic agents in patients with either high blood pressure or altered mental status, both of which are contraindications for thrombolytic therapy (see Chap. 10).

B. **Ventricular arrhythmias.** Some concern exists regarding the use of lidocaine to treat cocaine-induced arrhythmias, since the drugs have both proarrhythmic and proconvulsant effects mediated through sodium channel blockade. Although animal studies have yielded conflicting data regarding the safety of lidocaine use, limited human experience suggests that the use of lidocaine is safe several hours after cocaine use. Cautious use of lidocaine for the treatment of stable ventricular arrhythmias is reasonable. Unstable ventricular arrhythmias should receive defibrillation. Sodium bicarbonate reverses cocaine-induced QRS prolongation, and may therefore be useful, especially in the face of lactic acidosis.

C. **Hypertension.** Indications for treatment of acute hypertension remain the same as for patients with hypertension unrelated to cocaine; however, the hypertensive stimulus will disappear as cocaine is metabolized. Therefore, careful monitoring of patients receiving antihypertensive agents must occur. The great majority of hypertension secondary to cocaine can be managed conservatively in a quiet environment with adjuvant benzodiazepine administration. Additional pharmacologic treatment is usually not necessary because hypertension will resolve as cocaine is metabolized. Once again, beta-adrenergic blockade should be avoided.

D. Tachycardia. As with hypertension, sinus tachycardia will resolve with conservative management and benzodiazepine administration. Other pharmacotherapies, if necessary, should bear in mind the cautions noted above.

E. Anxiety and agitation. Agitated patients should receive liberal doses of benzodiazepines titrated until the desired sedation is achieved. Combative patients should be rapidly sedated because the use of patient restraints alone may exacerbate agitation, muscle activity, rhabdomyolysis, and hyperthermia. Haloperidol may lower the seizure threshold and is less effective than diazepam in multiple animal models.

F. Other. The treatment of pulmonary edema and other complications secondary to cocaine-induced myocardial ischemia has not been systematically studied, and these conditions are generally treated as recommended in other sections of this text (see Chap. 14), with additional emphasis on the treatment cautions noted above.

V. Complications. Cardiovascular complications secondary to cocaine-associated myocardial ischemia occur early in the hospital course. Patients free of complications at the time of ED arrival who do not sustain a myocardial infarction are unlikely to develop subsequent life-threatening arrhythmias, congestive heart failure, or cardiogenic shock. Approximately one-third of patients with cocaine-associated MI will develop complications; however, the great majority of complications occur within 12 hours of presentation.

Because of a low risk of late complications, patients with cocaine-associated chest pain may be ideal candidates for a 12-hour observation period, and acute myocardial infarction may be "ruled out" in the ED.

VI. Initial disposition. The disposition of patients with cocaine-associated chest pain is based on the patients' likelihood of having serious life-threatening disease and the risk of further complications. Most cases of aortic dissection, cardiac tamponade, congestive heart failure, acute vulvular insufficiency, and pulmonary embolism can be identified by history, physical examination, and diagnostic testing in the ED. Their treatment is discussed elsewhere in this text.

Patients with cocaine-associated chest pain without a clearly identified noncardiac explanation have a 20%–60% incidence of ischemic heart disease and a 6% frequency of myocardial infarction. Unfortunately, clinical parameters that could reliably predict or exclude AMI early in its course have not been identified. The location, duration, and quality of chest pain, as well as symptoms associated with chest pain, do not appear to be of use in predicting AMI. Since MI occurs in 4%–5% of patients with cocaine-associated chest pain and normal initial ECGs, a normal ECG does not significantly decrease the likelihood of MI. As a result of the difficulty in identifying patients with cocaine-associated chest pain at low risk for MI, most patients warrant prolonged observation or admission, with serial serum marker testing.

Patients with cocaine-associated chest discomfort who do not sustain an infarction are at very low risk for developing complications after hospital arrival. Patients with cocaine-associated chest pain have approximately a 6% incidence of myocardial infarction, and the likelihood of developing complications secondary to cocaine-associated MI is between 28% and 44%. Cocaine-associated AMI patients may be identified with 94%–100% accuracy by the combined use of electrocardiography, serial CK-MB levels, and a 12-hour observation period. Fewer than 2 out of 1000 patients with cocaine-associated chest discomfort are expected to develop cardiovascular complications not identified during a 12-hour observation period that includes cardiac isoenzyme determinations and ECG testing. Although this strategy has not thoroughly been tested in multicenter clinical trials, its advantages are obvious.

VII. **Long-term management.** Premature development of atherosclerosis may have important long-term implications for the management of patients with cocaine-associated myocardial ischemia. Analogies with unstable angina (unrelated to cocaine) have been made. Up to 40% of patients with cocaine-associated myocardial infarction report prior episodes of chest pain, and new-onset cocaine-associated chest pain predicts an increased risk for MI. Despite analogies, the long-term approach to the management of patients with cocaine-associated chest pain does not require the same level of intensity as the approach to patients with unstable angina unrelated to cocaine.

   A. **Long-term prognosis.** The long-term prognosis of patients with cocaine-associated chest pain is predominantly based on uderlying medical problems and the ability to stop using cocaine. The one-year actuarial survival of this cohort is 98%, with an incidence of late myocardial of 1%. Patients who continue to use cocaine are at increased risk for adverse events (recurrent chest pain, MI, and death) over the ensuing year, whereas patients who stop using cocaine do well.

   B. **Diagnostic testing.** Since patients with cocaine-associated chest pain are not at high risk for myocardial infarction or death over the ensuing year, urgent cardiac evaluation is probably not necessary for patients who "rule out" for MI. Evaluation for possible underlying coronary artery disease may be accomplished on a more elective basis.

      1. **Cardiac catheterization.** Studies of coronary artery anatomy have occurred predominantly in patients who have sustained myocardial infarctions secondary to cocaine. Between 31% and 67% of patients with cocaine-associated MI have underlying coronary artery disease, despite an average age in the 30s.

      2. **Exercise treadmill testing.** The prognostic value of exercise treadmill testing is unclear. An abnormal stress test predicts a greater than 90% likelihood of underlying coronary artery disease. Most patients with cocaine-associated chest pain have normal stress tests. However, a significant percentage of patients

with normal stress tests after cocaine-associated myocardial infarction have coronary artery disease. Abnormal exercise treadmill tests predict underlying coronary artery disease, but normal exercise treadmill tests do not exclude underlying disease.

C. Secondary prevention. Cessation of cocaine use is the hallmark of secondary prevention, because recurrent chest pain, myocardial infarction, and death are less frequent in these patients. Tobacco smoking enhances cocaine-induced coronary artery vasoconstriction and therefore should be avoided. Traditional cardiac risk factor modification may be useful. Because 60% of patients admit recurrent cocaine use over the next year, prophylactic beta blockade should be avoided.

Bibliography

Goldfrank LR, Hoffman RS. The cardiovascular effects of cocaine. *Ann Emerg Med* 20:165–175, 1991.

Hollander JE. Management of cocaine associated myocardial ischemia. *New Engl J Med* 333:1267–1272, 1995.

Hollander JE, Hoffman RS. Cocaine induced myocardial infarction: an analysis and review of the literature. *J Emerg Med* 10:169–177, 1992.

Hollander JE, et al. Cocaine associated myocardial infarction: mortality and complications. *Arch Intern Med* 155:1081–1086, 1995.

Hollander JE, et al. Prospective multicenter evaluation of cocaine associated chest pain. *Acad Emerg Med* 1:330–339, 1994.

Lange RA, et al. Potentiation of cocaine induced coronary vasoconstriction by beta-adrenergic blockade. *Ann Intern Med* 112:897–903, 1990.

Tricyclic Antidepressants

Michael T. Kelley

I. **Epidemiology.** Tricyclic antidepressants (TCA) continue to be the leading cause of morbidity and mortality for the intentional drug overdose. TCAs currently available are listed in Table 32-1. Although treatment of depression is the primary indication for cyclic antidepressants, there are a growing number of indications for these drugs not listed in the product labeling (see Table 32-2). Mortality from these drugs is primarily due to cardiac complications and cardiac arrest. When TCAs are taken in combination with other cardiac drugs, such as beta-blockers or calcium channel-blockers, profound effects on the heart are seen that are often very resistant to treatment.

II. **Mechanisms of toxicity**
   A. **Cardiovascular.** Death from TCA overdose is usually due to cardiac effects, hypotension, and cardiac arrhythmias. This cardiotoxicity is due to TCA-induced cardiac sodium channel blockade and subsequent antichronotropic, antiinotropic and antidromotropic effects. Hypotension is aggravated further by TCA induced alpha-adrenergic blockade.
   B. **Central nervous system.** TCAs inhibit the presynaptic neurotransmitter reuptake of various CNS catecholamines. This enhances seizure activity and altered mental status. TCAs inhibit the movement of chloride at the gamma-aminobutyric acid (GABA) receptor complex. This inhibition increases seizure activity. TCAs also inhibit central sympathetic reflexes.
   C. **Peripheral effects.** TCAs have anticholinergic, antihistaminic and anti-adrenergic effects. Therefore, patients present often with signs and symptoms of anticholinergic overdose (see Chap. 34).

III. **Clinical syndrome of TCA overdose**
   A. **Presentation**
      1. **History.** Along with identification of the TCA ingested, the time of ingestion is very important in the management and prediction of outcome. A large number of TCA overdose cases have trivial symptoms on presentation, but can progress to a major life-threatening event. Almost all life-threatening events occur within 6 hours after ingestion, and the majority occur within 2 hours. The typical scenario in TCA overdose is an intentional ingestion in a suicide attempt of someone who has been diagnosed with depression and recently started on TCA therapy.

      Initial symptoms of overdose are typically sedation, lethargy, stupor, altered mental status, and eventually coma, with or without seizures.
      2. **Physical examination.** Anticholinergic signs predominate early in patients with TCA overdose. Dilated pupils, warm, dry skin and dry mucus membranes, decreased or absent bowel sounds, hallucinations, sedation, and tachycardia are seen. The tachycardia can

Table 32-1. Currently available tricyclic antidepressants

Drug	Daily dose (mg)
Amitriptyline	75–200
Amoxipine	150–300
Clomipramine	100–250
Desipramine	75–200
Doxepine	75–300
Imipramine	75–200
Nortriptyline	75–150
Protriptyline	20–40
Trimipramine	75–200

rapidly progress to bradycardia, heart block, and asystole in serious ingestions. Hypotension accompanies the decreased cardiac output.

A decrease in mental status, respiratory depression, and seizures are seen in serious ingestions. Reflexes are usually brisk, and clonus is not uncommon. Amoxipine has a higher propensity to cause seizures with less cardiovascular symptoms, whereas amitriptyline hydrochloride causes more sedation and cardiovascular effects.

B. Assessment. TCA overdose should be expected in any patient who presents with prolonged QRS and CNS symptoms. However, the TCA amoxipine can cause seizures before widening of the QRS interval.

Table 32-2. Current indications for tricyclic antidepressant use

Indications
Depression
Obsessive-compulsive disorder
Panic disorder*
Enuresis
Attention deficit hyperactivity disorder*
Headache (prophylaxis)*
Peptic ulcer*
Narcolepsy*
Bulimia*
Cocaine withdrawal*
Urinary incontinence
Puritis

* Indications not included in product labeling.

1. **Laboratory.** Electrolytes, BUN, creatinine, glucose, creatinine phosphokinase, urine myoglobin, and pulse oximetry are useful but nonspecific tests.
2. **ECG findings.** The ECG is important for diagnosis and prognosis in a TCA overdose. Because of the anticholinergic effects, an initial tachycardia is seen. TCAs interfere with the movement of sodium ions through the sodium channel. All the intervals of the ECG are prolonged. Classically, a prolongation in QRS is seen. A QRS longer than 100 milliseconds is indicative of TCA ingestion. A QRS duration of 120 milliseconds or longer is a predictor of cardiac and neurologic toxicity. QRS duration greater than 160 milliseconds is predictive of cardiac dysrhythmias. A right axis deviation with a prominent R wave in avr also correlates with serious TCA intoxication. The ECG is more predictive of toxicity than the serum TCA level.
3. **Chest x-ray (CXR).** CXR is only needed for suspicion of aspiration, endotracheal tube (ETT) placement, or if signs and symptoms indicate another possible diagnosis.
4. **Tricyclic plasma levels.** The therapeutic concentration of TCA is 300 ng/ml. Serious toxicity usually is seen when the total TCA (patent compound and metabolite) is 1,000 ng/ml or greater. However, life-threatening toxicity can occur at levels less than 1,000 ng/ml. Plasma levels are usually not as predictive as the ECG of toxicity. No correlation between serum levels and QRS duration has been found. In the acute ingestion, it is not clinically useful to obtain TCA levels.
5. **Arterial blood gases (ABGs).** ABGs can be valuable in the management of intoxication. Maintenance of pH in the normal or slightly alkalotic range is an advantage in TCA overdose. As such, baseline ABGs are important, and in the patient with clinical deterioration, frequent ABGs are indicated.

C. **Management**
1. **Supportive care.** Securing the airway and maintaining vital signs are the initial therapeutic measures of choice. Respirations should be supported as necessary. Sudden onset of hypotension, seizures, and respiratory arrest can occur; therefore, IV access should be obtained early, preferably with an isotonic solution. Although hyperventilation can help to initially correct acidosis until bicarbonate can be administered, low PCO_2 may precipitate seizures.

   Continuous ECG monitoring is recommended. In serious overdoses the initial tachycardia can progress to bradycardia and asystole.
2. **Decontamination.** Because of the possibility of rapid deterioration and sudden onset of seizures, gastric lavage with a 36–40 French lavage tube and instillation of activated charcoal (10 times the ingested dose in grams) are the modalities of choice for decontamination. Syrup of ipecac is contraindicated.

3. **IV fluids.** One of the mainstays of treatment is to prevent hypotension. An initial bolus of 15–20 ml/kg (children) or 200–400 ml (adults) of normal saline is appropriate. However because TCAs are cardiac toxins and depress cardiac output, caution should be used to prevent overhydration. Pulmonary artery catheterization is useful to distinguish the extent of decreased peripheral vascular resistance and decreased cardiac output.

4. **Vasopressors.** Hypotension should be treated aggressively to prevent the formation of lactic acidosis. Acidosis increases the binding of TCAs to the cardiac sodium channel and increases cardiotoxicity. **Norepinephrine** (0.1–0.2 µg/kg/min initial dose, titrate continuous infusion to blood pressure) is the vasopressor of choice. It has direct action on the vasculature and minimal myocardial irritation. TCAs deplete norepinephrine from the presynaptic nerve terminal. Catecholamine stores are often depleted in patients with chronic TCA use. Therefore, dopamine, which acts by releasing presynaptic norepinephrine, may not be effective. Dopamine, owing to its beta-adrenergic stimulatory effects, may also increase myocardial irritability. If cardiac output is low despite adequate filling pressures, dobutamine may be beneficial.

5. **Sodium bicarbonate.** Hypertonic sodium bicarbonate and sodium lactate can reduce the prolongation of the ECG and help correct hypotension and cardiac arrhythmias. Sodium bicarbonate should be administered in patients with QRS prolongation, hypotension or arrhythmias. Bolus therapy (1–2 mEq/kg) is preferred and may be repeated as necessary to treat the symptoms and maintain the pH between 7.50 and 7.55. By mixing the sodium bicarbonate into a continuous drip, the hypertonic sodium effect of the bolus is lost. However, acidosis can aggravate the cardiotoxicity of the TCAs and a drip may be appropriate if the goal is to correct acidosis.

6. **Antiarrhythmics.** The treatment of choice is sodium bicarbonate. Specifically avoid the type Ia and Ic antiarrhythmics.

7. **Treatment of seizures.** Seizures should be treated aggressively to avoid formation of lactic acidosis that can worsen cardiotoxicity. Benzodiazapines and barbiturates are drugs of choice (diazepam 5–10 mg or lorazepam 1–2 mg repeated as necessary; phenobarbital 20 mg/kg infused over 30–60 minutes). Phenytoin has not been found to be helpful and in animal studies has increased the incidence of ventricular tachycardia. If the seizures cannot be readily controlled, paralysis is indicated to prevent acidosis. If the patient is paralyzed, continuous EEG monitoring is necessary.

8. **Other methods of drug elimination.** Hemodialysis and hemoperfusion are not effective for TCA overdoses. TCAs are highly bound to tissue and proteins and consequently have a large volume of distribution.

Encouraging animal experiments have been completed that demonstrate efficacy of TCA specific antibody **Fab fragments.** Currently these antibodies are not available for human treatment.

  9. **Physostigmine.** Physostigmine is contraindicated in the treatment of TCA overdose because it can increase cardiac toxicity.
D. **Patient disposition**
  1. **Admission criteria.** Patients with signs of intoxication should be admitted to a monitored bed for 24 hours. Serious delayed toxicity has only been reported in patients who have not received proper decontamination. If a patient is asymptomatic, with normal ECG, discharge or transfer to psychiatric care is safe at 24 hours.
  2. **Discharge criteria.** There is good evidence that the majority of serious events associated with TCA intoxication occur within 6 hours after ingestion. If the patient has received appropriate decontamination and there are no signs of intoxication (i.e., no anticholinergic signs, no ECG changes, including tachycardia), it is safe to assume the ingestion did not occur, was not serious, or was prevented by decontamination. These patients may be safely discharged to the care of a psychiatrist. However, psychiatric consultation should be obtained on all suicide attempts regardless of the seriousness of the attempt.

Bibliography

Baldessarini RJ. Drugs and the treatment of psychiatric disorders. In Gilman AG, et al. (eds.). *Goodman and Gilman's The Pharmacological Basis of Therapeutics* (8th ed.). New York: Pergamon Press, 1990.

Benowitz NL. Cyclic antidepressants. In Olsen KR (ed.). *Poisoning and Drug Overdose* (2nd ed.). Norwalk, CT: Appleton & Lange, 1994.

Hoffman JR, Votey SR, Bayer M, Silver L. Effect of hypertonic sodium bicarbonate in the treatment of moderate-to-severe cyclic antidepressant overdose. *Am J Emerg Med.* 11:336–341, 1993.

Liebelt EL, Francis PD, Woolf AD. ECG lead a VR versus QRS interval in predicting seizures and arrhythmias in acute tricyclic antidepressant toxicity. *Ann Emerg Med* 26:195–201, 1995.

Weisman RS, Howland MA, Hoffman RS, et al. Cyclic antidepressants. In Goldfrank LR, et al. (ed.). *Goldfrank's Toxicologic Emergencies* (5th ed.). Norwalk, CT: Appleton & Lange, 1994.

Calcium Channel Blocker and Beta-Blocker Toxicity

Colin G. Kaide

With the invention of many new types of calcium channel blockers (CCBs) and beta-adrenergic receptor blockers (BBs), and with the expanding roles they play in the practice of medicine, there has been an increase in the number of patients seen for accidental or intentional overdose of these medications. Along with the traditional roles they play in the treatment of hypertension and arrhythmias, both BBs and CCBs are employed in diverse, noncardiovascular disease states such as chronic pain, migraine headaches, schizophrenia, tremors, pheochromocytoma, glaucoma, and anxiety. Poisoning from these medications may result from intentional or accidental overdose or may occur with appropriate therapeutic dosing in a patient with intrinsic conduction system disease, preexisting cardiac pump dysfunction, and liver or renal failure. Some medications may predispose a patient to increased toxicity from smaller doses of CCBs and BBs. These may include concomitant use of ethanol, BBs/CCBs, and other cardiovascular medications.

According to the annual report of the American Association of Poison Control Centers, in 1993 there were 5063 exposures to BBs with 17 deaths, and 6730 CCB poisonings with 35 deaths. Of the 74 mortalities in 1993 associated with cardiovascular drugs, CCBs and BBs together accounted for 70%.

Understanding the principles of management for these drug toxicities is essential in a time when these agents have expanding roles in medical practice.

I. **Calcium channel blocker toxicity**
   A. **Pharmacology.** The calcium channel blockers are classified as class IV antiarrhythmic drugs. This group is comprised of chemically diverse compounds that all share the common action of inhibiting the influx of calcium across cell membranes of cardiac and smooth muscle through slow calcium channels. The most clinically important effects of this are the dose-dependent decrease in cardiac contractility and vascular smooth muscle tone and the slowing of conduction through the atrioventricular (AV) and sinoatrial (SA) nodes.

   There are three main chemical classes of CCB, each of which demonstrates slightly different pharmacologic effects based on subtle differences in receptor binding. They are the phenylalkylamines, benzothiazepines, and dihydropyridines, the prototypes of which are verapamil, diltiazem, and nifedipine, respectively. A fourth class, the phenylpiperizines, contains investigational drugs that are not in use clinically at this time (Table 33-1).

   The CCBs are all rapidly absorbed from the GI tract and have an onset of action as rapidly as 30 minutes. Sustained release preparations begin their action with similar rapidity, but their peak effect usually is delayed. All

Table 33-1. Calcium channel blockers

Generic name	Trade name	Class	Available preparation	Half-life (hours)	Duration of action	Sinus rate	Inotropy	AV node rate	Vascular tone
Verapamil	Calan*	PAA	PO, IV, SR	4	6–8	↔	↓↓	↓↓	→
Diltiazem	Cardizem	BTP	PO, IV, SR	4–6	6	→	↔/↓	→	↓↓↓
Nifedipine	Procardia**	DHP	PO, SL, SR	2	7	↔/↑	↔	↔	↓↓
Nimodipine	Nimotop	DHP	PO	1–2	4	↔/↑	↔	↔	↓↓
Amlodipine	Norvasc	DHP	PO	30–50	24	↔/↑	↔	↔	↓↓
Felodipine	Plendil	DHP	PO, SR	10	6–8	↔/↑	↔	↔	↓↓
Nicardipine	Cardene	DHP	PO, IV, SR	8–9	3	↔/↑	↔	↔	↓↓
Isradipine	Dynacirc	DHP	PO	8–16	12	↔/↑	↔	↔	↓↓
Bepridil	Vascor	***	PO	42	?	→	↓↓	→	→

* Also Isoptin.
** Also Adalat.
*** Not related to others; may prolong Q-T interval via membrane stabilizing effects.
↔ = No change.

three prototype drugs are protein-bound and lipid-soluble and undergo hepatic metabolism. Urinary excretion of verapamil and nifedipine and their metabolites plays a significant role in elimination. Diltiazem and its metabolites are excreted into bile and eliminated in feces.

B. **Pathophysiology.** The pathophysiologic changes seen in CCB overdose vary with the drug ingested. CCBs vary in their effect on target cells as a function of their receptor-binding characteristics; in overdose the subtleties of pharmacologic effects characteristic to a particular drug tend to be maintained.

1. **Verapamil.** Verapamil is a nonselective inhibitor of the slow calcium channel, exerting its effects on the conduction system, the heart muscle, and the vasculature. This results in a **slowing of AV node conduction,** decreased cardiac contractility, and **peripheral vasodilatation,** respectively. When compared to other CCBs, verapamil demonstrates the strongest effect on cardiac conduction. Verapamil overdoses manifest a much more severe effect at the AV node than any other CCB. Although verapamil (and diltiazem) have a depressant effect at the SA node, it usually is offset by reflex tachycardia. At high concentrations verapamil also can have an inhibitory effect on fast sodium channels producing effects reminiscent of Ia antidysrhythmics such as widening of the QRS complex or Q-T prolongation.

2. **Nifedipine.** Nifedipine is more selective than verapamil, blocking the slow calcium channels in some tissues while leaving others relatively unaffected. Nifedipine has its effects predominantly on vascular smooth muscle, causing decreases in systemic and coronary vascular resistance. The hypotension seen in overdoses results primarily from **vasodilatation.** Even at very high doses, nifedipine exerts little decrease in inotropy and AV conduction. Although the SA node is not directly affected, the vasodilatation caused by nifedipine may cause an increased heart rate via **reflex tachycardia.** Nimodipine, another dihydropyridine, is similar to nifedipine, but it has a particular affinity for vasodilatation of the cerebral vasculature and is used for that effect in the treatment of vasospasm seen in subarachnoid hemorrhages.

3. **Diltiazem.** Diltiazem shows similar effects to those of verapamil; however, it is much less potent. It has the ability to block slow and fast channels depending on the dose. Although it may have similar AV node blocking potential as verapamil, it shows less lengthening of AV refractoriness. It causes less vasodilatation than nifedipine.

C. **Presentation of CCB overdose**

1. **History.** The patient who is intoxicated with CCBs may present with a spectrum of illnesses ranging from few or no symptoms to complete cardiovascular collapse. Onset of symptoms after CCB intoxication can occur within minutes for IV dosing. With oral preparations, typical onset is 1–3 hours post ingestion. With

sustained release (SR) preparations, symptoms generally start later and have been reported to occur after more than 6 hours in up to 10% of patients.

In most cases, CNS symptoms seen with all classes of CCBs are due to cerebral hypoperfusion. These symptoms include lightheadedness, dizziness, syncope, altered mental status, lethargy, and coma. In contrast, some reports indicate that confusion and decreased level of consciousness may occur despite normal perfusion. In patients with underlying coronary artery disease, hypotension may trigger angina symptoms. Gastrointestinal side effects may include nausea, vomiting, and constipation from diminished GI motility.

In the diagnosis of CCB overdose, history and clinical suspicion will provide the most useful information to the clinician, since some of the characteristic findings of hypotension, bradycardia, and varying degrees of cardiac blockade are also characteristic of other drug overdoses (see sec **III.C.**). Elucidation of all underlying medical problems and other drugs that the patient uses or may have taken in overdose will be helpful in comprehensive management (Table 33-2).

2. **Physical examination.** Myocardial depression and hypotension are the hallmark signs of CCB intoxication. The typical bradycardia and bradyarrhythmias seen with verapamil and diltiazem (and others in their classes) may be overridden in nifedipine intoxication by the reflex tachycardia secondary to severe vasodilatation. Significant myocardial pump dysfunction can be seen with verapamil and diltiazem poisoning and may result in signs of congestive heart failure or angina.

Patients often appear lethargic, but not cold and

Table 33-2. Differential diagnosis of CCB and BB intoxication

Drugs	Poisons	Physical problems
Calcium channel blockers	Organophosphates	Myocardial infarction
Beta-blockers	Hydrogen sulfide	Sinus node disease
Digoxin	Cyanide	AV node disease
Clonidine		Hyperkalemia
Lidocaine		
Quinidine		
Procainamide		
Chloroquine		
Sedative hypnotics		
Narcotics		
End-stage tricyclics		
End-stage cocaine		

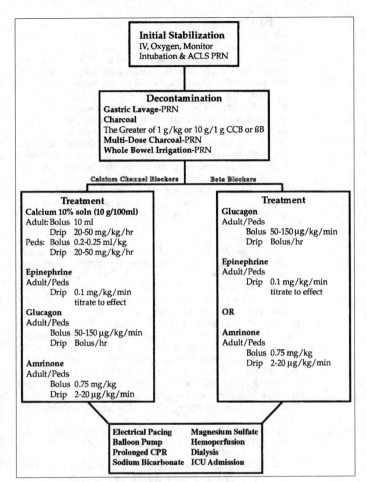

Initial Stabilization
IV, Oxygen, Monitor
Intubation & ACLS PRN

Decontamination
Gastric Lavage-PRN
Charcoal
The Greater of 1 g/kg or 10 g/1 g CCB or ßB
Multi-Dose Charcoal-PRN
Whole Bowel Irrigation-PRN

Calcium Channel Blockers

Treatment
Calcium 10% soln (10 g/100ml)
Adult: Bolus 10 ml
        Drip 20-50 mg/kg/hr
Peds: Bolus 0.2-0.25 ml/kg
        Drip 20-50 mg/kg/hr

Epinephrine
Adult/Peds
        Drip 0.1 mg/kg/min
              titrate to effect
Glucagon
Adult/Peds
        Bolus 50-150 µg/kg/min
        Drip Bolus/hr

Amrinone
Adult/Peds
        Bolus 0.75 mg/kg
        Drip 2-20 µg/kg/min

Beta Blockers

Treatment
Glucagon
Adult/Peds
        Bolus 50-150 µg/kg/min
        Drip Bolus/hr

Epinephrine
Adult/Peds
        Drip 0.1 mg/kg/min
              titrate to effect

OR

Amrinone
Adult/Peds
        Bolus 0.75 mg/kg
        Drip 2-20 µg/kg/min

Electrical Pacing	Magnesium Sulfate
Balloon Pump	Hemoperfusion
Prolonged CPR	Dialysis
Sodium Bicarbonate	ICU Admission

Fig. 33-1.   Algorithm for CCB and BB intoxication.

clammy, despite hypotension. Although rare, focal neurologic deficits have been reported.

D. Assessment
   1. Laboratory studies. Initial laboratory studies should include BUN, creatinine, electrolytes, glucose, calcium, and an ABG. A routine CBC and magnesium, phosphate, and liver function tests may be performed as needed. Alterations in glucose homeostasis with resultant hyperglycemia may be evident in the blockade of calcium-dependent release of insulin. Metabolic acidosis, possibly a result of hypoperfusion, can be found on routine screening labs.
   2. ECG. ECG tracings typically show a narrow complex junctional rhythm with CCBs that have strong AV

nodal blocking properties. Second- and third-degree AV block or sinus arrest with junctional escape rhythm may result in bradycardia. PR prolongation can be seen with verapamil (even with therapeutic doses). Reflex sinus tachycardia may be seen with nifedipine and amlodipine (a dihydropyridine). Inverted P waves, nonspecific ST and T wave changes, and even asystole have been reported. Ventricular tachyarrhythmias are rare and when seen should suggest primary cardiac disorders, electrolyte imbalances, and other drug toxicities. The exception to this is seen with bepridil (Vascor) and very high-dose verapamil, which have class Ia antiarrhythmic activity and can cause Q-T prolongation with resultant torsades de pointes.

   3. **Toxicology screening.** As in any intentional overdose, levels of salicylates and acetaminophen should be obtained since they are widely available and frequently appear as potentially lethal coingestants. Levels of other therapeutic medications such as digoxin should be sought to alleviate potential confusion caused by their untoward effects. Digoxin manifests cardiotoxic ECG effects similar to those manifested by CCBs. Drug levels of CCBs are not routinely available and have not been shown to correlate with the clinical picture or have prognostic significance.

E. **Management.** The goal of treatment in a CCB overdose is to improve perfusion to critical organ systems. Attempts to decrease the amount of absorbed drug, increase the heart rate and myocardial contractility, and improve vascular tone should be the mainstay of therapy. The propensity of the CCB poisoned patient to undergo rapid deterioration necessitates timely evaluation and treatment in the critical care area of the emergency department (ED).

   1. **Supportive care.** As in any cardiovascular emergency, stabilization of the airway, breathing, and circulation (ABCs) take the highest priority. The patient should be placed on a cardiac monitor with supplemental oxygen and have at least one large-bore IV line established. Obtunded patients, or those suspected of imminent cardiovascular collapse should have definitive airway control initiated with rapid sequence endotracheal intubation. Agents that may cause a further drop in blood pressure, such as thiopental and high-dose midazolam, should be avoided while performing the rapid-sequence intubation. Consider etomidate or ketamine with a paralytic agent to facilitate laryngoscopy and tube placement.

   2. **Decontamination.** In patients presenting to the ED within 1–2 hours of ingestion, orogastric lavage should be considered. A dose of activated charcoal is indicated after lavage in any patient with suspected overdose of CCBs. The larger of 1 g/kg body weight or 10 g/g CCB ingested should be administered. Repeat dosing of activated charcoal without cathartic (0.5 g/kg q4–6h) may help in overdoses of sustained release prepara-

tion CCB. In addition, for sustained release CCB overdoses, whole bowel irrigation may be considered with
solutions like Golytely (1–2 liter/hr for adults and 500
ml/h for children until all pills are accounted for or
clear diarrhea is produced). Because CCBs are highly
protein-bound and lipophilic and have a large volume
of distribution, dialysis and hemoperfusion are relatively ineffective in CCB overdose.

3. **Treatment of hypotension.** As the initial treatment
of hypotension, **fluid boluses** of isotonic saline may
be helpful (1 liter for adults and 20 ml/kg for children).
Care should be exercised to avoid injudicious fluid
overload and resultant pulmonary edema in patients
with impaired contractility. Further treatment of hypotension should include calcium and pressor therapy.

   a. **Calcium therapy.** Calcium salts are the mainstay
   of treatment of symptomatic CCB overdose. Calcium chloride is preferable to the gluconate or glu-
   cepate forms because it has been shown to produce
   more reliable increases in plasma-ionized calcium
   concentrations. The initial dose is a 1 g IV bolus
   (10 ml of 10% solution) or 0.1–0.2 ml/kg, followed
   by a continuous infusion. The effect of bolus dosing
   of calcium on blood pressure and cardiac output
   usually is only transient, suggesting that an infusion of 20–50 mg/kg/hr of calcium chloride in saline
   may provide a more sustained, effective treatment.
   The most prominent effect of calcium is on contractility with minimal effect on SA/AV nodal conduction or on vasodilatation. Measurement of calcium
   levels has been suggested at 30 minutes then every
   2 hours thereafter, but the need or usefulness of
   this has not yet been established. **Warning:** calcium treatment may have deleterious effects in patients who have overdosed on or who are using
   digoxin!

   b. **Catecholamines.** The choice of pressor agents
   should be based in part on the theoretical advantage of mixed alpha$_1$ and beta$_1$ agonists and in part
   on the clinician's familiarity with specific pressor
   agents. Both dopamine and epinephrine have
   these properties and have been used successfully.
   An important consideration with catecholamine
   use is that the amount of agonist drug needed may
   be much higher than usual and should be titrated
   to effect (e.g., adequate tissue perfusion, heart rate
   >60), and not limited to standard doses.

   c. **Glucagon.** Glucagon, the mainstay of treatment
   in BB toxicity, has been shown to be beneficial in
   treating CCBs as well. It enhances myocardial performance by increasing cyclic AMP just as catecholamines do, but it interacts with its own specific
   glucagon receptor. Because of the variable response to this treatment, a total dose of 10 mg
   should be given IV before moving on to another
   agent. One approach is to try 50–150 µg/kg

(3.5–10.5 mg in a 70-kg patient initially) and re-peat the dose if necessary. The effect of glucagon lasts only 15 minutes, and an infusion of 2–10 mg/hr (or the initial effective bolus dose given by drip/hr) is a reasonable place to start. No maxi-mum dose is yet defined for glucagon, and doses from 2–10 mg/hr for 26 hours have been reported. Nausea, vomiting, mild hypertension, hyper-glycemia, and transient hyperkalemia may be seen with high-dose glucagon. Serious side effects of glucagon administration are not described. The manufacturer uses phenol in the ready-to-mix preparation of glucagon. The drug should be resus-pended in saline or D5W to avoid phenol toxicity with these unusually high doses.

   d. Phosphodiesterase inhibitors. Amrinone, a phosphodiesterase inhibitor, is gaining popularity in CCB overdose treatment. It acts to inhibit the breakdown of cAMP, prolonging its effects on in-tracellular calcium. In canine models and in some studies of human CCB intoxication, it improved cardiac function. The loading dose is 0.75 mg/kg, followed by a titrated infusion of 2–20 µg/kg/min.

4. Treatment of bradycardia. The treatment for brady-cardia and hypotension often follow the same course. For instance, not only calcium therapy can reverse hy-potension, it also can reverse bradycardia and block as well. Atropine and pacing, however, are specific thera-pies aimed at the bradycardia in CCB overdose.

   a. Atropine. Up to 30% of patients with CCB over-dose and bradycardia may respond to atropine. The usual dose of 0.5 mg q2–3min may be repeated to a vagolytic dose of 3 mg (pediatric dose = 0.02 mg/kg; min = 0.15 mg, max = 3 mg).

   b. Electrical pacing. Transcutaneous or transve-nous pacing may be required in cases of refractory bradycardia. In CCB overdose the optimal rate for pacing is 50–60 bpm. Slower rates with higher cur-rent settings would provide the optimal pacer cap-ture range while avoiding a contractile deficit (negative Woodworth staircase effect).

5. Other treatment modalities. Extracorporeal circu-lation, aortic balloon pumps, and prolonged CPR have been employed with varying degrees of success. Treat-ment of rare malignant arrhythmias should follow standard ACLS protocols, such as infusion of magne-sium in the treatment of torsades de pointes.

F. Patient disposition. Patients who are initially asympto-matic and who subsequently begin to develop signs of tox-icity should be stabilized and admitted to an intensive care unit. In order to safely discharge a patient from the ED, blood pressures must be reassessed and orthostatic changes evaluated. Urine output should be assured, and a repeat ECG also should be checked. Patients with sus-pected CCB ingestion who remain asymptomatic through

8–10 hours of observation may be medically cleared of this ingestion and transferred to psychiatric care as needed.

II. Beta-adrenergic blocker toxicity

A. **Pharmacology.** Beta-adrenergic antagonists, or beta-blockers (BBs), are class II antiarrhythmic agents with a wide range of pharmacologic properties which include varying degrees of receptor selectivity, intrinsic agonist properties, membrane stabilizing effects, and lipid solubility. The ultimate results of these actions are to decrease heart rate, contractility. SA/AV nodal conduction, and blood pressure. In overdose these drugs may have the deleterious effect of inducing CNS depression and potentiating hypotension, hypoglycemia, and bronchospasm.

   The 20 or so BBs in existence today can be classified according to a number of parameters: receptor selectivity (blockade of $beta_1$ only), intrinsic agonist activity (stimulation of beta receptors), membrane stabilizing properties (sodium channel blockade), and lipid solubility. $Beta_1$ receptors are located in the myocardium, kidney, and eye; $beta_2$ receptors are found in adipose tissue, the pancreas, the liver, and smooth and skeletal muscle. At normal doses receptor selectivity is maintained; however, in overdose it is lost, and $beta_1$ and $beta_2$ receptors are affected almost equally (Table 33-3).

B. **Pathophysiology.** Poisoning from these medications may result from intentional or accidental overdose or may occur with appropriate therapeutic dosing in a patient with intrinsic conduction system disease or preexisting pump dysfunction. Some conditions or medications may predispose a patient to increased toxicity from smaller doses of BBs. These may include concomitant use of CCBs, congestive heart failure, and reactive airway disease. Although a rare occurrence, ocular instillation of aqueous BB may precipitate hypotension and/or bradycardia in sensitive individuals. The exact symptoms and signs may vary with the type of BB used, depending on whether it is $beta_1$ selective, has beta agonist properties, or is a vasodilator. For instance, labetolol has vasodilator properties and may cause more hypotension, whereas sotolol, which has class III antiarrhythmic effects, may potentiate ventricular arrhythmias.

C. **Clinical presentation**

   1. **History.** One of the most important features of BB overdose is the early, sudden onset of potentially life-threatening toxicity. The patient who is intoxicated with BBs may present with a spectrum of illness ranging from few or no symptoms to complete cardiovascular collapse. Onset of symptoms after BB intoxication can occur within minutes for IV dosing. With oral preparations, typical onset is 20 minutes to 4 hours postingestion. With sustained release (SR) preparations, peak effect may be significantly delayed.

      Symptoms are very similar to CCB overdose (see above). Changes in mental status are common, ranging from depression of consciousness to seizures. The

502 V. Toxicologic Cardiovascular Emergencies

Table 33-3. Beta-blockers

Generic name	Trade name	Available preparation	Half-life (hours)	Duration of action	Membrane stabilizing	Cardioselective	Lipid solubility	Partial agonist
Acebutolol	Sectral	PO	3–4	10–24	+	+	Mod	+
Atenolol	Tenormin	PO, IV	5–8	24	0	+	Low	0
Betaxolol	Betoptic	PO, OC	14	12–24	0	+	Low	0
Bisoprolol	Zebeta	PO	10–12	24	0	+	Low	0
Carteolol	Cartrol	PO	6	72	0	0	Low	++
Esmolol	Brevibloc	IV	8 min	20 min	0	+	Low	0
Labetalol	Normodyne*	PO, IV	4–6	8	0	0	Low	0
Levobunolol	Betagan	OC	5–6	8	0	0	Low	0
Metoprolol	Lopressor	PO, IV, SR	3–4	3–6	+/–	+	Mod	0
Nadolol	Corgard	PO	12–20	14–24	0	0	Low	0
Penbutolol	Levatol	PO	5	24	0	0	Low	+
Pindolol	Visken	PO	4	24	+	0	Mod	+++
Propranolol	Inderal	PO, IV, SR	4	4–8	++	0	High	0
Sotalol	Betapace	PO	7–18	24	0	0	Low	0
Timolol	Timoptic**	OC, PO	4	15	0	0	Low	+/–

* Also Trandate.
** Also Blocadren.

generalized tonic-clonic seizures tend to be brief in duration and respond to conventional therapy. The mechanism for these effects has not been fully elucidated but may result both indirectly from decreased CNS perfusion (myocardial depression) and from the direct effect of sodium channel blockade and membrane stabilization. Bronchospasm with resulting shortness of breath rarely can be seen in individuals who do not have underlying reactive airway disease.

2. **Physical examination.** Bradycardia and hypotension are the hallmark cardiac manifestations of severe BB intoxication. Unlike calcium channel blocker overdose, hypotension with BBs usually is not the result of direct vasodilatation. The exception to this is with labetalol, which exerts direct vasodilator effects through its alpha blocking properties.

D. **Assessment**

1. **Laboratory studies.** Initial laboratory studies should include an ECG, BUN, creatinine, electrolytes, glucose, and an ABG. A routine CBC and calcium, magnesium, phosphate, and liver function tests may be added as needed. Beta-blockers can cause hypoglycemia, especially in diabetics on insulin, due to inhibition of pancreatic islet cells. Acidosis is common due to hypoperfusion. Drug levels of BBs are not routinely available and are not shown to be necessary in early management of toxicity. Digoxin levels as indicated may help limit the differential diagnosis. Digoxin and BB overdose share similar cardiovascular features.

2. **ECG.** ECG findings may include sinus bradycardia (or rarely tachycardia), varying-degree AV nodal blockade, interventricular conduction delays (QRS widening), hemiblocks, and asystole. Drugs with prominent membrane-stabilizing effects are most likely to produce the Ia antiarrhythmic-like QRS widening. Although tachyarrhythmias are not common with most BBs, sotalol, owing to its class III effects, may produce ventricular tachycardia/fibrillation or torsades de pointes.

E. **Management.** The goal of treatment in a BB overdose is to improve perfusion to critical organ systems. Attempts to decrease the amount of absorbed drug, increase heart rate, and contractility and to improve vascular tone should be the mainstay of therapy.

1. **Supportive care.** The propensity of BB-poisoned patients to undergo rapid deterioration of their condition would necessitate timely evaluation and treatment in the critical care area of the ED. As in any emergency, stabilization of the ABCs take the highest priority. The patient should be placed on a cardiac monitor with supplemental oxygen and have large-bore IV lines established. The obtunded patient or a patient suspected of imminent cardiovascular collapse should have definitive airway control initiated with rapid-sequence endotracheal intubation.

2. **Decontamination.** In patients presenting to the ED within 1–2 hours of ingestion, orogastric lavage should

be considered. In some series pill fragments have been recovered up to 4–6 hours after ingestion. A dose of activated charcoal with cathartic is indicated after, or in place of, lavage in any patient with suspected overdose of BBs. In addition to repeated activated charcoal administration, for sustained release BB overdoses whole bowel irrigation may be considered with solutions like Golytely (1–2 liter/hr in adults and 500 ml/hr in children until all pills are accounted for or clear diarrhea is produced). Unlike overdoses of calcium channel blockers, certain BBs (those with a small volume of disribution and a long half-life) can be eliminated with hemoperfusion or hemodialysis (e.g., acebutolol, atenolol, nadolol, and sotalol).

3. **Treatment of hypotension**

   a. **IV fluids.** In contrast to CCB overdose, primary vasodilatation in BB overdose is not as much of a problem as a profound decrease in contractility. Care should be exercised to avoid injudicious fluid overload in patients with impaired contractility. Small fluid boluses of isotonic saline may be helpful as the initial treatment of mild hypotension. However, if bradycardia and decreased inotropy are the causes of the hypotension, these problems should be addressed directly.

   b. **Glucagon.** Glucagon has become first-line therapy in BB-intoxicated patients. Clinical experience has shown favorable success even in cases for which other modalities have failed. Glucagon stimulates the production of cAMP via nonadrenergic mechanisms and can enhance contractility, heart rate, and AV conduction. Glucagon should be given to adults at the dose of 3–5 mg boluses q5min until a response occurs, to a maximum dose of 10–15 mg. Pediatric dose is 50–150 µg/kg. Response should be seen in a few minutes but only lasts 10–20 minutes, usually requiring a glucagon drip. Optimal drip dosing has not been established, but 2–10 mg/hr (or the initial effective bolus dose given by drip/hr) is a reasonable place to start.

   c. **Catecholamines.** Beta-adrenergic agents are an integral part of BB overdose management, but failures have been seen using these agents alone. **Epinephrine** has strong beta$_1$ agonist properties and may be the pressor of choice. Successes have been reported with doses from 30 to greater than 100 µg/min. Isoproterenol also has strong beta$_1$ effects, but its beta$_2$ stimulation causes vasodilatation and may contribute to worsening hypotension. Agents with predominantly alpha-adrenergic properties may improve vascular tone, but they do not have much effect on inotropy and chronotropy and may decrease cardiac output by raising afterload. If isoproterenol is used, a logical combination may be to add an alpha agent like phenylephrine or norepinephrine to counteract the beta$_2$ mediated vasodilatation. **Dopamine,** a mixed alpha and beta agent, may be a reasonable choice at intermediate doses; however, as one approaches 20 µg/kg/min, alpha effects begin to predominate. An important consideration with catecholamine use is that the amount of beta agonist drug needed may be much higher than usual and should be titrated to effect (e.g., adequate tissue perfusion, heart rate >60) and not necessarily limited to standard doses.

   d. **Phosphodiesterase inhibitors.** Amrinone is becoming more popular in the literature as an adjunct to, or as a replacement for, catecholamine use in BB overdose. Its ability to inhibit cAMP breakdown by a pathway distinct from catecholamines makes it a good choice in the catecholamine-blocked patient. The loading dose is 0.75 mg/kg followed by a titrated infusion of 2–20 µg/kg/min.

4. **Treatment of bradycardia**
   a. **Atropine.** Atropine at standard doses may improve heart rate but only in up to 25% of patients.
   b. **Electrical pacing.** Pacing may be beneficial in BB overdose, especially for overdrive pacing in sotalol-induced torsades de pointes.
   c. **Sodium bicarbonate.** Sodium bicarbonate (as used in cyclic antidepressant overdoses) may be useful in treating the wide-complex tachycardia induced by BB with membrane-stabilizing properties.

5. **Other treatment modalities.** Extracorporeal circulation, aortic balloon pumps, and prolonged CPR have been employed with varying degrees of success. Treatment of malignant arrhythmias should follow standard ACLS protocols such as infusion of magnesium in the treatment of torsades de pointes.

F. **Patient disposition.** Patients with mild bradycardia (>50 bpm) and mild symptoms can be evaluated on an individual basis, but generally they should be admitted for observation due to the potentially prolonged effects of BB overdose. Patients who present initially asymptomatic and subsequently begin to develop signs of toxicity should be stabilized and admitted to an intensive care unit.

   In order to safely discharge a patient, blood pressures must be reassessed and orthostatic changes evaluated. Urine output and a repeat ECG should also be checked. Patients with suspected BB ingestion who remain asymptomatic through 8–10 hours of observation may be medically cleared of this ingestion and transferred to psychiatric care as needed.

Bibliography

Goldfrank LR, et al. *Goldfrank's Toxicologic Emergencies.* Norwalk, CT: Appleton & Lange, 1994.

Kerns W, Kline J, Ford M. Beta-Blocker and calcium channel blocker toxicity. In Ford M, Olshaker J (eds.), *Emergency Medicine Clinics of*

North America: Concepts and Controversies in Toxicology. Philadelphia: Saunders, 1994.

Smilkstein MJ. Common cardiac medications. In Rosen P, Barkin R (eds.), *Emergency Medicine: Concepts and Clinical Practice.* St. Louis: Mosby–Year Book, 1992.

Viccellio P, Henry M. Beta blockers and calcium channel blockers. In Tintinalli JE (ed.), *Emergency Medicine: A Comprehensive Study Guide.* New York: McGraw-Hill, Inc, 1992.

Wolf L, Spadafora M, Otten E. Use of amrinone and glucagon in a case of calcium channel blocker overdose. *Ann Emerg Med* 22:1225–1228, 1993.

Miscellaneous Drugs and Toxins

Michelle A. Flemmings

Almost all classes of medications have an effect on the cardiovascular system. Depending on the particular medication, these effects may be beneficial in therapeutic doses but undesirable and potentially life-threatening when taken in excessive or toxic doses.

It is important to always include the side effects and toxic effects of medications in the differential diagnosis of a patient with cardiovascular complaints. Increasing numbers of patients with underlying medical problems are prescribed several medications that, even at recommended doses, can adversely affect the cardiovascular system. Combinations of agents can potentiate adverse effects directly or by altering metabolism and elimination of the medications involved.

This chapter will discuss the cardiovascular effects of beta-adrenergic agonists, alpha-adrenergic agonists, methylxanthines, anticholinergics, stimulates, and cholinergic drug ingestions. Discussion will focus on their general presentation, assessment, and emergency department (ED) management.

I. **Beta-adrenergic agonists.** Beta-adrenergic agonist agents are most commonly used in the treatment of asthma and chronic obstructive pulmonary disease. In the treatment of acute exacerbation of bronchospasm, inhaled beta-agonist medications are considered first-line therapy because of their rapid onset of action, ease of delivery, and relative lack of adverse side effects. Table 34-1 lists some of the more commonly used agents.

The beta-adrenergic agonists are classified as selective (B_1 or B_2) or nonselective. B_1 receptors are primarily located in the myocardium and when stimulated result in tachycardia and increased inotropy. B_2 receptors, which are concentrated in bronchial and vascular smooth muscle, cause bronchodilatation and vasodilatation with reflex increase in heart rate when stimulated. B_2 receptors are also found in the genirourinary (GU) tract, GI tract, and skeletal muscle. The manifestations of beta-agonist ingestion will depend somewhat on relative receptor selectivity.

A. **Presentation**

1. **History.** The patient history is the most crucial portion of the assessment in any case of possible toxic ingestion. Questions should be asked regarding the medication regimen, including changes in dosage or frequency of use and addition of other medications, both prescription and over-the-counter. Patients should be questioned about their social habits, including the use of recreational drugs and alcohol. A past medical history emphasizing underlying illnesses will be helpful in anticipating possible complications of both the ingestion and therapeutic modalities applied.

   Because these agents are most commonly prescribed for the treatment of bronchospasm, the classic history

Table 34-1.   Commonly used beta-agonist medications

Drug	Route of administration	Therapeutic use
Terbutaline	PO, IV, SQ, aerosol	Bronchodilatation
Metaproterenol	Aerosol	Bronchodilatation
Albuterol	IV, aerosol	Bronchodilatation
Isoproterenol	IV	Increased inotropy, increased chronotropy, bronchodilatation

is a patient with asthma or chronic obstructive pulmonary disease (COPD) who is experiencing an acute exacerbation of bronchospasm unrelieved by several repeated doses of inhaled beta$_2$-agonist agents over the past several minutes to hours. Patients develop tolerance to the therapeutic effects of inhaled beta$_2$ agonists when these are taken in overdose. They complain of difficulty breathing and tremor followed by palpitations and dizziness. Gradual onset of rapid heart rate occurs and is associated with headache, gastrointestinal upset, and nausea. Patients with underlying cardiovascular disease may report sudden worsening of shortness of breath and anginal chest pain.

2. **Physical examination**
   a. **General appearance.** The general appearance is that of an anxious and agitated person. The patient will likely exhibit rapid shallow breathing with the use of accessory muscles and audible bilateral expiratory wheezes.
   b. **Pulmonary.** Tachypnea occurs in an attempt to maintain adequate oxygenation despite ventilation-perfusion mismatching. Further complicating acute bronchospasm, toxic doses of inhaled beta-adrenergic agonists can cause paradoxic bronchoconstriction, resulting in sudden worsening of relative hypoxia. This reaction is due to the propellant agents used and to the development of hypersensitivity within the bronchial tree. A silent chest, unequal breath sounds, or signs of impending respiratory failure indicate the need to postpone further physical examination in favor of definitive management of airway and breathing. In the elderly, rales may be audible because of congestive heart failure (CHF).
   c. **Cardiac.** Blood pressure typically is decreased, but may be increased. The pulse is rapid and regular, with occasional extrasystoles or irregular rhythm requiring further evaluation with a 12-lead ECG. Patients with a history of coronary artery disease can present with hemodynamic compromise because of their inability to compen-

sate for these physiologic alterations. Hypotension
with a thready pulse and cool extremities or distended neck veins, S3 gallop, and rales may be
noted.

d. GI. Although patients often complain of nausea
and may vomit, the abdominal examination is
usually unremarkable. Bowel sounds may be decreased.

e. Skin. The skin is often flushed and diaphoretic because of vasodilatation and the hyperdynamic
state of the cardiovascular system.

f. CNS. Tremors of the extremities are evident, often causing great concern to the patient. Because
beta agonists do not cross the blood-brain barrier,
central nervous system symptoms are uncharac-
teristic. Any patient suspected of ingesting a toxic
amount of a beta agonist who presents with an altered mental status should be evaluated regarding
possible coingestants, electrolyte or acid-base disturbance, and primary CNS pathology.

B. Assessment

1. Laboratory studies. Evaluation should include blood
for electrolytes, glucose, phosphate, and arterial blood
gases (ABGs). **Hypokalemia** is a common complication
of beta-agonist ingestion because of the beta-mediated
intracellular movement of potassium. Transient hyperkalemia may also be noted as potassium stores are released from the liver prior to entering skeletal muscle.
Hyperglycemia is commonly seen because of stimulation of glycogenolysis and gluconeogenesis and inhibition of the actions of insulin in peripheral tissues by
beta agonists. Diabetic ketoacidosis has been reported
with the intravenous use of albuterol. Arterial blood
gases may reveal hypoxia and mild metabolic acidosis
due to increased anaerobic metabolism and increased
serum lactate. Serum CK and CK-MB cardiac isoenzymes should be obtained in addition to the above-
mentioned lab values.

2. ECG. The most common finding on ECG is sinus
tachycardia due to direct beta$_1$-receptor stimulation.
Other rhythms may include supraventricular tachycardia (SVT), ventricular ectopy, ventricular tachycardia (VT), and ventricular fibrillation (VF). In patients
with underlying cardiac disease, the ECG can show
ST-segment and T-wave abnormalities indicative of
ischemia or infarction.

3. X-rays. Radiographs are rarely diagnostic in beta-
agonist intoxication but may demonstrate associated
complications, such as pneumothorax and congestive
failure.

C. Management

1. Supportive care. Airway, breathing, and circulation
(ABCs) should be secured. Continuous cardiac monitoring and oxygenation to maintain an adequate tissue saturation by pulse-oximetry are imperative. An
IV line should be started with isotonic fluid.

2. **Treatment of hypotension.** If hypotension is present, the initial treatment involves isotonic fluid loading, with appropriate care taken to avoid overhydration in children or in patients with underlying cardiovascular disease. If fluid loading is unsuccessful, dopamine 2–10 µg/kg/min or levarterenol 2–4 µg/min can be titrated to desired blood pressure response. Patients with coexistent congestive heart failure or myocardial infarction may benefit from dobutamine 2–10 µg/kg/min.

3. **Treatment of arrhythmias**
   a. **Sinus tachycardia (ST).** ST occurs in response to hypotension and requires no specific intervention other than the treatment of hypotension.
   b. **Supraventricular tachycardia (SVT).** SVT can cause hemodynamic compromise by decreasing cardiac output and worsening hypotension. The preferred treatment is cardioversion. SVT without hemodynamic compromise may be treated with **adenosine** 6 mg rapid IV push followed by a 30-ml normal saline bolus followed by two 12-mg rapid IV doses to a maximum 30-mg total dose or cessation of arrhythmia. **Verapamil** IV can cause severe hypotension and its use is **not** recommended. **Beta blockade** to treat tachyarrhythmias is **not** advised because this may worsen bronchospasm and congestive symptoms.
   c. **Ventricular ectopy** is frequently noted and can be attributed to multiple causes, including electrolyte imbalance (hypokalemia), hypoxia, or acid-base disturbance. Correction of these metabolic derangements is usually sufficient treatment.
   d. **Ventricular tachycardia (VT) and frequent multifocal premature ventricular contractions (PVCs).** Lidocaine 1 mg/kg IV bolus followed by continuous IV drip at 2–4 mg/min is recommended. **Defibrillation** is the treatment of choice in pulseless VT per advanced cardiac life support (ACLS) guidelines.

4. **GI decontamination.** Once the ABCs have been stabilized, the remainder of general management can be instituted. If the overdose was taken by mouth, GI decontamination with normal saline (NS) gastric lavage with a large-bore (36–40 French) lavage tube is indicated. Lavage should be followed by the administration of activated charcoal (10 g/g ingested) to absorb any residual drug in the stomach.

5. **Treatment of seizures.** Patients presenting with seizures should cause the clinician to search for possible coingestants, since seizures are uncommon in pure beta-agonist overdose. The first-line treatment of seizures is with **diazepam** 10–20 mg IV (0.1–0.2 mg/kg in children) or **lorazepam** 1–2 mg IV initially with repeat dosing as needed to acutely control seizure activity. A loading dose of **phenytoin** 17 mg/kg IV is then given—no faster than 50 mg/min in adults and 1–3 mg/kg/min

in neonates. The daily maintenance dose is 5 mg/kg/d in both adults and children. If seizures continue, **phenobarbital** 15–20 mg/kg initially and 60–200 mg daily in adults (3–6 mg/kg/d in children) can be added to prevent seizures. CT scan with and without contrast and lumbar puncture should be performed to rule out intracranial pathology.

D. Patient disposition

   1. Admission criteria. Patients who present with chest pain, rales, arrhythmias (other than ST), or persistent hypotension often require hospitalization for further treatment, as well as evaluation, including cardiac monitoring, in an intensive care setting. Bronchospasm that continues despite ED treatment or that requires intubation necessitates admission to the hospital. Seizures—even a single seizure—require admission for continued treatment and diagnostic evaluation regarding possible coingestants, associated metabolic imbalance, or primary CNS abnormality.

   2. Discharge criteria. Patients who present to the ED with beta-agonist intoxication and mild symptoms (e.g., tremor alone) may be discharged from the ED after evaluation and treatment with activated charcoal following 4–6 hours of observation and cardiac monitoring. On discharge, patients should be instructed on the proper use of their medications and cautioned that increased frequency of use may cause development of tolerance to the intended therapeutic effects and indicate the need to seek medical attention.

II. Alpha-adrenergic agonists. Alpha-adrenergic agonist medications cause release of epinephrine and norepinephrine, stimulating the sympathetic nervous system. Routes of administration include IV, PO, and SQ for medical therapeutic use, as well as snorting, smoking, skin popping, and orifice placement when used in a recreational manner. Maximum effect can be seen as soon as 30 minutes after transmucosal exposure and within a few hours after PO dosing. The duration of action is variable, depending on the agent, dosage, and use of coingestants.

There are few pure alpha-adrenergic agonists. Most agents primarily stimulate alpha receptors but also activate beta receptors to a variable degree. These medications, referred to as **sympathomimetics,** cause vasoconstriction with reflex bradycardia as well as tachycardia and hypertension, depending on the relative amounts of alpha- and beta-receptor stimulation. Tachyarrhythmias are common, and myocardial ischemia, infarction, and dysfunction can occur.

Alpha agonists have a wide range of therapeutic applications, including use in cold remedies, as decongestants, and as appetite suppressants (Table 34-2). **Ephedrine** and **pseudoephedrine** are naturally occurring alpha agonists that cause both direct and indirect stimulation of the sympathetic nervous system. Their onset of action is rapid, and ephedrine often causes elevated BP at recommended therapeutic doses. Complications of chronic ephedrine abuse include cerebral angiitis and congestive cardiomyopathy. **Phenylpropanol-**

Table 34-2.   Alpha-adrenergic agonist medications

Drug	Therapeutic use
Ephedrine	Decongestant, stimulant
Phenylephrine	Decongestant, stimulant
Phenylpropanolamine	Appetite suppressant, stimulant
Pseudoephedrine	Decongestant, stimulant
Methylphenidate	Stimulant
Ergot derivatives	Vascular headache prescriptions

amine can cause an increased QT interval with atrioventricular (AV) conduction blocks requiring pacemaker placement. Although most incidents of overdose are accidental, alpha agonists are often intentionally abused for increased wakefulness, alertness, and euphoria.

A. **Presentation**
   1. **History.** The symptoms of alpha-agonist overdose result from sympathetic overstimulation. A common ED presentation is an accidental overdose of over-the-counter decongestant, cold remedy, or appetite suppressant. Patients may complain of gradual onset of tremulousness followed by the sensation that their skin is crawling, or that they feel nervous and tense. Patients often report a rapid heartbeat with pounding beats or palpitations, often stating that their heart is beating in their head or ears. Complaints of chest pain, shortness of breath, and the sensation of impending doom are common. Subjective fever, numbness, and tingling of the fingers or perioral area, excessive thirst due to drying of the mucous membranes, headache, abdominal pain, diarrhea, insomnia, and realistic nightmares are also reported.

   Following intentional ingestion, symptoms vary depending on the agent ingested, the dosage, the route of administration, and coingestants, if any. Patients may exhibit paranoid behavior, making history taking and physical examination difficult, if not impossible. They often report feeling out of control and are often very restless, in almost continuous motion despite attempts at calming and reassurance.

   2. **Physical examination**
      a. **General appearance.** The general physical examination in mild overdose may reveal an upset, agitated patient with visible tremors of the extremities. **Vital signs** are remarkable for tachycardia, elevated blood pressure, and tachypnea. There may be a slight elevation of core body temperature, but hyperthermia is distinctly unusual in mild intoxication and warrants further investigation regarding coingestants or underlying medical conditions, such as hyperthyroidism or neuroleptic malignant

syndrome. The skin usually appears cool, clammy, and pale. The pupils are often dilated.

b. **Cardiopulmonary.** Tachypnea is common because of direct alpha-mediated stimulation of the CNS breathing centers, which results in rapid, shallow respirations. Severe tachypnea or dyspnea is seen because of cardiovascular compromise, pulmonary complications (e.g., emboli), and vasospasm, with associated ventilation and perfusion mismatching and hypoxia. Patients may also exhibit the use of accessory muscles of respiration, peripheral cyanosis, and eventually respiratory failure.

c. **GI.** Bowel sounds are often diminished. Certain overdoses can result in mesenteric ischemia, in which case a rectal examination can reveal guaiac-positive or bloody stools.

d. **CNS.** Symptoms of CNS toxicity run the gamut from anxiety, restlessness, and agitation to confusion, psychosis, seizure, and coma. Patients are highly aware of their environment and intensely fascinated with even simple objects in their midst. **Seizures** occurring in the course of alpha-agonist overdose are often a direct result of ischemia from cerebral vasospasm. However, seizures may also follow cerebrovascular accident (CVA) or ICH, especially in patients with focal neurologic findings.

B. **Assessment**

1. **Laboratory studies.** Laboratory studies are generally nonspecific, but should include a CBC and electrolytes. Elevated leukocyte count, possibly with increased shift to the left, is caused by sympathetic stimulation and demargination. Hemoconcentration with elevated hematocrit reflects dehydration due to increased fluid losses. **Hypokalemia** is due to excessive intracellular movement and increased fluid losses. If **hyperkalemia** is seen, this signals increased tissue destruction secondary to elevated body temperature, vasospasm, or seizures and can result in renal failure via rhabdomyolysis. A toxicology screen should be obtained, especially in patients who present with seizures or altered mental status or when no history is available. Sympathomimetics are detected on thin-layer chromatography or Enzyme-Multiplied Immunoassay Technique (EMIT).

2. **ECG.** ECG should be performed in all patients with suspected sympathomimetic intoxication. The most common rhythm noted is sinus tachycardia; however, supraventricular tachycardia, ventricular ectopy, ventricular tachycardia, and ventricular fibrillation may also be seen.

3. **X-rays.** Chest x-rays (CXRs) can demonstrate pulmonary vascular congestion, pulmonary hypertension, pneumothorax, pneumomediastinum, and pneumonitis. A CT scan should be performed in all patients with focal neurologic findings, status epilepticus, signs of

head trauma, or altered mental status. Findings on CT may include intracerebral hemorrhage, cerebral infarcts, and a foreign body.

C. Management

1. **Supportive care.** ABCs should be secured. Continuous cardiac monitoring and oxygenation to maintain an adequate tissue saturation by pulse-oximetry are imperative. An IV line should be started with isotonic fluid.

2. **Specific therapy**

    a. **Hypertension.** Systolic blood pressure above 170 mm Hg or diastolic pressure above 110 mm Hg is associated with an increased risk of intracerebral hemorrhage and the development of encephalopathy. The treatment of a hypertensive crisis requires effective lowering of blood pressure within 15 minutes of ED presentation. **Nitroprusside** begun at 0.3 µg/kg/min titrated to blood pressure response and no more than 10 µg/kg/min results in rapid, yet predictable, lowering of blood pressure within minutes. There is slight reflex tachycardia but no change in coronary artery blood flow. Patients with significant blockage may experience ischemia or infarction due to coronary steal, which is particularly common when clonidine is used in combined therapy. **Labetalol** 20 mg IV should be injected over 2 minutes with blood pressure checked at 5 and 10 minutes after injection, followed by additional doses of 40 mg and 80 mg given at 10-minute intervals until adequate response is obtained or a total 300-mg dose is given. Labetalol is an alpha$_1$ and nonselective beta blocker that lowers blood pressure by direct vasodilatation. Because it does not cause reflex tachycardia, it is well suited for use in treatment of catecholamine excess. Labetalol can also be given by continuous infusion at 2 mg/min until an adequate response is obtained. The rapidity of its therapeutic action is related to the rapidity of IV injection. Because of the urgent need to lower blood pressure, continuous IV dosing and oral dosing are **not** recommended. Caution should be exercised when labetalol is used in patients with a history of asthma, COPD, and CHF. Additionally, at low doses beta-blocker effects predominate and can cause worsening of hypertension because alpha stimulation persists. **Phentolamine** is an adrenergic-blocking agent that causes reduction in the total peripheral resistance and reflex tachycardia through arteriolar and venous dilatation. The initial dose is 2.5–3.0 mg IV q5min following blood pressure response. Adverse effects include prolonged hypotension and induction of cardiac arrhythmias.

    b. **Arrhythmias.** The most commonly noted arrhythmia is sinus tachycardia, which requires no specific therapy unless it occurs along with hypertension.

- (i) **SVT. Adenosine** 6 mg is the initial drug of choice for SVT, given as rapid IV push with a bolus of 30-ml normal saline followed by two 12-mg rapid IV doses to a maximum 30-mg dose or until the arrhythmia ceases. **Diltiazem** IV 0.25-mg/kg bolus can also be given over 2 minutes as an initial dose, followed by a 0.35-mg/kg IV bolus dose in 15 minutes if the response is inadequate. **Esmolol** can also be used, with a loading dose 0.5 mg/kg given over 1 minute followed by an infusion of 50 µg/kg/min. If the SVT does not respond, a repeat bolus is given. If the SVT terminates, the maintenance dose infusion is continued.

- (ii) **Ventricular arrhythmias.** Ventricular ectopy, ventricular tachycardia, and ventricular fibrillation can also occur. Single PVCs are often indicative of myocardial irritability due to hypoxia, acidosis, and hypokalemia; correction of these derangements is often sufficient therapy. Frequent PVCs (more than 6 per minute) or multifocal PVCs can be treated with **betablockers** or **calcium channel blockers.** Lidociane 1 mg/kg IV bolus with a continuous infusion of 2–4 mg/min can also be used.

c. **GI decontamination** with saline lavage and administration of activated charcoal is performed after stabilization of the ABCs. If blood pressure continues to be poorly controlled, neither lavage nor induced emesis is recommended because of the potential to worsen hypertension, increase intracranial pressure, and cause intracerebral complications.

d. **Treatment of complications**

- (i) **Seizures** are initially treated with benzodiazepines, which also assist in controlling the blood pressure. **Diazepam** 10–20 mg IV or **lorazepam** 2–6 mg IV will serve to acutely control seizure activity. **Phenytoin,** 15–20 mg/kg loading dose, given no faster than 50 mg/min is administered, followed by 300 mg/d maintenance therapy. Failure to adequately control seizures may require the addition of other agents, such as **phenobarbital** 15–20 mg/kg and 60–200 mg/d.

- (ii) **Hyperthermia** can occur and contribute to the development of seizures, status epilepticus, and rhabdomyolysis. Treatment should consist of cooling blankets, evaporation, iced saline gastric and bladder lavage, and benzodiazepines to decrease restlessness.

- (iii) **Vasospasm.** Overdose of ergot derivatives results in severe vasospasm, which requires treatment with low-molecular-weight dex-

tran and hyperbaric oxygen in order to preserve the tissues at risk.

D. Disposition. Patients presenting with mildly elevated
blood pressure and pulse rate can be discharged after 6
hours of evaluation and observation in the ED. If hypertension and tachycardia do not resolve quickly or require
specific therapy, the patient must be admitted. If the patient is hemodynamically stable without cardiovascular
complaint, admission to a telemetry unit is appropriate.
Those who are hemodynamically unstable, have cardiovascular complaints or a hisotry of underlying cardiovascular disease may benefit from admission to the intensive
care unit.

III. Stimulants. Stimulant drugs cause the release of catecholamine and noncatecholamine neurotransmitters and are
often referred to as sympathomimetics. Routes of administration include PO, IV, SQ, and insufflation (snorting). The maximum drug effect is noted within minutes if injected or
smoked, within 30 minutes if snorted, and from 30 minutes to
a few hours if taken IM or transcutaneously. A duration of action of up to 24–36 hours is seen (e.g., methamphetamine) but
varies with the agent dosage and the mode of administration.

The release of epinephrine and norepinephrine causes
stimulation of peripheral alpha and beta receptors, resulting
in tachycardia and hypertension. Stimulation of central alpha
receptors causes hypotension and bradycardia. $Beta_1$-adren-
ergic receptors are found primarily in the myocardium, and
cause increased inotropy and chronotropy when stimulated.
$Beta_2$ receptors are located in the smooth muscle of the vasculature, bronchial tree, and uterine wall and cause vasodilatation, bronchodilatation, and uterine wall relaxation. The
primary noncatecholamine neurotransmitters released by
stimulant agents are dopamine and serotonin, which are responsible for the sense of well-being and vivid hallucinations
experienced with stimulant use and desired by their abusers.

Stimulant agents are used for their anorectic properties as
appetite suppressants and in pep pills for their ability to increase wakefulness. Toxicity with amphetamines is very variable, with potentially life-threatening reactions occurring
after doses as small as 30 mg. Fatal reactions are seen following doses greater than 400 mg, but chronic use increases tolerance and hence the lethal dose. Phencyclidine (PCP) was
first used as an anesthetic and analgesic and was favored because of its relative lack of respiratory and myocardial depression. With time, however, it was found to cause severe
postanesthesia reactions, including hallucinations, agitation,
and violence, and its use was curtailed. At the present time,
the primary use is recreational because of its very desirable
mood-altering properties.

Sympathomimetics are rarely involved as single ingestions.
The most frequent combinations are with heroin, sedative-
hypnotics, and tranquilizing agents in attempt to balance
adrenergic overstimulation.

A. Presentation

   1. History. Signs and symptoms on presentation after
      sympathomimetic ingestion will depend on the pa-

tient's baseline health and the manner of use or abuse:
acute simple ingestion, acute overdose, or chronic
abuse. Acute simple intoxications usually occur when
over-the-counter medications (e.g., diet pills) are used
in excess in an attempt to achieve desired therapeutic
effects more rapidly. The dose ingested is usually
small, and serious clinical reactions are few. Patients
will complain of feeling nervous or jumpy and often
appear visibly agitated. Acute overdose causes both
central and peripheral symptoms leading to a combination of signs of adrenergic overstimulation with altered perception of self and surroundings. Initial
sympathetic stimulation gives way to myocardial, respiratory, and CNS depression, resulting in vasomotor
collapse and death.

Chronic abuse may present differently. Patients often give vague medical complaints with negative results on evaluation. Insomnia and restlessness with
weight loss are often reported along with development
of tolerance to the euphoric effects. Patients often
binge with ever-increasing doses to achieve desired effects, becoming caught in a cycle of worsening abuse.
However, patients do not develop tolerance to the
adrenergic effects and may present to the ED with a
hypertensive emergency or in cardiac arrest.

The diagnosis of stimulant intoxication should be
considered when patients present with a history of
substance abuse and symptoms consistent with adrenergic stimulation. Other diagnoses to be considered
include thyrotoxicosis, alcohol or sedative-hypnotic
withdrawal, anticholinergic ingestion, complication of
MAOI use, tricyclic antidepressant (TCA) overdose,
and CNS infection. Obtaining a thorough history is
crucial to the evaluation and treatment. In addition to
details regarding the stimulant ingested, a history of
use of other medications is important. A past medical
history is helpful in predicting and anticipating possible complications.

2. **Physical examination**
   a. **General appearance.** Tachycardia, increased res-
      piratory rate, and elevated blood pressure are seen
      as a result of adrenergic stimulation. Body tempera-
      ture may be slightly elevated, with skin diaphoretic
      and flushed. Severe hyperthermia has been re-
      ported, with associated development of hepatic
      necrosis and DIC occurring more often with amphet-
      amine, cocaine, and PCP intoxication. Pupils are di-
      lated but reactive, deep tendon reflexes are brisk,
      and tremors of the extremities are evident. The skin
      may demonstrate track marks in the case of IV drug
      abuse (IVDA) or skin popping.
   b. **Cardiopulmonary.** Pulses are rapid and bound-
      ing, yet heart rates over 130 are unusual in pure
      PCP ingestion, suggesting that possibly a coinges-
      tant or another stimulant (e.g., amphetamines)
      has been ingested. The lungs are clear, but rales

518 V. Toxicologic Cardiovascular Emergencies

may be audible with associated JVD and S3 gallop in patients with underlying cardiac disease. This is primarily due to increased heart rate, increased systemic vascular resistance with increased myocardial stress, and consequent increase in myocardial oxygen demand.

c. **Neurologic.** Dopamine and serotonin release causes an acute toxic psychosis consisting of auditory and visual hallucinations, delusions, and paranoid behavior. Patients often present to the ED as a result of bizarre or violent behavior and consequent trauma. Catatonia, mutism, dystonic posturing, and automatisms are common. Deep tendon reflexes (DTRs) are brisk and symmetric. Seizures occur and can be generalized or focal, with status epilepticus a frequent cause of morbidity.

B. Assessment

1. **Laboratory studies.** Blood should be sent for CBC, electrolytes, and toxicology screen. Leukocytosis is seen because of stress demargination and movement of WBCs into the circulation. Elevation of the hematocrit occurs through dehydration and hemoconcentration. Serum potassium may be decreased because of increased intracellular shift mediated by beta-adrenergic receptor stimulation. **Hyperkalemia** is seen when there is tissue destruction from seizures or increased body temperature. When rhabdomyolysis is present, acute renal failure intervenes and further increases in potassium are noted. Measurement of serum creatine phosphokinase (CPK) may aid in assesing the degree of rhabdomyolysis. **Metabolic acidosis** occurs because of the generation of excess lactate from increased muscle activity and seizures.

   Further laboratory studies should be obtained based on the history, complaints, and physical examination. If significant hyperthermia is present, LFTs and coagulation profile should be checked to look for indicators of liver necrosis and DIC. Patients with complaints of chest pain, severe shortness of breath, or signs and symptoms of cardiopulmonary dysfunction should have total serum CK and CK-MB cardiac isoenzymes evaluated for possible myocardial infarction.

   A toxicology screen should be sent on all patients who present without history and who are comatose or seizing. The diagnosis of PCP ingestion is difficult to make without a toxicology screen. A positive test indicates PCP use within the preceding 1–2 weeks but should not rule out the possibility of other drug ingestions.

2. **Ancillary tests.** X-rays are useful in the diagnosis of associated trauma, and ECG is helpful in the assessment of arrhythmias or the detection of myocardial ischemia.

C. Management

1. **Supportive care.** ABCs should be secured. Continuous cardiac monitoring and oxygenation to maintain

an adequate tissue saturation by pulse-oximetry are imperative. An IV line should be started with isotonic fluid. Frequent vital sign monitoring is needed to guide therapy as well as to detect hyperthermia.

2. **Observation.** Seizure precautions should be instituted. They consist mainly of placing the patient in an area where continuous visual observation is possible, padding the side rails of the stretcher, and removing any objects from the immediate vicinity that may cause bodily harm if contacted during a seizure. Restraints are often needed to limit self-destructive behavior or injuries.

3. **Specific therapies**

   a. **Hypertension.** Hypertension is the most frequently occurring cardiovascular toxic effect of stimulant ingestion. The blood pressure elevation is often severe and can be life threatening because of the increased myocardial work load and resultant dysfunction combined with the inability to compensate for the new hemodynamic state. BP elevations greater than 170 mm Hg systolic or 110 mm Hg diastolic are considered hypertensive emergencies because of their propensity to cause severe end-organ damage, and effective management is necessary to lower blood pressure within 15 minutes of initial ED presentation. The basis for hypertension is vasoconstriction, and therefore agents that cause reliable, controlled vasodilatation are most effective. **Nitroprusside** 0.5–3.0 μg/kg/min provides rapid, titratable therapy of severe hypertension and is recommended as first-line therapy. A potential drawback is the lack of effect on tachycardia and the theoretical risk of further increase in heart rate due to reflex tachycardia. **Labetalol** is an effective alpha and beta blocker used in the treatment of hypertension as well as tachyarrhythmias. The initial dose is 20 mg IV over 2 minutes and then 40–80 mg IV q10min until blood pressure is adequately controlled or a total of 300 mg has been administered. Continuous IV drip can be started after the initial 20-mg bolus if a blood pressure response is seen. The advantage of labetalol over Nipride is the added treatment of tachycardia. **Propranolol** given IV at 1 mg/min is effective in lowering blood pressure as well as in treating tachyarrhythmias. The dose can be increased q1–5min to a maximum of 0.15 mg/kg until the desired effect is obtained. As with labetalol, exacerbation of bronchospasm and CHF can be problematic. In addition, propranolol use results in beta blockade without alpha blockade. Unopposed alpha stimulation in the setting of stimulate ingestion can result in the development of a hypertensive crisis. Should this occur, **phentolamine,** an alpha blocker, can be used in doses of 2.5–5.0 mg IV q5min while monitoring blood pressure and heart rate for response. If there is an inadequate response, propranolol and phentolamine should be discontinued and either nitroprusside or labetalol should be substituted. Nitroglycerin IV results in vasodilatation and lowered blood pressure. Doses starting at 3 µg/min and titrating up to desired blood pressure levels are especially useful in patients who also have chest pain, pulmonary edema, and evidence of myocardial ischemia. If no IV access has been established, **nifedipine** 10 mg sublingually may be administered. The main disadvantages to this mode of therapy are the lack of titratability and the risk of precipitous decrease in blood pressure and hemodynamic instability.

b. **Hypotension.** Should cardiovascular collapse occur, the initial treatment consists of IV hydration with NS. Bolus therapy is reported through a large-bore line until a blood pressure increase is noted. Then the IV hydration can be continued at a rate sufficient to maintain adequate perfusion. If hydration alone is insufficient, pressor therapy should be added. **Dopamine** 10–20 µg/kg/min is often effective. **Dobutamine** 2–10 µg/kg/min (maximum dose 40 µg/kg/min) should be added if cardiovascular reevaluation indicates cardiogenic shock. **Caution** must be used in the setting of acute myocardial infarction, and contraindications include IHSS, aortic stenosis, and tachyarrhythmia.

c. **Arrhythmias.** A 12-lead ECG is essential to the management of the cardiovascular toxic effects of stimulant ingestion.

   (i) **ST.** Tachyarrhythmias are common, with ST occurring most frequently. As states previously, ST alone requires no specific therapy, but when associated with hypertension requires therapy in order to decrease myocardial work load. Agents such as propranolol and labetalol may be used in the previously recommended doses while heart rate and blood pressure are closely monitored.

   (ii) **SVT Adenosine** can be given as 6 mg IVP followed by two repeat doses of 12 mg IVP if sinus rhythm does not convert to normal after the initial dose. Each dose should be followed by a rapid IV bolus of 20–30 ml of NS. **Esmolol** can be given in an initial loading dose of 0.5 mg/kg over 1 minute followed by an infusion of 50 µg/kg/min if adenosine is unavailable or ineffective. **Verapamil,** 5 mg IVP q5min to a maximum dose or 20 mg in 30 minutes, may be effective in some patients. Verapamil is **not** recommended for use in patients with sick sinus syndrome, CHF, or pulmonary edema.

   (iii) **Ventricular dysrhythmias,** including PVCs, can occur in association with stimulant ingestion. Single infrequent PVCs may not require specific therapy. PVCs that are in couplets or that are multifocal in nature require therapy directed at correction of hypoxia, electrolyte, and acid-base abnormalities. **Esmolol** can be given in a 0.5-mg/kg/min bolus and then in continuous IV drip, 50 µg/kg/min for 4 minutes, with a repeat bolus and an increase in the IV drip rate until the arrhythmia ceases, hypotension or bradycardia develops, or a total dose of 200 µg/kg/min is reached. **Propranolol,** 1 mg/min IV and increased q1–5min to a maximum of 0.15 mg/kg, may be used with caution, since there is a greater risk of developing hypotension and bradycardia in addition to exacerbating bronchospasm and CHF.

- (iv) **VT** may be treated with **propranolol** in the above-mentioned doses. **Lidocaine,** 1 mg/kg IV bolus followed by continuous IV drip of 2–4 mg/min, can be given as standard therapy but is **not** recommended as first-line therapy because it has the propensity to lower the seizure threshold. VT unresponsive to antiarrhythmic agents is treated with **synchronous cardioversion.**
- (v) **Pulseless VT** is treated as ventricular fibrillation with CPR and **defibrillation** per ACLS protocols.

d. **Myocardial ischemia.** Myocardial ischemia occurring with stimulant overdose is multifactorial in nature. Direct vasoconstriction leading to increased peripheral vascular resistance and increased myocardial work, coronary vasospasm, and platelet aggregation all contribute to the development of ischemia. Myocardial damage is confirmed with continued chest pain, an abnormal ECG, increased CK and CK-MB values, or abnormal wall motion on imaging studies. Therapy using oxygen, nitrates, aspirin, and thrombolytic agents as indicated combined with effective therapy of arrhythmias and hypertension serves to reduce morbidity and mortality.

e. **GI decontamination** with saline lavage and administration of activated charcoal is performed after stabilization of the ABCs. If blood pressure continues to be poorly controlled, neither lavage nor induced emesis is recommended because of the potential to worsen hypertension, increase intracranial pressure, and cause intracerebral complications.

f. **Charcoal hemoperfusion.** If hemodynamic compromise is present, charcoal hemoperfusion can be instituted to speed the elimination of amphetamines. PCP is removed only in small amounts with hemoperfusion.

g. **Urinary acidification.** If amphetamines or PCP have been ingested, acidification of the urine may

theoretically increase elimination. However, this
may cause acid-base derangements and decrease
the solubility of myoglobin, thus favoring the development of renal failure.

h. **Other treatment considerations**

(i) **Seizures** should be treated initially with
benzodiazepines. Diazepam 10–20 mg IV or
lorazepam 2–6 mg IV may be used to control
seizure activity. This is followed by **phenytoin** in a 17–20 mg/kg IV loading dose (given
no faster than 50 mg/min) and in a maintenance dose of 5–6 mg/kg/d. **Phenobarbital,**
15–20 mg/kg initial dose and daily doses of
60–200 mg/d in adults and 3–6 mg/kg/d in
children, is given if seizures are not adequately controlled with phenytoin. Continued
refractory seizure activity requires treatment
with neuromuscular blockade, general anesthesia, or barbiturate coma and continuous
EEG monitoring. Refractory seizures as well
as focal neurologic findings or persistent
change in mental status require further evaluation. A CT scan of the brain and a lumbar
puncture should be performed to rule out intracranial pathology.

(ii) **Agitation** is best treated by offering reassurance and placing the patient in a quiet
area with minimal environmental stimulation. Patients should be kept under close observation at all times because of their
erratic behavior and the risk that they will
cause harm to themselves or others. PCP is
highly lipid-soluble and accumulates in the
brain and adipose tissue, providing a source
of prolonged intoxication. Benzodiazepines
are the first-line drug treatment for agitation and may also result in lowering of blood
pressure and heart rate. **Diazepam** or **lorazepam** in the previously mentioned doses
may be used and titrated to attain the desired effect. Other causes of persistent agitation warrant further evaluation. The use of
neuroleptic agents and phenothiazines is
not recommended because they interfere
with heat dissipation, increase the risk of
hypothermia and decrease the seizure
threshold.

(iii) **Hyperthermia** requires prompt therapy.
Intravenous hydration, removal of clothing,
ice packs in the axillae and groin, and cooling blankets all serve to increase heat dissipation and thereby decrease core body
temperature. Antipyretic agents such as acetaminophen and NSAIDs are not useful in
this setting because of the etiology of the increased temperature. Treatment of agitation

and seizures with benzodiazepines also contributes to lowering body temperature by decreasing muscle activity, as does neuromuscular blockade.

(iv) **Rhabdomyolysis.** If rhabdomyolysis is suspected based on the presence of dark-colored urine, elevated CPK, or renal failure, the initial treatment is alkalinization of the urine and aggressive fluid hydration to maintain an adequate urine output.

D. Disposition

1. **Admission criteria.** Patients who remain hypertensive or tachycardic or who are resistant to therapy must be admitted to a telemetry unit or intensive care unit for further treatment and evaluation. Those persons with chest pain or those who require continuous IV antihypertensive therapy, intubation, or ventilatory support require admission to an intensive care unit for continuous cardiorespiratory monitoring. Intensive care admission is also required for patients with persistent mental status changes, focal neurologic examination, or status epilepticus. Patients who have had a seizure, all pediatric patients, and patients suffering trauma associated with sympathomimetic ingestion also require hospitalization.

2. **Discharge criteria.** Patients who present with mild tachycardia and slight elevation of blood pressure may be discharged from the ED after treatment, evaluation, and 6 hours of observation if their clinical status remains stable and no arrhythmias are noted.

IV. Methylxanthines. Methylxanthines inhibit the action of the enzyme phosphodiesterase, thereby preventing the metabolism of cyclic adenosine monophosphate (cAMP). In addition, methylxanthines cause the release of epinephrine and norepinephrine. The effect of these two processes is the relaxation of smooth muscle, an increase in inotropy and chronotropy, and CNS stimulation.

The major methylxanthines are aminophylline, theophylline, and caffeine. Aminophylline and theophylline are used therapeutically in the treatment of bronchospasm and stimulation of the CNS respiratory centers in disease states such as sleep apnea. Caffeine is primarily a food additive and is often used in combination with stimulants such as phenylpropanolamine. Appetite suppressants using caffeine and amphetamine combinations were banned by the FDA in 1983.

The route of administration as well as the patient's own metabolism and elimination play major roles in the development of methylxanthine toxicity. IV dosing is most often associated with acute toxic side effects consisting of increased heart rate, palpitations, and tremor within minutes of administration. The rate of metabolism of methylxanthines is affected by the patient's age, underlying illnesses (e.g., cardiac and hepatic dysfunction), cigarette smoking, and the use of concomitant medications. The outcome of toxic ingestion also depends on the chronicity of the ingestion, with patients chronically treated with methylxanthine medications being more susceptible to the major causes of morbidity and mortality at lower serum levels.

A. **Presentation**

1. **History.** The manner in which patients with methylxanthine intoxication present varies depending on the route of administration, the duration of ingestion, and the patient's rate of metabolism of the medication. Most often, the patient will be newly started on the medication and will present to the ED with a history of bronchospasm treated with inhaled beta agonists as well as a methylxanthine. If the dose was given intravenously, within minutes of receiving a loading dose of theophylline (5–6 mg/kg) the patient will report feeling jumpy and nervous with palpitations. The onset of symptoms of toxicity is delayed in PO doses and in sustained-release preparations (1–2 hours and 6–8 hours, respectively. Patients with methyxanthine overdose present with persistent nausea and vomiting with a history of treatment for bronchospasm. The differential diagnosis list in patients with nausea, vomiting, and tachycardia should also include theophylline toxicity in addition to DKA, thyrotoxicosis, Addison's disease, alcohol withdrawal, beta-agonist intoxication, CNS infection, and salicylate overdose.

   Patients often present with agitation, tremors, lightheadedness, nervousness or palpitations. More seriously, chest pain indicative of myocardial ischemia may be a presenting complaint. Patients often report nausea and may vomit because of the combined effects of decreased lower esophageal sphincter pressure from smooth muscle relaxation and increased gastric acid secretion.

   Tremors are the most common symptoms of CNS toxicity but seizures are the most serious, accounting for up to 50% of deaths associated with methylxanthine overdose. The incidence of seizures is increased with higher drug levels; underlying diseases involving the kidneys, liver, lungs, or cardiovascular system (which can decrease the rate of metabolism); and an underlying CNS abnormality (e.g., CVA or seizure disorder).

   Patients presenting with chronic overdose most often complain of tremor and GI upset. The usual history is one of chronic methylxanthine use with a recent increase in dose; the addition of another medication that competes for cytochrome P-450 enzymes (e.g., cimetidine or erythromycin); or cigarette smoking, which decreases P-450 activity.

2. **Physical examination.** The physical examination will be notable for tachycardia and tachypnea. Blood pressure may be slightly decreased because of beta$_2$ stimulation resulting in vasodilatation. The pupils are dilated but reactive. Depending on the underlying pulmonary status, the lungs may be clear or reveal wheezing. The heart rate is rapid and may be regular or irregular based on the underlying rhythm diagnosed by 12-lead ECG or cardiac monitor rhythm strip

evaluation. Persons with underlying coronary artery disease (CAD) may present with audible rales, S3 gallop, and JVD consistent with CHF.

B. Assessment

1. **Laboratory studies.** The CBC is not diagnostic in methylxanthine overdose but may reveal leukocytosis in response to cathecholamine release. Hypokalemia is a frequent finding and is due to multiple causes, including beta-adrenergic-mediated intracellular movement of potassium as well as kaliuresis and increased potassium losses associated with vomiting. Volume contraction and hydrogen ion losses from vomiting result in metabolic alkalosis, which in turn contributes to hypokalemia. Respiratory alkalosis is seen resulting from tachypnea. Lactic acidosis, increased glycogenolysis, and increased gluconeogenesis are due to excess circulating catecholamines. A toxicology screen is helpful in diagnosing coingestants that may require directed therapy to prevent further morbidity.

2. **Theophylline level.** Drug levels should be obtained in methylxanthine intoxication. Although elevated levels are not necessary for patients to become symptomatic, toxic levels do correlate with different outcomes. Theophylline is thought to be therapeutic at levels between 10 and 20 g/ml. The initial theophylline level should be repeated q2h to help guide further therapeutic interventions. Above the level of 25 mg/liter the incidence of seizures increases. The theophylline level to some extent also dictates management in that charcoal hemoperfusion is indicated in the treatment of patients with levels above 90 mg/liter. However, the serum measurement of theophylline should not be considered separate from the patient; the same drug level in different patients may require different therapeutic modalities. Theophylline levels should serve as a guide, and the trend, rather than the absolute level, should be considered along with the clinical status of the patient.

3. **ECG.** A 12-lead ECG should be performed on all patients presenting with methylxanthine intoxication to allow for assessment of heart rhythm and changes indicative of ischemia or infarction that require specific therapy.

C. Management

1. **Supportive care.** Airway stabilization is essential to proper management. Patients presenting with a change in mental status or seizures often require immediate intubation to maintain a patent airway. Those persons with acute bronchospasm will require intensive therapy directed at relief of bronchoconstriction, including the use of inhaled beta$_2$ agonists, supplement oxygen, and steroids. If these measures fail to relieve bronchospasm and respiratory fatigue intercedes, the patient will also likely require endotrachael intubation. Patients should be continuously monitored by ECG and pulse-oximetry.

2. **Hemodynamic alterations.** An IV line should be started, and a fluid challenge with NS (500 ml–1 liter over 30–60 minutes) should be given in an attempt to expand the extracellular fluid volume and treat **hypotension.** If there is an inadequate response, a repeat bolus may be given. Lack of response to IV fluids indicates the need for treatment with alpha agonists or **beta-blocking agents.** Beta blockade is theoretically the most effective method of treatment; however, it can cause bronchospasm as well as contribute to a further decrease in blood pressure. **Esmolol,** 500 µg/kg IV over 1 minute and then 50 µg/kg/min continuous IV infusion, may be used. **Propranolol** 1 mg IV q5–10min can also be given, titrating the dose to blood pressure and heart rate response. The advantage of esmolol is that it is short-acting; once the IV drip is discontinued, the agent is metabolized within 5–10 minutes. Esmolol may still exacerbate bronchospasm.

3. **Antiarrhythmnic therapies.** Tachydysrhythmias are frequently seen associated with methylxanthine intoxication. Direct beta-adrenergic receptor stimulation accounts for the majority of cases; however, hypoxia, electrolyte imbalance, and acid-base abnormalities are other causes to be considered.

    a. **ST** is by far the most commonly noted rhythm disturbance and usually requires no specific therapy.

    b. **Atrial fibrillation and multifocal atrial tachycardia** are most often seen in patients with COPD and chronic methylxanthine poisoning. Fast atrial fibrillation is best treated with agents to achieve ventricular rate control. **Digoxin,** 0.6–1.0 mg IV over 1 hour and then 0.25–0.50 mg daily dosing, will often result in adequate rate control in 3–6 hours, which can limit its usefulness in the acute setting. **Diltiazem,** 0.25 mg/kg initial IV dose and then 0.35 mg/kg second IV dose if necessary, is probably a better choice. **Beta blockade** may also be effective in achieving rate control but is associated with the risk of exacerbation of COPD, bronchospasm, and CHF. Atrial fibrillation resulting in hemodynamic compromise is treated with cardioversion.

    c. **SVT** is also seen, occurring more often in children than in adults. Because methylxanthines interfere with adenosine receptor activity, adenosine is often **not** effective in treating SVT in this setting. **Diltiazem** and **propranolol** in the above-mentioned doses are recommended. SVT causing hemodynamic compromise is treated wtih **cardioversion.**

    d. **Ventricular arrhythmias.** Methylxanthines decrease the threshold for VF. However, ventricular arrhythmias, including VT and VF, are almost solely seen in patients with preexisting heart disease. The treatment for frequent or multifocal PVCs and VT with a pulse is **lidocaine,** 1 mg/kg IV loading dose and then continuous infusion at

2–4 mg/min, or **propranolol.** Pulseless VT is treated as VF with **defibrillation.**

4. **GI decontamination.** Following stabilization of the ABCs, GI decontamination is performed via an orogastric tube. This is especially important when sustained-release formulations were ingested, because it very quickly decreases the amount of medication remaining available for absorption. **Lavage** should be done as quickly as possible after ingestion when maximal amounts of medication are still present in the stomach and more easily removed. Larger, sustained-release preparations may not be as effectively removed as smaller tablets.

5. **Multidose activated charcoal.** Multidose activated charcoal is extremely effective in binding methylxanthines within the GI tract as well as those given intravenously. It can be used in both acute and chronic ingestions and is safe for use in children and the elderly. The use of charcoal in neonates is cautioned against because of risk of the development of necrotizing enterocolitis in an immature GI tract. The recommended dose is 1 g/kg q2–4h, aiming for a theophylline-to-charcoal ratio of 10:1 in milligrams, which results in a reliable decrease in theophylline level.

6. **Whole bowel irrigation.** Whole bowel irrigation is used when activated charcoal fails to decrease theophylline levels. Isotonic polyethylene glycol, 2 liter/hr (adults) or 0.5 liter/kg (children), can be given PO, NG, or OG until stools are clear. This method of clearance can be used in addition to activated charcoal in ingestions of large amounts of sustained-release tablets and can remove large amounts of medications even before absorption has occurred if given early in the course of treatment.

7. **Extracorporeal drug removal.** Extracorporeal methods of removal are indicated with single acute ingestions when the theophylline level is greater than 90 mg/liter or seizures or life-threatening arrhythmias are present. It is also recommended for use in the elderly with cardiac or hepatic dysfunction in whom metabolic rates are decreased. Other methods of elimination should still be instituted because it often takes time to establish extracorporeal methods, and valuable time is often wasted when no treatment is given. **Charcoal hemoperfusion** provides maximal elimination partly because of the high affinity of charcoal to the theophylline. Adverse effects of charcoal hemoperfusion include thrombocytopenia, hypocalcemia, and hemolysis, which can be decreased in incidence with the use of microencapsulated charcoal. Hemodynamic stability and anticoagulation with heparin are also required. The use of charcoal hemoperfusion is limited in neonates and small children by their size, and exchange transfusion is substituted. Peritoneal dialysis and hemodialysis are not nearly as effective as charcoal hemoperfusion.

528 V. Toxicologic Cardiovascular Emergencies

8. **Treatment of seizures.** Seizures associated with methylxanthine intoxication carry a 50% mortality. Immediate control of seizure activity is of utmost importance. Benzodiazepine therapy is first line. **Diazepam** 10–20 mg IV and **lorazepam** 2–6 mg IV may be effective in acutely controlling seizure activity. If seizures persist, phenobarbital 15–20 mg/kg initially and then 60–200 mg daily in adults or 3–6 mg/kg/d in children is given. Seizures that remain refractory require endotracheal intubation, in addition to the use of neuromuscular blockade, general anesthesia, and continuous EEG monitoring. Effective seizure control prevents the development of hypoxia, acidosis, and rhabdomyolysis, but seizures may often only be fully treated after adequate clearance of the methylxanthine.

D. **Disposition**
1. **Admission criteria.** All patients with significant methylxanthine ingestion with increased theophylline levels require admission for further evaluation and treatment. Intensive care admission is necessary for patients with seizures, chest pain, CHF, and life-threatening arrhythmias, and for those who require intubation and mechanical ventilation. Admission to a telemetry unit is essential for all other patients because arrhythmias may develop at any time during the course of the overdose treatment.
2. **Discharge criteria.** Patients may be discharged home after ED evaluation, treatment with activated charcoal, and 6 hours of observation if they meet certain criteria. They must present with mild symptoms (e.g., tremor only), be otherwise healthy, have a theophylline level in the high normal range (and decreasing), and have no arrhythmia other than mild ST. These patients require close outpatient follow-up, which is best arranged prior to ED discharge.

V. **Anticholinergics.** The mechanism of action of anticholinergic medications is via inhibition of the muscarinic acetylcholine receptors in the parasympathetic nervous system in smooth muscle, the GI tract, the genitourinary tract, the exocrine glands, and the eye. These receptors are also involved in transmissions via the vagus nerve, which affects heart rate and AV nodal conduction. Thus inhibition due to anticholinergics results in autonomic dysfunction, manifested as hyperthermia, tachycardia, mydriasis, a decrease in gastric motility, dry skin and mucous membranes, and urinary retention. CNS symptoms include seizures, coma, and movement abnormalities. There are few purely anticholinergic medications (e.g., atropine, ipratropium bromide), but there are several classes of medications that possess anticholinergic properties (Table 34-3).

Antihistamines are divided into H_1 and H_2 receptor antagonists. H_1 receptor antagonists are used in over-the-counter allergy and cold remedies and motion sickness medications. They are often combined with stimulants, analgesics, and sympathomimetics. Antihistamines may be administered IV,

Table 34-3. Commonly used anticholinergic medications

Drug	Therapeutic use
Atropine	Arrhythmia therapy, organophosphate toxicity
Benztropine	Antiparkinsonian drug
Chlorpheniramine	Antihistamine
Cyclobenzaprine	Muscle relaxant
Diphenhydramine	Antihistamine
Hydroxyzine	Antihistamine, antiemetic
Ipratropium	Bronchodilator
Meclizine	Antiemetic, therapy of motion sickness
Scopolamine	Antiemetic, therapy of motion sickness
Trihexyphenidyl	Antiparkinsonian drug

IM, PO, or TQ, with symptoms of overdose often noted within 30 minutes of ingestion. H_2 receptor antagonists cause a decrease in gastric acid secretion and are primarily used in the treatment of peptic ulcer disease. Parasympathetic blockade occurs, causing tremor, insomnia, and tachycardia, with children being more sensitive to these excitatory symptoms even at therapeutic doses. H_1 receptor antagonists also possess a quinidinelike effect in overdose, resulting in conduction abnormalities that can be life threatening.

There are several types of antipsychotic medications. Of these the phenothiazines, thioxanthines, and butyrophenones possess anticholinergic properties in addition to alpha blockade and antidopamine effects. In overdose, patients who ingest these medications present with decreased blood pressure due to vasodilatation and myocardial depression, initial sedation, and then agitation and movement disorders. They may also have hyperthermia due to impaired temperature regulation.

Common to all anticholinergic ingestions are signs of autonomic dysfunction. In patients with tachycardia, hyperthermia, and dry skin the clinician must also consider alpha-adrenergic overdose, thyrotoxicosis, and sympathomimetic overdose. Dry skin favors anticholinergic ingestion, but the other items may often only be diagnosed with diagnostic laboratory testing, including a toxicological screen and thyroid function testing.

A. Presentation

1. **History.** Patients presenting to the ED with an anticholinergic intoxication often give a history of having recently been prescribed a new medication, often for the treatment of nausea, psychiatric illness, or parkinsonism. In some cases, such as sleeping pill overdose (diphenhydramine), eyedrop overuse (atropine), or seed ingestion (jimson weed), the history may not be as easily obtainable. Depending on the medication, the dose, and the route of administration, within minutes

patients report the onset of symptoms consistent with autonomic dysfunction: often agitation, restlessness, nervousness, and tremor. Other neurologic symptoms include ataxia, confusion, hallucinations, delirium, and coma. Seizures are seen due to CNS stimulation and are more frequent in children, most often with tricyclic antidepressant overdose (see Chap. 32). Patients may have GI complaints, including nausea, dryness of the mouth, and a bitter taste in their mouth.

2. **Physical examination**
   a. **General examination.** Vital signs are remarkable for tachypnea, tachycardia, and a slight increase in core body temperature. The most striking of these is the tachycardia, which can often be to such an extent that it may cause hemodynamic compromise that can be life threatening. Blood pressure is normal to slightly decreased because of vasodilatation in response to the tachycardia, but may drop precipitously when tachycardia becomes extreme. An elevated temperature with warm, flushed skin is due directly to autonomic dysfunction associated with anticholinergic ingestion. Tachypnea occurs in an attempt to dissipate heat.

   Patients often appear dehydrated, with dry mucous membranes and skin due to inhibition of the muscarinic receptors in exocrine glands as well as to the increased insensible losses, increased body temperature, and lack of increased fluid intake to compensate. Pupils are dilated and may be either sluggishly reactive or nonreactive, causing patients to complain of blurred vision.

   b. **Cardiac.** As stated, tachycardia is common. On auscultation the rhythm is usually regular but may also reveal extrasystoles. Skipped beats and irregular heart rhythms may also be noted but occur infrequently.

   c. **GI.** Peristalsis is slowed, and there may be few, if any, bowel sounds. Urinary retention is common and the bladder is easily palpable, although this may not occur with inhaled ipratropium.

B. **Assessment**
   1. **Laboratory studies.** The CBC is typically normal and serves mainly to rule out infectious etiologies of hyperthermia and mental status change. Electrolytes are also usually normal but may demonstrate slight hyperkalemia associated with increased tissue breakdown due to increased muscle activity and elevated temperature. A total CK and urinalysis (dip and microscopic) should be sent to further evaluate the possibility of rhabdomyolysis. A baseline BUN and creatinine test should be obtained to assess renal function. An ABG test will evaluate for hypoxia and acid-base abnormalities as the cause of change in mental status. None of these tests are specific or diagnostic of anticholinergic overdose.

2. **ECG.** A 12-lead ECG with rhythm strip should be obtained in all patients with anticholinergic ingestion because of the high frequency of associated arrhythmias. The ECG most commonly reveals ST. In some anticholinergic overdoses, a prolonged QT interval and right-axis deviation can be seen. The finding of other arrhythmias indicates the possibility of massive overdose, electrolyte or acid-base abnormality, or hypoxia.

3. **X-rays.** A flat plate of the abdomen may illustrate radiopaque tablets (e.g., TCAs and phenothiazines). This is a nonspecific finding that can be seen with other medications, including chloral hydrate, iron supplements, enteric coated salicylate and potassium preparations, and iodides.

4. **Other diagnostic tests.** A toxicology screen including acetaminophen, salicylate, and alcohol levels should be obtained in all patients who present without a clear history or who are comatose or seizing. With the exception of TCAs, phenothiazines, and antihistamines, most true anticholinergics like atropine or jimson weed are not detected on a toxicology screen. In patients in whom TCA intoxication is suspected, a TCA level may be helpful (see Chap. 32).

C. **Management**

1. **Supportive care.** The airway must be secured as aggressively as possible. Intubation and ventilation are imperative in patients with coma and altered airway reflexes. Oxygenation to maintain an adequate saturation by pulse-oximetry should be administered by the appropriate route. Continuous ECG monitoring, frequent vital signs, and mental status checks should be instituted. An IV line with normal saline should be started. As in any comatose patient, dextrose, naloxone, and thiamine should be administered.

2. **Treatment of hypotension.** A bolus of 500–1000 ml of NS or lactated Ringer solution (LR) should be given over 30–60 minutes to treat hypotension, followed by continuous IV hydration at 2–3 times maintenance as indicated by vital signs and clinical examination. If there is no response, and if ABGs indicated the presence of acidosis, sodium bicarbonate therapy should be administered to maintain the pH in the normal range. Persistent hypotension despite fluid challenge may require the addition of pressor agent therapy. **Levarterenol** 2–4 µg/kg/min or **phenylephrine** infusion starting at 100–180 µg/min and titrating based on blood pressure and heart rate response are good options. The risk of using alpha agents to treat hypotension in the case of anticholinergic ingestion is sympathetic overstimulation with consequent cardiovascular collapse. **Dopamine is not recommended** because of beta effects and the risk of further vasodilatation with worsening hypotension, tachycardia, and increased myocardial oxygen consumption. **Dobutamine** will increase heart rate and myocardial work

load and may not adequately treat hypotension. A **Swan-Ganz catheter** may need to be placed to assist in the assessment of fluid status and cardiopulmonary hemodynamics to rule out cardiogenic shock as a possible etiology. **Intra-aortic balloon pumps** can also be inserted to augment cardiac output but can contribute to the development of arrhythmias.

3. **Treatment of hypertension.** Hypertension may also be seen and is best treated with **nitroprusside** 0.3 µg/kg/min titrated to blood pressure response. Beta blockade risks worsening hypertension because of unopposed alpha stimulation. Unresponsive hypertension is treated with **physostigmine.**

4. **Treatment of arrhythmias.** Arrhythmias are the leading cause of death in anticholinergic overdose, with VF as the most commonly seen lethal arrhythmia.

   a. **Atrial arrhythmias.** ST is commonly noted and usually requires no specific therapy. SVT may occur and is frequently associated with cardiovascular collapse, requiring treatment with cardioversion. Adenosine may be given in an attempt to treat when there is no immediate threat to life. Beta-blockers and calcium channel blockers should be avoided because they may precipitously worsen hypotension.

   b. **Ventricular arrhythmias.** The increases in the QRS width and QTc seen with anticholinergics are due to myocardial depression and are poor prognostic indicators. There is an associated increased risk of development of ventricular arrhythmias, including torsades de pointes, with a **QRS width greater than 120 milliseconds.** This rhythm requires placement of a temporary **pacemaker** and the use of prophylactic antiarrhythmics.

      (i) **VT.** The drug of choice for VT is **lidocaine** 1 mg/kg bolus and then 2–4 mg/kg/min continuous IV infusion. Procainamide, quinidine, and disopyramide are absolutely **contraindicated** because of the development of intractable VT and VF. Bretylium is **not** recommended because of initial catecholamine stimulation worsening cardiovascular status. VT associated with atrioventricular (AV) block may require **synchronous cardioversion** and temporary **pacemaker** placement **prior** to the use of lidocaine.

      (ii) **Pulseless VT** is treated as VF with **defibrillation,** and lidocaine is used to increase the likelihood of successful conversion to sinus rhythm.

5. **GI decontamination.** In patients in whom oral anticholinergic ingestion is suspected, GI decontamination by NS lavage through a 36–40 French lavage tube and instillation of oral activated charcoal are indicated.

6. **Physostigmine therapy.** Physostigmine is a reversible anticholinesterase inhibitor that allows acetyl-

choline to accumulate in the synapse in order to overcome the blockade caused by anticholinergic medications and neuromuscular blocking medications. Neostigmine and edrophonium are also anticholinesterase inhibitors but, unlike physostigmine, do not cross the blood-brain barrier. **Indications** for the use of physostigmine in the treatment of anticholinergic ingestion are the treatment of cardiac dysrhythmias resistant to treatment with lidocaine, unstable SVT, refractory seizures, prolonged CNS symptoms, and cases of ileus that prevent effective use of multidose activated charcoal. It is especially useful in the acute setting to confirm anticholinergic overdose as a diagnostic test. Because of its side-effects profile, many researchers advocate its use only as a diagnostic test, especially in the intentional overdose setting, where coingestants are likely.

Side effects of physostigmine include nausea, emesis, abdominal cramps, bradycardia, seizures, and bronchospasm. Physostigmine is **contraindicated** in patients with abnormal cardiac conduction pathways or possible TCA coingestion. Relative contraindications include seizures, diabetes mellitus, peripheral vascular disease, asthma, and mechanical obstruction of the GI or GU tracts.

A test dose of 0.02 mg/kg physostigmine is given **slow** IV push over 5 minutes. The dose in children is 0.02 mg/kg (maximum dose 0.5 mg/min), in the elderly 0.5 mg/min, and in adults 2 mg total (nor more than 1 mg/min). Three types of responses may be noted. The onset of action of physostigmine may be delayed 15–30 minutes, indicating possible massive anticholinergic ingestion, mixed overdose, or overdose complicated by acidosis or hypoxia. Treatment of massive overdose may require readministration of physostigmine for a longer period of time. Following the correction of acid-base abnormalities, a repeat trial dose should be given and a toxicology screen sent to rule out the presence of coingestants. An immediate response, within 5–15 minutes, may be seen, but these patients frequently need repeat dosing because the duration of action of the agent ingested is often longer than that of physostigmine. **Continuous IV administration is not recommended.** Lastly, patients may develop signs and symptoms of cholinergic toxicity, with lacrimation, salivation, urination, and defecation. This indicates that the patient's symptoms were **not** due to anticholinergic intoxication, and, if severe, these symptoms may be treated with **atropine** 0.5 mg IV per 1 mg of physostigmine given. Physostigmine is not recommended for routine use in anticholinergic overdose, and its use is an indication for admission to an intensive care setting for observation and evaluation.

7. **Other considerations**
   a. **Agitation.** Treatment of severe CNS stimulant effects in order to prevent hyperthermia and

seizures is a relative indication for the use of physostigmine. Agitation is best treated with benzodiazepines such as **diazepam** or **lorazepam**. Antipsychotic and neuroleptic medications should **not** be used because they possess anticholinergic properties that can potentially worsen agitation, impair thermoregulation, and lower the seizure threshold.

b. Hyperthermia must be treated aggressively with cooling and IV hydration because of the associated high morbidity.

c. Seizures due to anticholinergic overdose are treated with benzodiazepines and stabilization of the ABCs. Seizures refractory to conventional therapy, including phenytoin and phenobarbital, are an indication for the use of physostigmine.

D. Disposition

1. Admission criteria. Because of the high morbidity and mortality rates associated with significant anticholinergic ingestion, patients should be admitted to the hospital for further treatment and evaluation. Patients maintaining a near normal blood pressure and a normal ECG and who are without arrhythmia or a change in mental status during ED evaluation may be admitted to a telemetry unit for 12–24 hours. Those patients with an abnormal ECG, life-threatening arrhythmias, or labile blood pressure require intensive care admission for 12–24 hours or until the arrhythmias cease. All patients requiring treatment with physostigmine must be admitted to an intensive care setting.

2. Discharge criteria. Patients presenting to the ED after a small anticholinergic ingestion who are normotensive with slight tachycardia after ED evaluation may be discharged if they meet certain criteria. They must be treated with charcoal and observed for 4–6 hours, and they must not develop unstable vital signs, abnormal ECG changes, or a change in mental status. Psychiatric consultation should be obtained prior to discharge because many of these patients have underlying psychiatric illnesses or may have presented after a suicide attempt. In the case of pediatric ingestion, investigation of the home for safety and parental supervision is important, along with documentation of normal salicylate and acetaminophen levels.

VI. Cholinergics. Cholinergic receptors are of two types: muscarinic and nicotinic. Muscarinic receptors are located mainly in postganglionic parasympathetic nerves of exocrine glands, and nicotinic receptors are concentrated in the neuromuscular junction of skeletal muscle. Acetylcholine is the neurotransmitter released at these synapses. Cholinesterases within the synapse rapidly degrade any excess acetylcholine after release. Exposure to anticholinesterases results in the accumulation of acetylcholine in the synapse, resulting in excessive cholinergic stimulation.

These anticholinesterase-type agents are also referred to as parasympathomimetics. Pilocarpine, used in the treatment of glaucoma, causes miosis and a therapeutic decrease in intraocular pressure. Bethanechol causes contraction of the detrusor muscle with an increase in ureteral peristalsis, and is used to treat urinary retention. Organophosphates, first used in warfare as nerve gas, are used as insecticides. These agents bind irreversibly to acetylcholinesterase, resulting in prolonged toxic symptoms, including lacrimation, salivation, defecation, and emesis. Carbamate-type insecticides also bind acetylcholinesterase but spontaneously reverse after minutes to hours, resulting in a shorter duration of toxic activity. Organophosphates and carbamates are highly lipid-soluble, causing symptoms of toxicity after percutaneous and inhalational exposures. Symptoms of rebound toxicity can be seen up to several weeks following organophosphate exposure, despite therapy, because the agent within the adipose tissue moves into the bloodstream. Death following exposure can occur within 5 minutes or after 24 hours, depending on the agent, the type of exposure, and the patient's baseline health. Copious bronchial secretions that block the alveoli can cause hypoxia; this is the most common cause of death, followed by paralysis of the msucles of respiration.

A. Presentation

1. **History.** The manner in which patients present following cholinergic intoxication is dependent on the agent as well as the mode and duration of exposure. An overdose of bethanechol or pilocarpine can cause dyspnea, syncope, and complete heart block. In organophosphate overdose, the presentation differs and is based on occupational versus nonoccupational exposure. Occupational exposure is by far more common, with dermal exposure or inhalation being the most frequent routes of exposure. Nonoccupational exposure is often an oral intoxication.

   An agricultural or horticultural work history in a patient who presents with symptoms of excessive parasympathetic stimulation prompts a diagnosis of organophosphate exposure. Many cases, however, require a high degree of suspicion to arrive at the proper diagnosis.

   Symptoms vary between acute and chronic exposure, with the constellation of symptoms best summarized by the mnemonic SLUD—salivation, lacrimation, urination, defecation. Acute intoxication results in sudden onset of bronchospasm with associated bronchorrhea, rapidly leading to respiratory insufficiency. Weakness is generalized and is accompanied by involuntary muscle twitching, with the patient complaining of lack of control. Patients also complain of ocular pain and blurred vision, severe nausea, emesis, and diarrhea.

2. **Physical examination**
   a. **General physical examination.** Following acute exposure, the general appearance is that of an obviously ill person. Blood pressure is decreased, the heart rate is decreased, and there is an increased or decreased respiratory rate, depending

on the status of the CNS and respiratory muscle involvement. The skin is warm, flushed, moist, and diaphoretic. Miosis occurs almost immediately, accompanied by lacrimation. Conjunctivae are congested and corneal abrasions may be present, but funduscopic examination is unrevealing. There is copious discharge from the nostrils, and traces of the agent may be present in the nares if a large inhalational exposure has occurred. The mucous membranes are moist, and patients are often drooling from excessive salivation. Fasciculations of the tongue may be noted, and speech is slurred.

   b. Cardiopulmonary. Auscultation of the lung fields often reveals wheezing due to bronchoconstriction, but coarse rhonchi and rales may also be appreciated because of the large amounts of bronchial secretions. The heart rate is slow and regular.

   c. GI. The abdomen is often protuberant with increased bowel sounds due to intestinal hyperactivity and hypersecretion.

   d. Neurologic. Muscle weakness may be local or generalized and is associated with fasciculation. DTRs may be decreased or absent, and muscle paralysis can occur suddenly.

B. Assessment

   1. Laboratory examination. Blood should be drawn for CBC, electrolytes, glucose, BUN, and creatinine. Although results are not diagnostic in organophosphate exposure, they may help to exclude other diagnoses. Blood should be drawn for serum and RBC levels of **cholinesterase.** The diagnosis of organophosphate exposure is confirmed by **decreased** levels. In acute exposure, often the serum level will be the first to fall. Most medical facilities do not have the capability to perform these tests, and results from independent laboratories may require 24–48 hours. Treatment should **not** be withheld pending results if the clinical picture is consistent with cholinergic intoxication.

   In cases where no history is obtainable or the patient presents in coma or with seizures, a toxicologic screen should also be sent in an attempt to narrow the differential diagnosis list.

   2. ECG. A 12-lead ECG should be performed because arrhythmias including complete heart block may occur but are not pathognomonic.

   3. Radiographs. A chest x-ray will assist in the evaluation of lung fields for infiltrates and pulmonary vascular congestion. In severe cholinergic poisoning, alveolar infiltrates may be present.

C. Management

   1. Supportive care. Early stabilization of the airway is of the utmost importance. Respiratory failure associated with organophosphate exposure occurs because of copious bronchial secretions, muscle fatigue, and paralysis of the voluntary muscles of respiration. In some cases, treatment of respiratory insufficiency and the associated hypoxia may potentially treat hypotension and cardiac abnormalities. Patients should be oxygenated to maintain an adequate tissue saturation. IV access and continuous cardiac monitoring are mandatory.

2. **Atropine.** Following protection of the airway, adequate oxygenation, and cardiac monitoring, atropine can be administered. If given prior to the treatment of hypoxia, atropine administration may cause ventricular fibrillation. The adult dose is 2–5 mg IV (children, 0.05–0.10 mg/kg IV) q5–10min until hypersecretion ceases. Large initial doses are required and are followed by continuous IV drip of 50 mg/hr maintenance infusion for at least 48 hours and until cholinesterase levels are noted to be increasing for 3 consecutive days. Tachycardia and mydriasis may occur and may be extreme but should not dissuade one from further atropinization. The desired therapeutic end-point is decreased bronchorrhea, lacrimation, and salivation.

3. **Treatment of pulmonary complications.** The mainstay of treatment of pulmonary complications of cholinergic overdose is atropine, aggressive airway management, and ventilatory support. Continued bronchospasm and laryngospasm can be treated with epinephrine 1:1000 dilution, 0.1–1.0 mg SQ, and inhaled beta$_2$ agonists. Morphine, aminophylline, and theophylline use are **contraindicated,** and phenothiazine- or reserpine-type tranquilizers are to be avoided. **ARDS** may occur as a complication of cholinergic toxicity. Despite ventilator assistance, patients develop severe hypoxia, high airway pressures, and bilateral interstitial infiltrates on CXR. Treatment consists of continued mechanical assisted ventilation with positive end-expiratory pressure (PEEP) added to keep terminal bronchioles patent. Steroid therapy may be added but has not been shown to improve recovery of increase survival.

4. **Pralidoxime.** Because atropine only treats the muscarinic effects of cholinergic poisoning, pralidoxime, a cholinesterase reactivator, is used to treat the respiratory depression and skeletal muscle weakness. After atropinization and oxygenation, pralidoxime, 1–2 g/100ml NS IV (children, 25–40 mg/kg IV), is given over 15–30 minutes. A slow IV push administration, **not** exceeding 200 mg/min, may be used in cases where fluid overload poses significant risk. A repeat dose may be indicated after 1 hour if muscle weakness was not reversed with the initial dose. Additional doses should be given cautiously for recurrent weakness because of continued release of the organophosphate agent from lipid stores. Dosing may also be guided by repeat levels of cholinesterase, with a maximum daily dose of 6 g. There are no known medical contraindications to the use of pralidoxine. Adverse effects include blurred vision, dizziness, headache,

tachycardia, and hyperventilation. This agent is not indicated for use with carbamate pesticides because they possess a relatively short duration of action. Inappropriate use in this situation can result in increased toxicity due to direct neuromuscular blockade and anticholinesterase inhibition.

5. **Other considerations**
   a. **Hypotension** is treated initially with atropine, followed by bolus IV fluids. If hypotension remains problematic, therapy with pressor agents is added (e.g., **dopamine** 10–20 μg/kg/min, **dobutamine** 2–10 μg/kg/min, or **levarterenol** 2–4 μg/kg/min may be used and titrated to achieve desired blood pressure response). Patients who are persistently hypotensive should have **central venous pressure (CVP)** or a **Swan-Ganz catheter** placed to assist in further management of fluid resuscitation.
   b. **Cardiac arrhythmias** are common. **Sinus bradycardia** is most common and is often treated by reversing hypoxia and administrating **atropine.** **Complete heart block** also occurs and may require placement of a temporary **pacemaker** until it resolves with treatment of cholinergic toxicity. **VT** is treated with **lidocaine,** 1 mg/kg IV bolus and then 2–4 mg/min continuous IV drip. **VF** is treated with **defibrillation.**
   c. **Seizures** can occur because of hypoxia and the direct CNS stimulatory effects of organophosphates. Seizures **not** responsive to treatment with **atropine** may be cautiously treated with **diazepam** up to 20 mg in adults (0.1–0.2 mg/kg in children) in a slow IV push. **Phenytoin,** 17 mg/kg loading dose (given no faster than 50 mg/min IV), with continuous cardiac monitoring is given to provide continued seizure control. Seizures refractory to phenytoin are treated with **phenobarbital,** 15–20 mg/kg initially and then 60–200 mg/d in adults; 3–6 mg/kg/d in children.

6. **Decontamination.** The treatment of a patient with organophosphate exposure begins in the prehospital phase with decontamination. Prehospital personnel responding at the scene and health care workers treating the patient must be properly outfitted to not become victims themselves. Protective suits, gas masks, and gloves are advised.

   Areas used for treatment should be adequately ventilated while isolation from the main ED treatment areas is maintained to decrease the risk of inadvertent exposure of hospital staff and other patients to toxins. Areas exposed to the toxin in the course of patient transport and ED treatment must be thoroughly washed with soap and water and all bed linens and gowns disposed of in hazardous waste receptacles. Housekeeping personnel tending to this task should be outfitted in a manner similar to the health care workers.

It is important to not only remove the patient from the source of the compound but also to remove and properly dispose of clothing that may contain the pesticide residue. Skin and hair should be washed with alcohol and sodium bicarbonate as soon as possible. **GI decontamination** should then proceed with placement of an orogastric tube followed by NS lavage and **multidose activated charcoal.** This may not be necessary in patients with emesis and diarrhea or in patients with a strictly dermal exposure.

D. Disposition
1. **Admission criteria.** All patients with a clincially significant exposure to organophosphate or carbamate compounds require hospitalization and admission to an intensive care unit for at least 48–72 hours of continuous observation. Treatment with atropine and pralidoxime is continued as clinically indicated. Serum and RBC cholinesterase levels are followed during and after treatment with pralidoxime. Levels increasing for 3 consecutive days indicate adequate toxin elimination, and the patient may be transferred to a general patient care floor for further observation and stabilization prior to discharge. Decreasing levels of cholinesterase despite therapy may be seen because of continued release of organophosphate compounds from lipid storage sites and require continued therapy. Fatalities have resulted from such relapses.
2. **Discharge criteria.** Patients with normal or slightly decreased serum cholinesterase may be discharged after evaluation and observation for 24 hours with close outpatient follow-up. Patients with minor dermal exposure to organophosphates should be observed in the ED with continuous cardiac monitoring and pulse-oximetry for 6 hours following decontamination. Those remaining asymptomatic may be discharged home with instructions to return if they develop muscle twitching, diaphoresis, or ocular symptoms. Outpatient follow-up should be arranged, prior to ED discharge, for patients to be evaluated within 24 hours.

Bibliography

Cetaruk E, Aaron C. Hazards of nonprescription medications. *Emerg Med Clin North Am* 12:483–510, 1994.

Dilsaver SC, Votolato NA, Alessi NE. Complications of phenylpropanolamine. *Am Fam Practice* 39:201–206, 1989.

Goldfrank LR, Flomenbaum NE. *Goldfrank's Toxicologic Emergencies* (3rd ed.). Appleton-Century-Crofts, 1986.

Sidell FR. Clinical effects of organophosphate cholinesterase inhibitors. *J Appl Tox* 14:111–113, 1994.

Stork C, Howland A, Goldfrank L. Concepts and controversies of bronchodilator overdose. *Emerg Med Clin North Am* 12:415–436, 1994.

Truwit J. Toxic effects of bronchodilators. *Crit Care Clin North Am* 7:639–657, 1991.

Vascular Emergencies

35

Deep Venous Thrombosis

Daniel R. Martin

I. **Significance.** Although pulmonary embolism is one of the most common causes of death in the United States, recently more support has developed for the concept that these emboli are merely a complication of deep venous thromboses (DVTs), and that over 90% of pulmonary emboli originate from the lower extremities. Recent reports estimate that the incidence of DVT in the United States may be as high as 600,000 cases annually.

II. **Pathophysiology.** The pathophysiology of DVTs requires some knowledge of the formation of thrombi in the lower extremities. It is felt that the venous thrombus starts as a platelet nidus near venous valves and where turbulence in flow exists. As thrombogenic materials accumulate, a red fibrin thrombus forms, and this may grow as platelets and fibrin aggregate. If the thrombus does not detach and embolize, the endogenous thrombolytic system may dissolve the clot. If this does not occur or there is only partial dissolution, the thrombus can become organized and incorporated into the venous wall. These interruptions of the venous valves can cause future venous stasis.

Virchow emphasized that the triad of factors that predispose to DVT include **venous stasis, injury to the intima,** and **changes in the coagulation process** that favor thrombosis formation (hypercoagulable states).

Causes of venous stasis include prolonged lower extremity immobilization, prolonged bed rest, recent surgery, right-sided congestive heart failure, and pregnancy.

Causes of endothelial injury include previous DVT, trauma, and lower extremity surgery such as hip surgery. Although most postoperative DVTs arise in the calf, recent estimates are that 20% of patients undergoing general surgery and 40% to 50% with skeletal trauma may have thrombi that originate in the proximal veins. Although most calf thromboses are asymptomatic, 20% to 30% may extend into the proximal veins.

The hypercoagulable states have been recently divided into primary or inherited disorders (Table 35-1) amd secondary disorders (Table 35-2). Recently a factor V gene mutation (factor V Leiden mutation) causing resistance of factor V to activated protein C has been found to be one of the most common inherited causes of hypercoaguability. Although screening all patients for these disorders is not cost effective, it has been suggested that patients with recurrent, familial, or juvenile DVTs or thromboses in an unusual location be screened for inherited disorders. Diagnostic evaluation should include tests for antithrombin III, protein C, protein S, fibrinogen levels, and evaluation for factor V Leiden mutation.

III. **Clinical deep venous thrombosis**

A. **Presentation.** The accuracy of the clinical diagnosis of DVT is at best 50%. The most common symptoms of patients with DVTs include **pain, swelling,** and **erythema.**

Table 35-1.   Primary hypercoagulable states

Antithrombin III deficiency
Protein C deficiency
Protein S deficiency
Fibrinolytic abnormalities
Hypoplasminogenemia
Dysplasminogenemia
Tissue plasminogen activator release deficiency
Increased levels of plasminogen activator inhibitor
Dysfibrinogenemia
Homocystinuria
Heparin cofactor II deficiency
Increased levels of histidine-rich glycoprotein

Source: Nachman RL, Silverstein R. Hypercoagulable states. *Ann Intern Med* 119:819–827, 1993.

The most common physical findings include unilateral lower extremity edema, Homan's sign (calf pain with passive dorsiflexion of the foot), and palpation of a venous cord representing the actual clot. However, studies have demonstrated that Homan's sign and a palpable cord are present in 30% or fewer patients with documented DVTs and occur in a similar number of patients without a DVT. Other causes of lower extremity pain such as musculoskeletal causes, impaired venous or lymphatic flow, and popliteal inflammatory cysts (Bakers's cyst) should be

Table 35-2.   Secondary hypercoagulable states

Cancer
Pregnancy
Oral contraceptives
Nephrotic syndrome
Myeloproliferative disorders
Hyperlipidemia
Diabetes mellitus
Paroxysmal nocturnal hemoglobinuria
Postoperative states
Vasculitis
Antiphospholipid syndrome
Increased levels of factor VII and fibrinogen
Anticancer drugs
Heparin thrombocytopenia
Obesity

Source: Nachman RL, Silverstein R. Hypercoagulable states. *Ann Intern Med* 119:819–827, 1993.

considered. Because of the inaccuracy of the clinical diagnosis of DVTs, patients with any symptoms or signs of DVT that are not obviously explained by other diagnoses should undergo objective evaluation.

B. Assessment. Once the diagnosis of DVT is suspected, objective tests must be used to make the diagnosis. The most widely available tests include venography, duplex ultrasonography, and impedance plethysmography (IPG).

1. **Venography.** Venography has been considered the "gold standard" in diagnosing DVT. It is performed by injecting contrast into a vein on the surface of the foot. Because the diagnostic accuracy is sufficiently high (>95%), it is used as the gold standard to which other noninvasive tests are compared. Unlike many noninvasive tests, venography is accurate with DVTs below the knee. The disadvantages of venography are that it is expensive, requires technician support, interpretation by a radiologist, IV contrast administration, and is associated with a 1% to 3% incidence of inducing a thrombosis. Recent reports also claim that in up to 25% of patients requiring this test, it could either not be done or it could not be interpreted. In addition, repetitive tests are not practical.

2. **Impedance plethysmography (IPG).** IPG relies on the principle that venous return from the lower extremity is rapid after release of cuff-induced venous obstruction, but slow if large veins are obstructed by thromboses. The test is done with the patient supine and legs elevated (15 degrees). A thigh cuff is rapidly inflated and deflated, and the change in volume is measured using electrodes positioned around the calf. The sensitivity of IPG in patients with symptomatic DVTs has been found to be as high as 97% for DVTs above the knee, although recent studies have demonstrated a sensitivity less than 70%. The advantages of IPG are that it is inexpensive, convenient, can be done by technicians, and requires only basic equipment. The disadvantages of IPG include the recent reports of low sensitivity, its operator dependency, and the insensitivity to calf and nonocclusive proximal DVTs. In fact, the optimal timing of follow-up studies has not been established. Although the sensitivity in recent studies has been lower, the specificity remains high. This study, if positive for DVT, can be used to begin treatment without the use of more invasive studies as confirmation (venography). Because up to 15% of DVTs can be missed after only a single test the studies demonstrating the highest sensitivity performed were serial outpatient studies. False positive results have been described for patients with severe arterial disease and raised venous or intrathoracic pressure.

3. **Duplex ultrasonography.** Duplex ultrasonography (realtime B-mode), performed slightly better compared to serial IPGs (3 studies over 8 days) when performed in a serial manner. The test is performed by scanning the thigh and popliteal areas for clot, and it

requires that the vein be visualized and compressible. The sensitivity has been described to be in the 97%–99% range. The advantages and disadvantages of duplex ultrasound are similar to those for IPGs. The advantages of duplex scans are that they are inexpensive, convenient, can be done by technicians, and require only basic equipment, although they are more sophisticated than IPG. One disadvantage of duplex scanning is that it is technician-dependent. It is also insensitive to thromboses in calf veins, iliac veins, and thromboses in the superficial femoral veins within the adductor canal. The optimal timing of follow-up studies has not been established. When IPG and compression ultrasonography were recently compared head-to-head, realtime compression ultrasonography outperformed impedance plethysmography.

4. **Other tests.** Several other tests have also been used to diagnose deep venous thromboses. Computer-assisted tomography can diagnose thromboses in abdominal, pelvic, and the great veins, and also has the advantage of being able to detect other causes of extrinsic venous compression. Although recent trials of magnetic resonance imaging have demonstrated promising results, limited availability and prohibitive expense make this an unlikely test to gain widespread acceptance. Serologic tests such as monoclonal antibodies specific for cross-linked fibrin and D-dimer, a product of plasmin breakdown, may be sensitive but lack specificity and require confirmation by more specific noninvasive testing.

C. **Management.** The goals of therapy in the treatment of deep venous thrombosis are to prevent pulmonary embolus, restore venous patency and valvular function, and prevent the postphlebitic syndrome. The incidence of pulmonary embolism in untreated deep venous thrombosis is approximately 40% but less than approximately 10% with anticoagulation therapy.

1. **Anticoagulation therapy.** The treatment of choice for most DVTs is anticoagulation with IV **heparin.** Heparin's primary effect is to prevent thrombus growth as the endogenous fibrinolytic system is permitted to work. Heparin therapy should begin when the diagnosis of DVT is made. The activated partial-thromboplastin time should be maintained in the therapeutic range or 1.5 to 2.5 times the control value. Subcutaneous injections designed to maintain the partial thromboplastin time in this range have shown equal efficacy. If full anticoagulation is not achieved within 24 hours, the risk of recurrent thrombosis is 15 times higher. As outlined in Chap. 36, recent data has emphasized the need to deliver larger loading and maintenance doses of heparin rather than the standard 5,000 unit loading dose followed by 1,000 U/hr. Heparin delivered on a per weight basis has resulted in a shorter time to full anticoagulation. Oral anticoagu-

lation with the vitamin K antagonist **coumadin** should be started early in the hospital course.

The major complications of heparin therapy are bleeding and thrombocytopenia. Contraindications to heparin include intracranial bleeding, intracranial lesions prone to bleeding, active internal bleeding, or a history of heparin-induced thrombocytopenia (HAT). The risk of bleeding from heparin increases with age and the activated partial thromboplastin time (APTT).

Low-molecular weight heparin has the advantage of a longer half-life and fewer hemorrhagic complications. It may also lead to less antiheparin antibody formation. It is not yet widely available.

2. **Thrombolytic therapy.** Indications for thrombolytic therapy in patients with pulmonary emboli are discussed in Chap. 36. Thrombolytic therapy promotes the dissolution of newly formed clots. Although early trials have suggested that thrombolytic therapy with anticoagulation is more effective than anticoagulation alone at establishing early restoration of venous patency and preserving valvular function, pathologic studies suggest that evidence of the postphlebitic syndrome is just as pronounced with thrombolytic therapy as with anticoagulation. In addition, the fact that thrombolytic therapy confers no greater pulmonary embolism protection than anticoagulation alone at the expense of a twofold to fourfold increased risk of intracranial bleeding makes this therapy less attractive for the treatment of DVT.

Contraindications to thrombolytic therapy have been summarized and are usually classified into absolute and relative. Absolute contraindications to thrombolysis include active internal bleeding, recent cerebravascular accident (CVA), recent (previous 2 months) CNS surgery, and intraspinal or intracranial neoplasm.

Management of bleeding complications depends on the site and severity. For major bleeding such as intracranial, expanding groin hematomas, or gross hematuria, thrombolysis should be discontinued and consideration should be given to fresh frozen plasma, cryoprecipitate, and blood.

3. **Caval interruption.** Caval interruption (such as with a Greenfield filter) is discussed in the chapter on pulmonary embolism (Chap. 36) and is indicated for

   1. acute pulmonary embolus with absolute contraindications to anticoagulation.
   2. severe bleeding occurring during anticoagulation.
   3. recurrent pulmonary emboli despite adequate anticoagulation.

Other possible indications for caval interruption have been recently reviewed. Some researchers have recommended caval interruption for massive embolism due to the risk of death if there is a recurrence.

The most commonly used device for caval interruption is the **Greenfield filter,** which is a conical stainless steel wire filter. The filter is 4.6 cm in length and 3.0 cm in diameter at its base when fully expanded. Although inserting the filter is very safe, complications such as misplacement of the filter, filter migration, wound hematoma, air emboli, caval perforation, or early caval occlusion have been reported. Despite filter placement, recurrent pulmonary emboli occurred in 2.4% of cases in one series.

Although caval interruption protects the patient from pulmonary emboli, it has no effect on venous thrombosis. Anticoagulation remains the primary therapy if there are no contraindications.

4. **Surgical embolectomy.** Surgical therapy of acute DVT has been attempted with early restoration of venous patency, but the vein commonly reoccludes because of incomplete removal of the thrombus and endothelial damage. This form of therapy, however, has been recommended for the treatment of phlegmasia cerulea dolens. This extensive form of venous occlusion can compromise the arterial circulation and even a small increase in venous return may be limb-saving.

D. **Patient disposition.** Currently, the standard therapy for acute DVT includes admission, heparinization, and initiation of oral coumadin. Subcutaneous heparin and the use of low-molecular weight heparin may provide outpatient options for patients with acute DVT without comorbidity.

Although in past years patients suspected of having a DVT were admitted and studied the following day, currently patients are studied noninvasively at the time of presentation and followed closely as outpatients if studies are negative. Admitting patients for venography the next day is not cost effective.

IV. **Special situations**
   A. **Calf vein DVT.** Whether to treat isolated calf vein DVTs remains a topic of controversy. The argument for treatment emphasizes that at least 20% of calf vein DVTs will extend proximally to the thigh compared to less than 5% after anticoagulation therapy. The incidence of symptomatic pulmonary embolism from calf vein DVTs is less than 5% compared to over 20% for proximal vein DVTs. In addition, there are no clinical symptoms or signs that can be used to predict which patients are likely to develop proximal extension. Current recommendations are to treat patients with calf vein DVT unless contraindications exist.

   B. **Recurrent DVT.** Patients with recurring DVT should undergo evaluation as above with concerns that a past history of DVT or pulmonary emboli increases risk of DVT. Evaluation should include coagulation studies to rule out a hypercoagulable state in cases where the etiology of the DVT is unclear. Symptoms of the postphlebitic syndrome can cause recurrent symptoms suspicious for DVT as well.

   C. **Postphlebitic syndrome.** This condition occurs, in part, because of endothelial damage and valvular destruction caused by a previous DVT. The symptoms occur in the absence of acute DVT and include swelling, pain, and venous stasis dermatologic changes. The dermatologic changes include venous ulcerations located on the medial or lateral part of the leg around the ankle. These symptoms occur mainly because of venous stasis, chronic venous hypertension, and failure of the calf-muscle pump. However, the frequency of this condition is unclear and may occur in the absence of clinical DVTs.

D. Superficial thrombophlebitis. This diagnosis is the result of a combination of a thrombosis and inflammation of a superficial vein that is commonly caused by a hypercoagulable state, venous stasis, or injury. Although the diagnosis is made clinically by palpation of a palpable indurated tender cord, these cases may also need objective evaluation to rule out DVT. Treatment is often symptomatic with elevation, warm soaks, nonsteroidal anti-inflammatory agents, and antibiotics if infection is suspected.

Bibliography

Grant BJB. Noninvasive tests for acute venous thromboembolism. *Am J Respir Crit Care Med* 194:1044–1047, 1994.

Heijboer H, et al. A comparison of real-time compression ultrasonography with impedance plethysmography for the diagnosis of deep-vein thrombosis in symptomatic outpatients. *NEJM* 329:1365–1369, 1993.

Nachman RL, Silverstein R. Hypercoagulable states. *Ann Intern Med* 119:819–827, 1993.

Verstraete M. The diagnosis and treatment of deep-vein thrombosis. *NEJM* 329:1418–1420, 1993.

Weinman EE, Salzman EW. Deep-vein thrombosis. *NEJM* 331:1639–1641, 1994.

Pulmonary Embolism

Daniel R. Martin

Pulmonary embolism is one of the most common causes of death in the United States, affecting 50,000 to 100,000 patients per year. Treatment can reduce mortality for 26% to less than 10%. Autopsy series have reported that pulmonary emboli (PE) have been undiagnosed in over 30% to 40% of postmortem cases.

I. Etiology. Understanding the pathophysiology of these embolic events requires an understanding of the formation of thrombi in the extremities (Chap. 35), since it is estimated that over 90% of all pulmonary emboli originate from the lower extremities. Conversely, 30% of patients with acute pulmonary embolism may have negative studies of the lower extremities. Although the specific risks for clot formation in the lower extremities have been discussed, clearly, venous stasis, intimal injury, and hypercoagulation states account for the physiologic causes of most emboli. Emboli also may arise from the iliac system, such as the prostatic or uterine veins, or from renal veins, the right cardiac chambers, or veins in the upper extremities. Emboli from sources other than the lower extremities account for less than 10% of pulmonary emboli.

II. Pathophysiology. The consequences of pulmonary emboli are numerous. Total or partial vascular occlusion by emboli initially results in decreased or absent blood flow to peripheral lung tissue while ventilation persists. This results in increased alveolar dead space and a high ventilation/perfusion (V/Q) ratio. Another immediate consequence of this obstruction is pneumoconstriction due to local hypocapnia in affected alveoli. Arterial hypoxemia results from several mechanisms. Right ventricular decompensation and falling cardiac output result in an increased arterio-venous oxygen difference, and the low mixed venous oxygen saturation returning to the right ventricle increases the right-to-left shunt. Blood diverted by the obstruction to unaffected areas of the lung causes hyperperfusion of these areas without concomitant changes in ventilation resulting in low V/Q areas. These effects increase in proportion to the degree of vascular obstruction.

Other events occurring in this setting include the decrease in alveolar surfactant, which results in atelectasis and edema. This occurs due to the effects on the type II alveolar cells, usually after a day or so of vascular obstruction. As blood flow to the affected lung tissue improves, the resulting infiltrates resolve. Although infarction of pulmonary tissue may occur, because the lung has several sources of oxygen (airways, pulmonary arteries, bronchial arteries, and possibly some perfusion from the pulmonary venous circulation), it is rare. Pulmonary infarction is more common when preexisting pulmonary disease exists.

Hemodynamic consequences of pulmonary emboli result from a marked reduction in the pulmonary vascular bed.

This results in increased vascular resistance, increased right ventricular afterload, and if severe enough, right ventricular failure. Although the pulmonary vascular reserve in normal patients can tolerate large areas of obstructed pulmonary vasculature, if the vasculature is already compromised by chronic pulmonary diseases or by other diseases resulting in elevated pulmonary artery pressures, less obstruction can be tolerated, and the hemodynamic consequences will be more severe.

Pulmonary emboli and ensuing right ventricular failure may have other more dramatic consequences as well. As right ventricular work rises, the oxygen requirements and the dependence on coronary perfusion increases. Further decreases in systemic arterial pressure may lead to right venticular ischemia and fatal arrhythmias.

Recognition and treatment of pulmonary embolism are the most important factors when considering morbidity and mortality of pulmonary emboli. If pulmonary emboli are recognized and treated, the mortality is as low as 3%. Untreated, however, the mortality is 26%.

III. Clinical pulmonary embolus

A. Presentation. The symptoms of pulmonary emboli (PE) may be subtle or difficult to detect clinically. In one study, 40% of patients with deep venous thromboses had asymptomatic pulmonary emboli. The most common symptoms of PE are chest pain and dyspnea, and the most common sign is tachypnea. However, these symptoms and signs are far from 100% sensitive and 100% specific, which creates clinical diagnostic difficulties. Table 36-1 presents frequency ranges for presenting symptoms and signs of patients with pulmonary emboli that are based on data from the UPET and PIOPED trials.

Although individual symptoms and signs lack sensitivity, combinations of symptoms such as dyspnea, hemoptysis, and pleuritic chest pain were 94% sensitive. However, all three of these findings occurred in only 22% of PE patients. Similarly, dyspnea or tachypnea occurred in 96% of patients, and dyspnea, tachypnea, or suspicious phlebitis occurred in 99% of patients.

Several presentations of pulmonary emboli have been described, but most presentations can be divided into massive, submassive, or pulmonary infarction. The term **massive pulmonary emboli** implies significant arterial obstruction (some have defined this as blockage of an area of lung tissue perfused by more than two lobar arteries) causing increased right ventricular afterload and elevated pulmonary artery pressure. These patients commonly present with syncope, jugular venous distention, cyanosis, or cardiogenic shock. **Submassive pulmonary emboli** are defined as emboli that do not cause right ventricular or pulmonary artery pressure elevation (or blockage to lung tissue perfused by less than two lobar arteries). These patients are more likely to present with dyspnea and tachypnea. Patients with pulmonary infarction present with evidence of infarcted pulmonary tissue such as pleuritic chest pain, hemoptysis, or infiltrates on chest x-ray.

Table 36-1.   Presenting symptoms and signs of patients with pulmonary embolism

Symptoms	Percentage
Dyspnea	73–84
Pleuritic chest pain	66–74
Apprehension	57–59
Cough	37–53
Hemoptysis	13–30
Diaphoresis	27–36
Syncope	13

Signs	Percentage
Tachypnea (RR>16)	70–92
Rales	51–58
Increased P-2	23–53
Tachycardia (HR>100)	30–44
Fever	7–43
Phlebitis	11–32
Cyanosis	1–19

Source: Bell WR, Simon TL, and DeMets DL, The clinical features of submassive and massive pulmonary emboli, *Am J Med* 62:355–360, 1977; and Stein PD, et al., Clinical, laboratory, roentgenographic, and electrocardiographic findings in patients with acute pulmonary embolism and no preexisting cardiac or pulmonary disease, *Chest* 100:598–603, 1991.

B. **Assessment**
   1. **Arterial blood gases.** Arterial blood gas analysis may show hypoxia; however, PO_2 and PCO_2 have been found to be poorly predictive for diagnosing or excluding pulmonary emboli. In fact, one series showed that in patients without prior lung or cardiac disease, 26% of patients with pulmonary emboli had a PO_2 greater than 80 mm Hg. Similarly, the pulse oximetry used to measure the oxygen saturation can be expected to be normal in a high percentage of patients with pulmonary emboli because the PO_2 can fall to 60 mm Hg or 70 mm Hg before this value becomes abnormal. The alveolar-arterial (A-a gradient) oxygen gradient, which is defined as $FIO_2 \times$ (barometric pressure $- 47$ mm) $- (PaCO_2 \times 1.25) - PaO_2$, has been found to be abnormally widened in 90% to 95% of patients with pulmonary emboli. Although pulse oximetry is probably the least sensitive and of no help in diagnosing pulmonary emboli, between the PO_2, pulse oximetry, and A-a gradient, the A-a gradient is clearly the most sensitive. However, the A-a gradient is not very specific, especially in elderly patients. Therefore, although the pulse oximetry and PO_2 are of little or no help in diag-

nosing acute pulmonary embolus, a normal A-a gradient suggests the absence of an embolus, and an abnormal A-a gradient may be due to causes other than pulmonary emboli.

2. **Electrocardiogram.** Although over 70%–90% of patients with acute pulmonary emboli have electrocardiographic abnormalities, these are usually nonspecific. Although the most common abnormality may be sinus tachycardia, QRS and ST and T wave abnormalities also occur commonly. From the UPET trial, right and left axis deviation and complete and incomplete right bundle-branch block each occurred in 5%–10% of patients with pulmonary emboli. Of the patients presenting with massive pulmonary emboli, 32% had electrocardiographic evidence of acute cor pulmonale such as $S_1Q_3T_3$, right bundle-branch block, P pulmonale, or right axis deviation. An $S_1Q_3T_3$ occurred in only 11% of UPET patients. From both the UPET and PIOPED trials, nonspecific ST and T wave changes were the most common electrocardiographic abnormalities. Either T wave inversion or ST-segment elevation or depression occurred in 64% of patients in the UPET trial and in 49% of patients in the PIOPED trial. From these data the electrocardiogram cannot be used to diagnose or exclude an acute pulmonary embolus.

3. **Chest x-ray.** Although a normal chest x-ray is unusual in patients with acute pulmonary emboli, the chest x-ray abnormalities are usually nonspecific. Of those PIOPED patients without previous cardiac or pulmonary disease, 84% had abnormal chest x-rays. Atelectasis, parenchymal abnormalities, and pleural effusions were the most common findings. Among the UPET patients, evidence of consolidation or elevated hemidiaphragm were the most common abnormal radiographic findings. These parenchymal infiltrates may not be due to infarction as previously thought; they may instead be due to local pulmonary hemorrhage, which usually resolves on follow-up chest x-rays. Cardiomegaly and congestive heart failure were rarely seen. Classic findings such as Westermark's sign (focal oligemia due to pulmonary vascular obstruction) and Hampton's hump (pleural-based wedge-shaped density in the peripheral area of infarction with a rounded convex apex pointing toward the hilum) occurred rarely. Since the chest x-ray findings of pulmonary embolism are nonspecific, they are used only to support the diagnosis and to exclude other etiologies of acute chest pain.

4. **Ventilation/perfusion scan.** The lung scan remains the most widely used test to diagnose pulmonary embolus. The perfusion scan is done by using technetium Tc 99m macroaggregated albumen via a peripheral vein. The ventilation scan is accomplished using xenon 133. Advantages of the lung scan are that it is noninvasive, that it can be performed in critically ill patients without further risk to patients, and that it is

very sensitive at detecting emboli larger than 2 mm in diameter. The major disadvantage of the lung scan lies in its interpretation, which has the potential for variablility among institutions and readers. Although in the PIOPED trial high-probability and normal scans correlated well with subsequent angiograms (high-probability scans had higher than 90% positive angiograms, and normal scans had more than 95% negative angiograms), the majority of patients with acute pulmonary emboli fell into other diagnostic categories such as indeterminate, low probability, and very low probability.

Combining retrospective older studies with more recent prospective trials, accurate diagnostic conclusions regarding the interpretation of lung scans can be made. A **normal lung scan** (and near normal in the PIOPED) excludes clinically significant pulmonary emboli, and therefore these patients do not require anticoagulation. A **high-probability lung scan** has an 85% or greater chance of having a positive angiogram, and therefore these patients can be anticoagulated without subsequent angiography. The difficulty lies in those patients with a lung scan between high-probability and normal.

One study reported a 31% incidence of pulmonary embolism in patients with low-probability scans, whereas only 17% of low-probability scans had documented pulmonary emboli in the PIOPED trial. In the PIOPED trial over 40% of scans were interpreted as intermediate, and less than 25% of scans were normal, near normal, or high-probability. Of these intermediate scans, approximately 33% had subsequent positive angiograms. From these trials, although normal, near normal, or high-probability scans help the clinician in making a decision, the majority of the scans were low or intermediate probability, creating a diagnostic dilemma for the clinician.

In the PIOPED trial this dilemma was further studied using the clinician's estimate of the clinical probability of pulmonary embolism prior to obtaining the lung scan. The clinical assessment considered high likelihood of pulmonary embolism (80% to 100% likely), intermediate likelihood (20% to 79% likely), and low likelihood (<19% likely). In the PIOPED trial, if the clinical assessment was greater than 80% with a high-probability scan, 96% of these patients had positive angiograms, and if the clinical assessment was less than 20% with a low-probability scan, only 4% had positive angiograms. Although this clinical assessment was useful in those patients with a low clinical assessment and a low-probability scan, other clinical assessment categories with low-probability scans and the intermediate scans remained difficult to interpret and required further diagnostic testing (Table 36-2).

5. **Lower extremities noninvasive testing.** Additional noninvasive testing has included lower extrem-

Table 36-2. Predictive value of the V/Q scan (% of patients with pulmonary embolus)

V/Q scan probability	Clinical suspicion (%)		
	High	Intermediate	Low
High probability	96	88	56
Intermediate	66	28	16
Low probability	40	16	4

Source: PIOPED Investigators. Value of the ventilation/perfusion scan in acute pulmonary embolism, *Am Heart J* 92:700–706, 1976.

ity venous studies to evaluate for possible deep venous thrombosis. The basis for this evaluation is that most pulmonary emboli arise from this source. However, when venography was performed in patients with documented pulmonary emboli, the studies were positive in only 43% to 57% of patients. Further, when patients with nondiagnostic scans were managed without anticoagulation but followed with serial impedance plethysmography studies, less than 3% of patients developed deep vein thrombosis or pulmonary emboli.

6. **Pulmonary angiography.** Although pulmonary angiography is the most definitive test to diagnose pulmonary emboli, it is invasive, and difficulty with visualization occurs in up to 3% of patients. However, it is clearly the most accurate and reliable means of diagnosing pulmonary emboli. The complications are death in less than 0.5%, other major complications in 1%, and less significant complications in 5%.

7. **Combination testing.** The strategy for diagnosing pulmonary emboli using the lung scan, available lower extremity venous studies, and pulmonary angiography is outlined in Figs. 36-1 through 36-4.

8. **New testing modalities.** More recently, other lab tests have been considered in contributing to the diagnostic algorithm of patients suspected of having pulmonary emboli. During resolution of thromboses, plasmin-mediated degradation of cross-linked fibrin occurs, resulting in release of fibrin degradation products such as D-dimer and thrombin-antithrombin III complexes. A preliminary study has demonstrated that measuring D-dimer at the time of presentation is 98% sensitive but lacks specificity for pulmonary emboli (40%). Although it was believed that this test could aid in the evaluation of suspected pulmonary emboli patients and that it could be used in conjunction with lung scanning, many questions still remain. The duration of D-dimer in the circulation is not clear, and more data are needed on which patients have false negative or false positive results. Other tests such as circulating plasma DNA also are being considered to aid in the diagnostic algorithms for pulmonary emboli.

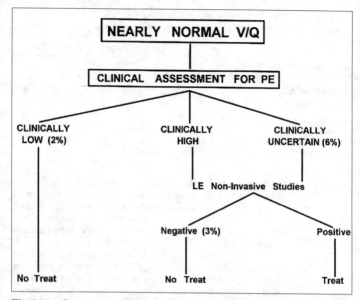

Fig. 36-1. Strategy for diagnosis of patients with "nearly normal V/Q scan" results. V/Q = ventilation/perfusion; PE = pulmonary embolus; LE noninvasive studies = lower extremity noninvasive studies referring to impedance plethysmography or ultrasound studies of the lower extremities; (%) refers to the percentage of patients having a pulmonary embolus in the PIOPED study. (Adapted with permission from Stein PD, et al., Strategy for diagnosis of patients with suspected acute pulmonary embolism, *Chest* 103:1550–1559, 1993.)

C. Management

1. **Anticoagulation therapy.** The treatment of choice for most cases of acute pulmonary emboli is anticoagulation with heparin. Heparin primarily prevents thrombosis growth as the endogenous fibrinolytic system is permitted to work. **Heparin** therapy should begin when the diagnosis of pulmonary emboli is suspected rather than delaying therapy unitl the diagnosis is certain.

A standard beginning regimen of anticoagulation consists of a 5000-unit heparin bolus followed by 1000 U/h with an activated partial thromboplastin time (APTT) goal of at least 1.5 to 2.5 times control. Some researchers have recommended a larger loading dose. One recent study recommends that the maintenance dose be started at 1300 U/h with the following recommendations based on the 4- to 6-hour APTT:

- If APTT is less than 45, rebolus with 5000 units, then increase rate by 240 U/hr;
- If APTT is 46 to 54, increase rate by 120 U/hr;
- If APTT is 55 to 85, continue current rate;

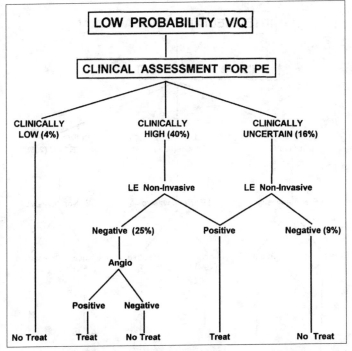

Fig. 36-2. Strategy for diagnosis of patients with a low probability V/Q scan. V/Q = ventilation/perfusion; PE = pulmonary embolus; LE noninvasive studies = lower extremity noninvasive studies referring to impedance plethysmography or ultrasound studies of the lower extremities; (%) refers to the percentage of patients having a pulmonary embolus in the PIOPED study; angio = pulmonary angiography. (Adapted with permission from Stein PD, et al., Strategy for diagnosis of patients with suspected acute pulmonary embolism, *Chest* 103:1550–1559, 1993.)

- If APTT is 86 to 110, stop infusion for 1 hour and decrease rate by 120 U/hr;
- If APTT is greater than 110, stop infusion for 1 hour and decrease rate by 240 U/hr.

More recently, heparin therapy has been recommended based on patient's weight. The bolus dose is 80 U/kg, then 18 U/kg/hr. With this regimen a greater percentage of patients achieved the therapeutic threshold within 24 hours compared to controls treated in standard fashion. Oral anticoagulation therapy (coumadin) therapy can be started on the same day as heparin. The starting dose of **coumadin** is 10 mg/d, with subsequent doses adjusted based on the international normalized ratio (INR).

The major complications of heparin therapy are bleeding and thrombocytopenia. Contraindications to heparin

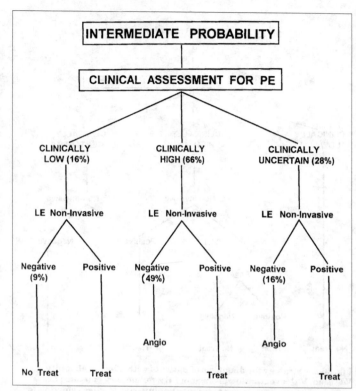

Fig. 36-3.   **Strategy for diagnosis of patients with an intermediate-probability V/Q scan. V/Q = ventilation/perfusion; PE = pulmonary embolus; LE noninvasive studies = lower extremity noninvasive studies referring to impedance plethysmography or ultrasound studies of the lower extremities; (%) refers to the percentage of patients having a pulmonary embolus in the PIOPED study; angio = pulmonary angiography. (Adapted with permission from Stein PD, et al., Strategy for diagnosis of patients with suspected acute pulmonary embolism,** *Chest* **103:1550–1559, 1993.)**

include intracranial bleeding, intracranial lesions prone to bleeding, active internal bleeding, and a history of heparin-induced thrombocytopenia (HAT). The risk of bleeding from heparin increases with age and the APTT, and a recent summary of heparin therapy estimated the risk of major bleeding to be between 1.6% and 7.1%. HAT occurs 3 to 15 days after heparin is begun.

Low-molecular weight heparin (LMWH) recently has been used in patients with deep venous thromboses and has the advantages of a longer half-life and a high bioavailability after subcutaneous injection. LMWH can be given every 24 hours and may result in fewer bleeding complications.

2. **Thrombolytic therapy.** Indications for thrombolytic therapy recently have been discussed. Thrombolytic

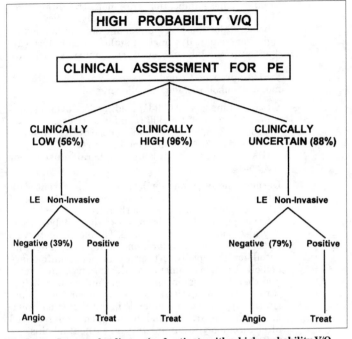

Fig. 36-4. Strategy for diagnosis of patients with a high-probability V/Q scan. V/Q = ventilation/perfusion; PE = pulmonary embolus; LE non-invasive studies = lower extremity noninvasive studies referring to impedance plethysmography or ultrasound studies of the lower extremities; (%) refers to the percentage of patients having a pulmonary embolus in the PIOPED study; angio = pulmonary angiography. (Adapted with permission from Stein PD, et al., Strategy for diagnosis of patients with suspected acute pulmonary embolism, *Chest* 103:1550–1559, 1993.)

therapy promotes the dissolution of newly formed clots. Although randomized trials have compared streptokinase or urokinase with heparin, none has demonstrated a clear mortality advantage.

The demonstrated advantages of thrombolytics, which have been summarized recently by Goldhaber, include accelerated clot lysis, rapid reduction in pulmonary artery pressure, improved pulmonary tissue reperfusion, and higher pulmonary capillary blood volume. Goldhaber also emphasized that pulmonary emboli patients treated with thrombolytics may have improved pulmonary hemodynamics compared to controls both at rest and with exertion.

The consensus indications for thrombolytic therapy in patients with acute pulmonary emboli have remained unchanged since 1980. They include (1) obstruction of blood flow to a lobe or multiple pulmonary segment, and (2) hemodynamic compromise, regardless of the pulmonary embolus's anatomic size. Unfortunately, these indications are not straightforward. Most texts recommend that thrombolytic therapy be considered for massive pulmonary emboli, defined as right ventricular dysfunction sufficient to reduce cardiac output, and that such pulmonary emboli are demonstrated angiographically.

FDA-approved thrombolytic regimens for acute pulmonary emboli include the following:

- Streptokinase: 250,000 IU loading dose over 30 minutes followed by 100,000 IU/h for 24 hours;
- Urokinase: 2,000 IU/lb loading dose over 10 minutes followed by 2,000 IU/lb/h for 12 hours;
- tPA 100 mg as a continuous peripheral infusion over 2 hours.

Despite these recommendations, more recent pulmonary emboli trials have used dosages of 100 mg of tPA over the initial 2 hours of therapy.

Other practical considerations of thrombolytic therapy also should be emphasized. Unlike thrombolysis in acute myocardial infarction, there is not a definite cutoff for thrombolytic therapy in acute pulmonary emboli. Dosage regimens for thrombolysis are fixed, and therefore coagulation tests are not needed during thrombolytic administration. Also, concomitant heparin therapy is not recommended, and if started previously, the heparin should be stopped and resumed after thrombolytic administration without a bolus.

Bleeding remains the most significant adverse effect of thrombolytic therapy. Studies comparing thrombolytic therapy to heparin have shown a higher incidence of major and minor bleeding compared to heparin therapy alone. Contraindications to thrombolytic therapy have been summarized and usually are classified into absolute and relative (see Chap. 10). Absolute contraindications to thrombolysis for acute pulmonary emboli include: active internal bleeding, recent cerebrovascular accident (CVA), recent (past 2 months) CNS surgery, and intraspinal or intracranial neoplasm.

Management of bleeding complications depends on the site and severity. For major bleeding such as intracranial, expanding groin hematomas, or gross hematuria, thrombolysis should be discontinued and consideration should be given to fresh frozen plasma, cryoprecipitate, and blood.

3. **Caval interruption.** Caval interruption (such as a Greenfield Filter) is indicated for:

   1. acute pulmonary embolus with absolute contraindications to anticoagulation.
   2. severe bleeding occurring during anticoagulation.
   3. recurrent pulmonary emboli despite adequate anticoagulation.

Other possible indications for caval interruption have been recently reviewed. Moser has recommended caval interruption for massive embolism due to the risk of death should a recurrence occur.

4. **Surgical interruption.** Emergent surgical embolectomy is generally recommended for documented (by angiogram or perfusion scan) massive pulmonary emboli with persistent hemodynamic compromise when thrombolysis or anticaogulation is contraindicated or if thrombolysis fails. The procedure is associated with a high mortality rate compared to more conservative approaches.

D. **Management of shock or cardiac arrest due to pulmonary embolus.** Clinically, this implies that elevations in right-sided pressures (pulmonary artery and right ventricular) and cardiac failure have occurred, resulting in hemodynamic compromise or cardiac arrest. Heparin therapy, designed to prevent clot propagation and permit the body's fibrinolytic mechanisms to work, is of little value in the setting of acute clinical deterioration. Clot lysis (thrombolytic therapy) or removal (embolectomy) is needed to restore circulation. The mortality in this setting is estimated to vary from 25% to greater than 50%.

The most logical approach for patients in cardiopulmonary shock or arrest, assuming that thrombosis has been documented either in the lungs by angiography/perfusion scan or in the lower extremities by venography or noninvasive studies, is to start **thrombolytic therapy** as soon as possible and to provide appropriate circulatory support with fluids and pressors.

If available, **cardiopulmonary bypass and embolectomy** also should be considered; it is the procedure of choice if thrombolysis is absolutely contraindicated or if thrombolysis fails. Although thrombolysis can be achieved peripherally with streptokinase, urokinase, or tPA, tPA has been given centrally (1 mg/kg) over 1 hour to patients with massive pulmonary embolism with prompt dissolution of thrombi and clinical improvement. Recently several case reports have described successful use of **percutaneous catheter fragmentation** combined with thrombolysis in patients with massive pulmonary emboli. In these cases large clots in central pulmonary arteries were fragmented and distributed to the peripheral pulmonary circulation, followed by thrombolysis. Clot fragmentation resulted in rapid improvement of hemodynamic compromise. Although performed mainly by cardiologists, it seems to be a simple technique to learn.

E. **Patient disposition.** Patients who are admitted to the hospital to rule out pulmonary embolus can be admitted to a monitored bed for anticoagulation and supportive care while awaiting their diagnostic studies. If hypotension, severe hypoxia, or cardiac arrhythmias are present, ICU admission is mandatory.

Patients subsequently diagnosed with acute pulmonary embolism require ICU admission as well. These patients are at risk for recurrent emboli, which could be fatal even if they appear clinically stable.

Bibliography

Bell WR, Simon TL, and DeMets DL. The clinical features of submassive and massive pulmonary emboli. *Am J Med* 62:355–360, 1977.

Moser KM. Venous thromboembolism. *Am Rev Respir Dis* 141:235–249, 1990.

PIOPED Investigators. Value of the ventilation/perfusion scan in acute pulmonary embolism. *JAMA* 263:2753–2759, 1990.

Stein PD, et al. Clinical, laboratory, roentgenographic, and electrocardiographic findings in patients with acute pulmonary embolism and no preexisting cardiac or pulmonary disease. *Chest* 100:598–603, 1991.

Stein PD, et al. Strategy for diagnosis of patients with suspected acute pulmonary embolism. *Chest* 103:1553–1559, 1993.

Urokinase Pulmonary Embolism Trial Study Group. Urokinase Pulmonary Embolism Trial. *JAMA* 214:2163–2172, 1970.

Acute Mesenteric Ischemia

Howard A. Werman

Acute mesenteric ischemia is a disease state that is caused by a structural or functional limitation in the splanchnic circulation. This results in both cellular hypoxia and intestinal acidosis. Acute mesenteric ischemia occurs in approximately 1 in 1000 hospital admissions. The incidence of the disease appears to be rising, partly because of the increasing age of the population and partly because acute mesenteric ischemia is replacing other curable complications of atherosclerotic heart disease as a cause of mortality. The causes of acute mesenteric ischemia are equally split between occlusive and nonocclusive varieties. The disease mortality is extremely high, varying from 50% to 90% depending on the population studied.

I. **Pathophysiology.** The blood supply to the gastrointestinal tract is derived from three sources: the celiac axis, the superior mesenteric artery, and the inferior mesenteric artery. The majority of splanchnic circulation is directed to the mucosal and submucosal regions of the gut. Normally, about one-quarter of the total cardiac output goes to the splanchnic circulation; however, this is highly variable. A variety of factors, including input from the autonomic circulation, hormones, and a variety of medications (Table 37-1) can alter the splanchnic blood flow. Ischemia develops when the splanchnic flow diminishes to 25% of its normal level and the delivery of oxygen and nutrients to the tissues exceeds the metabolic demands of the gut. Because the intestinal mucosa has a high metabolic rate, it is particularly sensitive to a hypoxic insult. The result is a shift to anaerobic metabolism with the resultant generation of lactic acid and production of excess CO_2.

Ultimately, bacterial pathogens invade the splanchnic, portal, and systemic circulations, leading to secondary sepsis. Finally, in cases where flow can be reestablished, reperfusion injury caused by oxygen free-radicals results with vasospasm and ischemia of the intestinal mucosa.

Acute mesenteric ischemia is frequently the result of an occlusive event. In 80% of these cases, arterial embolization is the cause. Valvular heart disease, atrial fibrillation, ventricular aneurysms, and cardiomyopathy are typically implicated. Less commonly, arterial thrombosis causes the ischemic event. In almost all cases, atherosclerotic vascular disease is the underlying etiology. Arterial thrombosis is typically preceded by symptoms of chronic intestinal angina such as postprandial pain and weight loss. Trauma to the mesenteric vessels, vasculitides, disseminated intravascular coagulation, volvulus, intussusception, and adhesive bands are often implicated. Mesenteric venous thrombosis occurs in 10% of all cases of acute mesenteric ischemia. In many cases, no cause is identified. Hypercoagulable states, oral contraceptives, sickle cell disease, thrombophlebitis, and inflammatory bowel disease have been implicated as causes in manyy cases.

Nonocclusive causes of acute mesenteric ischemia include

563

Table 37-1. Factors that reduce splanchnic blood flow

Alpha-adrenergic agents
  Phenylephrine
  Norepinephrine
  Epinephrine (high-dose)
  Dopamine (high-dose)
  Cocaine

Beta-adrenergic blocking agents

Hormones
  Vasopressin
  Serotonin (high-dose)

Leukotrienes
  Nonsteroidal anti-inflammatory drugs

Digitalis glycosides

Anesthetics
  Spinal anesthesia
  Halothane
  Enflurane
  Methoxyflurane
  Cyclopropane

Miscellaneous
  Calcium chloride
  Jejunal feeding
  Exercise
  Hemodialysis
  Pain
  Hypothermia

shock and other low-flow states, drugs (vasodilators, digitalis, catecholamines, cocaine, histamine, vasopressin), arteriovenous fistulae, hemodialysis, and cardiopulmonary bypass. In each case, a reduction of splanchnic blood flow below a critical level leads to ischemia.

The relationship between sepsis and acute mesenteric ischemia is confusing. The septic patient has reduced oxygen delivery, increased metabolic demands, and impaired oxygen utilization. These factors may lead to mesenteric ischemia. On the other hand, mesenteric ischemia may result in the introduction of bacteria and bacterial products into the circulation, initiating a clinical picture of sepsis. Ultimately, the patient develops multisystem organ failure.

II. **Differential diagnosis.** The differential diagnosis of acute mesenteric ischemia is quite broad, particularly because of the nonspecific nature of the patient's symptoms. Diseases such as diverticulitis, peritonitis, pancreatitis, cholecystitis, peptic ulcer disease, and acute appendicitis must be considered. Other entities with a more acute onset, such as ruptured abdominal aortic aneurysm, small bowel obstruction, renal colic, testicular or ovarian torsion, ruptured ectopic pregnancy, perforated viscus, and infarction of other abdominal organs, may be confused with acute mesenteric ischemia. Finally, extraintestinal disease states that present with abdominal complaints such as pneumonia, inferior myocardial infarction, diabetic ketoacidosis, acute intermittent porphyria, and other causes of sepsis must be included in the differential diagnosis.

A. Presentation

1. **History.** The presenting signs and symptoms in patients with acute mesenteric ischemia are highly variable and nonspecific. Therefore, establishing the diagnosis can be quite difficult. The most common complaint is abdominal pain, which is seen in 75%–90% of cases. Abdominal pain is frequently absent in the elderly, who often present with minimal findings. The pain typically develops over a period of days and may be either steadily progressive or intermittent. The pain is typically diffuse and poorly localized.

   Associated symptoms include nausea, vomiting, and a feeling of bloating. Fever is seen rarely. Other reported gastrointestinal symptoms include a change in bowel habits and bloody diarrhea.

   The key to establishing the diagnosis is to maintain a high index of suspicion in patients at risk for developing acute mesenteric ischemia (Table 37-2). The diagnosis should be considered in patients older than 50 years of age; those with valvular or atherosclerotic heart disease, artificial heart valves, atrial fibrillation, congestive heart failure, or sepsis; those using drugs such as vasodilators, digitalis, catecholamines, oral contraceptives, or cocaine; and those with sickle cell anemia, thrombophlebitis, vasculitis, or other diseases listed above. Acute mesenteric ischemia should also be

---

Table 37-2. Risk factors for development of acute mesenteric ischemia

---

Patients older than 50 years of age

Valvular or atherosclerotic heart disease

Artificial heart valves

Atrial fibrillation

Congestive heart failure

Sepsis

Low-flow states

Prior embolic disease

Use of drugs such as vasodilators, digitalis, catecholamines, oral contraceptives, or cocaine

Sickle cell anemia

Thrombophlebitis

Vasculitis

Dialysis

Recent decompression illness

Strenuous physical activity

considered in patients on dialysis, those with recent decompression illness, and those who have engaged in strenuous physical activity.

2. **Physical examination.** The physical examination is rather unimpressive and appears to be out of proportion to the patient's pain. Bowel sounds are often diminished. As the disease progresses and bowel perforation occurs, signs of peritonitis may be seen with involuntary guarding, rebound tenderness, and absence of bowel sounds. Rectal examination often demonstrates guaiac-positive stools, particularly when the more distal portions of the colon are involved.

In advanced cases, massive fluid losses into the bowel lumen produce signs of hypovolemia and hypoperfusion (hypotension, mental confusion, decreased urine output). As the disease process progresses, signs of neurologic dysfunction, myocardial depression, liver failure, renal failure, adult respiratory distress syndrome (ARDS), and clotting abnormalities all may be seen.

B. **Assessment**

1. **Laboratory tests.** Laboratory testing is performed hopefully to identify other causes of the patient's complaints. There are few laboratory findings that establish a firm diagnosis of acute mesenteric ischemia. The complete blood cell count often reveals a marked leukocytosis, often out of proportion to the patient's clinical appearance. An elevation in the hemoglobin and hematocrit is typically seen as a result of hemoconcentration from fluid losses. Electrolyte analysis is notable for an elevated serum potassium level. The patient's BUN also may be elevated because of fluid losses. Blood gas analysis reveals metabolic acidosis with a significant base deficit. An elevated serum amylase is frequently seen in acute mesenteric ischemia. Levels of serum creatinine phosphokinase (CPK), lactate dehydrogenase (LDH), serum glutamic oxaloacetic transaminase (SGOT), and serum glutamic pyruvic transaminase (SGPT) released from the gut submucosa are typically elevated. Finally, the serum lactate level may be increased because of underperfusion of the gut.

Patients with advanced disease present with laboratory findings consistent with multisystem organ failure, including respiratory acidosis and hypoxia, elevated BUN and creatinine levels, a clinical picture of disseminated intravascular coagulation, and elevations of liver function tests.

2. **Radiology.** Plain radiographs yield few clues to diagnose acute mesenteric ischemia. An acute abdominal series should be obtained to rule out other conditions such as perforated viscus, intestinal obstruction, or an abdominal aortic aneurysm. Demonstration of gas in the portal venous system, pneumotosis intestinalis, and "thumbprinting" of the bowel wall all suggest the diagnosis of acute mesenteric infarction but are seen

in only 20%–60% of cases. Both abdominal CT scanning and ultrasonography have limited value in establishing the diagnosis.

3. **Angiography.** Selective mesenteric angiography is the definitive study for establishing the diagnosis. Findings of vasospasm, arterial occlusion, and obstruction of venous flow are consistent with acute mesenteric ischemia. Mesenteric emboli are typically found at the origin of the middle colic artery, the first branch of the superior mesenteric artery. Mesenteric arterial thrombosis, on the other hand, is characteristically found at the origin of the superior mesenteric artery. Nonocclusive causes may present with segmental mesenteric vasospasm. However, the absence of these findings does not rule out the diagnosis, particularly when there is a nonocclusive cause. Other modalities, such as vascular duplex studies, endoscopy, and mucosal tonometry, are of limited value in the emergency setting.

C. **Management.** Acute mesenteric ischemia is a true medical emergency. The principles of initial management include establishing the diagnosis, initiating aggressive resuscitation and supportive therapy, and obtaining early surgical consultation.

Initial resuscitative efforts should focus on providing adequate oxygenation and aggressive fluid resuscitation. All patients with acute mesenteric ischemia should receive supplemental oxygen. For most patients, 100% oxygen via a nonrebreather mask is appropriate. Patients with more advanced disease who have depressed mental status, signs of respiratory failure, or hypotension require endotracheal intubation and ventilatory assistance. Electrocardiographic monitoring and continuous pulse-oximetry measurement should be instituted in all cases.

Attention to any underlying medical conditions is mandatory. Common interventions include correction of congestive heart failure, cardiac dysrhythmias, and volume deficits. Fluid requirements are usually significant in patients with acute mesenteric ischemia. Aggressive isotonic fluid resuscitation should be instituted with careful attention to the patient's mental status, pulse and blood pressure, and urinary output. In critically ill patients, particularly those with signs of cardiac compromise, Swan-Ganz catheter monitoring is imperative. The need for vasopressors such as dopamine or norepinephrine must be weighed against the reduction in splanchnic blood flow caused by these drugs. Broad-spectrum antibiotics should also be administered in patients with suspected mesenteric ischemia because of the coexistent sepsis in these patients. Coverage of enteric pathogens, especially gram-negative and anaerobic organisms, is imperative.

D. **Disposition.** Acute mesenteric ischemia carries a poor prognosis if not diagnosed and managed appropriately. These patients tend to be critically ill at the time of presentation. Admission to an intensive care setting is mandatory in almost all cases. Early surgical consultation is required for cases of suspected acute mesenteric thrombosis. Operative intervention is undertaken to determine the cause of the ischemic insult, to reestablish blood flow, to relieve obstruction, to remove nonviable bowel, and to drain infected tissue. With acute mesenteric embolic disease, an embolectomy typically is performed. A second-look operative procedure is carried out to ensure the viability of the remaining bowel. Acute mesenteric arterial thrombosis is often the result of atherosclerotic narrowing of the superior mesenteric artery. Bypass grafting is usually performed. In nonocclusive disease, management is typically based on treating the underlying cause of the ischemic insult. Selective infusions of vasodilators such as papaverine or glucagon have been used. Surgical intervention to remove nonviable intestine is undertaken when the patient is medically stabilized.

Bibliography

Benjamin E, Oropello JM, Iberti TJ. Acute mesenteric ischemia. *Disease-a-Month* 39:131–210, 1993.

Bergan JJ. Visceral ischemic syndromes: Obstruction of the superior mesenteric artery, celiac axis, and inferior mesenteric artery. In Sabiston DC (ed.). *Textbook of Surgery: The Biological Basis of Modern Surgical Practice.* Philadelphia: Saunders, 1991.

Green RM, Ouriel K. Peripheral arterial disease. In Schwartz SI, Shires GT, Spencer FC (eds.). *Principles of Surgery* (6th ed.). New York: McGraw-Hill, 1994.

Hockberger RS, Henneman PL, Boniface K. Disorders of the small intestine. In Rosen P, Barkin RM (eds.). *Emergency Medicine: Concepts and Clinical Practice.* St. Louis: Mosby–Year-Book, 1992.

Moore WM, Hollier LH. Mesenteric artery occlusive disease. *Cardiol Clin* 9:535–541, 1991.

Aortic Dissection

Michael D. Waite

Aortic dissection is the formation of a false lumen in the medial layer of the aortic wall by blood or hematoma. It is the most common aortic disaster, affecting 5 to 10 people per 100,000. This makes aortic dissection 2 to 3 times more common than the rupture of an abdominal aortic aneurysm. Acute aortic dissection carries a mortality of 50% over the first 48 hours. It is 2 to 3 times more common in men, and may occur more frequently in African Americans. The majority of those affected are between the ages of 50 and 70, but it may occur at any age.

I. **Pathophysiology and risk factors.** Medial injury due to accidental or iatrogenic trauma and medial degeneration are the most common etiologies of aortic dissection. Medial degeneration is now thought to be part of the natural aging process that is the result of the pulsatile aortic flow gradually weakening the intimal and medial layers of the aortic wall. This is often associated with aortic dilatation. This process is more advanced in people with **hypertension** in whom the hemodynamic forces are increased, and in those with **connective tissue disorders** such as Marfan's or Ehlers-Danlos syndrome type IV in whom the intimal and medial layers are weaker and less able to withstand the normal hemodynamic forces. Two-thirds of patients with aortic dissection have a history of hypertension, and as many as 75% of patients with Marfan's syndrome will develop aortic dissection. Aortic dissection is also more common in the third trimester of pregnancy, in patients with coarctation of the aorta or bicuspid aortic valves, and in those with aortic stenosis. It is also seen in patients who abuse cocaine, or it may be familial. The etiology is thought to be due to hormonal and hemodynamic changes in pregnant women, hypertension in patients with aortic valvular disease and cocaine abuse, and abnormalities in the procollagen III gene for patients with familial aortic dissection. Patients on steroid immunosuppression, especially those who are post-transplant, are also at risk for aortic dissection.

II. **Anatomy and classification.** Aortic dissection develops as the result of a transverse intimal tear in 95% of patients. Vasa vasorum hemorrhage may be the initiating event in rare instances. The intimal tear is located in the ascending aorta in 65% of patients, in the arch in 10% of patients, and in the upper descending aorta just distal to the left subclavian artery in 20% of patients. The dissection may propagate proximally or distally, and blood flow from the false lumen may reenter the true lumen at any point. The dissection terminates in the left iliac artery in 80% of patients.

Aortic dissection is classified on the basis of anatomy and acuity. In the **Debakey classification,** dissections affecting the ascending, arch, and descending portions of the aorta are type I, those involving only the ascending aorta are type II,

and those involving only the descending aorta are type III.
Type III dissections are classified further with those dissections involving only the supraphrenic aorta being type IIIa, and those extending into the subphrenic aorta being type IIIb (Fig. 38-1). A simplified system is the **Stanford classification** that classifies those dissections affecting the ascending aorta as type A, and those without ascending aortic involvement as type B (see Fig. 38-1). Patients with Marfan's syndrome most commonly suffer type II lesions that are often associated with fusiform aneurysms. The typical patients with type B lesions are older smokers with respiratory disease who have generalized atherosclerotic disease and hypertension.

Aortic dissections are considered to be acute if they have been present for less than 2 weeks. Those dissections of greater than 2 weeks duration are defined as chronic.

III. **Acute thoracic aortic dissection**
   A. **Patient presentation**
      1. **History.** Characteristically, patients will be between 50 and 70 years old, have a history of hypertension, and complain of the acute onset of pain that migrates. Most patients will have a history of one or more risk factors: hypertension, collagen vascular disease, pregnancy, aortic disease, cocaine abuse, strong family history of aortic dissection, recent cardiovascular procedure, or trauma.
         a. **Pain.** About 90% of patients complain of the acute onset of excruciating pain, often characterized as tearing. The pain may be located in the anterior chest with radiation to the neck, jaw, or arms (suggestive of ascending aortic involvement) or in the neck or jaw (suggestive of descending aortic involvement). Abdominal or flank pain mimicking pancreatitis, cholelithiasis, or nephrolithiasis may also occur. The pain may migrate from one area

Fig. 38-1. The Debakey (types I, II, and III) and Stanford (A and B) classifications of aortic dissections based on location of the dissection.

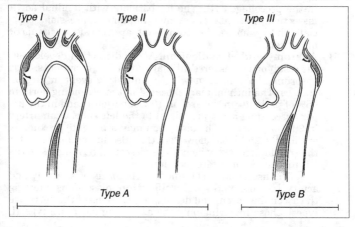

such as the anterior chest to the neck to the interscapular area, which is indicative of dissection originating in the ascending aorta and progressing to the descending aorta. The pain may subside without treatment over time, especially in patients with Marfan's syndrome. In patients taking steroids, aortic dissection may be painless. Additionally, the pain may start after vigorous exercise.

  b. **Vascular compromise and mediastinal compression.** In addition to pain, patients may have symptoms because of impaired flow through aortic branch vessels due to obstruction or compression or due to compression of mediastinal structures by an expanding false lumen. About 30% of patients will experience symptoms of impaired organ perfusion due to branch vessel compression or obstruction (Table 38-1). Additionally compromised blood flow to the kidneys may result in acute renal failure, hematuria, oliguria, and severe refractory hypertension. Symptoms of compromised perfusion may be transient because of reestablishment of flow through false lumen perfusion of the branch vessel or through reentry of the false lumen flow into the true lumen. The mediastinal structures that may be compressed and the symptoms to which they give rise are presented in Table 38-2.

  c. **Rupture.** The dissection may rupture into the heart resulting in an aortocardiac shunt, into the chest resulting in hemothorax, into the pericardium resulting in tamponade, or into the trachea or bronchi resulting in hemoptysis. It may also rupture into the esophagus resulting in hematemesis or melena, or into the abdomen resulting in hemoperitoneum or development of a retroperitoneal hematoma.

2. **Physical examination.** Patients appear uncomfortable and are typically distressed.

  a. **Vital signs.** Tachycardia is usually present, and signs of shock such as oliguria, decreased mental status, and cool diaphoretic skin may be present despite an elevated blood pressure. Blood pressure and pulse measurements should be obtained in all

Table 38-1. Symptoms due to compromised perfusion

Involved arteries	Symptoms	Incidence (%)
Coronary	Myocardial ischemic pain	3.0
Brachiocephalic, common carotid, intercostal, lumbar, or anterior spinal	Syncope, stroke, mental status changes, paraparesis	10.0
Brachiocephalic, subclavian, or iliac	Ischemic changes and pain in limb	13.0
Celiac or mesenteric	Abdominal angina	1.5

Table 38-2.   Symptoms due to compression of mediastinal structures

Involved structure	Symptoms
Recurrent laryngeal nerve	Hoarseness
Superior cervical ganglion	Horner's syndrome
Trachea or bronchi	Dyspnea, stridor
Esophagus	Dysphagia
Superior vena cava (SVC)	SVC syndrome
Cardiac conduction system	AV block

four extremities, and the carotid pulses should be evaluated. Hypertension is usually present. Pulse or blood pressure discrepancies in the upper limbs are present in 50% of patients with proximal dissections. Isolated hypotension may be present in one or more extremities due to arterial compromise. Pseudohypotension (extremity hypotension with adequate central arterial pressure) may be present. True hypotension is an ominous sign suggesting rupture or pericardial tamponade.

   b. Head and neck. The triad of Horner's syndrome—miosis, ptosis, and anhidrosis—may be present. Elevated jugulovenous distention (JVD) may be present and suggests congestive heart failure (CHF) or pericardial tamponade. Diminished carotid pulses or carotid bruits may be appreciated.

   c. Cardiac and pulmonary. Auscultation of the heart may reveal a diastolic murmur characteristic of aortic regurgitation due to aortic valve compromise, or an S_3 due to CHF. In rare instances, a harsh systolic murmur due to aortocardiac shunt may be present. Aortic regurgitation is present in 50% of patients in proximal dissections, and CHF is present in approximately 20% of patients. Signs of pericardial tamponade on examination include a pericardial rub, distant heart sounds, hypotension, pulsus paradoxus, and JVD. Pericardial tamponade is the leading cause of death in aortic dissection and must be recognized immediately. Crackles or rales may be present on auscultation of the chest, which is indicative of CHF. If the dissection has ruptured into the pleural space, decreased breath sounds and dullness on percussion of the chest may be present.

   d. Abdomen. The abdomen may be distended and rigid if intraperitoneal rupture has occurred. Tenderness may be present if mesenteric ischemia has occurred. Rectal examination may reveal blood due to bowel ischemia or rupture of the dissection into the gastrointestinal tract. Poor rectal tone indicates spinal cord ischemia or infarction.

e. **Extremities.** Signs of arterial compromise such as pallor, pulse discrepancies, or pain may be present.

f. **Neurologic.** Decreased mental status, hemiplegia, hemianesthesia, or paraparesis may be present. The eyes may be deviated towards the involved cerebral hemisphere.

B. **Patient assessment**

1. **Laboratory.** Laboratory tests obtained should include a complete blood count with platelet count, prothrombin time, partial thromboplastin time, electrolytes, BUN, creatinine, glucose, lactate, arterial blood gas, cardiac enzymes, liver function tests with amylase and lipase, haptoglobin, type and crossmatch, and urinalysis. Laboratory abnormalities may suggest hemorrhage or hemolysis; cardiac, renal, or mesenteric ischemia; or coagulopathy. Leukocytosis is commonly present.

2. **ECG.** The ECG may show ischemic changes or abnormalities of intracardiac conduction.

3. **Radiographic studies.** Every patient should have a chest x-ray. The choice of further studies will depend on institutional availability and preference as well as patient stability. Many surgeons require an angiogram prior to surgical repair, which necessitates discussing imaging options with the consulting surgeon early in the evaluation.

   a. **Chest x-ray.** From 80% to 90% will be abnormal. Three-fourths will have mediastinal widening. The aortic knob may be indistinct and intimal calcifications displaced inward. The esophagus may be displaced to the right, the left bronchus displaced downward, the right bronchus displaced upward, or there may be a pleural effusion (usually left-sided). The chest x-ray may show signs of aortic dissection when angiography, CT, and MRI are falsely negative.

   b. **Aortic angiography.** Angiography is the test of choice for unstable patients and when branch vessel involvement is a concern. Angiography also demonstrates aortic valve involvement and the extent of the dissection but is invasive and may not be readily available. Evaluation of the coronary arteries may also be performed. Angiography has a sensitivity of 88% and a specificity of 94% for dissection.

   c. **CT.** In most institutions, CT is the primary diagnostic technique, because it is readily available and the time required for the study is short. The diagnosis is confirmed by identification of two lumens separated by an intimal flap. The diagnosis is suggested by displacement of intimal calcifications/lumen compression or widening. CT shows pericardial or pleural effusions and may show a thrombosed false lumen that is not detected on angiography. CT has a sensitivity of 83% to 95% and a specificity of 87% to 100%, and is generally considered to be as accurate as angiography.

   d. MRI. MRI is most useful for chronic dissections or for very stable patients with acute dissections because the required prolonged study time precludes closely monitoring the patient during the study. MRI has a sensitivity and specificity of 100%.

   e. Echocardiography. Both transthoracic and transesophageal echocardiography (TEE) can be useful in the diagnosis of aortic dissection. TEE is easily and rapidly performed at the patient's bedside, and provides the most comprehensive information at a cost comparable to that of CT. However, the availability of a skilled reader is imperative, and distal dissections are not well studied by this method. Presently, the sensitivity of TEE is high (>98%), but specificity is low (68%–77%). The specificity is predicted to improve with the use of multiplanar probes and the development of more stringent diagnostic criteria.

C. Patient management

   1. Supportive care. Airway, breathing, and circulation (ABCs) should be secured as rapidly as possible. Continuous cardiac monitoring is essential. Two large-bore IV lines of isotonic fluid should be administered as needed to support blood pressure. Overhydration should be avoided. Central venous line monitoring should be used during administration of antihypertensive agents. A pulmonary artery catheter monitor is ideal. Pain should be controlled with IV narcotics.

   2. Blood pressure control. The blood pressure should be kept in the range of 100–120 mm Hg systolic, and the heart rate should be kept in the range of 60 to 80 bpm. The goal is to minimize dP/dt, because this is the force that produces propagation and rupture while maintaining adequate cardiac, cerebral, mesenteric, and renal perfusion. This is usually accomplished with use of a **beta-blocking** agent combined with **nitroprusside.** Propranolol is usually administered acutely as IV boluses of 1 mg q5min until the heart rate is between 60 and 70 bpm. Metoprolol as IV boluses of 5–10 mg q6h may be used in patients with bronchospasm or milder hypertension. Contraindications to and side effects of beta-blocking agents include bradycardia, atrioventricular (AV) block, hypotension, and severe bronchospasm. Nitroprusside is initially administered as a continuous IV infusion of 50 mg in 250 ml of a D_5W solution at 0.25–0.50 µg/kg/min. The infusion should be titrated in 0.25–0.50 µg/kg/min increments to obtain the desired blood pressure. Hypotension and headache are the major side effects of nitroprusside. Nitroprusside is contraindicated in patients with hypotension. Please see the chapter on hypertension for further discussion of the management of hypertension.

3. **Definitive therapy.** Surgical consultation should be obtained as soon as possible after diagnosis and classification to facilitate any surgical intervention. Definitive therapy varies with the type of dissection.
   a. **Type A or I and II.** Emergent surgery is indicated.
   b. **Type B or III.** Medical management is indicated unless pain or hypertension are uncontrolled, hemorrhage or arterial compromise is present, or if the dissection involves an aneurysm.

   Operative mortality is 5% to 10%. Five-year survival is approximately 60%. Acute mortality in patients treated medically is approximately 10%.

D. **Patient disposition.** All patients should be admitted to an ICU, either to an internist with surgical consultation, or to a vascular or thoracic surgeon capable of operative intervention.

   In patients who are treated medically or surgically, chronic therapy with a beta-blocking agent is indicated. Those being treated medically require chronic vasodilator therapy as well. Patients will require CTs performed three times/year during the first postdissection year, and then once or twice/year thereafter. About 20% to 40% of late deaths in patients treated both surgically and medically are due to recurrent dissection, rupture, or other complications of dissection.

Bibliography

Cigarroa JE, et al. Diagnostic imaging in the evaluation of suspected aortic dissection. *NEJM* 328:35–43, 1993.

Crawford ES. The diagnosis and management of aortic dissection. *JAMA* 264:2537–2541, 1990.

Rogove HJ, Moore KA. *Critical Care Medicines.* Columbus, OH: Contemporary Critical Care Resources, Inc., 1993.

Svensson LG, Crawford ES. Aortic dissection and aortic aneurysm surgery: clinical observations, experimental investigations, and statistical analyses, part II. *Curr Probl Surg* 29:923–987, 1992.

Treasure T, Raphael MJ. Investigation of suspected dissection of the thoracic aorta. *Lancet* 338:490–495, 1991.

Abdominal Aortic Aneurysm

Stephanie H. Conwell

I. **Epidemiology.** An aneurysm is defined as a focal dilation of the aorta involving an increase in diameter of at least 50%. The mean diameter of the abdominal aorta is 1.9 cm in women and 2.4 cm in men. CT and sonographic studies indicate that an elderly patient's abdominal aorta must exceed 3.0–3.3 cm in diameter to be considered aneurysmally dilated. In patients more than 50 years old, the normal abdominal aorta should not measure more than 2 cm in diameter. During the past 30 years, the age-and-sex-adjusted incidence of abdominal aortic aneurysms (AAAs) has tripled. More aneurysms of all sizes were diagnosed from 1971 through 1980 than in the previous two decades. Several recent studies suggest that the prevalence of AAAs may be more than twice as high as the traditionally reported value of 2% in men over the age of 60. These studies evaluated patients without known aortic disease who were referred for sonography and patients who agreed to undergo screening abdominal sonography. AAAs were detected in 4% of men and women between 65 and 80 years old and 11% of men 60 years or older. The infrarenal region is the most common location of AAAs.

The risk of rupture is significantly increased for aneurysms greater than 5 cm in diameter. AAAs were responsible for 14,982 deaths in the United States in 1988 among people 55 years of age or older. The reported mortality rates for emergency surgery for ruptured AAAs vary from 30% to 63%. The mortality rate for surgical repair of nonleaking AAAs is less than 5%.

See Fig. 39-1 for an illustration of the anatomy of the aorta.

II. **Etiology/Pathogenesis.** Aneurysms of the aorta were first thought to be atherosclerotic in origin. Currently, it is unclear whether atherosclerosis might be an incidental finding in patients with AAA, the consequence of aortic degeneration, or a causative factor of AAA.

Three theories of the etiology of AAAs have emerged: the genetic theory, the proteolytic enzyme theory, and the trace metal theory. The finding that men with a first-degree relative with an AAA experience a ten-fold increased risk of developing an AAA provides a strong argument for a genetic component. It has been reported that the genetic variation on chromosome 16 occurs in patients with AAA. This variation has been related to an increased activity of alpha$_2$ haptoglobin, leading to an acceleration of the hydrolysis of elastin fibers by elastase.

The second theory focuses on structural defects of the aortic wall caused by increased proteolysis. One study shows that there is a greater increase in proteolytic enzyme activity in patients who smoke.

A third theory, the trace metal theory, is based on the observation that in the blotchy mouse, aneurysm formation is related to an X-linked chromosome defect leading to an abnormality in copper metabolism. Copper is thought to play a

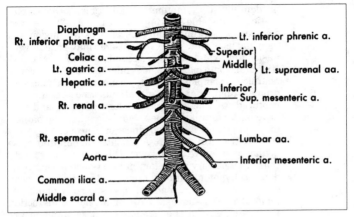

Fig. 39-1. Branches of the aorta. (From Rosen P.
Emergency Medicine: Concepts and Clinical Practice (3rd ed.). St. Louis: Mosby–Year Book, Inc., 1992.)

role in the cross linkages of collagen and elastin, which form
the extracellular matrix of the aortic wall.

Finally, it has been shown that the presence of an inflammatory infiltrate in the aortic wall correlates with aneurysmal enlargement in a rat model.

III. **Risk factors. Male** gender is one of the most important risk
factors for AAA. Hospital admissions for AAA occur three
times more often in men than in women. **Age** is clearly related to the risk of AAA. In men, a ten-fold increase in the incidence of AAA from age 55 to 85 has been reported. It has
also been suggested that **white males** have a higher mortality rate from AAA than nonwhite males. The prevalence of
AAA is higher among patients with **peripheral vascular
disease** than in patients without peripheral vascular disease. It is known also that patients with **hypertension** have
a significantly higher risk of AAA than patients without hypertension. O'Kelley and coworkers have calculated a fourfold risk of AAA for smokers compared to nonsmokers.
Cholesterol is another cardiovascular risk factor believed to
be associated with the occurrence of AAA. Several studies
support a **familial** occurrence of AAA. It is also noteworthy
that patients who do not have atherosclerosis and develop an
AAA have a higher incidence of aortic rupture and a stronger
family history of AAA.

Finally, several other factors have been related to the occurrence of AAA. These factors include body habitus, inguinal
hernia, chronic obstructive pulmonary disease, malignancies,
number of pregnancies, immunologic impairment, alcoholic
pancreatitis, trauma, and infections (mycotic aneurysms).

IV. **Clinical manifestations**
   A. **Presentation**
      1. **History.** Patients with AAA can be classified in one of
         three categories: (1) asymptomatic (diagnosis is made

incidentally), (2) symptomatic and stable, or (3) symptomatic and unstable (leaking or ruptured AAA). The most common presenting symptoms of AAA are abdominal pain and back pain. However, patients may present with misleading symptoms such as flank pain, anorexia, constipation, vomiting, urologic symptoms, lower extremity neurologic complaints, and peripheral ischemic syndromes. More than 90% of patients who present with ruptured AAA have sudden abdominal pain, and 50% have back pain. If the aneurysm is leaking, the patient may complain of lightheadedness or syncope.

2. **Physical examination.** A pulsatile abdominal mass is diagnostic of AAA. However, this finding may be obscured by obesity or abdominal distension. Tachycardia and hypotension may occur if blood loss has been significant. The presence of asymmetrical or absent femoral pulses suggests AAA or an aortic dissection that extends into the abdomen. These findings are rare because most aneurysms do not involve the iliac arteries. AAA should be considered in elderly patients who present with abdominal symptoms or signs (pain, tenderness, or distension) with or without the presence of hypotension.

B. **Assessment.** If a patient's presentation suggests leaking or ruptured AAA, the most important step is immediate surgical intervention. Diagnostic evaluations should be performed while the patient is being prepared for surgery, but surgery should not be delayed on the basis of outstanding diagnostic tests.

1. **Laboratory studies.** Laboratory studies do not directly aid in the diagnosis of AAA. Routine studies such as CBC, electrolytes, BUN, creatine, PT, PTT, and type and cross match are collected in anticipation of surgical intervention. In an acute hemorrhage, the hemoglobin and hematocrit may not be depressed, leading to a false sense of security on the part of the physician. The WBC can be elevated due to demargination, but the differential is usually normal. An ECG should be obtained to rule out the differential diagnosis of myocardial infarction, as well as myocardial ischemia from blood loss.

2. **X-rays, ultrasound, and CT.** Plain radiographs of the abdomen (anteroposterior and lateral views) detected abnormalities in 55% to 85% of patients with AAA in one study. The abnormalities included complete loss of one or both renal outlines (78%), soft tissue mass (67%), calcification of the aneurysm (65%), renal displacement (25%), and properitoneal flank stripe changes (19%). Plain films are unreliable as the sole diagnostic imaging modality for AAA. Ultrasound is currently the best method for diagnosing AAA at the bedside. In the emergency department, the sensitivity of ultrasound approaches 100%. However, the sensitivity of the CT scan is also near 100%, and the CT scan is more accurate than ultrasound in determining aortic diameter and presence of thrombus, defining ex-

tent of aneurysmal dilatation, and demonstrating suprarenal involvement. The advantages of CT over ultrasound include its ability to visualize the retroperitoneum and detect leaking from aneurysm. The CT scan also is not limited by the patient's obesity or the presence of overlying bowel gas, as is the case with ultrasound. The advantages of ultrasound over CT include cost efficiency, shorter study time, and no risk of complications from IV contrast administration. Both angiography and MRI are excellent modalities for imaging the aorta. However, both modalities are currently more costly and time-consuming than CT.

C. **Management.** Management of the suspected AAA in a symptomatic patient who is stable includes fluid resuscitation, surgical consultation, and a definitive diagnostic study (e.g., ultrasound or CT scan). If the patient begins to deteriorate before the diagnosis is confirmed, rapid surgical intervention must take place.

Management of the patient with an unstable presentation includes aggressive crystalloid followed by colloid fluid resuscitation, placement of MAST trousers, and preparation for surgery. At least two large-bore IV lines with isotonic solution should be placed empirically, even in the stable patient. Continuous cardiac monitoring and oxygenation should be initiated.

Surgical consultation should be obtained immediately and not delayed pending a definitive diagnostic test. Ten units of whole blood or packed cells and four units of fresh frozen plasma should be on hand for the unstable patient with suspected AAA.

D. **Patient disposition.** All unstable patients with suspected AAA should be taken immediately to surgery. The disposition of patients who are symptomatic but stable depends on the results of the ultrasound and CT scan. Many patients in this category are admitted to the surgical service and prepared for elective surgery.

Guidelines for the repair of asymptomatic AAAs are as follows: Aneurysms of 4 cm or greater should be repaired as soon as all necessary studies and treatment have been completed, and aneurysms 3–4 cm in size should be monitored closely for growth. Asymptomatic AAAs that cause distal emboli, visceral obstruction, or pain or tenderness or are caused by inflammation also should be repaired as soon as possible.

The surgical treatment of AAA includes immediate vascular control, evacuation of thrombotic material from within the aortic lumen, and placement of a synthetic graft.

Bibliography

Ernest CB. Abdominal aortic aneurysm. *N Engl J Med* 328:1167–1172, 1993.

Hallett JW. Abdominal aortic aneurysm: natural history and treatment. *Heart Dis Stroke* 1:303–308, 1992.

Pleumeekers HJCM, et al. Epidemiology of abdominal aortic aneurysms. *Eur J Vasc Surg* 8:119–128, 1994.

Rosen P, Barkin RM. *Emergency Medicine: Concepts and Clinical Practice.* St. Louis: Mosby–Year Book, 1993:1373–1383.

Siegel CL, Cohan RH. CT of abdominal aortic aneurysms. *Am J Roentgenol* 163:17–29, 1994.

Peripheral Vascular Insufficiency

J. Chadwick Tober

I. **Incidence.** Approximately 10% of the current population of the United States is 65 years of age or older, and it is estimated that this percentage will double soon after the year 2000. Present studies estimate a peripheral vascular insufficiency prevalence of 17% in populations aged 55 to 74 years of age. With an increasingly aging population, the incidence of vascular insufficiency will likely increase.

II. **Etiology.** Atherosclerosis, estimated to be the cause of vascular insufficiency in 90%–95% of cases, affects 1½ to 2 times as many men as women. It is linked to genetic and lifestyle factors. Hereditary factors such as diabetes mellitus, hyperlipidemia, hypercholesterolemia, hypertension, and hypercoagulable states, as well as lifestyle factors such as tobacco use, obesity, and sedentary lifestyle are associated with atherosclerosis. The majority of individuals present with symptomatic vascular insufficiency during and after the fifth decade of life. There is evidence that the atherosclerotic process is particularly aggressive in individuals diagnosed in the third and fourth decades of life.

   A. **Atherosclerosis.** The overwhelming cause of arterial insufficiency is atherosclerosis obliterans. Fatty deposits within the arterial wall are associated with inflammation and cytokine release, resulting in progressive medial and intimal proliferation. Areas of flow separation and dynamic wall shear changes, such as at arterial bifurcations, are particularly prone to these local dynamics. Hence atherosclerotic narrowing is often observed at the carotid, aortic, common femoral, and tibial bifurcations. When the arterial stenosis progresses beyond 75% of the vessel cross-sectional diameter, the reduction in flow and distal perfusion pressure becomes critical. Ischemia results when distal perfusion is insufficient to meet metabolic demands. **Claudication** results when exercising muscle groups become ischemic. **Rest pain** develops when distal peripheral nerves are hypoperfused. **Gangrene** develops when perfusion is impaired to the point of cellular death. In general, acute disruption of arterial perfusion is more poorly tolerated than gradual chronic ischemia. Other causes of vascular insufficiency are distal embolism, thrombosis of critical artery stenosis, trauma, vasculitis, and hypercoagulable conditions.

   B. **Embolism.** In contrast to chronic arterial insufficiency caused by progressive atherosclerotic narrowing, emboli generally present with severe extremity ischemia because collateral flow is poorly developed. Microthrombotic emboli or cholesterol embolization results in well-circumscribed infarction of the skin of the toes and feet despite strong proximal pulses. Emboli arise from the heart in 85% of patients. Another source of emboli is an atheromata-laden

581

arch and descending aorta or a mural thrombus layered in a descending abdominal aortic aneurysm. Paradoxic emboli arise from deep vein thrombi and embolize via cardiac septal defects such as a patent foramen ovale. True cryptogenic emboli for which no source can be identified are rare, since the use of transesophageal echocardiography is attributing an increasing number of these emboli to cardiac or aortic sources.

C. **Thrombosis.** In contrast to embolism, arterial thrombosis occurs primarily in chronically stenosed atherosclerotic arteries. Patients may present with a lesser degree of ischemia because collateral vessel flow has been recruited over time. Arterial trauma by missile penetration, blast effect, or crush injury may result in thrombosis because of intimal devitalization, intimal flaps, or stasis. Spontaneous arterial thrombosis is rare but can be found in hypercoagulable states such as antithrombin III deficiency, sensitivity to phospholipid antibody, primary vasculitis or vasculitis associated with connective tissue disorders, and paraneoplastic processes such as Trousseau's syndrome associated with ovarian, pancreatic, and pulmonary cancer.

III. **Acute peripheral vascular insufficiency**

A. **Patient presentation.** A thorough history and physical examination are the most important means of assessing a patient with suspected vascular insufficiency. Doppler studies, duplex imaging, a CT or magnetic resonance imaging/magnetic resonance angioplasty (MRI/MRA) scan, and angiography should be viewed as adjuncts in planning therapy subsequent to a well-performed history and physical examination.

1. **History of present illness**

a. **General.** In obtaining a history, one must ascertain the nature of the patient's pain, its duration, what exacerbates it, and whether there is a prior history of similar pain either in the affected or contralateral extremity. A contralateral extremity with similar or less intense symptoms is a good measure of the generalized disease process. A history of prior trauma or revascularization should be sought. Vasospastic disorders are suggested by pain or cyanosis of the digits in response to cold stimuli. New-onset severe chest pain radiating to the back or into the abdomen and accompanied by lower extremity ischemic complaints suggests arterial occlusion secondary to aortic dissection.

b. **Specific.** Patients with extremity arterial insufficiency will usually present with claudication, rest pain, pending tissue loss, or gangrene. **Intermittent claudication** is described as an aching or sharp pain in an exercised muscle group, usually the calf muscles. It is consistently instigated by the same degree of exercise, such as a distance walked, and is relieved by a rest of 5 or 10 minutes. Easy fatigability in an extremity may also be considered a sign of claudication. **Rest pain** occurs typically in the early morning hours and is described as an aching or sharp pain. Typical rest pain occurs at the distal forefoot at the level of the metatarsal heads, and is partially relieved by placing the foot in a dependent position. Walking often helps rest pain in its early stages, but severe constant pain at rest that is not improved by dependency, is an ominous warning of **impending tissue loss.** When extremity ischemia is severe enough to threaten the viability of the extremity, patients describe pain progressing to paresthesia and eventually paralysis (Table 40-1). A patient with the "five P's" is in danger of suffering limb loss. Irreversible muscle and nerve damage occurs 4 to 6 hours after onset of severe ischemia, although significant functional impairment has been documented with as little as 2 hours of severe ischemia. Rapid assessment and treatment of a patient with a cyanotic limb are essential to prevent these disastrous sequalae.

2. **Past medical history.** Details of **comorbidities** such as hypertension, coronary artery disease, cardiac arrhythmias, renal insufficiency, diabetes mellitus, blood dyscrasias, stroke, and connective tissue disorders should be sought. The amount and duration of tobacco abuse as well as whether there is a past history of illicit drug abuse also should be delineated. Because of the hereditary factors of atherosclerosis, a family history of similar symptoms or of "hardening of the arteries" is significant. The details of any premature deaths of family members should be elucidated.

A complete list of current **medications** should be made. Patients taking pentoxifylline or coumarin may have had a prior history of arterial insufficiency or thrombotic episodes. Patients taking immunosuppressive medications after organ transplantation may have an accelerated atherosclerotic process. Patients taking ergot alkaloids for migraine headaches may present with acute peripheral vascular insufficiency without a past history of insufficiency. Oral steroid compounds may have been prescribed to treat symptoms of vasculitis or connective tissue disorders. Vasodilatory medications such as nifedipine being taken

**Table 40-1. Signs and symptoms
of acute arterial occlusion: the five Ps**

Pain—may be the first sign

Pallor

Pulselessness

Parasthesias—severe progression of ischemia

Paralysis—usually late and ominous in ischemia
    (Poikilothermy)—assess in the context of the patient's
    syptoms

without a history of hypertension suggest treatment for vasospastic disorders. Oral contraceptive medications and estrogen replacement therapy are associated with spontaneous thrombosis in patients with hypercoagulable tendencies.

3. **Physical examination**
   a. **Extremity examination.** A diagnosis of **acute ischemia** is suggested not only by the history of sudden onset of extremity pain, but also by physical examination. An acutely ischemic limb will appear initially pale and gradually develop patchy violaceous discoloration that coalesces into generalized cyanosis as the ischemic insult continues. In cases of acute ischemia in previously unaffected extremities, the limb will appear developmentally normal except for this discoloration. The extremity will be anesthetic, and motor function will be decreased or absent. In advanced cases, thrombosis of the cutaneous venules may be observed, and prolonged infarction results in blister formation, epidermal sloughing, and possibly wet gangrene changes. The level of arterial occlusion is generally one arterial bifurcation or joint space level higher than the observed level of demarcation.

   Chronic ischemia is suggested by the prolonged presence of symptoms with mild or moderate progressive functional impairment of claudication or rest pain. The affected limb will demonstrate coolness, atrophy of the interosseous muscles of the hand or foot, thinning of the skin and subcuticular fat, alopecia, and brittle nails. Severe chronic ischemia is demonstrated by petechiae over the dorsum of the foot, well-circumscribed ulceration, or digit infarction. The symptoms of acute ischemia may be superimposed upon chronic ischemia. It is for this reason that a comparison of the contralateral extremity with the symptomatic extremity should be made.

   b. **Pulse examination.** A complete pulse examination is mandatory. The carotid, brachial, radial, ulnar, femoral, popliteal, posterior tibial, and dorsalis pedis pulses should be examined bilaterally and any change with position noted. The symmetry and strength of the pulses should be recorded: **normal** pulses are **+2, diminished** pulses are **+1, barely palpable** pulses are **trace,** and **absent** pulses are **0.** Very prominent pulses, particularly if unilateral or if found in the abdomen or in the popliteal fossa, should raise one's suspicion of aneurysmal disease. Diminished pulses in the contralateral asymptomatic extremity suggest a generalized disease process. Auscultation of bruits, particularly in the neck and epigastric regions, should be noted. A careful cardiac examination should note the presence of murmurs and heartbeat irregularity.

    c. **Doppler examination.** The use of a hand-held Doppler device augments the physical examination in that **ankle brachial indices** may be calculated and arterial flow may be confirmed if pulses are nonpalpable. Arterial flow at the ankle is occluded using a sphygmomanometer cuff, and resumption of arterial flow is listened for using the Doppler device as the cuff is deflated. The pressure at which flow resumes is noted, and the process is repeated in the arm. The ankle brachial index (ABI) is calculated by dividing the ankle pressure by the brachial pressure. The ABI correlates to the degree of arterial compromise (Fig. 40-1). Severely calcified vessels as in diabetes will falsely elevate the ABI because of noncompressibility of the vessel. The character of the Doppler signal, whether triphasic, biphasic, or monophasic, should be noted.

B. Patient assessment. The decision to pursue further diagnostic testing or begin management depends on the severity and duration of symptoms. Immediate consultation with a vascular surgeon should be sought in all cases of acute extremity ischemia. Time is of the essence, and tissue destruction will be minimized by a coordinated approach to diagnosis and management. Patients presenting

Fig. 40-1. Ankle brachial indices and symptoms.
(Modified from Yoa JST. Hemodynamic studies
in peripheral arterial disease. *Br J Surg* 57:761, 1970.)

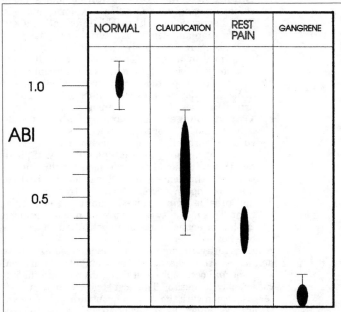

with chronic ischemia and without pending tissue loss may undergo a more complete workup prior to vascular consultation. Acquisition of the patient's past medical records will facilitate, but should not delay, workup and management.

1. **Laboratory studies.** Laboratory studies for all patients include tests for blood glucose, BUN/creatinine, CBC, and PT/PTT. In cases of recurrent thrombosis, vascular graft failure, or thrombosis in an otherwise healthy individual, a hypercoagulability profile for heparin antiplatelet antibody, protein C, and protein S levels, antithrombin III levels, and sensitivity to antiphospholipid antibody and anticardiolipid antibody should be obtained. An extra blood specimen should be obtained for possible typing and cross-matching of blood. An ECG should be obtained in all patients to ascertain the cardiac rhythm and look for evidence of prior myocardial infarction.

2. **Specialized vascular studies**
   a. **Segmental limb pressures/pulse volume recordings (SLPs/PVRs)** are performed in the vascular laboratory and are appropriate diagnostic studies in the workup of patients with stable ischemia when tissue loss is not imminent. These studies should include postexercise pressures in patients presenting with intermittent claudication. With this information the practitioner may more precisely define the level and degree of arterial stenosis.
   b. **Duplex arterial examination** combines ultrasound imaging with Doppler waveform analysis. This diagnostic modality yields information about the location and degree of arterial or bypass graft stenosis more accurately than SLPs/PVRs when performed by an experienced technician. It is the diagnostic modality of choice when screening patients with suspected carotid artery stenosis, and is useful in determining the caliber of the popliteal artery in cases of suspected aneurysm.
   c. **Transesophageal echocardiography** is the diagnostic modality of choice, since it is over 95% accurate if aortic dissection is suspected as the cause for acute extremity arterial insufficiency. If possible, this test should be performed for this indication in the emergency department (ED) to minimize delay, decrease patient transportation, and provide uninterrupted monitoring of the patient. This modality is also useful in determining a cardiac or aortic source of embolization on an elective basis.

3. **Angiography.** Angiography of the affected extremity delineates the character and extent of arterial stenoses and occlusions and is required before the initiation of lytic therapy. This test should be obtained after discussion with the vascular consultant. In cases of severe ischemia, the delay occurring while the an-

giogram is scheduled and performed may result in tissue loss.

C. Patient management

1. **Severe ischemia with impending tissue loss.** Whether caused by embolization or spontaneous thrombosis, treatment must be timely and involve early vascular consultation. Decisions about whether to anticoagulate and pursue further diagnostic testing or transport the patient to the operating suite depend on the extent and degree of ischemia and the anticipated delay before definitive therapy may be rendered.

   a. **Anticoagulation.** Heparin should be administered if evaluation by a vascular consultant is not readily available or if the patient must be transported to another facility for care. Anticoagulation should be considered if a substantial amount of the extremity is ischemic, particularly if there has been a delay in the arrival of the patient to the ED. Heparinization will prevent the administration of spinal or epidural anesthetic and hence should not be administered if the patient is to be transferred **immediately** to the surgical suite. Heparin should not be administered to patients with arterial insufficiency secondary to trauma. A relative contraindication exists for patients with a known history of GI bleeding or remote history of intracerebral hemorrhage. Patients with known heparin-induced thrombocytopenia should not routinely be administered heparin. Dosage is 5000 U IV followed by continuous IV infusion of 1000 U/hr to titrate the PTT between 60 and 80 seconds.

   b. **Antibiotic therapy.** Antibiotic therapy is recommended in cases of epidermal breakdown in ischemic extremities. For clean wounds, cephalexin 1 g IV q6h or ampicillin/sulbactam 1.5 g IV q8h is adequate initial therapy. In cases of sensitivity to cephalosporins, clindamycin 900 mg IV q8h or a single dose of vancomycin 1 g IV may be given. In cases of soiled wounds or wounds with necrotic tissue, the addition of an aminoglycoside is appropriate.

   c. **Lytic therapy.** In general, lysis of the thrombus or embolus is contraindicated in patients with severe, threatened tissue loss. This caveat may be modified by a vascular consultant for patients in whom no suitable surgical alternative exists.

   d. **Analgesia.** Adequate analgesia should be administered after the neurosensory examination has been documented. Narcotic analgesic levels should be titrated to allow serial examinations to be performed.

   e. **Definitive therapy.** Definitive therapy requires restoration of arterial flow either through extraction of the occluding thrombus or embolus or through bypass around the occluded segment of artery.

2. **Severe ischemia without impending tissue loss.**
   These patients require workup in the ED with the goal
   of establishing the cause of arterial insufficiency and if
   necessary admission for definitive therapy. Because
   these patients present with rest pain, a decision must
   be rendered as to whether tissue loss is probable before
   the patient can be followed up as an outpatient.
   ABIs and SLPs/PVSs are necessary, and in cases of
   rapid onset of rest pain, an angiogram may be requested
   while the patient is still in the ED with the expectation
   that the patient will be admitted for care as
   an inpatient. Early discusion with a vascular consultant
   will expedite care.

   a. **Anticoagulation.** In general, patients should not
      be anticoagulated routinely when presenting with
      this complaint. This recommendation should be
      modified when the rest pain is of rapid onset or the
      patient's workup, including angiogram, is for some
      reason to be delayed. Patients in whom a hypercoagulable
      state is known and in whom the coumarin
      dose is subtherapeutic should be heparinized.

   b. **Antibiotic therapy.** Patients with extremity cellulitis,
      necrotic tissue, or an elevated white cell
      count with or without an elevated blood glucose level
      require IV antibiotic coverage. Coverage should
      be broad-spectrum and may include ampicillin/
      sulbactam and an aminoglycoside, clindamycin and
      an aminoglycoside, or ciprofloxacin and an aminoglycoside.

   c. **Lytic therapy.** Catheter-directed lysis of an embolism
      or thrombus may be considered in cases of
      severe ischemia as long as no tissue loss is imminent.
      Systemically administered lytic agents have
      no role in clearing peripheral arterial thrombus.
      Lysis is an acceptable means of salvaging a thrombosed
      vascular bypass graft prior to surgical revision
      provided the thrombosis occurred within 3
      weeks of the patient's presentation. Patients in
      whom lytic therapy is planned should have a fibrinogen
      level added to their initial blood work.
      Urokinase is associated with a lower incidence of
      hemorrhage than either streptokinase or tissue
      plasminogen activator (t-PA). Heparinization
      should be delayed until an angiogram is obtained
      and the lytic agent is started. Arrangements must
      be made with vascular and radiologic consultants
      for this therapy, which commonly requires 24–48
      hours for completion.

   d. **Analgesia.** Analgesia should be titrated to the
      severity of the patient's symptoms. Oral analgesics
      should be avoided until the disposition of the patient
      is known because of the potential for aspiration
      during anesthetic induction.

   e. **Definitive therapy.** The majority of patients with
      severe rest pain will be admitted for complete di-

agnostic workup and therapy. Because most patients with this condition have multilevel arterial stenosis, and hence will require revascularization, vascular consultation is required to direct this workup once admission is arranged. Patients receiving intraarterial lytic therapy require admission to a monitored unit, often an intensive care unit.

3. **Mild to moderate ischemia without impending tissue loss.** Patients with mild to moderate arterial insufficiency will present with claudication or mild rest pain occurring briefly in the early mornings. Since these patients are generally not in danger of immediate tissue loss, hospitalization is uncommon. The degree of ischemia should be carefully documented before a discharge from the ED is made. Consultation with a vascular specialist is suggested to ensure that the patient receives appropriate therapy after discharge.

a. **Anticoagulation.** Patients presenting with mild to moderate arterial insufficiency do not require anticoagulation unless they are already taking coumarin. If the patient is chronically anticoagulated, one should obtain a prothrombin time (PT) to ensure that the dose is therapeutic. Coumarin dosage may be adjusted on an outpatient basis provided the PT is not excessive. There is no role for starting coumarin in the ED. Heparinization is required to counteract the procoagulant effect of coumarin, which decreases the vitamin K–dependent factors, protein C and protein S.

b. **Analgesia.** Pentoxifylline 400 mg tid PO may be started at this time. The patient should be advised that some improvement in ambulatory distance may be had with this medication. Since GI upset is common, this medication should be taken with food. Additionally, the patient should be advised to observe for the side effects of bruising, flushing, and mild dizziness. A mild, nonnarcotic analgesic should be recommended at this time.

c. **Definitive therapy.** Patients with ABIs over 0.5 usually rehabilitate without a revascularization procedure provided that tobacco use is ceased completely. An exercise program emphasizing progressive endurance training is also a key therapy for these patients. Treatment should be directed on an outpatient basis. Nonoperative therapy is the usual recommendation for patients with mild to moderate symptoms of vascular insufficiency. Angiography may be planned to determine whether angioplasty or other minimally invasive procedures should be included. As difficult as it may seem to the patient, cessation of smoking is mandatory. Referral to a physician accustomed to treating such patients is suggested.

Bibliography

Ey FS. Hypercoagulability in vascular surgery patients. In Porter JM, Taylor LM (eds.), *Basic Data Underlying Clinical Decision Making in Vascular Surgery*. New York: Quality Medical Publishing, 1994.

Fowkes F, Housley E, Prescott R. Edinburgh artery study: prevalence of asymptomatic and symptomatic peripheral arterial disease in the general population. *Int J Epidemiol* 20:384, 1991.

Gardner AW, Poehlman ET. Exercise rehabilitation programs for the treatment of claudication pain. *JAMA* 274:975, 1995.

Ouriel K, Camerota AJ. Thrombolytic therapy in the management of peripheral arterial occlusion. In Ouriel K (ed.), *Lower Extremity Vascular Disease*. St. Louis: Saunders, 1995.

Rutherford RB (ed.). *Vascular Surgery*. St. Louis: Saunders, 1995.

Vogt M, Wolfson S, Kuller L. Lower extremity arterial disease and the aging process: a review. *J Clin Epidemiol* 45:529, 1992.

Hemodynamic Alterations

VII

Hemodynamic Alterations

41

Hemorrhagic Shock

Charles Little

Hemorrhagic shock is a serious clinical entity requiring rapid treatment to avoid complications such as multiple system organ failure or death. Although there are multiple etiologies of hemorrhagic shock, the end result is the same. Decreased cardiac output secondary to hemorrhage causes decreased blood pressure, tissue hypoperfusion and hypoxia, lactic acidosis, and multisystem failure with subsequent death.

I. **Pathophysiology.** Shock is a state of inadequate tissue perfusion. In hemorrhagic shock inadequate circulating blood volume is present to meet cellular needs, particularly for oxygen. As cellular hypoxia occurs, conversion to anaerobic metabolism begins and lactic acid is produced. The production of lactate frees up hydrogen ions from NADH and $NADPH_2$ allowing further anaerobic metabolism but causing progressive metabolic acidosis. With prolonged shock, accumulation of waste products occurs and a progressive oxygen debt ensues. Neutrophil activation and release of inflammatory mediators may cause widespread tissue damage leading to multiple system organ damage. Eventually, without treatment, waste products accumulate to the point that autoregulation of tissue blood flow fails. When this happens arteriolar smooth muscle vascular tone is lost and precapillary sphincters open. This leads to widespread capillary pooling of blood volume and capillary sludging. Eventually, clinically "irreversible shock" occurs when tissue damage becomes so great it cannot be reversed.

II. **Differential diagnosis of shock states.** Conceptually, shock can be thought of in three broad categories.

1. Hypovolemic with inadequate circulating blood volume. Hemorrhagic shock is a form of hypovolemic shock.
2. Cardiogenic with impairment of cardiac function or venous return to the heart.
3. Distributive with loss of control of arteriolar tone and precapillary sphincter function.

It is important to recognize that these categories of shock may overlap. For example, an elderly patient with heart disease and the onset of gastrointestinal bleeding may have components of both cardiogenic and hypovolemic shock.

III. **Clinical hemorrhagic shock**
   A. **Presentation**
      1. **History.** Patient history may indicate obvious causes of shock such as trauma. Extensive questioning may be required with occult cases of blood loss such as gastrointestinal bleeding or ruptured ectopic pregnancy. There are numerous causes of hemorrhagic shock, but the common pathway is the loss of blood from the cardiovascular system.
      2. **Physical examination.** With the onset of uncontrolled blood loss, many compensatory mechanisms

are activated. Initially, CNS response and vasopressin (antidiuretic hormone) secretion causes decreases in urinary output and compensatory thirst. Intrathoracic constriction of venous capacitance vessels shunts blood into circulation. With any decrease in capillary hydrostatic pressure, transcapillary fluid shifts occur from interstitial fluid into the capillary bed. Physical findings vary depending on the degree of blood loss, as illustrated below.

a. **Mild to moderate shock (classes I and II).** With continued volume loss, the sympathetic nervous system is activated, which leads to most of the objective signs of hemorrhagic shock. A progressive **tachycardia** occurs depending on the severity of the volume loss. Vasoconstriction shunts blood to vital organs and away from skeletal muscle and skin resulting in **pale cool skin,** especially in the extremities. The diastolic blood pressure initially increases, reflecting increased arteriolar tone and resulting in a **decreased pulse pressure** (the difference between the systolic and diastolic blood pressure). Sympathetic activation of the CNS leads to **restlessness** or agitation. Activation of the sweat glands leads to moist "clammy" skin.

b. **Severe shock (classes III and IV).** As volume loss continues, compensatory mechanisms begin to fail and the systolic and mean arterial **blood pressures fall.** Confusion progressing to coma occurs as cerebral perfusion declines. Maximal **tachycardia** with heart rates of greater than 140 bpm occurs followed by bradycardia as a preterminal event.

The amount of blood loss and degree of shock can be roughly estimated based on physical examination (Table 41-1). It is important to note that this exact presentation will not occur in all patients. The elderly and the very young may progress to significant degrees of shock with little compensatory changes. In addition, medications such as beta-blockers and preexisting medical problems may prevent reflex tachycardia or other signs of shock.

B. **Assessment.** The general degree of acute blood loss can be estimated by physical examination (see Table 41-1). Blood pressure, heart rate, and urine output should be closely monitored. In complicated cases, invasive monitoring with central venous lines or a pulmonary artery catheter may be needed (see Chap. 5).

1. **Laboratory studies.** Laboratory studies may not initially reflect the degree of blood loss. The **hemoglobin** and **hematocrit** will not fall with acute hemorrhage until significant transcapillary fluid shifts occur. This usually requires 1 to 2 hours to become apparent and 24 to 36 hours to equilibrate. The hematocrit will fall as crystalloid fluid administration occurs. **Arterial blood gases** and **serum lactate** levels help assess

Table 41-1. Estimated fluid and blood losses based on patient's initial presentation (for a 70-kg male)

| | Hemorrhage class | | | |
	Class I	Class II	Class III	Class IV
Blood loss (ml)	<750	750–1500	1,500–2,000	>2,000
Blood loss (% blood volume)	<15	15–30	30–40	>40
Pulse rate	<100	>100	>120	>140
BP (mm Hg)	Normal	Normal	Decreased	Decreased
Capillary refill	Normal	Decreased	Decreased	Decreased
Respiratory rate	14–20	20–30	30–40	>35
Urine output (ml/hr)	>30	20–30	5–15	0
Mental status	Slightly anxious	Mildly anxious	Anxious and confused	Confused and lethargic
Fluid replacement (crystalloid to blood in a ratio of 3:1)	Crystalloid	Crystalloid	Crystalloid + blood	Crystalloid + blood

Source: ACS Committee on Trauma, *Advanced Trauma Life Support® Student Manual* [1993 edition]. Chicago: American College of Surgeons, 1993.

the degree of acidosis present and guide oxygen and ventilatory support. A persistently elevated lactate level reflects continued tissue hypoperfusion. The platelet count, prothrombin, and partial thromboplastin times should be followed to allow replacement therapy if a coagulopathy develops. Female patients should have pregnancy tests.

Further assessment according to the cause of hemorrhage is indicated. See specific shock states below.

2. **ECG.** The ECG is not diagnostic for hemorrhagic shock, but ECG changes consistent with ischemia can be seen, especially in patients with underlying coronary disease who are stressed by the hyperdynamic shock state.

C. **Management**
   1. **Supportive care.** Assessment of the airway and breathing is critical. Endotracheal intubation of patients unable to protect their airway or ventilate adequately is indicated. Supplemental high-flow oxygen by mask is indicated in all patients in shock. External bleeding sites require control with direct pressure. Patients should be placed on a continuous cardiac monitor, and frequent vital signs should be performed. Blood for laboratory analysis and blood **typing and crossmatching** should be obtained with vascular access. In addition, placement of a Foley catheter to monitor urine output and a nasogastric (NG) tube to decompress the stomach and prevent aspiration is helpful.
   2. **Intravenous fluid therapy.** Vascular access should be obtained with a minimal of two large-bore peripheral IV catheters, 14–16 gauge. If peripheral IV access fails, cutdowns or placement of a large-bore pulmonary artery introducer catheter is indicated. Routine central venous catheters are unsuitable because their length severely limits flow rates.

      An initial fluid bolus of 1 to 2 liters of normal saline or lactated Ringer's solution should be rapidly administered (20 ml/kg in children). If the patient does not improve or if the patient is in obvious class III or IV hemorrhagic shock, 1–2 units of packed **red cells** or whole blood (10 ml/kg in children) should be administered. Crystalloid and blood should continue to be administered in roughly a 3:1 ratio of crystalloid to blood until the patient's vital signs normalize and urine output improves. This 3:1 ratio is necessary to replace transcapillary fluid shifts and to allow obligatory cellular and interstitial fluid accumulation to occur. Critically ill patients should be given Type O Rh-negative blood on arrival. More stable patients can wait for type-specific blood (10- to 20-minute availability) or crossmatched blood (30- to 60-minute availability).

      Controversy has persisted for years about the use of **colloids** (albumin, dextran, and hydroxyethylstarch) in resuscitation. Studies suggest that colloids may be detrimental in traumatic hypovolemic shock but are beneficial in other forms of hemorrhagic shock. Because of their cost and potential for side effects, colloids generally should be withheld unless specifically indicated.

If signs of tissue hypoperfusion persist (hypotension, persistent lactic acidosis, poor urine output, cerebral or myocardial dysfunction) invasive monitoring with a pulmonary artery catheter and arterial pressure catheter is indicated. Volume loading to a pulmonary capillary wedge pressure (PCWP) of 16 with a hematocrit greater than 30% should be performed. Measurement of cardiac index and calculation of systemic vascular resistance should be done to guide appropriate vasopressor therapy.

3. **Treatment of complications.** Coagulopathies from trauma, hypothermia, and dilution should be corrected according to laboratory values. Metabolic acidosis with pH less than 7.20 should be corrected with sodium bicarbonate.

   After severe or prolonged shock, widespread tissue injury and inflammation may occur causing organ system failures. Renal damage may lead to **acute tubular necrosis** and renal failure. This requires optimization of fluid volume. A trial of furosemide diuresis and low-dose dopamine may convert oliguric renal failure to nonoliguric failure. Dialysis may be needed.

   Pulmonary injury may lead to **adult respiratory distress syndrome (ARDS).** Supplemental oxygen and often prolonged mechanical ventilation may be needed.

   Immunologic function is depressed following shock. Heightened awareness and early response to fever and leukocytosis with cultures and broad-spectrum antibiotics is warranted.

D. **Patient disposition.** Patients with true hemorrhagic shock are rarely discharged from the hospital. An exception might be a healthy patient who lacerated a superficial artery that is easily treated with suturing and 1 to 2 liters of crystalloid.

   Patients who have a correctable bleeding site (e.g., splenic injury or ectopic pregnancy) are managed with surgery and, if uncomplicated, may be managed in a non-ICU setting.

   Patients with significant or prolonged shock, serious underlying medical problems, or continued bleeding should be managed in an ICU.

IV. **Management of specific causes of shock**
   A. **Traumatic shock**
      1. **Presentation.** The mechanism of injury is usually obvious, but patients can appear initially quite stable with significant underlying injury.
      2. **Assessment and management.** Rapid assessment and stabilization are performed the same as in the general management of hemorrhagic shock. General surgery should be consulted early in significantly injured patients. Specific diagnostic tests depend on the mechanism and area of injury.

It should be ensured that there is no cause of shock in addition to hemorrhage such as tension pneumothorax, pericardial tamponade, or neurogenic shock from spinal cord injury.

Rapidly developing hemorrhagic shock in trauma almost always indicates a major chest, abdominal, or pelvic injury. Head injury alone does **not** cause shock.

In the setting of blunt trauma, the cervical spine and long bone fractures should be stabilized.

B. Gastrointestinal bleeding

1. **Presentation.** Patients with GI bleeding may present with dizziness, weakness, syncope, or other vague complaints. Generally, with significant acute blood loss hematemesis or hematochezia is present. With chronic blood loss, coffee ground emesis or tarry stools may be reported.

2. **Assessment and management.** Initial assessment and stabilization should be performed as described in sec. **III.B.** A rectal exam to check for blood and nasogastric tube placement are required.

   a. **Upper GI (UGI) bleeding.** Bleeding from the nasogastric tube generally indicates a bleeding source proximal to the ligament of Trietz. Conversely, lack of blood from the NG tube could occur with duodenal bleeding without reflux into the stomach. In clinical practice, if UGI bleeding is fast enough to cause shock, a lack of bloody NG output is unlikely. In UGI bleeding, NG lavage until the lavage fluid clears may slow bleeding, and is necessary to permit endoscopy to reveal and potentially cauterize the bleeding site. Lavage through a large orogastric tube may be required to remove blood clots.

   b. **Lower GI (LGI) bleeding.** With rapid bleeding at rates above 1 ml/min, angiography may be used to reveal and possibly embolize the bleeding site. At slower rates, radionuclide scans may reveal the source of bleeding. In stable patients, colonoscopy may reveal the source of bleeding.

      If the patient is easily stabilized, further workup and treatment can be done medically. If the patient is unstable or if there is rapid persistent bleeding, emergent surgery may be needed.

C. Ruptured ectopic pregnancy

1. **Presentation.** Bleeding from a ruptured ectopic pregnancy may present as syncope or vague abdominal complaints. Generally, with bleeding that is sufficient to cause shock, abdominal pain and tenderness are present. The combination of vaginal bleeding with abdominal pain in the setting of pregnancy suggests ectopic pregnancy. All females of child-bearing potential with abdominal pain or vaginal bleeding should have pregnancy testing performed.

2. **Assessment and management.** Initial assessment and resuscitation should be performed as in the therapy of general hemorrhage (see sec. **III.B.**). A pelvic

examination should be done to check for bleeding and adnexal masses or tenderness. Abdominal or transvaginal ultrasound will rapidly allow assessment of adnexal masses and reveal free intraperitoneal blood. Culdocentesis may be used to check for intraperitoneal blood if ultrasound is unavailable. Immediate consultation with gynecology or general surgery will hasten operative management. In a patient with shock from a ruptured ectopic pregnancy, operative intervention with laparoscopy or laparotomy is indicated.

Bibliography

ACS Committee on Trauma. *Advanced Trauma Life Support Student Manual.* (1993 Ed.) Chicago: American College of Surgeons, 1993.
Geller ER. *Shock and Resuscitation.* New York: McGraw-Hill, 1993.

Septic Shock

Philliph I. Bialecki and Karla R. Haversperger

Septic shock is the leading cause of death among ICU patients, with a mortality rate approaching 60%. The continuum of disease pathology that begins with sepsis provides many early clues that may allow prompt recognition and treatment of the underlying septic condition before the development of frank septic shock. Prompt recognition and early institution of monitoring and therapies is crucial to reduce mortality and morbidity from septic shock. The incidence of sepsis is approximately 400,000 cases annually in the United States, with 50% of those going on to develop septic shock. Sepsis is the thirteenth leading cause of death overall and accounts for 5 to 10 billion dollars in health care costs per year.

I. **Definition.** There is now a consensus on the terminology used to define sepsis. Sepsis is the systemic response to infection with two or more of the following: temperature greater than 38°C or less than 36°C, tachycardia, tachypnea, WBC count over 12,000/mm^3 or under 4,000/mm^3, or greater than 10% band forms. Severe sepsis occurs with organ dysfunction, hypoperfusion (e.g., lactic acidosis, oliguria, altered mental status), or hypotension (systolic BP greater than 90 mm Hg or a reduction of 40 mm Hg from baseline). Septic shock is sepsis-induced hypotension despite adequate fluid resuscitation along with organ perfusion abnormalities.

II. **Pathophysiology.** Sepsis begins with a nidus of infection. The most common source is gram-negative bacteremia from a urinary source, accounting for 34% of all cases. Peritonitis or an abscess in the GI tract (14%), pneumonia (9%), and skin or soft tissue (7%) are all sources; no source is found in 36% of the cases. Organisms vary depending on age, source of infection, and immune status of the patient (Table 42-1). Approximately 60% of all cases arise from gram-negative bacteria, 35% from gram-positive bacteria, and 5% from fungi and other etiologies. Identifying the source helps in directing antimicrobial therapy.

A common pathway in the pathogenesis of septic shock, no matter what the source, has been elucidated. Release of endogenous mediators from mononuclear phagocytes and other cells, including endothelial cells, is central to the development of the clinical manifestations of sepsis. **Endotoxin** (a component of the gram-negative cell wall) in gram-negative sepsis, peptidoglycans in gram-positive sepsis, and various other exotoxins such as toxic shock syndrome toxin-1 and pseudomonas exotoxin A all have been implicated. These mediators cause vasodilatation, loss of vascular integrity, and myocardial dysfunction, all of which contribute to the development of the clinical picture of septic shock.

Early septic shock is characterized by vasodilatation, decreased systemic vascular resistance, and increased cardiac output. Pulmonary vascular resistance is increased early in septic shock, leading to pulmonary hypertension, impaired

Table 42-1. Empiric antibiotic recommendations for sepsis

Neonates	*Enterobacteriaceae, Listeria,* Group B streptococci, enterococci	Ampicillin and either cefotaxime or gentamicin, ± nafcillin
Children	*Pneumococcus, H. influenzae, meningococcus, Streptococcus*	Cefotaxime or ceftriaxone, ± nafcillin
Adults		
Community acquired	*Enterobacteriaceae, S. aureus, streptococcus*	Ceftriaxone and aminoglycoside
IVDU (endocarditis)	*S. aureus,* gram-negative, *enterococci*	Penicillin, gentamicin, and nafcillin
Immunocompromised, neutropenic (all ages)	Gram-negative including *P. aeruginosa, S. aureus, Streptococcus epidermidis*	Ceftazidime and aminoglycoside ± vancomycin or Piperacillin/tazobactam and aminoglycoside Imipenem
Source Known		
Abdominal/pelvic	*Enterobacteriaceae,* anaerobes, *enterococci*	Ampicillin/sulbactam and aminoglycoside, or Ampicillin, metronidazole, and aminoglycoside
Urinary	*Enterobacteriaceae, enterococci*	Ampicillin and aminoglycoside or third-generation cephalosporin and aminoglycoside (if gram-negative)
Petechial rash		
Children	*Meningococcus, H. influenzae*	Cefotaxime or ceftriaxone
Adult	*Meningococcus,* gram-negative sepsis/DIC	Third-generation cephalosporin (ceftazidime if *Pseudomonas* suspected) and an aminoglycoside
If RMSF suspected (even if rash not present)		Chloramphenicol

RMSF = Rocky Mountain spotted fever.

oxygen diffusion, increased microvascular permeability, and pulmonary edema. Late septic shock is characterized by myocardial dysfunction leading to further hypoperfusion, oliguria, and tissue ischemia. This leads to adult respiratory distress syndrome (ARDS) up to 70% of the time. ARDS increases mortality to 80%–90%. The leading cause of death in septic shock is multiorgan dysfunction syndrome (MODS), which results from irreparable tissue ischemia of vital organs.

III. **Adult septic shock**

A. **Patient presentation.** Questions to the patient should be directed at finding a possible source of infection. Complicating factors, such as a history of alcohol abuse, cancer, recent surgeries, or nursing home or assisted living, should be obtained. If the patient's mental status is altered, caretakers and family should be contacted for the answers to these important questions. A thorough physical examination is essential to not overlook potential sites of infection.

1. **Early sepsis.** Signs of early sepsis include **tachycardia** (heart rate >100) and **tachypnea** (respiratory rate >20), but **fever** remains the hallmark of infection. Hypothermia is often present in the elderly and those with chronic underlying diseases such as alcoholism or uremia. Patients immunocompromised secondary to chemotherapeutics, immunosuppressant drugs, or steroids may blunt the febrile response. Shaking chills are predictive of bacteremia. Confusion or other mental status changes are often apparent in this early state. The initial cardiovascular response to sepsis is a decline in systemic vascular resistance (SVR) to 500 dyne/sec/ch^2, resulting in an increased cardiac output (warm or hyperdynamic shock). The end result is hypoperfusion even in early septic shock. The skin remains warm in these patients despite hypotension.

2. **Late sepsis.** The skin now becomes cold and clammy, with increasing **tachycardia, pallor,** and **cyanosis.** As shock evolves, the SVR rises (to 800–1000 dyne/sec/ch^2) leading to normal or diminished cardiac output due to the release of various myocardial depressant factors. The result is decreased organ perfusion and further ischemia. **Oliguria** and hypotension not responsive to fluids or pressors follow.

B. **Assessment**

1. **Laboratory studies.** Laboratory studies in these patients should include, at a minimum, a CBC, electrolytes, BUN/CK, glucose, PT/PTT, liver function tests, lactate, arterial blood gas, chest x-ray, and cultures of the blood, urine, and sputum. Further testing can be based on potential infectious sources as dictated by the clinical presentation. Sepsis usually is accompanied by a **leukocytosis,** with a large percentage of neutrophils (a "left shift"). Overwhelming bacteremia in the elderly, debilitated, or immunocompromised can manifest a relative leukopenia. **Thrombocytopenia** occurs as a prelude to **disseminated intravascular coagulation (DIC),** which is an ominous complication in late sepsis.

Lactic acidosis occurs early in septic shock and serves as an excellent marker of tissue perfusion. Increased lactate levels are associated with increased mortality, and clearance correlates with enhanced survival. Acute tubular necrosis with resultant renal failure is not uncommon. Hyperbilirubinemia with acute cholestatic jaundice may precede bacteremia.

2. **Search for a source of sepsis.** As previously described, a thorough physical examination is essential to prevent missing a possible source for infection. Perirectal abscess, infected decubitus ulcers, and abdominal abscess can be missed, especially in the debilitated patient. In patients with in-dwelling lines or catheters, these lines should be considered as likely sources and, if possible, should be removed or at the very least cultured. Again, **cultures** from all possible sources including blood, urine, sputum, cerebrospinal fluid, and wounds should be attained. A **chest x-ray** should be attained on all patients since the elderly and immunodeficient often hide a pneumonia without the usual signs or symptoms. Obtaining a **urinalysis** is crucial since the urinary tract is the most common known source of septic shock. **CT scan** of the head, chest, or abdomen should be guided by clinical suspicion. In 36% of all cases no source is found.

C. **Management**
   1. **Supportive care.** As always, the airway, breathing, and circulation (ABCs) come first. Optimizing oxygen delivery by decreasing hypoperfusion and minimizing oxygen consumption is the goal. To accomplish this the patient needs a patent airway. The decision to intubate a septic patient should be guided by an assessment of the patient's ability to protect the airway, factoring in the patient's mental status, work of breathing, and ability to effectively oxygenate and blow off CO_2. All patients experiencing hypotension should have two large-bore IV lines placed, supplemental oxygen to keep the SaO_2 greater than 92%, and continuous saturation monitoring.
   2. **ECG and pressure monitoring.** ECG monitoring is essential for all patients suspected of sepsis, as is close blood pressure monitoring. Patients in need of pressor therapy should have an arterial line placed for continuous blood pressure monitoring. Central venous pressures (CVP) should be used to guide fluid resuscitation in the patient with septic shock (goal CVP = 8 mm Hg). If pressors are needed, a Swan-Ganz catheter should be placed to optimize fluid and pressor management. The goal PCWP should be 10–15 mm Hg (see Chap. 8 for further information on hemodynamic monitoring).
   3. **Fluid replacement.** The first line of treatment for hypotension in the patient with severe sepsis is isotonic IV fluids. Either lactated Ringer's (LR) or normal saline (NS) are appropriate IV fluids. An initial fluid challenge of 1000 ml is generally safe with close monitoring. If there are any signs of pulmonary compro-

mise (increasing dyspnea, tachypnea, tachycardia, or decreasing SaO_2) during this bolus, it should be stopped and pressor therapy instituted to optimize tissue perfusion. The decision to use pressors generally comes after at least 1000–1500 ml of crystalloid have been infused in an average-size adult. There is debate over the best time to institute colloid (blood, albumin, heptastarch) use, but it generally is agreed that the hemoglobin should be kept above 10 g/dl.

4. **Pressor therapy**
   a. **Dopamine** generally is used as the first-line pressor in patients without a Swan-Ganz catheter in place. Dopamine activates dopaminergic receptors in the kidney at small doses (<5 µg/kg/min), increasing renal perfusion. At higher doses (5–20 µg/kg/min) it activates alpha$_1$ receptors and acts as an inotrope and vasopressor. Starting dosage in septic shock not responsive to fluids is 5–10 µg/kg/min. Above 20 µg/kg/min another pressor should be added.
   b. **Norepinephrine** is a resonable choice for a second-line agent since it works as a very potent alpha agonist and is therefore a very potent vasoconstrictor. Starting dose is 2 µg/min, titrating to desired response.
   c. **Dobutamine** is a beta$_1$ and beta$_2$ adrenergic agent that is used as an inotrope and vasodilator to augment cardiac output. Its use should be reserved for late sepsis when the SVR is higher and myocardial depressants are most active. Initial dose is 2–10 µg/kg/min, with a maximum dose of 40 µg/kg/min. The goal of pressor therapy is to maintain perfusion as indicated by mental status, urinary output, and skin perfusion at the lowest possible dose. Generally a systolic blood pressure above 90–110 mm Hg is necessary to maintain adequate tissue perfusion.

5. **Antibiotics.** Timely use of an appropriate antibiotic regimen has been shown to improve survival and decrease the frequency of shock. Antibiotic choice should be guided by the presumed site of infection, as well as by the age and immune status of the patient (see Table 42-1). When possible, cultures should be gathered prior to antibiotic treatment; however, patients in extremis should not have antibiotics withheld pending delays for diagnostic testing. Typically 2–3 drug coverage is recommended for sepsis. Studies support the use of a third-generation cephalosporin and an antipseudomonal penicillin. Many experts also recommend the addition of an aminoglycoside. Doses should be adjusted for renal or hepatic failure, and antibiotic choice should be reassessed if culture results are available. A failure to respond to antibiotic therapy suggests the presence of an abscess.

6. **New therapeutic approaches.** Future therapy for sepsis will surround blunting the effect of exogenous

mediators. Steroids have not been shown to be beneficial in sepsis, and they may increase mortality due to
secondary infection. **Monoclonal antiendotoxins,**
antitumor necrosis factor (TNF), and interleukin-1
(IL-1) receptor antagonists have shown some promise
in limited studies. However, results have been limited,
and the studies themselves are plagued with design
difficulties. In addition, the cost of these products is
considerable (most are about $4,000 per treatment).

D. Patient disposition. All patients with sepsis need to be
admitted to the hospital. Those who are elderly, debilitated, or immunocompromised should be admitted if sepsis is suspected, since these patients can clinically
deteriorate quickly. Patients who have hemodynamic compromise that does not respond to initial fluid challenge
need admission to an intensive care unit.

Immunocompetent, young, otherwise healthy patients
who have close follow-up and no hemodynamic compromise may be discharged to home in certain circumstances.
A dose of IV antibiotics, followed by oral antibiotics
at home is reasonable; however, the patient's primary
care provider should be contacted and close follow-up
arranged.

IV. Pediatric septic shock. There are a number of differences
between adults and children regarding septic shock. History
and physical findings differ according to the age of the child,
as do the likely pathogens and choice of antibiotic therapy.
Common sources for bacterial pathogens in children are the
gastrointestinal tract, genitourinary tract, and upper respiratory tract. Bacteremia occurs when local infection seeds the
bloodstream. Resolution of bacteremia depends directly on
the load and virulence of the bacteria and is also a function of
the overall health of the child as well as appropriate timing of
therapy. As with adults, actually isolating a pathogen is often
difficult in children. Bacteremia that goes unchecked by either endogenous or exogenous means becomes sepsis.

Symptoms and signs of sepsis result from the body's physiologic response to cytokines activated by pathogens (in children, pathogens are often bacterial but can also be viral).
Fever, vasodilation, tachycardia, and white cell abnormalities are all hallmarks of early sepsis in children. Systemic vascular resistance decreases, which manifests as
relative hypovolemia. Heart rate increases to improve cardiac output and thus preserve oxygen delivery to vital tissues.
As oxygen demand exceeds delivery, end-organ damage occurs as evidenced by hypoxemia, lactic acidosis secondary to
anaerobic metabolism, changes in mental state (irritability or
lethargy, decreased or increased sleepiness), and decreases in
splanchnic perfusion. **Hypotension** is a late and ominous
sign in children with septic shock.

A. Presentation. A complete head-to-toe assessment is essential. Mental status evaluation in children is often difficult, especially in nonverbal children. The most obvious
sign will be irritability or lethargy. Meningeal signs are
not reliable in children under the age of 18–24 months.
Fever, tachycardia, and **tachypnea** also will be present

in early sepsis. Skin color and perfusion will be altered. Color can vary from ruddy to pale to ashen. **Mottling** is usually present. Capillary refill, although used frequently, is not always reliable and can vary with environmental temperature. Examination of the skin for rashes or petechial lesions is of utmost importance.

B. Assessment

    1. Laboratory studies. The typical basics of a workup for sepsis in children without clear focus for infection are a CBC and differential, glucose, electrolytes, BUN, creatinine, blood culture, catheterized urine culture, and cerebral spinal fluid studies if the child is stable. Other studies, such as arterial blood gas, coagulation studies, liver function tests, and plasma lactic acid, tend to be helpful but are not essential. In children, sepsis may be associated with **leukocytosis** and **bandemia;** however, in the very young or immunocompromised patient, there can be a relative leukopenia. Relative thrombocytopenia also can exist with sepsis. Elevated plasma lactate levels occur whenever systemic perfusion is compromised, but the measurement of such does not replace the physical examination, which can be assessed rapidly and followed through therapeutic interventions. Certain children with inborn errors of metabolism often can present with a shock-like picture; it is in these children that more extensive lab studies should be obtained as early in presentation as possible, since it may be the only time that chemical abnormalities will be detected.

    As in adults, a chest X-ray, urinalysis, and body fluid cultures should be obtained to search for a source. In infants younger than 2 years, this should include a cerebrospinal fluid analysis to rule out meningitis.

C. Management

    1. Supportive care. Respiratory compromise in ill children can be common. Assessment of the airway should include the nose because infants are obligate nasal breathers. The pediatric airway is narrower and more pliable than in adults, and therefore patency may be difficult for the septic child to maintain. Endotracheal intubation should be performed by persons experienced in the procedure. Supplemental oxygen should not be withheld from children. IV access is essential with the largest caliber angiocath possible, at least 22-gauge. If IV access cannot be established within 60–90 seconds, an intraosseous (IO) needle should be placed in the proximal tibia. This procedure is usually successful in children less than 8 years old. The IO needle system can be used to administer isotonic fluids, blood products, dextrose, catecholamines, and antibiotics.

    2. ECG and pressure monitoring. Cardiorespiratory monitoring with oxygen saturation is crucial in the child with sepsis. Blood pressure monitoring is also essential, but it should be remembered that blood pressure changes are late events in pediatric septic shock.

Patients who are admitted to pediatric intensive care units will be monitored continuously for arterial blood pressure and central venous pressure. Pulmonary artery catheterization is not used in all pediatric centers. Invasive hemodynamic monitoring is used less frequently in pediatrics because of limitations in equipment sizes and risks associated with its use.

3. **Fluid replacement.** Isotonic fluid, either NS or LR, should be administered promptly in the child with sepsis as boluses of 20 ml/kg up to 60–80 ml/kg. Reassessment of overall patient status and vital signs after each bolus is essential. If 3 to 4 isotonic fluid boluses have been administered and perfusion is still compromised, colloids such as 5% albumin should be used next, again in boluses of 20 ml/kg. The goal of fluid therapy is to improve mental status, urinary output, and skin perfusion. Most pediatricians trained in emergency medicine or critical care would begin vasopressors after 100–120 ml/kg total fluids if symptoms persist.

4. **Pressor therapy.** In infants, a systolic blood pressure above 77 mm Hg is desirable. In toddlers and older children, the systolic blood pressure should be maintained above 99 mm Hg. For tissue perfusion to be maintained, a diastolic blood pressure greater than 40 mm Hg in infants and 50 mm Hg in children is sufficient. When used, the sequence of vasopressors will typically start with **dopamine** in dosages of 10–20 µg/kg of ideal body weight. Dobutamine often is added if there is evidence of myocardial depression. However if the patient is in extremis with myocardial depression, epinephrine at dosages of 0.1–1.0 µg/kg will be administered. When myocardial depression is absent and potent vasoconstriction is still needed despite dopamine, norepinephrine is given at infusion of 0.05–1.0 µg/kg.

5. **Antibiotic therapy.** Choice of antibiotics should be based on the age of the child, since pathogens tend to be age-specific. **Newborns** (0–28 days) are typically infected with group B streptococcus, enterococcus species, *Listeria monocytogenes,* and gram-negative bacilli and should be treated with ampicillin and gentamicin or ampicillin and ceftriaxone. **Infants** (1–3 months) usually are infected by all of the newborn agents and *Streptococcus pneumoniae, Haemophilus influenzae,* and *Neisseria meningitidis* and should therefore be treated with ampicillin and ceftriaxone. **Children** 3 months to 5 years old will be infected with *S. pneumoniae, N. meningitidis,* and *H. influenzae* (although immunization programs have dramatically decreased the incidence of disease caused by this agent); treatment for this age group should be with ceftriaxone until CNS involvement is ruled out.

If *S. pneumoniae* in an institution is resistant to penicillins and meningitis is suspected, vancomycin must be added pending complete sensitivities. Chil-

dren over the age of 5 years are additionally susceptible to community-acquired agents, and therefore
broad-spectrum coverage needs to include activity
against *Mycoplasma pneumoniae.* Any infant or child
with nosocomially acquired infection or who is im-
munosuppressed or who has a device for permanent
vascular access should be treated with vancomycin
plus an aminoglycoside or third-generation cephalosporin. The clinical condition can often worsen in the
initial period following antibiotic administration secondary to release of cytotoxic agents and endotoxins
upon death of bacteria.

D. Patient disposition. All infants and children presenting
with septic shock should be admitted to a hospital or
transferred to a tertiary pediatric medical center. Children with sepsis but not septic shock can be managed
based on their clinical condition.

In children over 1 month of age suspected of having only
bacteremia, with improvement after relative minimal IV
fluid therapy, a single dose of third-generation cephalosporin can be given, oral antibiotics prescribed, and the
patient discharged with instructions to follow up with a
physician the next day. Contact telephone numbers with
the patient's family should be verified. Notification of the
patient's primary care provider at or before time of discharge will help to assure the follow-up process.

Bibliography

Baraff L, et al. Practice guideline for the management of infants and
  children 0 to 36 months of age with fever without source. *Pediatrics*
  92:1–12, 1993.
Salez-Llorens, McCracken. Sepsis syndrome and septic shock in pediatrics: current concepts of terminology, pathophysiology, and management. *J Pediatr* 123:497–508, 1993.

Anaphylactic Shock

Ellen C. Corey

I. **Definition.** The term anaphylaxis has been used traditionally to describe an IgE-mediated, antigen-induced immunologic event. Preformed IgE is activated by antigen exposure and induces chemical mediator release from mast cells in previously sensitized individuals. The chemical mediators are responsible for the systemic symptoms in anaphylactic events. Recently, other pathophysiologic mechanisms, such as anaphylactoid reactions, have been identified as capable of causing the same clinical syndrome as classic IgE-mediated events. Contemporary usage of the term anaphylaxis defines the clinical syndrome rather than the etiologic agents or biochemical mediators. Thus, anaphylactic shock is an immediate, life-threatening clinical syndrome with multiorgan system involvement. Systemic features of anaphylactic shock include dermatologic, respiratory, cardiovascular, and gastrointestinal involvement. Anaphylactic shock is classified pathophysiologically as distributive shock, although fluid losses due to capillary leak may lead to true hypovolemic shock.

II. **Scope of the problem.** At least 400–800 deaths per year occur in the United States because of anaphylactic shock. The rate of fatal anaphylaxis from any cause has been estimated to be 0.4 case per million individuals.

III. **Causative agents.** The leading cause of fatal anaphylaxis is penicillin allergy, with an estimated 100–500 deaths per year in the United States. Similarly, an anaphylactic reaction occurs in about 1–5 per 10,000 administrations of beta-lactam antibiotics. Radiocontrast-induced anaphylaxis has been responsible for as many as 500 deaths annually. The rate for anaphylactic reactions to these two agents, penicillin and radiocontrast, is approximately 1 reaction per 5000 exposures. Hymenoptera envenomations cause 40–80 deaths per year in the United States. Food exposures are also common causes of fatal reactions (Table 43-1).

IV. **Mortality.** Fewer than 10% of anaphylactic reactions are fatal. In beta-lactam reactions, 10% are life threatening and 1% are fatal. The leading causes of death from anaphylactic shock are respiratory complications (70%) and cardiovascular dysfunction (24%).

V. **Recurrence.** Various estimates exist for the risk of recurrent reactions. Individuals who are reexposed to penicillin after a nonfatal anaphylactic reaction have a 10%–20% risk for anaphylaxis, and the risk is 20%–40% for radiocontrast agents and 40%–60% for Hymenoptera stings. Cross-reactivity of agents is also clinically important. Cross-reactivity rates ranging from 5% to 30% between penicillin and other beta-lactam antibiotics have been reported. If a subsequent reaction does occur, it will generally be more serious than the previous one.

VI. **Pathophysiology of anaphylactic shock**

    A. **Classic anaphylaxis.** Classic anaphylaxis is typically seen in response to penicillin, food, Hymenoptera stings,

Table 43-1. Common causes of anaphylactic shock

Drugs	Hymenoptera stings	Foods and food additives	Medical agents
Penicillin	Yellow jackets	Milk	Radiographic contrast material
Beta-lactams	Honeybees	Eggs	Latex
Vancomycin	Hornets	Fish and shellfish	Foreign proteins
Aspirin and NSAIDs	Wasps	Nuts	
Sulfa agents	Bumblebees	Monosodium glutamate	
Angiotensin-converting enzyme inhibitors	Imported fire ants	Fruits	

airborne allergens, and some parasites. Three processes are necessary for IgE-mediated anaphylaxis to occur:

1. Initial exposure to an antigen leads to formation of IgE antibodies.
2. A latent period after the initial exposure is necessary for sensitization of the mast cells by the IgE antibody to occur.
3. Reexposure to the antigen leads to cross-linking of the IgE antibody that is fixed to the mast cell or basophil membrane. This leads to mast cell and basophil activation, which causes the release of preformed and rapidly generated chemical mediators.

B. **Chemical mediators.** A variety of biologically active mediators are released from the mast cells. These mediators are capable of activating an inflammatory cascade.

1. **Histamine** is a preformed mediator that is the most important mediator of anaphylaxis. It has both vasogenic and smooth muscle spasmodic effects and a very short half-life. There are three histamine receptors. The H_1 receptor activation by the histamine released from the mast cells is responsible for the majority of clinical signs and symptoms of anaphylaxis. H_1 receptor activation causes coronary artery vasoconstriction, bronchoconstriction, cutaneous vascular permeability, and intestinal smooth muscle contraction. The H_2 receptor stimulates ventricular and atrial inotropy, atrial chronotropy, coronary vasodilation, and gastric acid secretion. The H_3 receptor inhibits central and peripheral nervous system neurotransmitter release and may inhibit further histamine formation.

2. **Tryptase** is a preformed protease present in mast cells that is responsible for proteolysis and complement activation. Tryptase has a half-life of several

hours and may be useful for biochemical determinations of an anaphylactic event.

3. **Leukotrienes** are formed via the arachidonic acid cycle from lipids from cell membranes. These chemical mediators are orders of magnitude more spasmogenic than histamine, with up to 6000 times the bronchoconstricting potential of histamine. Aspirin inhibits the conversion of arachidonic acid via the cyclooxygenase pathway and may lead to increased production of the leukotrienes. The leukotrienes have also been known as the slow-reacting substance of anaphylaxis.

4. **Chemotactic factors** such as eosinophil chemotactic factor and neutrophil chemotactic factor recruit additional immune response to the site of organ system involvement. These cells in turn are responsible for the rebound of symptoms, which may occur in 7%–20% of patients (Fig. 43-1).

C. **Non–IgE-mediated reactions.** These include a diverse group of etiologies that do not involve IgE induction of the chemical mediators or anaphylaxis.

1. Direct **mast cell release** of the chemical mediators of anaphylaxis has been termed an "anaphylactoid" reaction. These reactions are generally nonimmunologically mediated and do not involve the classical IgE mechanism. Causative agents include radiocontrast media and drugs such as morphine.

2. **Complement activation (C3a, C5a)** can occur with exposure to foreign proteins such as blood products or gamma globulin.

3. Other mechanisms that may lead to anaphylaxis are the activation of the **arachidonic acid cycle** via aspirin and nonsteroidal anti-inflammatory medication ingestions. Cholinergic anaphylaxis and idiopathic

Fig. 43-1. Natural history of anaphylactic reactions.

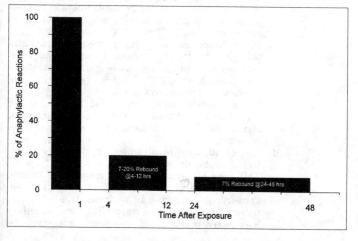

anaphylaxis are also possible and are of unknown causes.

VII. Clinical presentation and management of anaphylactic shock

A. Presentation

1. **History**

   a. The **abrupt onset** of systemic symptoms following exposure to an inciting agent is the hallmark of anaphylactic reactions. The vast majority of patients develop symptoms within 30–60 minutes of exposure to the inciting agent. The history of exposure to a potential causative agent is an important aid to the diagnosis of anaphylaxis.

   b. The **route of administration** of the causative agent will correlate with the severity of the reaction. Intravenous and intramuscular exposures are more serious.

   c. The **quantity** of antigen is proportional to the severity of the reaction.

   d. Patients with a **past medical history** of cardiac or respiratory disease are at higher risk for severe reactions.

   e. The use of **beta-blockers** can lead to more severe reactions.

   f. An **atopic individual** is not at greater risk than a person without atopy for the development of classic IgE-mediated anaphylaxis.

   g. A past history of **allergies** to medications, foods, or environmental allergens should be determined in the assessment of all patients with anaphylaxis.

2. **Physical findings, signs, and symptoms** (Table 43-2)

   a. **Individual variation** exists in the onset, manifestations, and clinical course of anaphylactic shock. Anaphylaxis involves multiple organ systems, including the airway and respiratory system, the cardiovascular system, the skin, and the gastrointestinal system. Early involvement of the respiratory and cardiovascular systems heralds a severe reaction.

   b. Early clinical manifestions are frequently **dermatologic.** Pruritus, generalized flushing, and urticaria are common. Dermatologic manifestations are present in 90% of cases. Nonpruritic angioedema may also occur.

   c. **Upper airway** edema may lead to a subjective sensation of tightness in the throat, hoarseness, stridor, drooling, or difficulty in handling oral secretions.

   d. **Lower airway** involvement is generally manifested by cough, wheeze, and subjective dyspnea. This may progress rapidly to respiratory failure.

   e. **Cardiovascular** involvement may result in severe hypotension due to peripheral vasodilation, increased capillary permeability, and capillary leak. Activation of the H_2 receptor by histamine release and the development of acidosis may be responsible for arrhythmias such as ventricular fibrillation and cardiovascular collapse.

f. **Gastrointestinal** symptoms may result from smooth muscle contractions and capillary leak leading to mucosal edema. Symptoms may include nausea, vomiting, abdominal cramping, diarrhea, and tenesmus.

g. **Neurologic** signs such as syncope, altered mental status, and seizures may occur as a result of other pathophysiologic processes.

h. **Gynecologic** manifestations of smooth muscle contractions may cause pelvic pain and cramping.

B. **Assessment.** A focused primary and secondary survey evaluating for airway, breathing, and circulatory compromise must be rapidly performed and simultaneous management of any compromise in these areas implemented. Assessment for skin and gastrointestinal signs will be helpful in making the diagnosis and distinguishing anaphylaxis from other disorders included in the differential diagnosis of anaphylaxis (Table 43-3).

1. **Routine laboratory studies.** There are no pathognomonic laboratory tests to establish the diagnosis of anaphylaxis. Arterial blood gases (ABGs) should not be used to make decisions regarding a patient's respiratory status—upper airway edema is not adequately measured by ABGs, and respiratory failure will be apparent clinically.

2. **ECG.** Baseline ECG changes may include nonspecific ST-T wave changes. Patients should be continuously monitored for arrhythmias that may result from the primary insult or as a side effect of agents used to treat the anaphylactic reaction.

3. **Diagnostic adjuncts.** Pulse-oximetry should be used to continuously monitor oxygenation. An indwelling urinary catheter should be used to monitor urine output. A Swan-Ganz catheter or CAP line readings may be useful for guiding the management of patients who are persistently hypotensive despite IV fluids and epinephrine.

4. **Esoteric tests.** Tryptase and histamine levels may be useful retrospectively to confirm the diagnosis of anaphylaxis. Tryptase has a half-life of several hours, and serum drawn up to 6 hours after the event may demonstrate an elevated level. Histamine has a much shorter half-life and must be drawn within 10–60 minutes of the event to be clinically useful. These tests may be used by medical examiners to determine the cause of death.

C. **Management**

1. **Airway management.** Conservative management with suctioning and hyperextension of the neck with chin lift or jaw thrust may provide temporizing measures, but definitive management of upper airway edema and obstruction is crucial. Early oral endotracheal intubation with direct visualization of the

Table 43-2. Clinical manifestations of anaphylaxis and related pathophysiology

Organ system	Reaction	Symptoms	Signs	Pathophysiology
Respiratory tract Upper	Rhinitis	Nasal congestion Nasal itching Sneezing	Nasal mucosal edema Rhinorrhea	Increased vascular permeability Vasodilatation Stimulation of nerve endings
	Laryngeal edema	Dyspnea Hoarseness Throat tightness Hypersalivation	Laryngeal stridor Supraglottic and glottic edema	As above, plus increased exocrine gland secretions
Lower	Bronchospasm	Cough Wheezing Retrosternal tightness Dyspnea	Cough Wheeze, rhonchi, Tachypnea Respiratory distress Cyanosis	As above, plus bronchiole smooth muscle contraction
Cardiovascular system	Circulatory collapse	Lightheadedness Generalized weakness Syncope Ischemic chest pain	Tachycardia Hypotension Shock	Increased vascular permeability Vasodilation Loss of vasomotor tone Increased venous capacitance Decreased cardiac output Direct mediator-induced myocardial suppression Decreased effective plasma volume Decreased preload Decreased afterload Hypoxia and ischemia Dysrhythmias Iatrogenic effects of drugs used in treatment Preexisting heart disease
	Dysrhythmias	As above, plus palpitations	ECG changes: Tachycardia Nonspecific and ischemic ST-T wave changes Right ventricular strain Premature atrial and ventricular contractions Nodal rhythm Atrial fibrillation	

System	Manifestation	Symptoms	Signs	Mechanism
	Cardiac arrest		Pulseless ECG changes: Ventricular fibrillation, Asystole	
Skin	Urticaria	Pruritus, Tingling and warmth, Flushing, Hives	Urticaria, Diffuse erythema	Increased vascular permeability, Vasodilation
	Angioedema	Nonpruritic extremity, periorbital and perioral swelling	Nonpitting edema, frequently asymmetrical	Increased vascular permeability, Vasodilation
Eye	Conjunctivitis	Ocular itching, Increased lacrimation, Red eye	Conjunctival inflammation	Increased vascular permeability, Vasodilation, Stimulation of nerve endings
Gastrointestinal tract		Dysphagia, Cramping abdominal pain, Nausea and vomiting, Diarrhea (rarely bloody), Tenesmus	Nonspecific	Increased mucous secretions, Gastrointestinal smooth muscle contraction
Miscellaneous CNS		Apprehension, Sense of impending doom, Headache, Confusion	Anxiety, Seizures (rarely), Coma (late); Nonspecific	Secondary to cerebral hypoxia and hypoperfusion, Vasodilation
Hematologic	Fibrinolysis and DIC	Abnormal bleeding and bruising	Mucous membrane bleeding DIC	Mediator recruitment and activation, Uterine smooth muscle contraction
Genitourinary		Pelvic pain, Vaginal bleeding, Urinary incontinence	Increased uterine tone, Vaginal bleeding, Urinary incontinence	Bladder smooth muscle contraction

Source: Lindzon RL, Silvers WS. Allergy, hypersensitivity, and anaphylaxis. In Rosen P (ed.), *Emergency Medicine: Concepts and Clinical Practice* (3rd ed.). St. Louis: Mosby–Year Book, 1992.

Table 43-3.   Differential diagnosis of anaphylactic shock

Upper airway obstruction
Foreign body aspiration
Supraglottitis
Croup

Lower respiratory obstruction
Status asthmaticus

Cardiogenic shock
Acute myocardial infarction

Cutaneous disorders
Carcinoid syndrome
Mastocytosis
Stevens-Johnson syndrome
Monosodium glutamate syndrome
Scromboid

Neurologic disorders
Vasovagal syncope
Seizure disorder

Other forms of distributive shock
Neurogenic shock
Septic shock

airway before edema formation obscures it is the preferred method of airway management. Intubation for lower airway obstruction (bronchospasm) can usually be delayed for a trial of pharmacologic therapies. The use of a rigid stylet, smaller endotracheal tube, and fiberoptic bronchoscopic intubation may be helpful. If endotracheal intubation is impossible, a cricothyrotomy or transtracheal jet ventilation should be performed. Several pharmacologic agents may be useful to treat upper airway edema (see sec. **6.** below) but should not replace aggressive early management of the airway.

2. **Oxygenation.** Adjunctive oxygen therapy and assisted ventilation should be delivered as indicated by the patient's condition. High-flow oxygen via a nonrebreather mask is prudent during the early assessment and management phase.
3. **CPR** should be performed if indicated.
4. **IV fluid replacement.** The rapid administration of a fluid bolus via large-bore IV lines with crystalloid solutions such as lactated Ringer or normal saline may initially be helpful in treating hypotension. Persistent hypotension despite initial pharmacologic agents and

fluid replacement is an indication for the use of pressor agents.

5. Frequent **monitoring** for vital signs and cardiac arrhythmias and an ECG for ST-segment changes will help to determine the response to therapy. Because of the biphasic clinical syndrome in 7%–20% of patients, continuous monitoring is vital (see Fig. 43-1).

6. **Pharmacologic agents.** Pharmacologic agents used to treat anaphylaxis either reverse the effects of mediators on target tissues or inhibit further release (Table 43-4).

    a. **Epinephrine** is the mainstay of therapy for anaphylaxis. The alpha-agonist effects of epinephrine increase peripheral vascular resistance and reverse peripheral vasodilation, vascular permeability, and systemic hypotension. The beta-agonist effects produce much-needed bronchodilation and improve cardiac inotropy and chronotropy. Other beneficial effects of epinephrine include the stabilization of cell membranes and the reduction in further chemical mediator release. Side effects of epinephrine include hypertension, tachycardia including tachydysrhythmias, and increased myocardial oxygen consumption, which can lead to myocardial ischemia. This agent must be used with caution in the elderly and in patients with a history of coronary artery disease. Relative contraindications to the use of epinephrine include hypertension, coronary artery disease, and pregnancy.

    b. **Glugacon** is the agent of choice when epinephrine is relatively contraindicated, making it particularly useful in anaphylactic patients on beta-blockers, patients with known coronary artery disease, pregnant women, and patients with severe hypertension. In addition, it may be a useful adjunct in patients who are refractory to epinephrine therapy. Glucagon enhances cyclic adenosine monophosphate (cAMP) synthesis within the heart and GI tracts, leading to positive inotropy and chronotropy and smooth muscle relaxation. Side effects may include nausea, vomiting, hypokalemia, hyperglycemia, and occasional cases of Stevens-Johnson syndrome.

    c. **Antihistamine** agents are classified as H_1 blockers or H_2 blockers and competitively block the corresponding receptors. Agents from both classes are standard in the therapy of anaphylaxis. H_1 blockers, such as diphenhydramine, will block further histamine effects at the H_1 receptor responsible for bronchoconstriction, cutaneous vascular permeability, and intestinal smooth muscle contractions. This may prevent further histamine-mediated deterioration of the patient's condition. Antihistamines do not decrease the amount of histamine released by the mast cells, but they block hista-

Table 43-4.   Pharmacologic therapy of anaphylaxis

Severity of reaction	Agent	Route	Adult dose	Pediatric dose
Severe	Epinephrine (1:10,000 solution)	IV (over 5 minutes)	0.3–0.5 mg (3–5 ml)	0.1 µg/kg (0.1 ml/kg)
	Glucagon	IV	1–5 mg bolus, 2 mg/hr	1–2 mg bolus, 1–2 mg/hr
	Diphenhydramine	IV	25–50 mg	0.5–1.0 mg/kg
	Cimetidine	IV	300 mg	5–10 mg/kg
	Ranitidine	IV	50 mg	0.5 mg/kg
	Methylprednisolone	IV	125–250 mg	1–2 mg/kg
	Hydrocortisone	IV	250 mg	4–8 mg/kg
	Racemic epinephrine	Nebulized	0.5–0.75 ml in 2.5 ml normal saline	0.5 ml
	Albuterol	Nebulized	0.5 ml in 2.5 ml normal saline	0.01 ml/kg
	Aminophylline	IV	6 mg/kg loading dose, 0.5 mg/kg/hr	6 mg/kg loading dose, 0.9 mg/kg/hr
	Epinephrine infusion (1 ml of 1:1000 solution in 500 ml D5W)	IV	0.25–2.50 ml/min	0.25–2.50 ml/min
	Isoproterenol	IV	0.5–5.0 µg/min	0.1 µg/kg/min
	Dopamine	IV	4–10 µg/kg/min	4–10 µg/kg/min

	Drug	Route	Adult dose	Pediatric dose
Moderate	Epinephrine (1:1000 solution)	SQ or IM	0.3–0.5 ml	0.01 ml/kg
	Glucagon	IM	1 mg	0.5–1.0 mg
	Diphenhydramine	IM or IV	25–50 mg	1 mg/kg
	Cimetidine	IV	300 mg	5–10 mg/kg
	Ranitidine	IV	50 mg	0.5 mg/kg
	Methylprednisolone	IV	50–125 mg	1–2 mg/kg
	Hydrocortisone	IV	250 mg	4–8 mg/kg
	Albuterol	Nebulized	0.5 ml in 2.5 ml normal saline	0.01 ml/kg
Mild	Epinephrine) (1:1000 solution)	SQ	0.3 ml	0.01 ml/kg
	Glucagon	SQ	1 mg	0.5 mg
	Diphenhydramine	PO or IM	25–50 mg	1 mg/kg
	Cimetidine	PO	300 mg	5–10 mg/kg
	Ranitidine	PO	150 mg	1–2 mg/kg
	Prednisone	PO	60 mg	20–40 mg

mine effects at the target tissues. The side effects of antihistamines include dizziness, sedation, blurred vision, tachycardia, palpitations, hypotension, urinary retention, and seizures. Antihistamines may also precipitate blindness in patients with glaucoma. H_2 blockers are somewhat controversial since the H_2 receptor has some coronary artery vasodilatory effects. Many clinicians have effectively used H_2 agents in anaphylactic reactions, including ranitidine and cimetidine.

d. **Corticosteroids** are commonly employed in allergic and anaphylactic reactions. In a critically ill, unstable patient, the use of these agents will have no immediate effectiveness since they have an onset of action of 4–6 hours. These agents may blunt the biphasic reaction and may be useful in the treatment of refractory bronchospasm. The exact mechanism of action of steroids is unclear.

e. **Vasopressor** agents such as dopamine, isoproterenol, and epinephrine infusions may be necessary for patients with hypotension that does not respond to epinephrine and IV fluids.

f. **Aminophylline** may provide useful additional bronchodilation in patients with refractory bronchospasm. By increasing cAMP levels, aminophylline directly relaxes smooth muscle. Risks associaated with aminophylline use include gastrointestinal, cardiovascular, and central nervous system toxicities. Aminophylline should be used with caution in patients with cardiac disease, liver disease, and congestive heart failure.

7. **Respiratory agents**

a. **Albuterol** and other beta$_2$ agonists for aerosolization act relatively selectively on the beta$_2$-adrenergic receptors for the treatment of bronchospasm and have become the bronchodilators of choice for bronchospasm. Adverse effects may include tremor, headache, tachycardia, palpitations, muscle cramps, nausea, and weakness. Hypokalemia is also a common side effect of beta$_2$ agonist use.

b. **Aerosolized epinephrine** may be useful in the prehospital setting via metered dose inhalers. With 15–20 doses the patient will receive 1.5–3.0 mg of epinephrine, similar to the doses received by subcutaneous or intravenous routes.

c. **Terbutaline** may be used for bronchospasm in a subcutaneous dose of 0.25 mg and may be repeated every 15–30 minutes. This agent is less beta$_2$-specific than the other agents and may have more cardiac side effects.

d. **Isoproterenol** causes potent beta$_1$- and beta$_2$-adrenergic activity. It can produce bronchodilation, peripheral vasodilation, increased inotropy, and chronotropy.

8. **Alternative and adjunctive therapies**
   a. Removing a stinger by flicking it out of the skin (do not squeeze the stinger, which may then express additional antigenic material) may limit further antigen exposure.
   b. A loosely applied venous tourniquet proximal to the site and placement of the limb in a dependent position may help limit antigen absorption. Similarly, the application of ice to areas of exposure for 15 minutes every half-hour may help decrease the antigen load.
   c. Local infiltration of epinephrine 0.1–0.2 ml, 1:1000 solution, at the site of antigen exposure may reduce the absorption of antigen.
D. **Patient disposition.** Admission to the hospital is prudent for all patients who are refractory to epinephrine, on beta-blockers, or exhibit significant rebound during the initial observation period. Patients with upper airway obstruction or hypotension should be considered for admission even if these conditions are clinically resolved after treatment.

   Observation units or short stay units are useful for patients with significant underlying cardiac or pulmonary disease, elderly patients, or patients with borderline severity.

   Discharge to home after 2–6 hours of observation is appropriate for most patients and should include the following home-going instructions or plan:
   1. **Referral** to an allergist for desensitization if possible. Discontinuation or avoidance of inciting antigen (e.g., antibiotics or foods) should also be encouraged.
   2. A regimen of 48–72 hours of **antihistamines** is prudent to help prevent relapse. An oral agent such as diphenhydramine 25–50 mg q6h is indicated. An H_2 receptor blocker like cimetidine 300 mg q6h PO can be considered as well.
   3. A short course of **steroids** (taper) may be useful for patients who experience difficult bronchospasm and hypotension, or for patients with persistent bronchospasm who required steroids during their initial management. A short, tapering course (7–10 days) of oral prednisone is standard.
   4. **Inhaled beta agonists** are useful in patients with bronchospasm. An outpatient metered-dose inhaler of albuterol should be used for bronchospasm that may occur for at least 48–72 hours after the anaphylactic event.
   5. Prefilled **epinephrine syringes** are commercially available for patient use outside the hospital environment. Patients with anaphylaxis should be given a prescription for these devices and have them available for self-injection in the event of a future exposure.
   6. It is also prudent to advise patients to carry **identification** that indicates their known allergies or

anaphylactic sensitivities, such as a medical identification bracelet.

Bibliography

Barsan WG. Respiratory drugs. In Barsan WG, Syverud SA, Jastremski MS (eds.), *Emergency Drug Therapy*. Philadelphia: Saunders, 1991:352–371.

Bochner BS, Lichtenstein LM. Anaphylaxis. *N Engl J Med* 324:1785–1790, 1991.

Heilpern K. The treacherous clinical spectrum of allergic emergencies: diagnosis, treatment and prevention. *Emerg Med Rep* 15:211–222, 1994.

Lindzon RD, Silvers WS. Allergy, hypersensitivity and anaphylaxis. In Rosen P (ed.), *Emergency Medicine: Concepts and Clinical Practice*. St. Louis: Mosby–Year Book, 1992:1042–1065.

Solomone JA. Anaphylaxis and acute allergic reactions. In Tintinalli JE (ed.), *Emergency Medicine: A Comprehensive Study Guide*. New York: McGraw-Hill, 1992:901–903.

Wasserman SI, Marquardt DL. Anaphylaxis. In Middleton EM Jr, et al. (eds.), *Allergy: Principles and Practice* (3rd ed.). St. Louis: Mosby–Year Book, 1988:1365–1377.

44

Neurogenic Shock

Michael P. Sotak

Neurogenic shock is an acute life-threatening complication of spinal cord and brainstem trauma or high spinal anesthesia. Neurogenic shock is often confused with spinal shock, which is the nervous tissue dysfunction that is seen after spinal cord injury. Neurogenic shock is characterized by hypotension and bradycardia caused by an interruption of the sympathetic nervous system and unopposed parasympathetic activity and vagal tone.

I. **Scope of the problem, its incidence and mortality.** Spinal cord injury affects 30–50 people per million annually with 7,500 to 12,500 new injuries yearly in the United States alone. About 80% of injuries occur in males and 60% of injuries occur between the ages of 10 to 30 years. Motor vehicle accidents account for most spinal cord injuries (41%), followed by falls (13%), firearms injuries (9%), and recreation injuries (5%). A case fatality rate of 48% of spinal cord injury victims has been reported, with 79% occurring in the field.

II. **Common causes.** Neurogenic shock is seen almost exclusively in cervical or high thoracic spinal cord injuries. It is common in complete cervical and upper thoracic cord lesions and becomes less common as more motor function is preserved below the level of the lesion. It can also be seen in high spinal anesthesia.

III. **Pathophysiology.** Neurogenic shock results from the loss of sympathetic tone and unopposed parasympathetic and vagal tone to the heart and on the arterioles and venules below the level of the spinal cord lesion. The loss of sympathetic tone is caused by disruption of the descending sympathetic pathways in the spinal cord.

   A. **Cardiac.** Bradycardia may be seen along with hypotension, but the extent to which the bradycardia may contribute to the hypotension is not known. Although the exact mechanism is not known, cardiac abnormalities most likely arise from disruption of the sympathetic fibers leaving the first through the fourth thoracic level that innervate the heart. Evidence for this includes the frequent association of bradyarrhythmias with cervical lesions but not with thoracic or lumbar lesions.

   B. **Vascular.** The loss of sympathetic tone on the vasculature and unopposed parasympathetic tone causes vasodilatation of the arterioles and venules. This results in intravascular pooling of blood below the level of the spinal cord lesion and consequent hypotension.

IV. **Differential diagnosis of neurogenic versus other shock states.** Shock is defined as an abnormality of the circulatory system that results in inadequate organ perfusion. The causes of shock can be divided into three broad categories: hypovolemic, cardiogenic, and vasogenic, which can be differentiated by Swan-Ganz monitor placement (Table 44-1). Neurogenic shock is a diagnosis of exclusion. Only after all

**Table 44-1.   Hemodynamic parameters differen-
tiating neurogenic shock from other causes of shock**

	Cardiac output	Wedge pressure	Systemic vascular resistance
Cardiogenic	Decreased	Increased	Increased
Hypovolemic	Decreased	Decreased	Increased
Septic	Variable	Decreased	Decreased
Anaphylactic	Decreased	Decreased	Decreased
Neurogenic	Increased	Decreased	Decreased

other causes of shock (such as hypovolemic, cardiogenic, anaphylactic, septic and mechanical distributive shock) have
been ruled out, can the diagnosis be safely made.

V. **Clinical aspects of neurogenic shock**

 A. **Presentation.** The typical patient with neurogenic shock
will have sustained some type of blunt or penetrating
trauma that causes brainstem or spinal cord injury. The
patient will also have a history of sensorimotor loss with
hypotension, usually without tachycardia.

   1. **History.** A description of how the patient sustained the
injury is important to understand the mechanism of injury and the potential for further injury. Ambulance
personnel are invaluable in providing information
about paralysis immediately after the accident or the
deterioration of sensorimotor status since the accident.
This information allows the examiner to assess and
document the site, extent of injury, and whether paralysis is present. If the patient is awake, a history of neck
or back pain and weakness or loss of sensation in the
extremities is critical. As a general rule, any patient
sustaining an injury above the collar bone or a head injury resulting in an unconscious state should be suspected of sustaining a cervical spine injury. Any patient
involved in a high-speed motor vehicle accident also
should be suspected of having incurred a spine or
spinal cord injury. An unconscious patient who was involved in a fall or motor vehicle accident has a 5% to
10% chance of sustaining a cervical spine injury.

   2. **Physical examination.** The diagnosis of neurogenic
shock is made in a patient with sensorimotor defects
and **hypotension.** The patient may have associated
bradycardia, but this is not absolute. The awake patient with paralysis is usually able to identify the site
of pain at the site of injury, because the loss of sensation is below this level. If the patient is unconscious,
clinical findings suggesting a spinal cord injury include:

     a. Flaccid areflexia, especially with a flaccid rectal
sphincter, below the level of the injury.
     b. Diaphragmatic breathing.
     c. Ability to flex, but not extend, at the elbow (typical
for low cervical lesions).

    d. Grimaces to pain above, but not below, the collar bone.

    e. Priapism, an uncommon but characteristic sign.

B. Assessment

  1. Laboratory. The diagnosis or treatment of neurogenic shock is not dependent on laboratory tests, and these tests should be centered on the management of the associated injuries of the trauma patient with neurogenic shock. Laboratory tests should include all of the routine trauma labs such as CBC with platelets, PT/PTT, electrolytes, BUN, creatinine, glucose, liver function tests, amylase, lipase, blood alcohol, blood and urine toxicology screen, and arterial blood gases.

  2. X-rays. X-rays should include:

    a. A complete cervical spine series with a lateral view that visualizes all seven cervical vertebrae, an odontoid view, an anteroposterior view, and oblique or pillar views.

    b. Anteroposterior and lateral views of the thoracic, lumbar, and sacral spine.

    c. Chest and pelvic x-rays.

    d. Other spine x-rays such as tomograms, oblique views, and CT scans as needed.

    A more complete listing of the common cervical spine fractures is included below.

  3. Hemodynamic monitoring. Central venous pressure (CVP) or Swan-Ganz monitoring should be performed in the patient suspected of having neurogenic shock. In a young and previously healthy person, central venous monitoring should be adequate to insure that proper volume replacement has occurred, prior to starting vasopressors. Swan-Ganz monitoring is more invasive, but gives more information on the patient's cardiovascular status (see Chap. 8). As discussed above, Swan-Ganz monitoring will also assist in distinguishing different types of shock.

C. Management. The patient with neurogenic shock needs a complete history and physical examination as detailed above. Because most patients will have a history of trauma, a systematic approach such as that taught in the Advanced Trauma Life Support Course should be used. This begins with assessing the airway, breathing, circulation, directed neurologic exam, and exposure (ABCDEs) in the primary survey.

  1. Airway with cervical spine control. If not already done, a secure airway and cervical spine immobilization should be quickly accomplished by securing the head, chest, and pelvis on a backboard with a hard cervical collar. If needed, endotracheal intubation of the patient is best done by the orotracheal route after removal of the cervical collar, with the head immobilized by an assistant (see Chap. 2). Rapid sequence intubation with paralysis and sedation is preferred to avoid further cervical trauma.

  2. Breathing. The patient should be ventilated if not breathing. All cervical spine trauma patients should be placed on 100% nonrebreather masks, with careful attention given to their pattern of respirations, since respiratory acidosis is common with diaphragmatic breathing. Pulse oximetry and continuous transcutaneous CO_2 monitoring are also helpful in assessing ongoing changes in respiratory status.

3. **Circulation.** Ongoing blood loss should be halted when possible. The patient should be placed on a cardiac monitor, and two large-bore IV lines should be established. Fluid resuscitation with isotonic fluids such as lactated Ringer's solution or normal saline should be initiated.

4. **Directed neurologic exam.** Level of consciousness, pupillary response, and motor response should be assessed.

5. **Exposure.** The patient should be completely undressed.

6. **Secondary assessment.** After the primary survey is done, a complete examination from head to toe should be performed, including a thorough neurologic exam. Particular attention should be paid to evidence of spinal column injury, such as midline tenderness, crepitance, or palpable step offs on the neck and back.

   Patients with spinal cord injury are at increased risk for heat loss from vasodilatation. Warm crystalloid and blankets should be used liberally.

7. **Assessment of other injuries.** In patients who have a neurologic deficit, the abdominal exam is not reliable for diagnosing intraabdominal injury. Either a diagnostic peritoneal lavage or abdominal CT scan is required if the mechanism of injury warrants evaluation of the abdomen. Orthopedic, pulmonary, and neurologic injuries should be assessed and cared for in the usual manner.

8. **Steroid therapy.** Patients suffering spinal cord injuries can be treated with high-dose steroids to limit cervical spine damage, although their use is controversial and not universally accepted. Treatment should begin within 8 hours of the injury with methylprednisolone 30 mg/kg IVP followed by a continuous infusion of methylprednisolone at 5.4 mg/kg/hr.

9. **Treatment of hypotension.** In the patient with evidence of spinal cord injury, warm extremities, and persistent hypotension despite fluid resuscitation, the diagnosis of neurogenic shock should be considered. Bradycardia may or may not be present. Some type of central monitoring should be established and adequate fluid replacement assured before starting a vasopressor agent. If the patient's central venous pressures are low despite 2 liters of crystalloid replacement, then a source of occult blood loss should be reevaluated. At this point, transfusion of packed red blood cells also should be considered. It should be noted that relatively large amounts of crystalloid infusion are often needed

to maximize the CVP in patients with neurogenic shock.

If the patient's central venous pressure is normal or elevated, then a vasopressor agent should be considered. There is no literature to suggest that one vasopressor agent is better than another. Table 44-2 lists vasopressors and doses that can be used. The systolic blood pressure should be corrected to above 100 mm Hg or as clinically indicated by mental status or urine output.

Treatment of bradycardia has not been well studied in neurogenic shock. A parasympathetic dose of 0.4 mg/kg of atropine may be used to treat bradycardia, but usually no treatment is needed.

D. **Patient disposition.** All patients with neurogenic shock will need either orthopedic or neurosurgical consultation as soon as possible and ICU admission. A plan of care involving the trauma surgeon and the orthopedic or neurosurgical consultant should be made. Transfer to a tertiary care center with a neurosurgical intensive care unit is recommended. Neurogenic shock usually resolves in two to

Table 44-2. Vasopressors and their doses in neurogenic shock

Vasopressor agent	Adult dose	Pediatric dose
Ephedrine	5 mg IV bolus to increase pressure as needed.	Not recommended
Phenylephrine	10 mg in 250 ml start with 100 to 180 µg/min and decrease to a maintenance infusion of 40–60 µg/min after hypotension corrected. May also be given as 0.1–0.5 mg IV bolus q10–15min.	1 mg in 5 ml. Dilute 0.6 mg/kg with D5W to total 100 ml (0.1 µg/kg/min = 1 ml/hr). Start at 2 ml/hr. Range 0.1–1.0 µg/kg/min.
Dopamine	200 mg in 250 ml start with 4 µg/kg/min and titrate to effect. Range 0.5–20 µg/kg/min.	200 mg in 5 ml. Dilute 6.0 mg/kg with D5W to total 100 ml (1 µg/kg/min = 1 ml/hr). Start at 2 ml/hr. Range 2–20 µg/kg/min
Dobutamine	250 mg in 250 ml start with 0.5 µg/kg/min and titrate to effect. Range 0.5–10 µg/kg/min.	250 mg in 5 ml. Dilute 6.0 mg/kg with D5W to total 100 ml (1 µg/kg/min = 1 ml/hr). Start at 5 ml/hr. Range 5–15 µg/kg/min.

three weeks. The patient should remain in a monitored setting until the vital signs have normalized.

The most common complication with acute spinal cord injury is pneumonia. All patients need aggressive respiratory care to prevent this complication. During the initial weeks of hospitalization, the orthopedist or neurosurgeon needs to assess the spinal column for stability. If the spinal column is unstable, either bed rest or an operative procedure may be needed.

VI. **Common cervical and thoracic spine fractures**
   A. **Cervical spine fractures and spinal cord injury.** Injury to the cervical spine or spinal cord results from one or more of the following mechanisms: (1) axial loading, (2) flexion, (3) extension, (4) lateral bending, (5) rotation, and (6) distraction. A complete series of cervical spine films should contain a lateral view that includes all seven cervical vertebrae, an odontoid view, an anteroposterior view, and oblique or pedicle views. Injuries to the spinal cord can occur with any cervical spine fracture, even stable ones, because the vertebral body may collapse posteriorly and injure the spinal cord. When the lateral cervical spine film is examined, a prevertebral soft tissue swelling is a sign of hematoma and fracture.

   1. The distance between the pharynx and the anterior/inferior border of C-3 should be less than 5 mm. An increase in this distance is indirect evidence of a cervical spine fracture, commonly associated with minimally displaced C-2 fractures.
   2. The prevertebral space in children is normally two-thirds the width of the C-2 vertebral body. This distance varies with inspiration and expiration, so an assessment for a hematoma in this area will not be reliable in crying children.
   3. Below the larynx, the tracheal air shadow is further from the anterior cervical spine. In this area, the prevertebral space should be less than the width of the vertebral body.

   B. **Common cervical spine fractures**
   1. **C-1 (atlas).** A fracture of the atlas usually involves a blowout fracture of the ring (Jefferson fracture). Axial loading is the common mechanism. It is seen as a fracture of the lamina on the lateral view and as asymmetry or widening of the lateral masses on the odontoid view. One-third of these fractures are associated with a C-2 (axis) fracture. These fractures usually are not associated with cord injuries but should be considered unstable.
   2. **C-2 (axis)-dislocation of C-2.** The transverse ligament attaches the odontoid to the anterior ring of C-1. Injuries to the transverse ligament may displace the odontoid process posteriorly into the spinal canal. The injury to the transverse ligament may occur without bony injury. The diagnosis should be considered when the space between the odontoid and the anterior ring of C-1 is wider than 5 mm in an adult. Displacement of

the odontoid can occur without spinal cord injury. This is because the odontoid occupies one-third of the ring of C-1 and the spinal cord occupies one-third of the ring, which leaves approximately one-third of the space in the ring empty for movement of the odontoid. All suspected transverse ligament injuries should be treated as unstable.

3. **C-2 (axis)-odontoid fractures.** Three different types of fractures may be associated with the odontoid. These may be difficult to see on x-ray and, if suspected, should be further investigated with CT.
    a. **Type I.** Type I fractures usually occur above the base of the odontoid and are most often stable.
    b. **Type II.** Type II fractures, which occur at the base of the odontoid, are usually unstable. In children younger than 6 years of age, the epiphysis may appear as a fracture at this level.
    c. **Type III.** Type III fractures extend into the vertebral body.

4. **Rotary subluxation-odontoid.** This injury is most often seen in children. The ring of C-1 rotates around the odontoid, causing one of the lateral masses to appear larger than the other. This is seen on the odontoid view, and can be differentiated from rotation by examining the symmetry of the basilar skull structures.

5. **C-2 posterior element fractures.** The "Hangman's fracture" involves the posterior elements of C-2. C-2 is subluxed forward on C-3. The mechanism of injury is extension and distraction or extension and axial load. This is an unstable fracture.

6. **C-3 through C-7 fractures.** Injury to this part of the cervical spine is associated with various fractures and dislocations. The mechanism in stable cervical spine fractures is usually flexion/axial loading, extension/axial loading, or flexion/rotation. Unstable vertebral fractures in this area include:
    a. Fractures identified by disruption of the anterior and all of the posterior elements.
    b. Fractures identified by overriding of a superior vertebral body by more than 3.5 mm.
    c. Fractures identified by angulation between two adjacent vertebral bodies of more than 11 degrees.

7. **Facet dislocations.** Facet dislocations may produce an unstable injury. This is especially true in bilateral facet dislocations. On the lateral cervical spine film, a unilateral facet dislocation should be considered if the superior vertebral body is displaced more than 25% over the inferior vertebral body. A bilateral jumped facet should be considered if the superior vertebral body is overriding by 50% or more. On the anteroposterior film, misalignment of the cervical spinous processes is suggestive of a unilateral facet dislocation.

8. **Teardrop fractures.** A bony avulsion off the anterior superior aspect of the cervical spine vertebral body usually indicates an extension-type injury. These are

almost always stable and not associated with spinal cord injury. A teardrop fracture of the anterior inferior vertebral body is an ominous radiographic sign. Spinal cord injuries are often associated with this flexion injury. This sign may be associated with displacement of the intervertebral disc or posterior fragments of the vertebral body into the spinal canal, causing spinal cord injury.

C. **Thoracic spine fractures and spinal cord injury.** Fractures in this region are most commonly the result of hyperflexion with resultant wedge compression of the vertebral body. The amount of wedging is usually small with less than 25% difference between the anterior and posterior portions of the vertebral body. The rigidity of the rib cage makes most of these stable fractures. Unfortunately, the spinal canal is narrow in this region, and spinal cord injuries with these fractures are usually complete lesions.

Bibliography

American College of Surgeons. *Advanced Trauma Life Support Student Manual.* United States, 1991.

Lehmann KG, et al. Cardiovascular abnormalities accompanying acute spinal cord injury in humans: incidence, time course, and severity. *J. Am Coll Cardiol* 10:46–52, 1987.

Levi L, et al. Hemodynamic parameters in patients with acute cervical cord trauma: description, intervention, and prediction of outcome. *Neurosurgery* 33:1007–1017, 1993.

Tibbs PA, et al. Diagnosis of acute abdominal injuries in patients with spinal shock: value of diagnostic peritoneal lavage. *J Trauma* 20:55–57, 1980.

Tintinalli JE, Krome RL, Ruiz E (eds.). *Emergency Medicine: A Comprehensive Study Guide.* New York: McGraw-Hill, 1992.

45

Hypertensive Emergencies and Urgencies

Robert L. Levine

In 1983, more than 57 million people were hypertensive, with 25% of the population having a diastolic blood pressure at least 90 mm Hg and with up to 50% of the population becoming hypertensive by the sixth decade of life. Hypertension directly and indirectly contributes to over half of all deaths in the United States through its effects on the heart, brain, and kidneys. Hypertension is one of the major risk factors for ischemic heart disease, and it is the major risk factor for cerebrovascular accidents and end-stage renal disease.

The rate of ischemic heart disease increases in relation to both the systolic and diastolic pressures. This occurs because hypertension increases stress, which results in left ventricular hypertrophy, accelerated atherosclerosis, and mismatch of myocardial oxygen supply and demand. These abnormalities manifest clinically as an increased risk for myocardial infarction (MI), congestive heart failure (CHF), and sudden death from arrhythmias. The risk of developing a stroke or renal failure also is directly related to the diastolic and systolic pressures. Renal insufficiency and uremia ultimately develop in 10%–20% of hypertensive patients; in fact, hypertension is the most common cause of end-stage renal failure requiring dialysis in the United States!

As a major contributing factor to over half the deaths in the United States, and as one of the few risk factors directly amenable to treatment, hypertension and its treatment have assumed a key role in the prevention of heart, brain, and kidney disease.

I. **Definition.** Hypertensive emergencies and urgencies are differentiated by the presence of acute end-organ damage. The new classification of hypertension and the schedule for follow-up are presented in Tables 45-1 and 45-2. Hypertensive emergencies are a particular subgroup (subgroup 4) defined clinically as a marked elevation of blood pressure accompanied by end-organ damage. Urgencies manifest elevated pressures without acute changes in pressure-sensitive systems. The organ systems involved include the cardiovascular system, brain, and kidneys. End-organ manifestations are presented in Table 45-3. Hypertension in the absence of these changes represents a condition requiring urgent but not emergent therapy. In fact, aggressive therapy of hypertensive urgencies can lead to increased morbidity, in addition to adding time and expense to the patient's emergency department (ED) course.

Transient elevations of blood pressure are commonly noted in the general population. These elevations are usually mild to moderate in severity and have no associated complications. In fact, about 10% of patients with mild-to-moderate hypertension will normalize their pressures with no treatment at all. This is not meant to imply, however, that hypertension is ever truly uncomplicated. Patients with transient hypertension are at risk of eventually going on to develop chronic

**Table 45-1.   Classification of blood
pressure for adults age 18 years and older***

Category	Systolic (mm Hg)	Diastolic (mm Hg)
Normal†	<130	<85
High normal	130–139	85–89
Hypertension‡		
Stage 1 (mild)	140–159	90–99
Stage 2 (moderate)	160–179	100–109
Stage 3 (severe)	180–209	110–119
Stage 4 (very severe)	≥210	≥120

* Not taking antihypertensive drugs and not acutely ill. When systolic and diastolic pressures fall into different categories, the higher category should be selected to classify the individual's blood pressure status. For instance, 160/92 mm Hg should be classified as stage 2, and 180/120 mm Hg should be classified as stage 4. Isolated systolic hypertension (ISH) is defined as systolic BP≥140 mm Hg and diastolic BP<90 mm Hg and staged appropriately (e.g., 170/85 mm Hg is defined as stage 2 ISH).

† Optimal blood pressure with respect to cardiovascular risk is systolic BP<120 mm Hg and diastolic BP<80 mm Hg. However, unusually low readings should be evaluated for clinical significance.

‡ Based on the average of two or more readings taken at each of two or more visits following an initial screening.

Note: In addition to classifying stages of hypertension based on average blood-pressure levels, the clinician should specify presence or absence of target-organ disease and additional risk factors. For example, a patient with diabetes and a blood pressure of 142/94 mm Hg plus left ventricular hypertrophy should be classified as "stage 1 hypertension with target-organ disease (left ventricular hypertrophy) and with another major risk factor (diabetes.)" This specificity is important for risk classification and management.

Source: *The Fifth Report of the Joint National Committee on Detection, Evaluation, and Treatment of High Blood Pressure,* National Institutes of Health, National Heart, Lung, and Blood Institute, January 1993.

hypertension. As mentioned previously, even mild, persistent elevations of pressure are associated with increased risk of coronary disease and stroke. However, chronic mild hypertension is not associated with acute complications and therefore does not need to be treated in the ED. Mild-to-moderate hypertension, noted in the ED, usually should be referred to a primary care physician for confirmation and treatment of persistent hypertension.

II.   **Complications.** Untreated systolic and diastolic hypertension significantly increases the risk of MI, cerebrovascular accident (stroke), and renal failure. However, this understates the acute impact of malignant hypertension (hypertensive crisis) on mortality. The natural history of untreated hypertensive crises is that patients die rapidly from stroke or renal failure with late deaths due to coronary artery disease. In older studies, less than 25% of patients with malignant hypertension survived one year without treatment. Only 1% survived five years. With simple treatment (guanethidine, an agent that works by producing sympathetic ganglionic blockade), survival dramatically increased. With treatment today,

**Table 45-2.   Recommendations for follow-up
based on the initial set of blood presure
measurements for adults age 18 and older**

Initial screening of blood pressure (mm Hg)*		Follow-up recommended†
Systolic	Diastolic	
<130	<85	Recheck in 2 years.
130–139	85–89	Recheck in 1 year.‡
140–159	90–99	Confirm within 2 months.
160–179	100–109	Evaluate or refer to source of care within 1 month.
180–209	110–119	Evaluate or refer to source of care within 1 week.
≥210	≥120	Evaluate or refer to source of care immediately.

* If the systolic and diastolic categories are different, follow recommendation for
the more immediate follow-up (e.g., 160/85 mm Hg should be evaluated or referred
to source of care within 1 month).
† The scheduling of follow-up should be modified by reliable information about
past blood pressure measurements, other cardiovascular risk factors, or target-
organ disease.
‡ Consider providing advice about lifestyle modifications.
Source: *The Fifth Report of the Joint National Committee on Detection, Evaluation, and Treatment of High Blood Pressure,* National Institutes of Health, National Heart, Lung, and Blood Institute, January 1993.

over 90% of patients survive one year and 80% survive five
years. Thus, the importance of aggressive treatment cannot
be overemphasized.

III. **Pathophysiology.** Hypertensive emergencies are defined by
the acute development of end-organ damage, characteristically manifested in three pressure-sensitive systems. These
systems include the central nervous system, the cardiovascular system, and the kidneys. Hypertension causes a characteristic arteriopathy with thickening of the medial walls of
the medium-sized arteries and with arteriolar necrosis. This
results in ischemic damage to the systems affected and also
can cause bleeding into these organ systems. The effect of hypertension on these systems is summarized in Table 45-3.
   The rapidity with which the pressure becomes elevated is
directly related to the extent of the damage. When the blood
pressure is chronically elevated, pressure-sensitive systems
have time to adapt, with arteriolar hypertrophy protecting
from further pressure-related damage. For example, under
normal circumstances the brain maintains perfusion (au-
toregulates) over a mean arterial pressure ranging from 60 to
120 mm Hg. When subjected to chronic hypertension, autoregulation shifts so that perfusion is maintained over mean
pressures from 110 to 180 mm Hg. This adaptive "shift to the
right" does not occur when the pressure is acutely elevated. In

Table 45-3.   Systemic manifestations of hypertensive emergencies

Cardiovascular effects
Acute pulmonary edema
New onset S_3
Chest pain
Ischemic changes on ECG

Central nervous system effects
Grade 3 and 4 retinal changes
  Hemorrhages and exudates
  Papilledema
Seizures
Focal deficits
  Cerebrovascular accidents
  Transient ischemic events
Coma

Renal effects
Hematuria
Progressive renal insufficiency

---

this circumstance, the blood vessels are overwhelmed, resulting in cerebral edema and encephalopathy. Retinal, renal, and cardiac changes also may be seen. An important corollary to the fact that acute changes of the pressure cause more damage than do chronic, slowly developing changes are seen when acutely lowering chronically elevated pressure to normal levels in patients in whom the "shift to the right" has occurred. Ischemic strokes and renal and cardiac insufficiency may ensue from the inappropriate, rapid normalization of pressure. Thus, the treatment of hypertension must take into account both the rapidity with which the pressure elevation occurred and the specific situation associated with the pressure elevation. Inappropriately aggressive therapy (i.e., too aggressive or not aggressive enough) can increase morbidity and mortality.

Most often hypertensive emergencies develop in patients with long-standing, poorly controlled chronic hypertension. Most patients have a history of hypertension for 10 years or longer and of noncompliance with medications. Chronic manifestations of hypertension such as left ventricular hypertrophy may be present; chronic changes are not considered defining events for hypertensive crisis. As mentioned above, the acute elevation of pressure superimposed on chronic hypertension ovewhelms the body's compensatory mechanisms. This results in the development of acute end-organ damage as defined above and warrants immediate treatment.

In the typical hypertensive crisis, elevated blood pressure causes acute organ damage, thus defining the emergency. However, in other circumstances the presence of specific, predisposing conditions places the patient at risk of morbidity and mortality if severe hypertension develops. These situations can develop with lower pressures than those usually seen with hypertensive crises because adaptive mechanisms cannot operate over such a short time period. Examples of these situations are listed in Table 45-4. These situations warrant aggressive therapy to lower the pressure. Preeclampsia and eclampsia are discussed later in this chapter.

IV. **Hypertensive emergencies**

A. **Patient presentation.** The typical patient with a hypertensive emergency has an acute elevation of blood pressure superimposed on poorly controlled hypertension (usually due to noncompliance with medications). Presenting signs and symptoms are related to the organ systems that suffer acutely (i.e., the heart, brain, and kidneys).

1. **Hypertensive encephalopathy.** The brain is the organ system that is most dramatically and acutely affected. Presenting **complaints** related to hypertensive encephalopathy range from severe headache, vomiting, drowsiness, and confusion to depressed consciousness, seizures, blindness, and coma. The **physical examination** is usually nonfocal, but on occasion focal findings may be observed and the course can still be reversible. Once focal findings are noted, one must be concerned with progression to irreversible brain damage. Early hypertensive encephalopathy is associated with microscopic hemorrhages or infarcts that are not obvious on CT but may present clinically as multiple focal deficits that are nonanatomic in their distribution. Retinal examination may demonstrate exudates and hemorrhages (grade 3 changes) or papilledema (grade 4), reflecting changes that are occurring in the brain.

Table 45-4. Situational hypertensive emergencies

Preeclampsia-eclampsia

Postoperative hypertension (especially cardiovascular and vascular surgery)

Bleeding from postoperative sites

Intracranial bleeding and other forms of cerebrovascular accidents

Myocardial infarction and hypertension

Acute left ventricular failure

Severe burns

Dissecting aneurysms

Severe epistaxis

Acute head injury

Acute excess of catecholamines

   Pheochromocytoma

   Monoamine oxidase inhibitor crisis

2. **Cardiac involvement.** Cardiac manifestations of hypertensive crisis include **angina** and acute **congestive heart failure (CHF).** Presenting complaints are chest pain and/or shortness of breath. On **examination** patients appear apprehensive and usually sit upright. Tachypnea is evident though cyanosis rarely develops. When cyanosis is seen, it may be peripheral in distribution and is due to peripheral vasoconstriction. Signs of heart failure may be noted, including jugular venous distention, a new S_3 or S_4 gallop, and crackles (rales) bilaterally in the lungs. Peripheral edema may not be present if heart failure develops acutely without being superimposed on chronic failure.

3. **Acute renal failure.** There are usually no signs or symptoms associated with the development of renal failure. Rather, laboratory evaluation including urinalysis and serum chemistries reveal the presence of hematuria and proteinuria associated with an acute increase in the serum creatinine. As with other manifestations of hypertensive crisis, these changes may be reversible with aggressive therapy.

B. **Patient assessment**
1. **Laboratory studies.** Routine laboratory tests to evaluate hypertensive emergencies include a CBC, serum chemistries including electrolytes, BUN, creatinine, and glucose. A urinalysis is also part of the routine workup. Cardiac enzymes are obtained if clinically indicated by the presence of chest pain or ECG changes.
2. **Chest x-ray (CXR).** The CXR may demonstrate a normal or enlarged heart. Evidence of pulmonary edema may range from vascular redistribution and interstitial edema through the typical "bat-winged" appearance of alveolar edema in patients with cardiac involvement.
3. **ECG.** Cardiac ischemia is manifested as ST depression or elevation on the ECG. These changes are reversible if the hypertensive crisis is successfully treated before the patient infarcts.
4. **CT scan.** CT scans should be obtained in all patients with presumed hypertensive encephalopathy or stroke. CT scans are usually normal early in the course of hypertensive encephalopathy. As the cerebral damage progresses, abnormalities noted on CT include cerebral edema, infarcts, and intracerebral hemorrhage. Chronic hypertensive bleeds usually are noted at the level of the internal capsule and result from rupture of the penetrating branches of the thalamostriate vessels.

C. **Management**
1. **Supportive care.** Routine management of hypertensive crises starts with securing the airway, breathing, and circulation (ABCs), the establishment of an IV line, O_2, and placement of the patient on a cardiac monitor. As part of the initial evaluation, pulse oximetry may help determine that the patient is adequately oxygenating.
2. **Antihypertensive therapy.** Once routine measures have been performed and the diagnosis of hypertensive

crisis has been confirmed clinically, antihypertensive therapy is initiated with the goal of lowering the blood pressure to an acceptable range (not normalizing) over the next hour. In general, the goal is to decrease the diastolic pressure by about 20%. As discussed, too rapid normalization of pressure can result in iatrogenic complications. Also, certain specific situations warrant slower reductions of pressure [e.g., cerebrovascular accidents (thrombotic) associated with hypertension and severe hypertension with no objective findings diagnostic of an emergency].

Nitroprusside (NTP) is the drug of choice for most hypertensive emergencies. However, newer agents may change our general approach to hypertensive crises, and certain situations may warrant starting therapy with other agents, for example, chest pain associated with hypertension. Pharmacotherapy, including discussion of the drugs commonly used to treat hypertensive emergencies and urgencies follows.

D. Pharmacotherapy of hypertensive emergencies. Hypertensive emergencies usually are treated with direct vasodilators whereas urgencies can be treated with vasodilators and other classes of agents. Vasodilators that rapidly lower the blood pressure can be divided further into groups of drugs with immediate onset and offset of action and those with longer half-lives and therefore more gradual onset and offset of effect. These agents are listed in Table 45-5 in groups based on rapidity of onset and offset of action and in Table 45-6 based on their predominant mechanism of action. They are discussed in more detail below.

1. Sodium nitroprusside. Sodium nitroprusside (nitroprusside or NTP) is the drug of choice for hypertensive

Table 45-5. Pharmacotherapy of hypertensive emergencies

Immediate
Sodium nitroprusside
Trimethaphan
Nitroglycerin

Very rapid
Nicardipine
Diazoxide*

Rapid
Labetolol
Enaloprilat
Esmolol
Nifedipine*
Hydralazine*

* Can be unpredictable.

Table 45-6. Pharmacological agents and their mechanisms

Direct vasodilators
Sodium nitroprusside
Nitroglycerin
Diazoxide
Hydralazine

Adrenergic inhibitors
Phentolamine (alpha blockade)
Trimethaphan camsylate (ganglionic blockade)
Labetolol [alpha and beta blockade (3:1 beta:alpha), oral and IV forms available]
Methyldopa (CNS blockade)
Clonidine (CNS blockade)

Calcium channel blockers
Nicardipine (oral and IV forms available)
Nifedipine

ACE inhibitors
Captopril
Enalopril (oral and IV forms available)

Pharmacologic therapy of hypertensive urgencies
Labetolol
Nifedipine
Enaloprilat
Clonidine

emergencies. Nitroprusside is a direct vasodilator with greater arteriolar dilatation than venodilatation. It is a highly potent and effective drug administered intravenously with an immediate onset and offset of effect. It can be titrated to any desired blood pressure, including hypotensive levels. Due to its potency and rapid onset and offset of effect, it requires frequent adjustment to avoid inducing iatrogenic hypotension with resultant complications (which can be disastrous). To prevent this from happening, intra-arterial blood pressure monitoring is used to provide immediate feedback. Alarm limits can be adjusted to notify medical personnel of potentially hazardous pressures. In some circumstances therapy may be started using a noninvasive pressure-measuring device, though this is not ideal when using nitroprusside.

Although NTP is usually the drug of choice for hypertensive crises, several situations exist where nitroprusside is either not optimal or must be used with other agents to control the pressure. For example, hypertension with chest pain is often best treated with IV nitroglycerin. Similarly, since use of NTP can be associated with an increase of intracranial pressure (ICP), it must be used with caution in situations in which ICP may be increased, such as a cerebrovascular accident (CVA). Trimethaphan lowers ICP and may be a better drug for this situation, though experience with this agent has become increasingly limited with the availability of the newer agents. Another hypertensive crisis in which trimethaphan may be better than NTP is acute aortic dissection. In this situation NTP must be used in conjunction with a beta-blocking agent (usually propranolol) to lower the pressure and simultaneously decrease the dP/dT. This is done to avoid increasing the shearing effect in the aorta. Trimethaphan lowers the pressure and, through its effect on cardiac sympathetics, simultaneously lowers the dP/dT.

Nitroprusside's major **side effect** is hypotension. However, several troubling but rare side effects may develop through the metabolism of NTP. Nitroprusside is metabolized to thiocyanate and finally cyanide. If used in high doses for a prolonged period of time—and especially in the presence of renal insufficiency—thiocyanate toxicity can develop. This presents as unexplained confusion and acidosis in a critically ill patient. When nitroprusside is used correctly, thiocyanate and cyanide toxicity are very rare complications because once nitroprusside therapy is begun, other agents are added expeditiously, allowing nitroprusside to be rapidly weaned. Finally, a common mistake is to institute therapy with nitroprusside after the pressure has been lowered to a desirable range with other agents. As with any therapy, as the situation changes, the therapeutic approach must be tailored to the situation at that time.

Dosage: Mix: 50 mg in 250 ml D5W (200 μg/ml)
Dose: 0.25 μg/kg/min to start, up to 10 μg/kg/min

2. **Trimethaphan camsylate.** Trimethaphan is an old drug that works by blocking sympathetic transmission in the spinal ganglia. Administered intravenously, it diminishes arteriolar and venular tone equally, partly through an orthostatic effect. Therefore, the head of the patient's bed needs to be elevated for trimethaphan to fully manifest its effects. Through blockade of the cardiac sympathetics, it decreases myocardial dP/dT, an effect that is beneficial in the treatment of dissecting aortic aneurysms. Trimethaphan also lowers ICP; in the past it was the drug of choice for neurosurgical emergencies associated with hypertension and an elevated ICP. Although highly effective, it is not very potent, and therefore large doses must be used (mg/min). Currently, this drug has been relegated to a second-line role for the treatment of hypertension because of its problems, including tachyphylaxis and gastric and urinary atony.

Dosage: Mix: 500 mg in 500 ml D5W (1 mg/ml)
    Dose: 0.3–6.0 mg/min

3. **Nitroglycerin.** Nitroglycerin is predominantly a venodilator with secondary, lesser effects on the arterioles. Its most common use is for the relief of angina, but in larger doses it causes hypotension. Nitroglycerin's hemodynamic effects render it an excellent choice for the treatment of hypertension associated with angina or congestive heart failure. It is a poor choice for primary hypertensive crises due not to cardiac disease but secondary to arteriolar constriction. In this circumstance, the intravascular volume may be normal or even low, a situation in which nitroglycerin can have adverse consequences. Several different IV preparations are available with different concentrations of drug/ml. It can be dosed as µg/min or µg/kg/min. Similar to nitroprusside, it is administered as an IV drip and titrated to effect, for example, for either relief of chest pain or achievement of a desired blood pressure.

Dosage: Dose: 5 µg/min–350 µg/min (0.5–5.0 µg/kg/min)

4. **Nicardipine.** Nicardipine belongs to the dihydropyridine class of calcium channel antagonists. It is related to nifedipine but has the advantage of being available in both oral and IV forms. Also, nifedipine has unpredictable blood pressure–lowering effects when administered orally, an effect not seen with intravenous nicardipine. Hypotension due to the administration of nifedipine can be profound. It can cause cerebrovascular accidents and MIs, problems not associated with intravenous nicardipine. Nicardipine, in its intravenous form, has major advantages over nifedipine and may even have advantages over nitroprusside. Nicardipine has an alpha half-life ($t_{\frac{1}{2}}\alpha$) of approximately 2.7 minutes, resulting in a very rapid but not immediate onset and offset of effect. Nicardipine onset develops gradually over several minutes, resulting in a predictable lowering of the systolic and diastolic pressures. With its intermediate half-life ($t_{\frac{1}{2}}\beta$) of 45 minutes, it requires few adjustments and rarely causes hypotension—two common problems with nitroprusside. Because its effects are predictable and less abrupt in onset, it can be administered without invasive arterial monitoring. These characteristics may make nicardipine the drug of choice for emergency department management of hypertensive crises. As a dihydropyridine, nicardipine shares the classes' cerebroprotective effects and is useful in hypertension associated with subarachnoid hemorrhages.

Nicardipine's **side effects** include hypotension and tachycardia, both of which are uncommon, are usually mild, and respond rapidly to discontinuation of the drug. Cardiac depressant effects are not a problem with this drug.

Dosage: Mix: 25 mg in 240 ml of dextrose or saline-
based fluid
Dose: 5–15 mg/hr continuous infusion

5. **Esmolol.** Esmolol is a beta-blocking drug that has a
very rapid onset and offset of action. Given by IV infusion, it can be titrated to desired effect. Though beta-
blocking agents can lower the blood pressure, they also
have the potential of producing a paradoxical increase
of pressure by unmasking unopposed alpha effects of
catecholamines. This can be particularly hazardous
with catecholamine excess. Despite this, esmolol can be
safely administered to many hypertensive patients. It
causes negative inotropic effects similar to other beta-
blockers and should be used cautiously if at all in patients with heart failure or bradycardia.

Dosage: Mix: 5 g in a compatible solution (most routine IV solutions)
Dose: 80 mg IV over 30 seconds followed by
an infusion of 150 μg/kg/min up to 300
μg/kg/min

6. **Diazoxide.** Diazoxide is a potent vasodilator with a
rapid onset (15 minutes) and a duration of effect as
long as 6 hours. Unfortunately, in its original dose of
300 mg intravenously, it often resulted in prolonged
hypotension. In smaller, 50-mg boluses it is a safe
drug, rarely causing hypotension. However, due to the
original experience with the larger dose and the availability of other agents, it has fallen out of favor.
   Labetolol, nifedipine, clonidine, and enaloprilat, all
of which have utility in the emergency management of
hypertension, are discussed in sec. **V.** Their beneficial
effects and role in the treatment of hypertensive crises
are discussed in that section. Hydralazine is reviewed
in the section on pregnancy-associated hypertension.
Phentolamine, used to treat hyperadrenergic crisis, is
not discussed in this chapter.

E. **Patient disposition.** True hypertensive emergencies
should be admitted to the intensive care unit (ICU) for
further treatment and stabilization. The goal of initial
treatment in the ED and in the ICU is to lower the pressure approximately 20% from the initial pressure. In most
cases the diastolic pressure should not be allowed to drop
below 120 mm Hg in the first 24 hours to avoid iatrogenic
complications. Once this level of pressure control has been
achieved, institution of oral therapy should commence
with the goal to change the patient from parenteral to oral
therapy over the next 24 hours.
   During the initial period of stabilization, **complications** may develop either related to the underlying hypertensive state or as an iatrogenic effect due to initiation of
antihypertensive therapy. These complications include
CVAs, MIs, and renal failure. When the patient presents
with these problems, treatment should be directed toward
lowering the pressure. When these problems arise after

the institution of therapy (especially new onset of CNS problems or deterioration of the renal function) consideration must be given to reducing the aggressiveness of therapy and allowing the blood pressure to rise. If the problems clear, subsequent antihypertensive therapy should be instituted in a more gradual manner with careful monitoring of the function of these systems.

V. **Hypertensive urgencies.** Severe elevations of systolic and diastolic pressures in the absence of acute end-organ damage leads to the diagnosis of hypertensive urgency. A systolic pressure of 250 mm Hg or a diastolic pressure of 160 mm Hg in the absence of acute complications is an urgent situation, perhaps requiring therapy to lower the pressure over the next 24–72 hours. Clearly, hypertension of this degree, if allowed to persist, will lead to increased cardiovascular, renal, and neurologic damage. However, with hypertensive urgencies, no acute damage exists at the time the patient presents. In this situation a window of opportunity exists within which the pressure can be gradually lowered. The most important goal is to avoid iatrogenic complications. Therefore, the goal is to lower the pressure gradually. In patients with very severe pressure elevations, therapy may be started in the ED to achieve a small (10%–20%) reduction in pressure after which therapy should be instituted with oral agents in the outpatient environment. Controversy exists over the need for ED therapy at all. One study comparing therapy begun in the ED with oral agents started after the patient had been discharged from the ED showed no difference in pressure at the time of follow-up three days later. More expense, more time spent in the ED, and more iatrogenic complications were seen in the acutely treated patients than in the outpatient group. This suggests that ED treatment of hypertensive urgencies should be reserved for those patients the clinician truly believes need acute therapy, either because of extreme elevation of pressure or because of compliance or education issues. Otherwise, hypertension should be treated with oral agents started in the patient's home.

A. **Patient presentation.** Hypertensive urgencies, similar to emergencies, usually are seen in patients with long-standing hypertension who are noncompliant with their medications. The patient may present with nonspecific complaints such as headache or atypical chest pain. The physical examination is nonspecific and is used to rule out the presence of an emergency.

B. **Patient assessment.** The ED evaluation should include whatever tests are necessary to confirm the absence of an emergent condition. The usual laboratory work-up includes the same tests as for emergencies: serum chemistries, CBC, urinalysis, and possibly an ECG and chest x-ray. The yield for these tests is not high unless there is new onset hypertension, symptoms related to a possible hypertensive emergency, or long-standing hypertension that was left untreated. Many patients may be managed without any laboratory or ancillary testing.

C. **Patient management.** As discussed above, the goal is to begin treatment in a manner that gradually lowers the pressure while avoiding iatrogenic complications. Therefore, **oral agents** usually are used for treatment, though several parenteral agents are useful as well (see sec. **D.**). In addition, many of the agents discussed in sec. **IV.** can be used to safely treat severe elevations in pressure.

D. **Pharmacotherapy of hypertensive urgencies**

1. **Labetolol.** Labetolol is a mixed alpha- and beta-blocking agent. In fact, the beta-blocking effect of intravenously administered labetolol predominates with a ratio of beta:alpha effects of 3:1. When compared to the other beta-blocking drugs available, this drug demonstrates a much more balanced blockade and is therefore useful for most hypertensive urgencies. It even has been used for hypertensive crisis, though its onset of effect is much slower than the drugs listed for hypertensive emergencies (see sec. **IV.D.**) It is also more difficult to titrate due to its long terminal half-life. When used for hypertensive crisis, the usual starting **dose** is 10–20 mg administered as an IV bolus, with doubling of the dose every 20–30 minutes until the desired effect is seen, or with repeat doses of 40–80 mg to a maximum of 300 mg. Most studies show that approximately 200 mg or more is needed for hypertensive crisis, requiring 1 to 2 hours to achieve. It is a remarkably safe drug despite its mixed alpha and beta effects. **Side effects** including bradycardia, heart block, congestive heart failure, and precipitation of bronchospasm, beta-blockade-associated side-effects are rarely seen with labetolol. Unopposed α effects resulting in exacerbation of pressure in situations of catecholamine excess also rarely occur.

2. **Nifedipine.** This agent is one of the most commonly used drugs for hypertensive crisis and urgency. However, it can be unpredictable in effect. Nifedipine is a calcium channel blocking agent of the dihydropyridine class. Its **dose** is 10 mg given as a capsule that the patient can either bite and swallow or just swallow. Onset of effect usually is seen 10–15 minutes after administration. If necessary, the dose can be repeated. Unfortunately, there is no way to predict who will or will not respond to nifedipine. Of those who respond, some patients have excessive drops in pressure resulting in iatrogenic complications. Nifedipine administration also causes tachycardia that can exacerbate ischemic heart disease. For this reason, many clinicians are moving from nifedipine to other agents. When therapy needs to be instituted and a calcium channel antagonist is selected, nicardipine (see sec. **IV.D.4.**) given intravenously has a more predictable onset, is easier to titrate, and rarely causes tachycardia. It probably should be used to replace nifedipine.

3. **Enaloprilat.** Enaloprilat belongs to the angiotensin-converting enzyme–inhibiting group of drugs (ACE inhibitors). It is given intravenously with a fairly rapid (15–30 minutes) onset of effect. The usual starting **dose** is 0.625–1.250 mg given q6h as an IV infusion.

As an ACE inhibitor its beneficial effects are mediated through vasodilatation. Therefore, it is beneficial in hypertensive states, especially hypertension assocaited with low cardiac output. Used infrequently in the ED, it may find its greatest usage in the ICU where it can be given acutely; as the patient improves, it can be changed to the oral form for continued therapy. Once oral therapy is instituted, enalopril, captopril, and other ACE inhibitors are equally effective. **Side effects** common to ACE inhibitors include elevation of the serum potassium, cough, angioedema, and renal shutdown when given to patients with bilateral renal artery stenosis. Fortunately, all of these side effects are reversible when the agent is discontinued. Newer agents that directly antagonize the angiotensin II type 1 receptor soon will be available clinically. Initially available as oral agents, they will probably have similar roles as the current ACE inhibitor class, but perhaps with fewer side effects.

4. **Clonidine.** Clonidine is a central nervous system alpha$_2$ receptor stimulant. Through this stimulation, it indirectly decreases blood pressure by diminishing CNS sympathetic output. Its onset of effect is not as rapid as most of the other agents discussed in this chapter. Given orally as **dose** of a 0.2-mg load followed by 0.1 mg hourly to a maximum of 1.2 mg, most hypertensive urgencies can be controlled over a 2- to 6-hour period. Doses greater than 1.2 mg/d probably should not be used. In this range, clonidine's alpha$_1$ stimulation causes the blood pressure to increase, negating its beneficial alpha$_2$ effects. Its major **side effects** are sedation and dry mouth—both alpha$_2$ effects. Clonidine, and to a lesser extent other alpha$_2$ stimulants such as guanabenz, cause a "rebound" syndrome when stopped abruptly. Although this syndrome may not cause pressures to overshoot pretreatment levels, the sudden increase in sympathetic outflow certainly can raise the pressure and become problematic, especially for patients taking more than 1.2 mg/d. Therefore, these agents should never be discontinued abruptly.

E. **Patient disposition.** Patients with hypertensive urgencies do not require admission to the hospital for their blood pressure. If other complicating conditions warrant admission, the pressure can be treated while in the hospital but should still be lowered gradually. For the vast majority of these patients, the discharge instructions should explicitly list the discharge medications and the regimen prescribed (dose and dosage interval). Common side effects should be noted, and the importance of therapy and adequate follow-up for long-term control of the blood pressure should be emphasized. A follow-up visit to have the blood pressure checked at 24–48 hours is a good idea for several reasons. First, it stresses the importance of treatment of hypertension, a silent killer. Next, it allows the pressure to be checked to avoid complications of over-aggressive therapy. Finally, it establishes a relationship between a primary care physician and a patient that requires lifelong therapy.

VI. **Hypertension in the pregnant patient**

A. **Patient presentation.** Hypertension in the pregnant patient can be divided into four categories: (1) chronic hypertension, (2) preeclampsia-eclampsia (PEE), (3) chronic hypertension with superimposed preeclampsia, and (4) transient hypertension.

Women with **chronic hypertension,** that is, hypertension diagnosed before pregnancy or before the twentieth week of pregnancy, rarely present a problem for the ED physician. In general, these patients should be maintained on their antihypertensive regimen throughout pregnancy. ACE inhibitors should be avoided during pregnancy, and beta-blockers can be problematic both in the beginning and end stages of pregnancy. Otherwise, diuretics, methyldopa, beta-blockers, and most antihypertensives are safe for use during pregnancy.

The onset of mild pressure elevations, such as systolic pressure greater than 140 mm Hg and diastolic pressure greater than 90 mm Hg represent profound derangements in the pregnant patient. Similarly, an increase in systolic pressure of 30 mm Hg or a diastolic rise of 15 mm Hg from the patient's baseline represents **pregnancy-induced hypertension (PIH).** For women presenting with PIH after the twentieth week of pregnancy, proteinuria and edema (preeclampsia) and seizures or coma (eclampsia) are true emergencies. Rapid, aggressive control of the pressure and underlying disease is necessary to avoid maternal and fetal morbidity and mortality. Risk factors for **preeclampsia-eclampsia (PEE)** include age more than 20 years, primigravida, twin or molar pregnancies, and a family history of PEE. PEE is associated with vasospasm, placental infarction and abruption, and fetal demise. Maternal effects include the constellation described above that defines PEE; headache and visual disturbances, ultimately ending in ischemic and hemorrhagic strokes; renal insufficiency; pulmonary edema; abdominal pain; and liver dysfunction. A microangiopathic hemolytic anemia and thrombocytopenia may be seen, especially in severe cases of pregnancy-induced hypertension. These findings may be part of the HELLP syndrome that presents in preeclamptic patients with hemolysis, elevated liver enzymes, and low platelets. Hepatic and splenic rupture can lead to maternal demise in this severe form of PIH. The development of seizures or coma marks the transition between preeclampsia and eclampsia. Hyperactive reflexes with clonus may be premonitory for eclampsia. Maternal and fetal mortality is increased with PIH and especially with eclampsia. Maternal mortality is currently less than 1%, but fetal mortality is at least 12% in eclamptics.

B. **Patient assessment.** The ED evaluation should include all the tests mentioned in sec. **V.B.** as well as a CBC, platelet count and coagulation studies, serum chemistries including an evaluation of renal and liver function, and a baseline magnesium level. **Fetal monitoring** should be instituted. In patients with altered mental status, a CT scan of the head should be obtained.

C. **Patient management.** Therapy should begin with stabilization of the ABCs and establishment of an IV line. Aspirin has been used experimentally to try to prevent prostaglandin-induced vasospasm. It may be useful, but it is not considered standard therapy at this time. Seizures usually are controlled with magnesium given intravenously and intramuscularly. **Magnesium** administration is continued until the reflexes become depressed (1+). Dosage of magnesium is 4–8 g IVP over 20 minutes, followed by an infusion of 1–3 g/hr. Complete loss of reflex activity antedates respiratory depression and can be used as a guide for serum magnesium levels. Diazepam and phenytoin also can be used to treat seizures, though the loading dose for phenytoin is decreased. Antihypertensive therapy has traditionally consisted of **hydralazine** in 5-mg IV bolules or by constant infusion. Hydralazine is not always available, and other alternatives such as nitroprusside and labetolol may need to be considered. **Nitroprusside** has been used successfully to treat eclampsia, and some high-risk obstetricians consider it to be the drug of choice for this condition. Concerns about cyanide toxicity in the fetus appear unwarranted and may be outweighed by the advantage of better blood-pressure control. **Labetolol** also has been used safely with good results. In the patient requiring such aggressive therapy, invasive hemodynamic monitoring may be indicated, including arterial and pulmonary artery pressure monitoring. Finally, in patients whose seizures cannot be controlled or those with life-threatening complications, emergency fetal delivery by Cesarean section should be considered.

D. **Patient disposition.** All patients with PEE should be admitted to the hospital for aggressive control of the pressure and the prophylaxis and treatment of seizures. An obstetrician should be consulted to see the patient and manage her on the ward (preeclamptic) or in the ICU (eclamptic). As already mentioned, maternal outcome is usually good with less than 1% mortality. Fetal mortality remains high, emphasizing the need for care throughout pregnancy.

Bibliography

The Fifth Report of the Joint National Committee on Detection, Evaluation, and Treatment of High Blood Pressure. NIH Publication No. 93-1088, January 1993.

Grossman W, Braunwald E. Pulmonary Hypertension. In Braunwald E (ed.). *Heart Disease: A Textbook of Cardiovascular Medicine* (4th ed.). Philadelphia: Saunders, 1992:790–816.

Hood DD. Hypertension Disorders of Pregnancy: Preeclampsia and Eclampsia. In Civetta JM, Taylor RW, Kirby RR (eds.). *Critical Care.* Philadelphia: Lippincott, 1988:1349–1357.

Kaplan NM. Systemic Hypertension: Mechanisms and Diagnosis. In Braunwald E (ed.). *Heart Disease: A Textbook of Cardiovascular Medicine* (4th ed.). Philadelphia: Saunders, 1992:817–851.

Kaplan NM. Systemic Hypertension: Therapy. In Braunwald E (ed.). *Heart Disease: A Textbook of Cardiovascular Medicine* (4th ed.). Philadelphia: Saunders, 1992:852–874.

Lucas MJ, Leveno KJ, Cunningham FG. A comparison of magnesium sulfate with phenytoin for the prevention of eclampsia. *New Engl J Med* 333:201–205, 1995.

Index

Page numbers followed by f *indicate figures; those followed by* t *indicate tables.*